Guide to
Nursing Leadership and Management: Theories, Processes and Practice

Chapter Motivation inspirational quotes begin each chapter

CHAPTER MOTIVATION

"Without continual growth and progress, such words as improvement, achievement, and success have no meaning."

Benjamin Franklin (1706–1790)

CHAPTER MOTIVES

- Define nursing informatics.
- Compare and contrast the nursing process and standards of informatics practice.
- Describe the role of information system standards in supporting communication between practitioners.
- Discuss the implications of nursing terminology to future nursing practice.
- Identify the six goals of information systems in the 21st century.
- Identify ways in which nursing informatics influences clinical practice.
- Identify personal accountabilities with regard to informatics.

Chapter Motives identify the key information that follows in the chapter

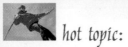

hot topic:

Health-Care Rationing

Rationing is one method that society uses to balance demands with limited resources. Even though the United States is viewed as a world leader in both scientific and technological aspects of medical care, not all citizens have access to basic health-care services. Current issues providing the context for rationing of health care are as follows:

1. Health-care services are restricted to individuals with sufficient financial resources (Cypher, 2003).

2. Health-care providers can choose not to accept certain forms of insurance, such as Medicaid or HMO plans, due to low payment (Cypher, 2003).

3. High deductibles and increasing insurance premiums are forcing many middle-income families to forego health-care coverage. In addition, small businesses are unable to supplement the cost of premiums for employees or even offer health-care coverage (Cypher, 2003).

4. Individuals with preexisting medical conditions are restricted in their access to health-care coverage.

5. P

The
limit
for i
not c

nies using a managed care system ration services through such methods as primary care gatekeeping, financial incentives to physicians, utilization review of services, and capitation. Primary care physicians serve as the point of access, or gatekeeper, to specialists, hospitalization, and other services. Limiting services or having consumers choose less costly treatments or simply no treatment at all is a primary objective of the managed care system. Physicians receive incentives that encourage them to ration health-care services. In addition, most managed care systems have a utilization review process in place, which requires prior authorization before a nonroutine service can be provided to a patient. Traditional insurance programs also attempt to ration services by not covering certain services in their policies. Often customers will avoid these procedures because they have to pay for them from their personal finances. Patients likewise self-ration their use of services when they do not have insurance coverage. This is often referred to as price-based rationing, because the patient has to evaluate the cost of receiving the services versus the perceived benefits of care (Baur, W___ & Fitzgerald, 1996).

___ntial legal and ethical issues surrounding the abil-
___zens to receive needed health-care services is a
___rsial topic without an easy solution. It is clear that
___nt system is in need of a dramatic reform to cor-
___e inequalities.

Practice Proof 7-1

Popularity of new drug-coated stents exceed supply. *Cardiovascular Watch*, July 21, 2003, p. 15.

Stents have been used since 1987 in conjunction with angioplasties to help prevent arteries from reclosing from plaque buildup. In the spring of 2003, Cordis Corporation released a new stent that was coated with the drug sirolimus. Research indicates that the drug-coated stents prevent scar tissue from reclogging the artery, which often results in another angioplasty within a year of the first procedure. Demand for the new stents is outpacing supply. At the time of this article, Cordis Corporation F__ the only drug-coated stent on the market. It is anticipa__ that Boston Scientific will receive approval from the Federal Drug Administration (FDA) within the next yea__ offer its own drug-coated stent. In addition, the Cordi__ stents sell for approximately $2,100 more than the ba__ metal stents, which is creating financial losses for som__ hospitals on these procedures.

1. What are the factors driving the demand for the drug-coated stents?

2. What are the possible rationing issues as a result of the shortage? What are possible solutions to this dilemma?

3. Explain the potential reimbursement ramifications from the new stents.

chapter star

Curricular Changes and Chaos Theory

Faculty members are increasingly embracing chaos theory as the framework within which decisions are made. The faculty at one nursing school adopted the shared governance model as the modus operandi. That organization has moved over the past 5 years from a quasi-participative model to a true shared governance approach. As this change occurred, faculty became more inclusive of divergent viewpoints among faculty members, more accepting of student input, and more comfortable with the faculty role.

This faculty "owns" the curriculum. Over the past 3 years and probably before that time, faculty began to work with the notion that changes needed to occur within the second senior semester of the curriculum. "Nudges" came from faculty members who were concerned with the amount of time devoted to and the character of the management clinical experiences. At that time, the course was a seven-semester credit course encompassing 4 lecture and 9 clinical hours each week. Nudges also came from students who expressed the same concerns as the faculty when offered the opportunity to voice experiences during exit interviews. The clinical decision-making course, which was at that time a three-semester credit hour lecture-only course, was intended to be the critical thinking culminating capstone experience in the last semester. Faculty members were concerned that there was not a clinical component associated with the course and that there was no medica

surgical clinical component during the last semester of study. Additionally, this factor was thought to influence NCLEX-RN first-time pass rates. These nudges found voice through faculty discussion occurring in various venues, some of which occurred in the copy room, over lunch, and in nursing faculty organization meetings. Faculty involved in the courses issued a proposal to transfer 2 semester credit hours (6 clinical clock hours) from the management course to the clinical decision-making course. The proposal was brought to the faculty as a whole for formal approval through the Undergraduate Curriculum Committee, where it found unanimous approval. The process by which this change occurred was characteristic of chaos theory in that all the members of the communities of interest had been involved in discussions. The change emanated from multiple sources and was guided by the mission and goals of the school of nursing, which serves as the attractor to keep the organization focused on a "student-centered, collegial environment." It is important to note that this school has long relied on the principles of shared governance that are congruent with chaos theory, parti-

Practice to Strive For 5-1

Catalano (1991); Guido (1997); and Mitchell & Grippando (1993) all point out Best Practices for Reducing the Risk of Malpractice Litigation:

I. *Maintain good communication with the clients in your care. This means being courteous and respectful; listening carefully; not making value judgments; assessing the ability of your client to follow and understand and then explaining treatments, orders, and medications at the level of understanding and in the language the client understands. Always verify and clarify telephone orders; optimally, do not take any telephone orders or give instructions or advice over the phone.*

II. *Always keep your knowledge and skills up to date. Do not administer any medication with which you are not familiar, and always practice within the professional standards and statutory span of your practice.*

III. *Follow and know your institution's policies and procedures, and always pay close attention to your clients' changing health status. Keep close attention to all details surrounding your clients, and document thoroughly, accurately, objectively, and in a timely manner.*

IV. *Always seek attention for a client's changing health status, and question physician orders if they are unclear or not in keeping with the client's condition. Remember to challenge policies or bureaucratic structures that may threaten your client's welfare.*

All Good Things...

Nursing informatics is a new and important part of the nursing care arsenal. Working in partnership with the other members of the team, informaticists help the team define the clinical, administrative, and research outcomes and how those outcomes can be supported with comprehensive clinical data. Informaticists assist in creating an infrastructure that supports clear communication through the design of documentation consisting of nonredundant data elements with nonambiguous definitions. Nurse informaticists guide nursing leaders through the selection of a terminology system that meets the clinical and strategic goals of nursing practice and supports patient care. Nurse informaticists actively participate with clinical and information systems leadership in designing the strategic direction of the EMR system, ensuring the practice needs and imperatives of nursing are incorporated.

Nursing informaticists also communicate and interpret the role of nursing informatics to the nursing community. Effective staff training in effective use of information systems is an ongoing focus of nurse informaticists. An important facet of their role is translation of key accountabilities of practicing nurses as they use information systems and assisting the nursing community to perceive and understand the importance of its ongoing engagement and input to the work of nursing informaticists.

Let's Talk

1. Discuss the interrelationship of law and ethics.

2. Discuss federal laws affecting nursing and their impact on the profession.

3. Describe the difference between the two types of common law.

4. Discuss the elements of malpractice, and give an example of each.

5. Give an example of the criminalization of negligence.

6. What are the three components of intentional torts?

7. Give an example of an intentional tort of battery.

8. Give one example of a best practice for reducing the risk of malpractice litigation.

9. Discuss advance directives and claims that may be lodged for not following them.

10. Give an example of each of the seven ethical principles.

11. Discuss the five steps of ethical decision making [MO]RAL model.

References give you the information you need to further research a topic of interest found in the chapter

REFERENCES

Altaffer, A. (1998, July). First line managers: Measuring their span of control. *Nursing Management*, 36–40.

Anthony, M. (2004). Shared governance models: The theory, practice, and evidence. *Online Journal of Issues in Nursing, 9*(1)1–10.

Bolman, L., & Deal, T. (2003). *Reframing organizations: Artistry, choice, and leadership.* San Francisco: Jossey-Bass.

Crowell, D. (1998, May). Organizations are relationships, a new view of management. *Nursing Management*, 28–29.

Effken, J., & Stetler, C. (1997). Impact of organizational redesign. *Journal of Nursing Administration. 27*(7/8), 23–32.

Erickson, J., Hamilton, G., Jones, D., & Ditomassi, M. (2003). The value of governance/staff empowerment. *Journal of Nursing Administration, 33*(2), 96–104.

_____e, P., Bakken. S., & Larson, E. (2004). _____rganizational culture and climate in health-_____ursing Administration, 34*(1), 33–39.

_____eadership and nursing care management* (2nd _____: W.B. Saunders.

_____an, R. (2000). Organizational culture and _____ournal of Nursing Administration, 30*(12),

_____tarius, T. (2001). Managed care evolution—_____ne from and where is it going? In Kelly-_____rsing leadership and management.* Australia: _____ Learning.

_____on, C. (2003). Leadership roles and manage-_____n nursing. Theory & application* (4th ed.). _____incott Williams & Wilkins.

_____. (2000). Guide to nursing management and _____l.). St. Louis: Mosby.

_____September). Do integrated delivery systems

NCLEX Questions

1. A nursing competency:
   A. Is a skill that the nurse has to perform.
   B. Is a specific behavior that a nurse must demonstrate.
   C. A and B.
   D. Is the proficiency level that the nurse must obtain.

2. A standard of care:
   A. Requires use of the nursing process.
   B. Is the degree of care, expertise, and judgment exercised by nurses under similar circumstances.
   C. A and B.
   D. Is the number of patients that a competent nurse can care for on any given shift.

3. What affects nursing regulation?
   A. A state nurse practice act.
   B. Accreditation by an official body.
   C. Policies and procedures.
   D. All of the above.

4. The goal of state and federal legislation is to:
   A. Protect the public.
   B. Regulate nursing education.

NCLEX-style Test Questions round out every chapter to reinforce the content and help you prepare for the exam

Additional Resources included on the enclosed CD-ROM and available free online at DavisPlus —

Complete the learning package.

On CD-ROM

- **Leading by Example** case studies with critical thinking questions
- **Interactive Learning Exercises**
- **Flash cards and study notes**
- **Links to popular websites**
- **And much more!**

On DavisPlus

- **Additional NCLEX-style questions**
- **Resume Builder**
- **Links to popular websites**

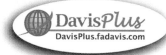
DavisPlus.fadavis.com

Nursing
Leadership
and
Management

Theories, Processes and Practice

Nursing

Leadership

and

Management

Theories, Processes and Practice

Rebecca A. Patronis Jones, DNSc, RN, CNAA, BC

Chancellor and Professor
West Suburban College of Nursing
Oak Park, IL

F. A. DAVIS COMPANY • Philadelphia

F.A. Davis Company
1915 Arch Street
Philadelphia, PA 19103
www.fadavis.com

Printed in the United States of America

Last digit indicates print number: 10 9 8 7 6 5 4 3 2 1

Publisher: Joanne P. DaCunha, RN, MSN
Developmental Editor: Caryn Abramowitz
Project Manager: Kristin L. Kern
Manager of Art & Design: Carolyn O'Brien

As new scientific information becomes available through basic and clinical research, recommended treatments and drug therapies undergo changes. The author(s) and publisher have done everything possible to make this book accurate, up to date, and in accord with accepted standards at the time of publication. The authors, editors, and publisher are not responsible for errors or omissions or for consequences from application of the book, and make no warranty, expressed or implied, in regard to the contents of the book. Any practice described in this book should be applied by the reader in accordance with professional standards of care used in regard to the unique circumstances that may apply in each situation. The reader is advised always to check product information (package inserts) for changes and new information regarding dose and contraindications before administering any drug. Caution is especially urged when using new or infrequently ordered drugs.

Library of Congress Cataloging-in-Publication Data

Jones, Rebecca A. Patronis.

  Nursing leadership and management : theories, processes, and practice / by Rebecca Patronis Jones.
     p. ; cm.
  Includes bibliographical references and index.
  ISBN-13: 978-0-8036-1362-1 (pbk. : alk. paper)
  1. Nursing services—Administration. 2. Nurse administrators. 3. Leadership. I. Title.
  [DNLM: 1. Leadership—Problems and Exercises. 2. Nursing, Supervisory—Problems and Exercises. 3. Nursing Care—organization & administration—Problems and Exercises. WY 105 J78n 2007]
  RT89.J645 2007
  610.68—dc22   2006034670

dedication

To all of the chapter authors for their diligence in going the extra mile to create both student and instructor learning materials that enhance the content of this book. To my husband Robert, daughter Aislan, and parents Jim and Ada Lee for their words of encouragement; and to the nurses from three generations of my family, Alice, Zelma, Jean, Patty, and Ginger, who have provided numerous stories about nursing. And last to Abbie, who provided nursing care to all of the members of our family in need.

preface

Introduction

Nurses lead and manage nursing care for patients, families, aggregates, and communities in a variety of settings, ranging from ambulatory to community to inpatient. Nurses also lead and manage care across the health-care continuum, including primary health promotion and prevention; secondary skilled, long term, and rehabilitative; and tertiary: emergent, urgent, and acute care. Strategies are drawn from both leadership and management theories. Leadership involves both the leader and the follower. In this text, we have defined **Leadership** as the process of envisioning a new and better world, communicating that vision to others, motivating others and enticing them to join in efforts to realize the vision, thinking in a different way, challenging the status quo, taking risks, and facilitating change (Valiga and Grossman). **Effective Followers** are individuals who work with and support leaders in their efforts to realize a vision by being engaged rather than alienated, suggesting new ideas and options, providing critical feedback on the ideas of others (including the leader), promoting positive relationships within the group, and acting as potential "leaders-in-waiting" (Valiga and Grossman). **Management**, one of the responsibilities of leadership, is a five-step process that comprises planning, organizing, directing, coordinating, and controlling (Garrison, Morgan, and Johnson).

The nurse's approach to leadership and management reflects the dynamic state of nursing practice and health care. Leadership has evolved from theories of the past, which pronounced that only great and noble men could be leaders, to more current theories that look at leadership as a learned process or a changing role depending on the situation. Management has evolved from competing managerial activities in a hierarchical, bureaucratic organization to complexity theory involving both the physical and social sciences. We have included a discussion of each of these concepts and theories in this textbook.

Purpose

The book is based on the philosophy that all nurses are leaders who use creative decision making, entrepreneurship, and life-long learning to create a work environment that is efficient, cost-effective, and committed to quality care. With that in mind, the primary goal for the textbook is to provide broad and comprehensive coverage of leadership and management theories and processes by synthesizing information from nursing, health care, general administration and management, and leadership literature and applying it to nursing. The book should engage readers with learning activities that will teach them how to research decision-making data (participatory action research process) and analyze and make reliable choices in managing their work environment. The content is based on research from several disciplines and provides a theory-based scholarly, yet practical, approach that is consistent with higher education.

Each chapter synthesizes information from nursing, health care, general administration and management, and leadership literature and incorporates relevant examples, case studies, vignettes, and best practices from leading experts in these fields.

Specific Objectives

The nurse is viewed as a proactive decision maker and problem solver engaged in critical thinking. Thus, the first specific objective of the book is to keep the student engaged in the learning process. The second goal of the book is to guide students toward applying the theory to practice and integrating evidence-based practice. Chapters require the student to participate in current research and analysis of the literature to become an active learner. Research briefs occur throughout various chapters to assist the student with application to practice and evidence-based practice to reach the second specific objective of the textbook. The third specific objective of the book is to help faculty keep students engaged in the learning process by providing the instructor with numerous elements on which to build the evaluation.

Key Features

Pedagogy included in the chapters follows:

- Chapter Motivation (a quotation representative of the chapter's content)
- Chapter Motives (measurable objectives for the chapter)
- Hot Topic (brief discussion of something currently at the forefront of the topic of a chapter)
- Chapter Star (description of a real-life person performing services that apply to the chapter in an exceptional way)
- Practice to Strive For (box focusing on best practices in the area of the chapter)
- Practice Proof (description of research study, with questions, to encourage thinking about evidence-based practice)
- All Good Things (summary of the chapter)
- Let's Talk (discussion and thought questions regarding the chapter content and related areas)
- Names of Web sites
- References
- NCLEX-style Test Questions
  An Instructor's CD package includes:
- Chapter objectives
- Glossary of terms used throughout the book
- Case studies with discussion questions and answers
- Learning exercises
- Names of Web sites
- PowerPoint slide presentation with key points for each chapter
- Image bank
- A test bank with multiple-choice and short-answer essay questions

A student CD will accompany each book and include:

- Chapter objectives
- Study notes (PowerPoint slides of key points for each chapter)

- Group/individual interactive learning exercises or clinical scenarios that require students to gather data and apply theory to solve problems
- Discussion questions
- Case studies
- Interactive self-assessment exercises
- Résumé help
- Games
- Names of Web sites
- A practice test bank

Tour of the Units and Chapters

The text is divided into five major parts with corresponding chapters. Part 1 focuses on understanding the theories of leading, following, and managing. The first three chapters are devoted to these topics and theories. The third chapter focuses on motivational theory. Part 2 provides information to aid readers in understanding organizations. Chapters 4 through 9 describe organizational structures and cover legal, ethical, and economic issues and influences related to the regulation of nursing care. This part also offers information on communication, both organizational and through the use of computers, or informatics. Part 3 discusses the skills needed to be an effective leader. Chapters 10 through 13 provide the reader with the latest decision-making and problem-solving theories and strategies. Part 3 also covers the concepts of change, team building, power, politics, and influence, along with tips for the new nurse leader on how to use these concepts. Part 4 focuses on the skills for being an effective manager. Chapters 14 through 21 cover the nuts and bolts of management. The theoretical base, principles, techniques, and strategies for the day-to-day management of nursing care are described in detail. Readers will learn how to plan, manage quality and risk, budget, staff and schedule, deal with conflict, and delegate to manage nursing care. The concept of culture is also discussed. Part 5 changes the focus to the skills new nurses need for a successful career. In Chapters 22 through 25, the reader will learn how to manage one's self and how to obtain the important first job.

contributors

NANCY HOWELL AGEE, RN, MN
Chief Operating Officer/Executive Vice President
Carilion Health System
Roanoke, VA

SHARON BATOR, MSN, RN
Assistant Professor
Southern University School of Nursing
Baton Rouge, LA

CONNIE J. BOERST, MSN, RN, BC
Assistant Professor
Bellin College of Nursing
Green Bay, WI

BARBARA B. BREWER, MALS, MBA, PHD, RN
Director of Professional Practice
John C. Lincoln North Mountain Hospital
Phoenix, AZ

CAROLINE CAMUÑAS, EDD, RN
Adjunct Associate Professor
Teachers College, Columbia University
New York, NY
Research Coordinator
J. J. Peters VA Medical Center
Bronx, NY

THERESA L. CARROLL, RN, PHD, CNAA
Professor, Department of Nursing Systems
University of Texas School of Nursing at Houston
Houston, TX

BARBARA SHELDEN CZERWINSKI, PHD, RN, CNAA-BC, FAAN
The Ohio State University Medical Center
Clinical Nurse Scientist
Columbus, OH

JUDY A. DAVIS, MS, MPH, APN, CNP
Clinical Faculty
University of Illinois at Chicago
Chicago, IL

MARY E. HORTON, ELLIOTT, DNSC, RN
Associate Professor
West Suburban College of Nursing
Oak Park, IL

BETSY FRANK, RN, PHD
Professor
Indiana State University College of Nursing
Terre Haute, IN

ELIZABETH GANEY-CODE, MSN, RN
Patient Care Nurse Manager
University of Texas MD Anderson Cancer Center
Houston, TX

SHIRLEY GARICK, PHD, RN MSN, ABQARP DIPLOMATE, LEGAL NURSE CONSULTANT (LNC)
Associate Professor
College of Health & Behavioral Sciences
Texas A&M University
Texarkana, TX

DEBORAH R. GARRISON, PHD, RN
Associate Professor
Associate Dean, Graduate Nursing Programs
University of Toledo
Toledo, OH

SHEILA C. GROSSMAN, PHD, APRN-BC
Professor and Director of Family Nurse Practitioner Program
Fairfield University School of Nursing
Fairfield, CT

MICHELLE B. HAGADORN, MA, CPA
Masters of Accountancy
Assistant Professor of Business Administration and Economics
Roanoke College
Salem, VA

EMILY HARMAN, MSN, RN
Assistant Professor and Associate Director of the RN to BSN PRogram
Ohio University School of Nursing
Athens, OH

PATRICIA M. HAYNOR, DNSC, RN, NHA
Villanova University
Villanova, PA

JACQUELINE J. HILL, PHD, RN, CRRN
Associate Professor
Interim Chair, Undergraduate Nursing Program
Southern University School of Nursing
Baton Rouge, LA

STACY GRANT HOHENLEITNER, MSN, RN, CNA, NHA
Villanova University
Villanova, PA

DEBORAH A. JASOVSKY, MSN, PHD, RN, CNAA, BC
Director of Nursing—Special Projects and Magnet Project Director
Raritan Bay Medical Center
Perth Amboy, NJ

JEWETT J. JOHNSON, MS, RN
Assistant Professor
Wilson School of Nursing
Midwestern State University
Wichita Falls, TX

ESPERANZA VILLANUEVA JOYCE, EDD, CNS, RN
Professor
School of Nursing
New Mexico State University
Athens, OH

JOSEPHINE KAHLER, EDD, RN, CS
Dean/Professor
College of Health & Behavioral Sciences
Texas A&M University-Texarkana
Texarkana, TX

MARY KAMIENSKI, PHD, RN, APRN-C, FAEN
Assistant Dean Graduate Nursing Programs
University of Medicine and Dentistry
Newark, NJ

PATRICIA MARTINEZ, MD
Chief Quality Officer
Asante Health System
Medford, OR

SHARON MCLANE, MBA, RN, BC
Director Nursing Informatics
University of Texas MD Anderson Cancer Center
Houston, TX

DEBRA A. MORGAN, EDD, RN
Assistant Professor and Coordinator of the RN to BSN and RN to MSN Programs
Wilson School of Nursing
Midwestern State University
Wichita Falls, TX

CAROLE A. MUTZEBAUGH, EDD, NP, CNS
Consultant, Care Management Associates
Director, Foundation for Care Management
Foundation for Care Management
Vashon, WA

MARY E. O'KEEFE, RN, PHD, JD
Legal Nurse Consultant
Mills Shirley L.L.P.
Galveston, TX

CARLA G. PHILIPS, PHD, RN
Ohio University School of Nursing
Athens, OH

DENISE TOP RHINE, MED, RN, CEN
Professor
Oakton College
Des Plaines, IL

CAROL SEAVOR, EDD, RN
President
Jefferson College of Health Sciences
Roanoke, VA

SUSAN SPORTSMAN, PHD, RN
Dean
College of Health Sciences and Human Services
Midwestern State University
Wichita Falls, TX

GEORGIANNA THOMAS, EDD, RN
Dean and Associate Professor
West Suburban College of Nursing
Oak Park, IL

THERESA M. VALIGA, EDD, RN, FAAN
Chief Program Officer
National League for Nursing
New York, NY

SHARON WALKER, MA
Career Planning Specialist
Our Lady of the Lake College
Baton Rouge, LA

reviewers

JOAN MANNING BAKER, RN, MSN, CCRN
Assistant Professor
Molloy College
Rockville Centre, NY

THOMAS BEEMAN, RN, PHD
Director, Undergraduate Nursing
University of Texas
El Paso, TX

MARY HILL, RN, DSN
Associate Professor
University of Mississippi
Jackson, MS

SUSAN MEYER, RN, MSN
Assistant Professor
Mount St. Mary's College
Los Angeles, CA

KAY MUGGENBURG, RN, PHD
Assistant Professor
University of Kentucky
Lexington, KY

VIVIAN SCHRADER, PHD, RN
Associate Professor
Boise State University
Boise, ID

PAMELA WHEELER, RN, PHD
Associate Professor
Linfield College
Portland, OR

JOYCE M. WOODS, RN, PHD
Nursing Instructor
Mount Royal College
Calgary, AB, Canada

POLLY GERBER ZIMMERMANN, RN, MS, MBA, CEN
Assistant Professor, Department of Nursing
Harry S Truman College
Chicago, IL

acknowledgments

A special thanks to Caryn Abramowitz and Mary Horton Elliott, DNSc, RN, Associate Professor, West Suburban College of Nursing, Oak Park, IL, for their assistance in the development of the ancillary materials.

contents

UNDERSTANDING THE THEORY OF LEADING, FOLLOWING, AND MANAGING

chapter 1

Leadership and Followership

THERESA M. VALIGA, EDD, RN, FAAN
SHEILA GROSSMAN, PHD, APRN-BC

CHAPTER MOTIVATION

"Cautious, careful people always casting about to preserve their reputation and social standing, never can bring about a reform. Those who are really in earnest must be willing to be anything or nothing in the world's estimation."

Susan B. Anthony

CHAPTER MOTIVES

- Distinguish between leadership and management.
- Compare characteristics of effective followers with those of leaders.
- Discuss how all nurses can provide leadership in and for the profession.

Today's climate demands individuals who are flexible, creative, and able to empower others to be flexible and creative. With the nursing shortage, managed care, higher patient acuity, fewer resources, highly diverse demographics, and outside influences, nurses need to be more effective leaders than ever as they manage patients in various settings.

But what is an effective leader without effective followers? This is also a time when nurses need to be effective followers, knowing who to follow, when to follow, how to follow, and how to use the follower role most powerfully. Because most of us are followers more often than we are leaders, the art of followership is a concept that needs to be explored in any contemporary discussion of leadership and management.

Burns (2003) viewed leadership as "a master discipline that illuminates some of the toughest problems of human needs and social change" (p. 3). Others suggest that leadership is about having a vision and getting people to follow, using the art of persuasion. Then there are some who equate leadership with management and use the words interchangeably. Bennis and Nanus (1985) described the phenomenon of leadership as well studied, with each interpretation providing a sliver of insight but none providing a holistic and adequate explanation. Sashkin and Sashkin (2003) took a rather simplistic, but helpful, perspective on leadership, stating that leadership that matters is the critical factor that makes a difference in people's lives and organizations' success.

Many experts have described leadership as encompassing the leader's personality, the leader's behavior, the talents of the followers, and the situational context in which leadership takes place. These experts also tend to agree that leadership can be learned. Knowing that leaders are not necessarily born but made, therefore, is an important concept when one considers that all nurses must be looked to as leaders in and for the profession.

Nursing's focus today is on delivering quality and cost-effective patient care rather than on accomplishing a list of nursing tasks. This focus requires that nurses fulfill both leadership and follower roles effectively. This chapter will explore the concepts of leadership and followership and discuss how nurses can improve their abilities to lead and follow.

Leadership Theories— Past and Contemporary

In order to understand the phenomenon of leadership and how contemporary perspectives shape leadership behaviors, it is helpful to know how views about leaders and leadership have changed over time. A brief outline of several of the more significant leadership theories provides such a context.

GREAT MAN THEORY

Just by reading the name of this theory, Great Man, one can imagine that it is not widely accepted today. Yet this was precisely how the world thought of leaders for many years. This theory assumed that all leaders were men and all were great (i.e., of the noble class). Thus, those who assumed leadership roles were determined by their genetic and social inheritance. It was not conceivable that those from the "working class" could be leaders, that leadership could be learned, or that women could be leaders.

TRAIT THEORIES

During the early part of the 20th century, several researchers studied the behaviors and traits of individuals thought to be effective leaders. Studies revealed that these leaders possessed multiple characteristics. Although there were commonalities among them (e.g., they tended to be taller, be more articulate, or exude self-confidence), there was no standard list that fit everyone or that could be used to predict or identify who was or could be an effective leader.

SITUATIONAL OR CONTINGENCY THEORIES

These theories embodied the idea that the right thing to do depended on the situation the leader was facing. The most well-known and used situational theory involves assessing the nature of the task and the follower's motivation or readiness to learn and using that to determine the particular style the leader should use. Despite widespread discussion and use of this theory, however, little research exists to support its validity.

TRANSFORMATIONAL THEORY

A new way of thinking about leadership emerged in the mid-1970s when James McGregor Burns asserted that the true nature of leadership is not the ability to motivate people to work hard for their pay but the ability to transform followers to become more self-directed in all they do. Transformational leaders, therefore, "look for potential motives in followers, seek to satisfy higher needs, and engage the full person of the follower. The result is a relationship of mutual stimulation and elevation that converts followers into leaders and may convert leaders into moral agents" (Burns, 1978, p. 4).

Barker (1990) asserted that transformational leaders need to have a heightened self-awareness and a plan for self-development. This positive self-regard satisfies the leader's self-esteem needs and tends to result in "self-confidence, worth, strength, capability, adequacy, and being useful and necessary" (Barker, 1990, p. 159).

NEW SCIENCE LEADERSHIP

Wheatley (1999) took this paradigm a step further when she described leadership as a method of thinking in a different way, a way that is not standard, orderly, or goal-oriented, Instead, she suggests we think about leadership in a way that reflects naturally occurring events: free-flowing, dynamic, and accepting of an anything-can-happen philosophy. She recommended we think of leadership through a new perspective. Leadership comprises naturally occurring events in which leaders have knowledge and serve as leaders when needed. Thus, there is no need for others to direct and control what we do.

Practice to Strive For 1-1

Nurses who function as leaders in clinical practice are not necessarily in positions of authority. They are not necessarily the charge nurses, nurse managers, or chief nursing officers, although they may very well be in such positions.

Nurse leaders, regardless of the position they hold in an organization, are the individuals who continually question the status quo, offer suggestions about how to improve patient care, and entice (not demand or require) colleagues to work toward a new level of excellence. These individuals are familiar with what is being written by experts in the field and draw on this literature to formulate a vision for improving their own area of practice (e.g., care of cancer patients, the homeless, patients undergoing surgery, or poor children in school). These individuals have a high degree of energy and are passionate about practice. In other words, they never give up. They challenge our thinking, propose alternative approaches to care, and are creative.

In many ways, nurse leaders make people uncomfortable because they do not allow others to remain in their "safe little corner of the world." Instead, they challenge others to grow, seek out new experiences, strive for excellence in the care they provide, and expand their horizons (e.g., working with an interdisciplinary team, serving on institutional committees, or proposing new legislation). But leaders also help and support colleagues as they face these new challenges and opportunities.

These are the practices to strive for if nursing is to secure its rightful place in health care. Every nurse has the potential to provide leadership. We simply need to stop putting limits on ourselves and our nurse colleagues.

Leadership Practices and Tasks

Kouzes and Posner (1995) asserted that leaders should follow five practices of leadership to assist in transforming followers to realize their own visions and become more self-directed: challenging the status quo, inspiring a shared vision, enabling others to act rather than to react, being a role model, and encouraging the heart. These practices were identified from an analysis of the memoirs of hundreds of managers, who were asked to reflect on what they perceived as their own best leadership experience. The findings from this research were similar to Bennis and Nanus' (1985) notions of what constituted leadership strategies: the management of risk; the management of attention; the management of communication; the management of trust, or credibility; and the management of respect. In addition, the work of Kouzes and Posner and Bennis and Nanus is consistent with that of Sashkin and Sashkin (2003) who, after 20 years of research, designed a four-dimensional model of transformational leadership that addresses communication leadership, credible leadership, caring leadership, and risk leadership (a concept they later renamed: creating opportunities).

Gardner (1990) also researched the concept of leadership and identified several tasks that leaders perform. Those tasks are as follows:

- *Envisioning goals*—pointing the group in a new direction or asserting a vision.
- *Affirming values*—reminding the group members of the norms and expectations they share.
- *Motivating*—promoting positive attitudes.
- *Managing*—keeping the system functioning and the group moving toward realizing the vision.
- *Achieving a workable unity*—managing the conflict that inevitably accompanies change and growth.
- *Explaining*—teaching followers and helping them understand why they are being asked to do certain things.
- *Serving as a symbol*—acting in ways that convey the values of the group and its goals.
- *Representing the group*—speaking on behalf of the group.
- *Renewing*—bringing members of the group to new levels.

These tasks provide specific guidelines for people interested in increasing their leadership ability, and they highlight the importance of leaders working closely with followers.

Perspectives on Followership

Although Gardner (1990) and others have acknowledged the importance of leaders and followers working together in order to realize a vision, the literature typically pays little attention to the concept of followership, and there are no "theories" of followership.

Perhaps one of the earliest discussions of followership was presented by Kelley (1992, 1998), who outlined four types of followers: sheep, "yes" people, alienated followers, and effective or exemplary followers. Sheep are passive individuals who comply with whatever the leader or manager directs but are not actively engaged in the work of the group. "Yes" people, in comparison, are actively involved in the group's work and eagerly support the leader; they do not, however, initiate ideas or think for themselves. Alienated followers do think for themselves and often are critical of what the leader is doing; they do not, however, share those ideas openly, they seem disengaged, and they "rarely invest time or energy to suggest alternative solutions or other approaches" (Grossman & Valiga, 2005, p. 47). The individuals who are engaged, sug-

gest new ideas, share criticisms with the leader, and invest time and energy in the work of the group are referred to as effective or exemplary followers.

Pittman, Rosenbach, and Potter (1998) also described four types of followers: subordinates, contributors, politicians, and partners. Subordinates are similar to Kelley's "sheep," doing what they are told but not actively involved. Contributors are like Kelley's "yes people," supportive, involved, and doing a good job, but not willing to challenge the ideas of the leader. Politicians are willing to give honest feedback and support the leader, but they may neglect the job and have poor performance levels. Like Kelley's effective or exemplary followers, the partners described by Pittman, et al. (1998) are highly involved, perform at a high level, promote positive relationships within the group, and are seen as "leaders-in-waiting" (p. 118).

Because leaders cannot be leaders unless they have followers, the role of the follower is extremely important in any discussion of leadership. In addition, the characteristics that describe effective/exemplary followers or partners are quite similar to those outlined for effective leaders themselves. Although the term "follower" "conjures up images of docility, conformity, weakness, and failure to excel" (Chaleff, 1995, p. 3), those who are effective in the role are independent, critical thinkers, innovative, actively engaged, able and willing to think for themselves, willing to assume ownership, self-starters, and able and willing to give honest feedback and constructive criticism (adapted from Grossman & Valiga, 2005, pp. 49–50).

Effective followers are not employees who simply "follow the rules" and accept whatever management decides. In fact, the concept of effective followers may not even be compatible with perspectives on management that assume a complacent, nonquestioning employee. But it is clearly aligned with the concept of leadership, because effective followers are seen as partners with the leader, working collaboratively to realize the vision they share. Thus, it is helpful to outline the differences between leadership and management.

Differences Between Leadership and Management

Leadership and management are related phenomena but they are not the same. It is important to realize that (a) not all individuals in management positions are necessarily leaders, and (b) leadership is not necessarily tied to a position of authority. While only those in management positions are expected to be managers, leadership can and needs to be exercised by each of us wherever we may be. In other words, even though an individual does not hold a management position, she can still be a leader on a clinical unit, in an institution, in her community, or in the profession as a whole.

In a classic article written in 1977, Zaleznik asserted that "leaders and managers are very different kinds of people: they differ in their motivations, in their personal history, and in how they think and act; they differ in their orientation toward goals, work, human relations, and themselves; and they differ in their worldviews" (Zaleznik, as quoted in Grossman & Valiga, 2005, p. 5). For example, leaders are creative, innovative, and risk-takers; managers often are more concerned with maintaining the status quo and taking few risks. In addition, managers often have a short-range perspective and are concerned about the "bottom line," whereas leaders have a long-range, visionary perspective and are concerned about moving toward realization of that vision.

It is important to remember that these distinctions point out the extremes of perspectives to illustrate the points that not all managers are leaders and not all leaders are managers. Despite the differences outlined by Zaleznik and others, however, many individuals are able to function as both leaders and managers simultaneously and effectively.

Indeed, our practice world is greatly enhanced when leaders are able to manage and managers are able to lead. Bennis and Nanus (1985, p. 21) have been quoted often as saying "leaders do the right thing, and managers do things right." In nursing practice, we must both do the right thing and do that thing right. For example, we apply standards of care to our practice that must be followed and acuity quotients that, in most cases, must be assessed in order to make decisions about staffing, admissions, and supports needed. Thus, we must do the thing right. But perhaps we also need to ensure that we are doing the right thing by evaluating if the standards fit our patient population and if the acuity and staffing ratios are relevant to our needs. If they are not, leaders need to step forward to create standards that do fit and that are relevant.

All nurses need to lead and manage effectively in patient care settings in order to accomplish tasks

hot topic:
Leader vs. Manager

Zaleznik (1977) wrote a classic piece on the comparison of leaders and managers, in which he described how each relates to other people, the organizations in which they work, and their goals. These differences are explained in terms of how managers and leaders view work, solitary activity, conflict, and the status quo.

He concludes that managers are generally viewed in terms of the organization they represent and are influenced by others' opinions. Leaders are more individualistic and really do not "belong" to organizations. He does, however, agree that leaders can be managers, and managers can be leaders.

Grossman and Valiga (2005, p. 7) summarize the differences between an "ideal" leader and an extremely "organization-focused" manager in terms of the following: position, power base, goals/vision, innovative ideas, risk level, degree of order, nature of activities, focus, perspective, degree of freedom, and actions.

and achieve maximum care quality. All need to share their visions of how patient care can be improved, and all need to learn from the leaders who have gone before them.

Nursing Leaders

The nursing profession claims many true leaders. They have expressed bold visions, invested enormous amounts of energy to realize those visions, effectively engaged followers in the quest, been passionate about the futures they hoped to create, and absorbed criticism, setbacks, and opposition on the road to success.

Florence Nightingale, for example, demonstrated how a healthful environment could promote healing and recovery, fought for the proper care of soldiers, and provided careful documentation of interventions and outcomes that laid a foundation for future research activities. Lillian Wald, who literally walked the rooftops of New York tenement buildings to provide care to the poor and helpless, created the concept of public health and demonstrated how nursing care could make a significant difference in the lives and well-being of individuals and communities. In nursing education, Isabel Stewart was a leader in establishing standards of quality for educational programs and instrumental in creating a program of study to prepare individuals for the teaching or faculty role.

In more recent years, nursing leaders have helped us establish ourselves as researchers, expert clinicians, influencers of public policy, theorists, and entrepreneurs. The development of nursing theories occurred through the passionate work of individuals such as Hildegard Peplau, Ida Jean Orlando, Dorothea Orem, Betty Neumann, Jean Watson, Imogene King, and Martha Rogers. Madeleine Leininger has enhanced cultural awareness and competence of all nurses. The creation of associate degree nursing programs was the result of research conducted by Mildred Montag, and its widespread implementation was realized through her efforts and those of individuals like Verle Waters and Elaine Tagliareni. The ability of nurses to influence public policy evolved from the leadership provided by Shirley Chater, Jessie Scott, Doris Block, Mary Wakefield, and Ada Sue Hinshaw.

Our profession has developed the science of nursing practice through the efforts of such individuals as Mary Naylor, Donna Diers, Nancy Fugate Woods, and Dorothy Brooten. The science of nursing education has been advanced through the sustained work of Nancy Diekelmann, Pamela Ironside, Marilyn Oermann, and Chris Tanner.

In nursing administration, the following individuals have provided significant leadership in changing the work environment for nurses: Leah Curtin, Barbara Donoho, and Joyce Clifford. Our nursing organizations have been successful in charting preferred futures for our profession through the leadership of their officers, including Lucille Joel, Nancy Langston, Sr. Rosemary Donnelly, and Angela Barron McBride.

We know the names and accomplishments of these talented nurses because each of them articulated a vision of a better future, was passionate about working to realize that preferred future, was successful in enlisting nurses in the effort, was willing to take risks, accepted criticism and suggestions, spoke eloquently, exhibited enormous amounts of energy, and was unwilling to accept the status quo or settle for "second best." In other words, each of these individuals was a leader. None of them started out as leaders, but their vision and passion helped

Practice Proof 1-1

May (2001) conducted a study of 508 women in the Houston area to identify the skills and attributes those women believed would be needed to succeed in leadership positions in the 21st century. Data from the 263 women who responded to the questionnaire, 137 of whom completed both the first and second rounds of the study, yielded six skills (listed in order of importance to the respondents) seen as the most important skills and attributes of leaders: personal integrity, strategic vision/action orientation, team building/communication skills, management and technical competencies, people skills, and personal survival skills (e.g., political sensitivity, self-direction, courage).

QUESTIONS:
1. To what extent are the skills and attributes needed by leaders in the 21st century that have been identified by participants in May's study consistent with those needed by nurses?
2. For those who do not possess these six strengths or need some assistance in improving their skills, how could nurses develop and/or improve them?

them become leaders. This same opportunity awaits each of us.

It we have a vision, if we are passionate about realizing it, and if we invest a great deal of energy to create our preferred future, then each one of us might be included in a list of "nursing's leaders" at some point in the future. We do not need to be in positions of authority right now. We do not need to hold a doctorate. We do not need to be published researchers with major grants. We do not need to be over the age of 50 or teach in a university. What we do need, however, is to exhibit the qualities of a leader.

Leadership Qualities

Gardner (1990) identified several attributes of leaders, including physical vitality and stamina, intelligence, good judgment, willingness to accept responsibilities, task competence (i.e., knowing what needs to be done), understanding of followers' needs, ability to work effectively with others, a need to achieve, ability to motivate others, and courage.

COMPETENCIES

In a presentation at the April 2004 American Society of Association Executives Foundation Forum, one of the most influential individuals in the area of leadership, Warren Bennis, offered his ideas about exemplary leaders. He asserted that leaders have the following six competencies:

1. **Leaders must foster a clear vision with an endowed purpose that is owned by the people involved with the leader**. To illustrate this competency, Bennis gave the following example of how Howard Schultz, founder of the Starbucks Coffee conglomeration, views his company's vision: "We aren't in the coffee business serving people; we're in the people business serving coffee."
2. Getting people to support a vision or mission takes work. **Leaders must "keep reminding people of what is important [because] people really can forget what they are there for."** Followers also need regular recognition in order to maintain their engagement with and commitment to the vision.
3. **Leaders must be optimistic and see possibilities**. Leaders must be adaptive to the constant change in our society, which "takes a hardiness attitude that allows [them] to face challenges and adapt all of it in a way that results in alignment."
4. **Leaders must create a culture of candor**. Bennis asserted that such a culture requires integrity, which evolves from a balance of ambition, competence, and having "a moral compass." When ambition surpasses competence or overrides one's moral compass, for example, integrity is lost, a culture of candor cannot be created, and one cannot be an effective leader.
5. **Leaders must mentor others and acknowledge their ideas and accomplishments**. Bennis said, "Drawing out the leadership qualities [of others] is the way of the true leader."
6. **Good leaders must be in tune to getting results**. Bennis shared a conversation he had with Jack Welch, previous CEO of General Electric. This highly successful corporate manager and leader noted that "getting results depends on customer satisfaction, employee satisfaction, and cash flow. If I have those three measurements, I can win." Thus, vision, good intentions, and strong desires are not enough; leaders are leaders because they make things happen.

GENDER DIFFERENCES

Today there are more women than ever before who are effective leaders, and it is expected that the number of women leaders, particularly those from minority groups, will continue to increase (Bennis, Spreitzer, & Cummings, 2003). There are more women governors, senators, and representatives. There are more women leaders in sports, science, business, education, and many other fields than ever before. In nursing, women have always led the profession toward change and development.

It is reported that women have different styles than men in many things, and because of these differences, it is assumed that women are better at some things (e.g., child-rearing, nursing) and men are better at others (e.g., sales, construction work). But when it comes to leadership, the styles of men and women allow both to be successful, particularly if stereotypical maleness is combined with stereotypical femaleness. A more androgynous perspective on leadership—one that combines the best of "femaleness" and the best of "maleness" and draws on the strengths of each style—therefore, is most helpful. The androgynous leader "blends dominance, assertiveness and competitiveness [often thought to be "male" characteristics] . . . with concern for relationships, cooperativeness, and humanitarian values [often associated with a "female" style]" (Grossman & Valiga, 2005, p. 112). Such a combination is critical in a world characterized by declining resources and increasing chaos and uncertainty.

GAINING POWER

McClelland and Burnham (1976) determined that power is a definitive aspect of leadership because it motivates individuals and contributes to their charisma. The concept of power is discussed more fully in Chapter 13 so it will not be examined in depth here. But it is important to look at power as a component of leadership.

The two primary sources of power are one's position in an organization and one's personal qualities. McClelland and Burnham (1976) asserted that hierarchical power, or the amount of authority one has in an organization, and the ability to provide rewards or "punishments" to others are used to attain organizational goals. They also noted that personal power, deriving from one's knowledge, competence, and trustworthiness, or from followers' respect for and desire to be associated with the leader, is used to influence others.

It is only when one's personal power is well established that one can exert transformational leadership. Transformational leaders with highly developed power are comfortable with themselves, have high self-efficacy, and empower followers to attain their own goals and, ultimately, the goals of the group or organization. We are well aware of the many disadvantages of people abusing their power, but when power is used in the service of others, positive results are realized. Greenleaf (1977) and Block (1993) used the term stewardship to describe the phenomenon of directing one's power toward the service of others, and they asserted that such a quality is essential in leaders. Stewardship is "the willingness to be accountable for the well-being of the larger organization by operating in service, rather than in control, of those around us" (Block, 1993).

Similar notions of building relationships through nurturing and empowerment, gaining power through community networking, and leading groups based on values of cooperation were offered by Chinn (2004). Chinn advocated for building one's personal power base so that it can be used to enhance the group's ability to achieve its goals and realize its vision, thereby using it to fulfill the leader role.

BECOMING A NURSE LEADER

Nurses need to view themselves as leaders, develop their leadership abilities, and embrace the challenges that face them in health care today (Grossman & Valiga, 2005). In order to become leaders, however, nurses must learn about leadership in their academic programs (Fagin, 2000), through on-the-job experiences, through mentors, or through other avenues. In order to develop their leadership skills, it is imperative for nurses to observe expert leaders, work hand-in-hand with such individuals, and receive constructive feedback on their performance. Having a "shadowing," or preceptor, experience with a leader, for example, allows nursing students to understand the context of an organization, develop their negotiation skills, think more broadly, communicate more effectively, collaborate more effectively, and be empowered (Grossman, 2005). Personal involvement, immersion in a situation, learning by doing, and practicing in the clinical setting with an experienced nurse have been cited as important to learning generally. They are also strategies to be used to help individuals learn how to be leaders.

Bennis and Thomas (2002) reinforced the notion that in order to become an effective leader an individual must be able to define her uniqueness or what makes her special. She must then continually grow and increase her expertise in that unique area so that she can be a leader who influences policy development, evidence-based practice, and dissemination of new understandings.

Many health-care organizations have leadership programs for their managers and those aspiring to become managers. Leadership skills can also be learned as part of the professional development of all nurses. Many professional organizations have leadership institutes and seminars at their annual conferences. When the nursing profession realizes that nurses need leadership skills as much as patient care and management skills and that every nurse, from the entry-level staff nurse to the chief executive nurse, needs to become an effective leader, we can expect that patient care outcomes will be enhanced and that nursing will most effectively influence health care.

All Good Things . . .

The mantle of leadership does not fall to only a few. Indeed, all nurses must think of themselves as a leader, act as a leader, and take on the challenges of a leadership role. All leaders are not managers or organizational office holders; many of them are staff nurses, faculty, and individuals on the "front lines" of patient care. By the same token, all managers are not leaders. Nurses also need to be effective followers, knowing who to follow, when to follow, and how to follow. It is only through the exercise of leadership and effective followership that nurses will be able to influence health care and create a preferred future for the profession.

Those of us who are leaders in the field must guide, support, and encourage those who aspire to this role. Those who aspire to genuine leadership must learn about this role, take the risks associated with expressing and moving forward to achieve a vision, and allow passions to drive actions. The patients, families, and communities we serve deserve nothing less.

Let's Talk

1. How can one be a leader as a staff nurse?

2. Suppose you are often dissatisfied with the way things are done in your institution but are afraid to speak up or propose alternative ways of doing things. Does this mean you can never be a leader in nursing?

3. It seems that leaders and effective followers may be more alike than leaders and managers. Is that so?

NCLEX Questions

1. Great Man leadership theory assumes that:
   A. All leaders are great men.
   B. Leadership is determined by genetic and social inheritance.
   C. Leaders are from the working class
   D. A and B.

2. Situational and Contingency theory:
   A. Embodies the idea that the leader does the right thing based on the situation.
   B. Involves assessing the nature of the task and the follower's motivation to determine the particular style the leader should use.
   C. Involves assessing contingent courses of action.
   D. Is based on the concept that leader characteristics must fit the situation.

3. Transformational leadership theory:
   A. Was developed in the mid-1970s by Warren Bennis
   B. Is the ability to transform followers to become more self-directed in all they do.

   C. Involves leaders who look for potential motive in followers, seek to satisfy higher needs, and engage the full person of the follower.
   D. B and C.

4. New Science leadership:
   A. Thinks of leadership through a new perspective of naturally occurring events.
   B. Is based on ethics, biology, and chemistry.
   C. Involves leading based on the situation.
   D. Involves a laissez-faire leadership style.

5. Kouzes and Posner (1995) asserted that leaders use the following practice(s) of leadership:
   A. Challenging the status quo.
   B. Inspiring a shared vision.
   C. Enabling others to act rather than to react.
   D. All of the above.

6. Gardner (1990) identified the following tasks that leaders perform:
   A. Representing the group by speaking on its behalf.
   B. serving as a symbol by acting in ways that convey the values of the group and its goals.
   C. Motivating and promoting positive attitudes.
   D. All of the above.

7. Kelley (1992, 1998) outlined types of followers as:
   A. Sheep, or "yes," people.
   B. Alienated followers.
   C. Effective, or exemplary, followers.
   D. All of the above.

8. Pittman, Rosenbach, and Potter (1998) described types of followers as:
   A. Subordinates who do what they are told but who are not actively involved.
   B. Contributors who are supportive, involved, and doing a good job but who are not willing to challenge the ideas of the leaders.
   C. Politicians willing to give honest feedback and support the leader.
   D. All of the above.

9. Gardner identified several attributes of leaders as:
   A. Including physical vitality and stamina.
   B. Intelligence and good judgment.
   C. Understanding followers' needs.
   D. All of the above.

10. Warren Bennis asserted that leaders have the following competencies:
    A. Foster a clear vision with an endowed purpose that is owned by the people involved with the leader.
    B. Must keep reminding people of what is important because people really can forget what they are there for.
    C. Must mentor others and acknowledge their ideas and accomplishments.
    D. All of the above.

REFERENCES

Barker, A. (1990). *Transformational nursing leadership: A vision for the future.* Baltimore: Williams & Wilkins.

Bennis, W. (2004). Highlights of "A leadership discussion with Warren Bennis." American Society of Association Executives Forum, www.asaenet.org/foundation

Bennis, W., & Nanus, B. (1985). *Leaders: The strategies for taking charge.* New York: Harper & Row.

Bennis, W., Spreitzer, G., & Cummings, T. (Eds.). (2003). *The future of leadership: Today's top leadership thinkers speak to tomorrow's leaders.* San Francisco: Jossey-Bass.

Bennis, W., & Thomas, R. (2002). *Geeks and geezers: How era, values, and defining moments shape leaders.* Cambridge, MA: Harvard Business School Press.

Block, P. (1993). *Stewardship: Choosing service over self-interest.* San Francisco: Berrett-Koehler Publishers.

Burns, J. (1978). *Leadership.* New York: Harpers.

Burns, J. (2003). *Transforming leadership: A new pursuit of happiness.* New York: Atlantic Monthly Press.

Chaleff, I. (1995). *The courageous follower: Standing up to and for our leaders.* San Francisco: Berrett-Koehler Publishers.

Chinn, P. (2004). *Peace and poser: Creative leadership for building community* (6th ed.). Sudbury, MA: Jones and Bartlett Publishers.

Fagin, C. (2000). Preparing students for leadership. In C. Fagin (Ed.), *Essays on nursing leadership.* New York: Springer Publishing.

Gardner, J. (1990). *On leadership.* New York: Free Press.

Greenleaf, R.K. (1977). *Servant leadership: A journey into the nature of legitimate power and greatness.* New York: Paulist Press.

Grossman, S. (2005). Developing leadership through shadowing a leader in health care. In H. Feldman & M. Greenburg (Eds.), *Educating for leadership* (pp. 266–278). New York: Springer Publishing.

Grossman, S., & Valiga, T.M. (2005). *The new leadership challenge: Creating the future of nursing* (2nd ed.). Philadelphia: F.A. Davis.

Kelley, R. (1992). *The power of followership: How to create leaders people want to follow and followers who lead themselves.* New York: Doubleday Currency.

Kelley, R. (1998). In praise of followers. In W.E. Rosenbach & R.L. Taylor (Eds.), *Contemporary issues in leadership* (4th ed., pp. 96–106). Boulder, CO: Westview Press.

Kouzes, J., & Posner, B. (1995). *The leadership challenge: How to keep getting extraordinary things done in organizations* (2nd ed.). San Francisco: Jossey-Bass.

May, L.K. (2001). *Leadership skills and attributes for Houston women in the 21st century.* Bellaire, TX: Greater Houston Women's Foundation.

McClelland, D., & Burnham, D. (1976). Power is the great motivator. *Harvard Business Review, 54*(2), 100–110.

Pittman, T.S., Rosenbach, W.E., & Potter, E.H., III. (1998). Followers as partners: Taking the initiative for action. In W.E. Rosenbach & R.L. Taylor (Eds.), *Contemporary issues in leadership* (4th ed., pp. 107–120). Boulder, CO: Westview Press.

Sashkin, M., & Sashkin, M. (2003). *Leadership that matters: The critical factors for making a difference in people's lives and organizations' success.* San Francisco: Berrett-Koehler Publishers.

Wheatley, M. (1999). *Leadership and new science: Discovering order in a chaotic world* (2nd ed.). San Francisco: Berrett-Koehler Publishers.

Zaleznik, A. (1977). Managers and leaders: Are they different? *Harvard Business Review, 55*(3), 67–78.

Management Theory

DEBORAH R. GARRISON, PHD, RN
DEBRA A. MORGAN, EDD, RN
JEWETT G. JOHNSON, MSN, RN

CHAPTER MOTIVATION

"The first and paramount responsibility of anyone who purports to manage is to manage self: one's own integrity, character, ethics, knowledge, wisdom, temperament, words, and acts. It is a complex, unending, and incredibly difficult, oft-shunned task."

Dee Hock, 2000, *in* The Art of Chaordic Leadership

CHAPTER MOTIVES

- Discuss the evolution of management theories and their relevance to nursing.
- Use selected management theories to develop strategies for managing challenges inherent in the charge nurse, clinical manager, and other leadership roles.
- Compare the strategies for managing nursing units from the perspectives of scientific management and chaos theory, noting the different approaches that would be used.
- Describe the roles assumed by nurse leaders.
- Practice decision making, communicating, negotiating, and delegating through the learning activities suggested in the chapter and its supplementary materials.

Nurses manage care for individual clients, families, and communities in hospitals, outpatient settings, clinics, health departments, home health agencies, long-term care facilities, and rehabilitation centers as well as in other specialized health-care organizations. The strategies they use to organize care are drawn from **leadership** and **management** theories. The approaches to leadership and management reflect the dynamic state of health-care delivery as nurse managers and leaders strive to empower nurses to provide care that produces optimal outcomes. Management and leadership have evolved and continue to evolve from a hierarchical structure based in early management theory to a more flattened and inclusive approach that incorporates concepts from the physical and social sciences. In the early 1900s, these theories drew from newtonian science that viewed the world from a mechanistic, functional point of view. From the late 1980s until the present, the scientific view has shifted to include chaos theory and complexity science. **Complexity science** is based upon discoveries in physics and biology that emphasize emergent relationships and recognize the self-organization inherent in complex, adaptive systems. Management theorists have been incorporating these concepts into new approaches to the complex world of business and health care. This chapter provides a chronology of this evolution and presents a foundation for nurse leaders in the 21st century.

Managers have traditionally been responsible for the control of resources required to accomplish organizational goals. These responsibilities include budgeting, staffing, and maintaining the functions of the organization while simultaneously balancing fiduciary responsibility for the resources of the organization. Rowland and Rowland (1997) define management as a five-step process:

1. Planning
2. Organizing
3. Directing
4. Coordinating
5. Controlling

The manager is employed by an organization and given the responsibility to accomplish specified goals for the organization. Managers are expected to teach workers the best way to perform the job; match the employee to the job; provide motivational incentives to workers; see that time, energy, and materials are used efficiently, and ensure that the organization fulfills its objectives. At the same time, managers seek to enhance efficiency, develop resources required to reach the goals of the organization's strategic plan, and manage across boundaries in the organization (Huber, 2000).

Nursing management roles in the hospital vary, and the work to be accomplished depends on the span of authority inherent in a particular position. Nurses occupy such positions as chief nursing officer, vice president for patient care, and director of nursing, and are sought to serve on the executive councils of hospitals, public health organizations, and other places that deliver or impact patient care. In many cases they are responsible not only for the nursing units in the organization but also for those areas that support patient care, such as pharmacy, respiratory care, physical therapy, cardiac rehabilitation, and other such departments. The span of control for nurses in these roles is broad, encompassing supervision of other nurse managers who focus on delivery of care within patient units as well as of managers in other disciplines who direct the delivery of care in ancillary departments important to overall patient care. Collaboration with other professionals on the patient care delivery team is an important part of these management roles.

Newly graduated staff nurses assume responsibility for leading a team of direct care providers and, therefore, need to know how to manage a patient care team effectively. This team often includes nursing assistants, patient care technicians, licensed vocational/practical nurses, and other registered nurses. In this role of team leader, the nurse is responsible for identifying outcomes that must be reached by the end of the shift and assigning work that is appropriate to the preparation, scope of practice, and expertise of those on the patient care team. Within a few months of graduation, new nurses are likely to find themselves in the role of charge nurse, in which they must employ management skills to ensure delivery of care to an entire patient unit. All nurses, with few exceptions, will find themselves in positions in which accomplishment of their functions requires coordinated effort of a team that they must lead.

Nursing students often conceptualize management roles as those of clinical manager, head nurse, director of nurses, or chief nursing officer and do not envision themselves in such positions of leadership. Although it is true that students do not immediately occupy these roles, the roles newly graduating nurses will assume do require knowledge and application of management and leadership strategies. Therefore, students should examine management principles very carefully, learn how to use them effectively, and implement them upon graduation and entry into practice. This chapter presents the evolution of management theories, their application to nursing practice, and the roles that nurse managers assume in managing time, money, and people to accomplish the mission and goals of the organization.

Management and Leadership Revisited

During the late 1980s and early 1990s, a debate began regarding whether management or leadership was the better approach to accomplishing the goals of an organization. In reality, management and leadership are two sides of the same coin. There is no doubt that management is an important function of any leadership position; both are required for the organization to function effectively. There is a lack of consensus about whether management is a subset of **leadership** or whether leadership is a subset of management. Often, leadership is conceptualized as the broader of the two concepts, with managing including such tasks as controlling resources, budgeting, and staffing. It is apparent that nurses in leadership positions are responsible for such activities, but their most important role involves the development of mission and goals for their areas of responsibility that support those of the organization. Development of mission and goals is necessarily a collaborative effort, and the leader must engender support for their development. Once developed, the leader must cast the vision in such a way that it garners support from the staff. **Effective leadership** calls to mind the notion of a manager with vision, who uses power in positive ways, challenges others to join with the team to accomplish the vision or mission, and creates a synergistic environment.

In his book *On Becoming a Leader,* Warren Bennis contrasts the concepts of management and leadership in this way:

- The manager administers; the leader innovates.
- The manager maintains; the leader develops.
- The manager focuses on systems and structure; the leader focuses on people.
- The manager relies on control; the leader inspires trust.
- The manager has a short-range view; the leader has a long-range perspective.
- The manager asks how and when; the leader asks what and why.
- The manager has his eye on the bottom line; the leader has his eye on the horizon.
- The manager imitates; the leader originates.
- The manager accepts the status quo; the leader challenges it.
- The manager is the classic good soldier; the leader is his own person.
- The manager does things right; the leader does the right thing (Bennis, 1994, p. 45).

Whereas Bennis sees leadership and management as two distinct concepts, with leadership being the more desirable, it is our belief that both management and leadership are essential to organizational life and growth and frequently reside within the same individual. The juxtaposition of the manager as being "bottom line–oriented" with the leader as "vision oriented" can and must occur simultaneously to keep the organization healthy. For example, one cannot ignore the budget and the available resources in favor of developing new strategies for meeting organizational needs. Both are necessary.

The principles required to achieve the goals of organizations are continuing to evolve as our society and our knowledge of the principles of our universe expand. Table 2-1 examines Bennis' juxtaposed ideas to see how they could be combined in light of knowledge in the 21st century.

The current state of health-care delivery in the United States clearly calls for innovation and the development of original solutions that challenge the status quo. Complexity theory, which will be discussed later in the chapter, recognizes that small changes "nudge" organizations in the right direction. As this transformation of the health-care delivery system takes place, it remains vitally important that nurse leaders manage resources to foster the adaptation that must occur to sustain the current systems that support patient care.

TABLE 2-1	Management and Leadership: 21st-Century View
The manager administers; the leader innovates.	All participants in the organization can be innovators who contribute to meeting the goals of the organization.
The manager maintains; the leader develops.	At the same time that new developments are occurring, there are existing processes that must be maintained. Effective leaders and managers are involved in both.
The manager focuses on systems and structure; the leader focuses on people.	People are a part of systems, and they must be considered together.
The manager relies on control; the leader inspires trust.	These must coexist within an organization; for example, expenses must be controlled to allow for financial solvency, but there must be trust that the funding will be present for required expenses.
The manager has a short-range view; the leader has a long-range perspective.	Managing an organization is similar to driving a car: one must be cognizant of other cars with which a collision could occur while making sure one's car is on the right road to reach the desired destination. To be effective leaders, managers must possess both long- and short-term perspectives.
The manager asks how and when; the leader asks what and why.	When the "what" and "why" have been determined, then the "how" and "when" become imperative to accomplishing the vision.
The manager has his eye on the bottom line; the leader has his eye on the horizon.	If one keeps one's eye only on the horizon, then the bottom line may go into negative numbers.
The manager accepts the status quo; the leader challenges it.	Chaos theory suggests that equilibrium, much the same as the status quo, is a stage preceding the demise of the organism. Living means that things are changing continuously. To manage effectively, managers must be open to change.
The manager is the classic good soldier; the leader is his own person.	Members of an organization at all levels need to seek authenticity.
The manager does things right; the leader does the right thing.	It is important not only to do the right things but to do them in the right way once a course of action is determined.

To get a better sense of the essence of leadership and management and their interaction with one another, knowledge of management theory is essential. Understanding current management thought requires an appreciation for the development of management theory across the time span of the late 18th, 19th, 20th, and early 21st centuries. The next section will paint a broad picture of the evolution of management theory.

Drucker (2001) makes the following comment about leadership in the 21st century: "One does not 'manage' people. The task is to lead people. The goal is to make productive the specific strengths and knowledge of each individual" (p. 81). He believes that this perspective is necessary to creating a climate that supports the productivity of the **"knowledge worker."** Rather than being subordinates, knowledge workers are associates; for the organization to work effectively, the knowledge workers must actually know more about their own jobs than their boss knows. The desired relationship is more like that between an orchestra conductor and the musicians than the traditional concept of the "superior-subordinate" dyad. In his book *The Essential Drucker* (Drucker, 2001), Drucker contrasts this current opinion of management with that in his 1954 book *The Practice of Management*. The assumption he held at that time was, "There is one right way to manage people—or at least there should be" (p. 77), which he now believes is at odds with reality and productivity. How is it possible that one of the most respected management theorists changed his view so drastically? This question is best answered by examining from a historical perspective the changes that have occurred in management theory.

TRADITIONAL MANAGEMENT METHODS

Prior to the mid-19th century, in preindustrial times, skilled artisans or craftsmen oversaw their trades. They accepted apprentices to work with them and taught them the skills of the trade. The master craftsmen made decisions about how and when to initiate and complete work. The master was in charge of the work, which typically was conducted in what became known as "cottage industries," in which only a few people worked together to create goods. Once the industrial age arrived in the mid-1800s, this worldview of work began to change (Nixon, 2003). Three genres of traditional management theory have evolved: scientific management, general administrative management, and bureaucratic management.

The Scientific Management Movement

Frederick Winslow Taylor (1856–1915) is known as the father of scientific management. He detailed his principles on increasing the productivity of workers in the Midvale Steel Works plant in Pennsylvania (Taylor, 1911). His principles included the ideas that:

1. a worker's job could be measured with scientific accuracy;
2. workers' characteristics could be selected scientifically and could be developed to investigate the causes of and solutions to work problems;
3. productivity would be improved through scientific selection of and progressive development of the worker; and
4. there should be continuing cooperation of management and workers (Inman, 2000).

The Industrial Revolution gave rise to large factories and created the need to organize the efforts of the supervisors and workers in the factories. Management theory developed to organize and teach work process in a scientific manner, fulfilling the all-important desire for profit (Taylor, 1911). Taylor's scientific management principles were based on managing time, materials, and work specialization. For example, he developed the concept of the time and motion study, with the idea that wasted time and effort could and should be eliminated. He analyzed workflow and created an inventory of stored materials. By controlling these variables, he was able to decrease production costs and increase productivity. These strategies are highly effective for managing task-oriented work. In the early 1980s, hospital facilities sought to use time and motion studies to determine patient:nurse ratios and staffing needs. Nurses and other healthcare workers were shadowed by analysts who tried to determine the amount of time required to provide patient care. However, the application to a profession such as nursing failed to capture the critical thinking, decision making, and judgment required for patient care.

Taylor believed that organizational function was optimal when the roles of individuals were designed to be highly specialized, thereby taking advantage of a particular skill set that existed within a worker. To achieve this level of specialization, he implemented the concept of functional foremanship, in which each worker would fall under a foreman responsible for each area of specialization. This emphasis on specialization was an early impetus for the development of specialty certification in nursing and was really an extension of the master apprentice paradigm.

General Administrative Theory

Henri Fayol (1841–1925) was a Frenchman who is remembered for the development of general administrative theory. He developed his management strategies in the mining industry and was writing at about the same time as Taylor. Management, according to Fayol's work, includes five overriding concepts: (1) prevoyance, or the anticipation of the future and the development of a plan of action to deal with it; (2) organization of people and materials; (3) command of the activity among personnel; (4) coordination of the parts of the organization into a unified whole; and (5) control through application of rules and procedures. In order for an organization to be productive, leaders must participate actively in all five of these areas.

Fayol is remembered for his 14 principles of management, which he felt supported the accomplishment of the overriding concepts. Although he did not specify which of the principles he believed to be directly related to each of the concepts, we have developed a table to illustrate how these principles help accomplish each of the required concepts. See Table 2-2 (Inman, 2000).

TABLE 2-2	The Relationship Between Fayol's Concepts and Principles of Management	
CONCEPT	**PRINCIPLE**	**RATIONALE**
Prevoyance	Subordination of the individual interest to the corporate good	The goals of the organization are of paramount importance and take precedence over the individual's particular needs.
	Esprit de corps	Development of high morale is important, and it is the responsibility of the manager at the top to have a vision and to communicate it to the employees in a way that motivates them to achieve it.
	Initiative	Employees should be able to develop and implement plans on their own.
Organization of people and materials	Division of work	Division of work was emphasized to increase workers' efficiency levels.
	Order	Both employees and materials need to be at the right place at the right time.
Command of activity among personnel	Unity of command	Fayol advocated having only one manager, with no conflicting line of command.
	Unity of direction	There must be one agreed-upon plan both up and down the hierarchy.
Coordination of parts into a unified whole	Centralization/ decentralization	This decision should be made based on organizational needs.
	Stability of tenure of personnel	The more stable the personnel and the managerial structures, the more successful the business.
Control through rules and procedures	Authority	Authority gives the "right" to issue commands and includes responsibility for the consequences.
	Discipline	Employees must obey and respect the rules that govern the organization. Good discipline involves the judicious use of penalties for breaking the rules.
	Scalar chain	The line of authority is drawn from highest management to lowest ranks, and communication moves up and down this line.
	Remuneration	Money is an important motivator, and a fair wage is to be paid for work performed.
	Equity	Justice and understanding are important to developing a fair and equitable system.

These principles introduced some ideas that continue to be used. For example, in the 21st century, hospital personnel departments continue to have a pay scale that strives to provide fair remuneration based on educational preparation and years of experience. Every organization strives to retain its staff because of the cost of recruiting, training, and orienting new employees. The development of "esprit de corps," or team spirit, continues to be important in today's workplace. Teamwork remains essential to providing optimal patient care, and high morale is conducive to the levels of collaboration and teamwork that are required in the complex health-care environment. Patient care is delivered by a collaborative team of knowledge workers including nurses, physicians, and therapists from a variety of disciplines, all of whom are necessary to the outcome of optimal patient care.

Bureaucratic Management

Max Weber (1846–1920) was a German sociologist who developed what was known as the "ideal bureaucracy." The ideal bureaucracy includes the concepts of division of labor, authority hierarchy, formal selection, formal rules and regulations, impersonality, and career orientation. He recognized that it would be impossible for people to be completely impersonal in their relationships at work, but he believed that impersonality would be optimal and would remove favoritism. Weber believed that the more impersonal, rational, and regulated the work environment, the more likely the employees were to be treated fairly, and the more likely the organization was to reach its objectives. Weber focused on what it was that made people respond to authority. He perceived that only through concentrating power in the hands of a few people in a hierarchical structure could an organization be managed effectively and efficiently. While he did not necessarily agree that bureaucracy was the best strategy, because it removed autonomy from the individual, he believed it was the only way to assure the overall success of an organization (Inman, 2000).

During the early 20th century when Taylor, Fayol, and Weber developed these approaches to management, the worldview was still based upon 17th-century science science. Classical physics had been established as Newton synthesized the work of Copernicus, Galileo, and Kepler. Newton's laws of motion and universal gravitation, along with the development of calculus to compute planetary orbits, set the stage for a framework of cause and effect and a reliance on prediction through formulae (Whittemore, 1999). It was from this perspective that the early management theorists developed their management strategies for the Industrial Age. The emphasis of management was to master the world of work through controls designed using the principles of classical physics and science as they were understood at that time.

Within health-care organizations today, one sees the continuing influence of traditional management theory in, for example, job descriptions that outline the responsibilities of each person, thereby dividing the labor, and in organization charts that depict the hierarchical structure and the areas of authority for particular positions. Job descriptions emphasize the functions to be associated with each job, and one of the functions of the manager is to avoid overlap between positions and to delineate clearly the functions expected. These methods are helpful in that job descriptions let workers know the expectations and responsibilities associated with the positions they occupy. However, it is also true that work would not get done if the only functions carried out

each day were limited to those outlined on the job description. The work to be accomplished is too complex to be listed in a document of any reasonable length. In addition, the complexity of the health-care environment is such that people need to be treated as knowledge workers and allowed to have both the responsibility and the authority to make decisions about operational issues.

In general, traditional management styles have their advantages and disadvantages. The prime advantage is that they enhance the organization and efficiency of industry. The disadvantages of traditional management include rigid rules, top-down decision making, and authoritarianism. In other words, traditional management theory created an environment that was less optimal from a humanistic perspective. Thus, at the end of the 1920s, the stage was set for the era of behavioral management. The pendulum would swing from an emphasis on the structure and organization of management to a focus on the people who work in the organization.

THE BEHAVIORAL MANAGEMENT MOVEMENT

The recognized beginning of the behavioral movement was a much cited study that lent its name to the **Hawthorne Effect.** Elton Mayo (1887–1957), a clinical psychologist working at the Harvard Business School, conducted studies at the Hawthorne plant of the Western Electric Company from 1927 to 1932. Mayo designed a study in which light levels in the workplace were first increased, during which time worker productivity increased. Subsequently, he lowered the light levels, and yet worker productivity continued to improve. His conclusion was that the environmental changes were not responsible for the increasing level of productivity but rather the fact that the workers received attention from the experimenters, which increased levels of self-esteem and group pride, which led to increased production. It was from this study that Mayo concluded that management must be concerned with preserving the dignity of the workers, demonstrating appreciation for their accomplishments and, in general, recognizing workers as social beings with social needs (Mayo, 1953). This has great implications for research because it is always possible that results may be altered by the very acts of observation and increased attention. This threat to validity has become known as the Hawthorne

Effect, after the name of the company where Mayo conducted his research.

Another well-known behavioral theorist, Douglas McGregor (1960), developed Theory X and Theory Y. Theory X represented the traditional viewpoints of management, which hold managers responsible for organizing money, materials, equipment, and people as well as for directing workers' efforts and motivating workers, controlling their actions, and modifying their behavior to fit the needs of the organization. Theory X suggests that, without active intervention by management, workers would be passive and nonproductive in their roles in the organization. Theory Y assumes that the desire to work is just as natural as the desire to play or rest, that external control and threat or punishment are not required to achieve organizational objectives because workers are self-motivated, and that the capacity to work creatively to solve problems is widely distributed in the workforce. McGregor believed that these were the two major managerial attitudes about employees and that these approaches directly affect how the employee responds to managerial leadership (Marquis & Huston, 2006).

THEORY Z: JAPANESE MANAGEMENT STYLE

In 1981 William G. Ouchi wrote a book on Japanese management style, entitled *Theory Z*. In this book he discussed the management methodologies used by Japanese corporations. This approach to management relied on principles that were diametrically opposed to those used in businesses in the West, including America, England, and Europe. Employment in the Japanese corporation is described as being lifelong, dependent upon the development of consensus, collaborative work, incentives for group work, and pride in the product or service being developed or provided.

See Table 2-3 for a comparison of the principles of the Japanese management style with Western management style.

Henry Mintzberg (1999) chairs an international Masters of Practicing Management program in which Japanese professors teach a module entitled *Managing People: The Collaborative Mind-Set*. The module emphasizes gaining contributions from all the people in the organization and on reaching consensus. Ouchi (1981) says that there are three com-

TABLE 2-3	Comparison of Japanese and Western Management Styles	
JAPANESE MANAGEMENT	**WESTERN MANAGEMENT**
Lifetime employment	Short-term employment
Slow evaluation and promotion	Rapid evaluation and promotion
Nonhierarchical	Hierarchical
Nonspecialized career paths	Specialized career paths
Implicit control mechanisms	Explicit control mechanisms
Collective decision making	Individual decision making
Collective responsibility	Individual responsibility
Holistic concern for employees	Segmented concern

Ouchi, 1981, pp. 48–49.

ponents to a valid consensus: (1) I believe that you have heard and understand me, (2) I have heard and understand your point of view, and (3) I can support the decision we have made together.

In Japan, the word **kaizen** refers to the principle of encouraging all people in the organization to contribute improvement ideas on a biweekly basis (Bodeck, 2002). This results in 24 improvement ideas per employee each year, compared with one idea per employee per year in the United States and one idea per 6 years, on average, in the United Kingdom. Organizational growth has been shown to be directly related to innovation. The more leadership encourages participation and ownership among the employees, the more productive the organization becomes. Ouchi (1981) discusses the importance of encouraging group contributions. In Japan, individuals rarely desire personal recognition because they believe that nothing is possible without everyone's contributions. Although in the United States the predominant values focus on individual accomplishments, it is increasingly recognized that shared governance, which recognizes the importance of contributions from every employee, is the desired model. The American

chapter star

Curricular Changes and Chaos Theory

Faculty members are increasingly embracing chaos theory as the framework within which decisions are made. The faculty at one nursing school adopted the shared governance model as the modus operandi. That organization has moved over the past 5 years from a quasi-participative model to a true shared governance approach. As this change occurred, faculty became more inclusive of divergent viewpoints among faculty members, more accepting of student input, and more comfortable with the faculty role.

This faculty "owns" the curriculum. Over the past 3 years and probably before that time, faculty began to work with the notion that changes needed to occur within the second senior semester of the curriculum. "Nudges" came from faculty members who were concerned with the amount of time devoted to and the character of the management clinical experiences. At that time, the course was a seven-semester credit course encompassing 4 lecture and 9 clinical hours each week. Nudges also came from students who expressed the same concerns as the faculty when offered the opportunity to voice experiences during exit interviews. The clinical decision-making course, which was at that time a three-semester credit hour lecture-only course, was intended to be the critical thinking culminating capstone experience in the last semester. Faculty members were concerned that there was not a clinical component associated with the course and that there was no medical-

surgical clinical component during the last semester of study. Additionally, this factor was thought to influence NCLEX-RN first-time pass rates. These nudges found voice through faculty discussion occurring in various venues, some of which occurred in the copy room, over lunch, and in nursing faculty organization meetings. Faculty involved in the courses issued a proposal to transfer 2 semester credit hours (6 clinical clock hours) from the management course to the clinical decision-making course. The proposal was brought to the faculty as a whole for formal approval through the Undergraduate Curriculum Committee, where it found unanimous approval. The process by which this change occurred was characteristic of chaos theory in that all the members of the communities of interest had been involved in discussions. The change emanated from multiple sources and was guided by the mission and goals of the school of nursing, which serves as the attractor to keep the organization focused on a "student-centered, collegial environment." It is important to note that this school has long relied on the principles of shared governance that are congruent with chaos theory, particularly with the concept of self-organization. Because all communities of interest had input and participated in the decision-making process through both formal and informal venues, the change was readily embraced. This change has produced excellent outcomes both in NCLEX-RN first-time pass rates as well as faculty and student satisfaction.

Nurses Credentialing Center (ANCC) has emphasized the importance of shared governance through its Magnet Hospital program. This type of management is becoming more acceptable for the knowledge worker in the nursing profession in the United States.

21ST-CENTURY MANAGEMENT THOUGHT

Management theory in the first decade of the 21st century is influenced by a new worldview, which has, once again, had its roots in the physical sciences. Managers are beginning to recognize that the direct cause and effect relationships, to which they held in the past, frequently do not exist in reality. Additionally, management theories are being promulgated in more complex systems and in professional systems, in contrast to the earlier

management theories that began to emerge during the manufacturing environment of the 17th century. During that time, the worldview incorporated the strict "cause and effect" ideas that originated from newtonian science. Chaos theory and complexity theory, which have emerged from quantum physics, now underscore our understanding and interpretation of the work people do in organizations. Hock (2000) has even coined a new term for management based in complexity science: chaordic (kay-ordic). The word borrows the first syllable of the word *chaos* and the word *order*. He defines the term **chaord** as "any self-organizing, self-governing, adaptive, nonlinear, complex organism, organization, community or system, whether physical, biological or social, the behavior of which blends characteristics of both chaos and order" (p. 22). Organizations have elements of both chaos and order, with innovation and progress occurring "at the edge of chaos."

Complexity science "is not a single theory. It is the study of complex adaptive systems—the patterns of relationships within them, how they are sustained, how they self-organize, and how outcomes emerge. Within the science there are many theories and concepts. . . . Complexity science is highly interdisciplinary including biologists, anthropologists, economists, sociologists, management theorists and many others in a quest to answer some fundamental questions about living, adaptable, changeable systems" (Zimmerman, Lindberg, and Plsek, 2001, p. 5.) The idea that systems in nature are self-organizing lends support for the knowledge worker supported by Drucker in that individuals within an organization can build a better system, bringing order out of chaos, when allowed to self-organize. Small changes occur that move the system into ever-evolving patterns. Ideas from complexity theory, such as chunking, attractors, self-organization, distributed control, and leveraging incremental changes, can be used in health-care organizations. See Table 2-4 for terms used in complexity science.

Application of complexity science represents a significant divergence from the traditional management notion that employees are "machines" to be controlled by management through specific job descriptions and charts. Organizations become "living entities" encompassing all of the traits and foibles of the individuals of which they are composed. Employees, managers, and organizations are rapidly changing and becoming more flexible in their interactions with each other. As stated earlier, it has been long understood that if an employee adhered rigidly to a job description, over half of the work to be accomplished would be left undone. Unstated in a job description is the expectation that the employee engage in the critical thinking, innovation, and interpersonal relationships required to accomplish the goals and objectives of the position. This shift is evidenced through the changes in Peter Drucker's perception of management referenced in the beginning of the chapter. He originally thought that there was one and only one way to manage people. He revised his thinking to recognize that in the 21st century employees are actually "knowledge workers" who necessarily know more about their area of responsibility than do their managers. The knowledge worker must be able to make

TABLE 2-4	The Language of Complexity Science
Attractor	The attractor, or strange attractor, brings organization to chaos. As a mission statement is embraced by individuals within an organization, it can form a strange attractor that resonates throughout the system.
Self-organization	The components of a living system (including people in a health-care organization) are capable of organizing themselves to create change that moves the organization toward growth and accomplishment of the mission.
Edge of chaos	The state between stasis and chaos is "the edge of chaos." It is at this place that the organization is at its most open to innovation.
Distributed control	Control leads to stasis and maintenance of the status quo. Distribution of information, power, and control to the individual members of the organization brings innovation and adaptation.
Leveraging incremental changes	Small changes can generate big effects.
Bifurcation	Tendency of systems to move from one attractor to another.
Fractals	Complex, repeating, self-similar patterns.

decisions and implement strategies that work; these changes can be made more effectively and efficiently at the point of contact of the worker with the environment than by management removed by several layers.

If employees are self-organizing, what does this leave the manager to do? Hock (2000) says managers first must manage themselves to ensure their own integrity, character, ethics, knowledge, wisdom, words, and acts. He thinks this should take about 50% of managers' time. Second, Hock says that 25% of managers' time should be spent managing the people who have authority over them to ensure that they will have higher-up support. The support and consent of those managers above are vital for achieving goals and desired results. Third, 25% of managers' time must be spent managing peers, competitors, and customers. This is done through developing collaborative relationships that result in outcomes that are good for all and tailored to meet the needs of peers and customers. This leaves no time for the people over whom the manager has authority. Hock's idea is that managers should hire ethical people who are in tune with the goals of the organization and then unleash them to do what they were hired to do. This idea matches well with the concept of a knowledge worker who is the specialist in the designated area of work. Complexity theory does not disregard previous management theories; instead, it borrows concepts from many theories, modifying them as part of the evolutionary process. Management using complexity theory is neither totally mechanistic nor behaviorist. Instead, it is a new, ever-changing process.

The manager has much in common with the artistic director of a ballet production who choreographs the dance moves, selects the music, and plans lighting and scenery. During the production, however, the dancers make the magic of the movements come to life. The entire performance is much more than the sum of the individual movements and roles. Another analogy is found in the coach of a team who works day after day to make a game plan that, at the time of the game, must be acted out and adjusted by the players on the field in response to the opposing team (Hock, 2000).

It is clear that management has moved beyond the mechanistic views of organizations and people that characterized management theories in the Industrial Age. The application of complexity theory, with its reliance on self-organization, offers solutions for nursing and today's health-care organizations. Strategies for applying this new science will continue to evolve. The next section of the chapter applies some of management concepts to the identified roles of managers.

Box 2-1

In their article, *The Five Minds of a Manager* (2003), Gosling and Mintzberg include the ideas that:

1. Managing yourself relies on a reflective mind-set. The manager has to take time to think about the patterns seen to gain a perspective on the work environment. Reflective journaling facilitates this strategy (Morgan, Johnson, & Garrison, 2005).

2. Managing your organization requires an analytical mind-set. The manager needs to seek to really understand what is going on within the organization. The goal is to look at the needs of the organization from new perspectives so as to identify issues and move the organization toward action and change. Data collection and analysis are parts of this mind-set, but data must be interpreted in light of the mission, goals, and relationships within the organization.

3. Managing your context depends on a worldly mind-set. Seek to understand the organization and its relationship to the community and world from diverse perspectives. This means that the manager needs to spend time outside the organization looking at the environment in which it exists and at the role it needs to fulfill.

4. Managing relationships requires a collaborative mind-set. The manager's job is not to manage people as individuals. Rather, it is to create structures and portray an attitude that encourages teamwork.

5. Managing change calls for an action mind-set. The manager first identifies pertinent factors within and outside the organization and then needs to communicate these factors in ways that move the organization in the right direction to accomplish its mission and goals.

Management for Nurses

The nurse manager has many varied formal and informal roles, which involve team building, decision making, communication, negotiation, delegation, and mentorship. Whether managing a group of patients or functioning in the role of charge nurse, clinical manager, director of nursing, vice president of patient care, or president of the local chapter of the American Nurses Association, nurses fulfill these tasks in order to lead and manage successfully.

TEAM BUILDER

In order to lead and manage effectively, a nurse must be able to build a strong team. The delivery of health care is a team activity, involving professionals and unlicensed personnel from a variety of disciplines. Based on traditional management models, the emphasis was on individuals in the workplace and was more likely to value individual performance. New management strategies emphasize the importance of self-organizing teams and the value of group activity. In the complex world of health-care delivery, each individual's participation as a team member is a requirement; failure to work as a team creates fragmentation of patient care.

Managers must first recognize that the workers they "supervise" are knowledge workers who can and will make the right contributions to patient care. Managers must communicate to all team members their belief in the ability of the team to work well together. Because health-care systems have traditionally been very hierarchical, employees may not be accustomed to being allowed to organize their own work or solve their own problems. When members of a team indicate their unwillingness to participate or their lack of faith in other team members, the leader must listen carefully and avoid saying too much. The objective is to help the concerned individuals assess their own contributions to the team and their expectations of other team members. Then, the manager must communicate a strong belief in the team's contributions to the goals of the organization. This conversation serves the purpose of empowering each team member to contribute fully to the work that is to be accomplished. Chaos theory supports the notion that small inputs can create a ripple effect with far-reaching consequences. Each input affects the system, and the system is altered in response to each input. The team leader, rather than being the purveyor of change, has the responsibility of ensuring that the changes are aligned with the organization's mission, goals, and objectives.

The mission and goals of the organization unify the team and should reflect the goals of the members of the organization. A mission of "providing excellent care to the patients on the ABC unit" is a good starting point. For example, through the use of attractors, the leader can help the team focus and move forward in the use of the knowledge and expertise of its members.

Practice to Strive For 2-1

- All participants in the organization are innovators who contribute to meeting the goals of the organization.

- Leaders/managers are involved in new developments while existing processes are maintained.

- People are a part of the systems, and they must be considered together.

- Revenues and expenses must coexist within an organization; for example, expenses must be controlled to allow for financial solvency, but there must be trust that the funding will be present for required expenses.

- To be effective leaders, managers must possess both long- and short-term perspectives. They must manage daily operations while planning for the future.

- Leaders/managers determine the "what and why"; thus, the "how and when" follow naturally to accomplish the organization's vision.

- Leaders/managers must be open to change and manage change effectively.

- Leaders/managers must always seek authenticity.

- Leaders/managers do the right things in the right way once a course of action has been determined.

- Leaders/managers lead people.

- Leaders/managers manage peers, competitors, and customers by developing collaborative relationships that result in outcomes that are positive for all yet tailored to meet the needs of the constituent groups.

- Leaders/managers use reflective journaling to facilitate reflection and think about patterns to gain a perspective of the work environment.

- Leaders/managers have an analytical mind-set. Data are collected and interpreted in the light of the organization's mission, goals, and relationships.

- Leaders/managers have a worldly mind-set by understanding the organization and its relationship to the community and world from diverse perspectives.

DECISION MAKER

The leader is well served to recall Drucker's (2001) comments about the knowledge worker of the 21st century. The individual who does the work of the organization is the one who knows the most about it. **Participative** and **transformational** leaders enter into relationships with the professionals in their organizations. They share information, discuss values, and collaborate on decisions. The self-esteem of team members correlates with involvement with decision making.

Sometimes decisions need to be made quickly, but even in those circumstances the leader is ill-advised to make the decision without gaining input from those who will be affected by the decision. If the decision will involve the need for change, the greater the number of people whose views have been considered, the greater will be the support for the change. A paradox that exists within organizations is that frequently there is an artificial time constraint placed on decision making, supposedly to move the organization along more rapidly. A decision made quickly without adequate consideration and input can often result in an excessive amount of time being required to respond to the problems associated with rapid, uninformed change. A wise leader negotiates for the time to make a well-informed decision and thus avoids the frustration and time associated with negative outcomes of hasty decision making.

COMMUNICATOR

Information is power. Current literature recognizes the importance of keeping the members of an organization informed about issues with which they are involved. Many health-care organizations function around the clock, which can make the role of communicator more complex. Personal face-to-face communication is optimal, so managers must make every effort to stagger their hours in the organization to allow this communication on a regular basis. Both formal and informal communication is important. Managers who make time for informal communication will have a more accurate understanding of the issues with which the knowledge workers are dealing; will develop more open, trusting relationships within the organization; as well as a greater understanding of factors affecting morale.

In the past, communication books were used as a way to enhance **"asynchronous"** communication among various shifts of workers. Today's computer technology supports communication through listserves, e-mail, and discussion boards. If an organization is not taking advantage of the technology that is available, the manager should investigate the availability and understanding of that technology.

An important aspect of communication is that it must be mutual. In bureaucratic organizations information often flows only downward, and there is a propensity for the information to fail to reach the unit level. Moreover, information rarely moves from the unit level up the hierarchy, leaving the higher-ups out of touch. This type of communication is a sure recipe for disaster. Under these circumstances, the knowledge workers on the unit are lacking important information about their environment, and their contributions cannot be fully informed. Likewise, individuals responsible for guiding the overall vision of the organization are uninformed about day-to-day happenings, which makes it difficult to create realistic strategies.

NEGOTIATOR

The nurse manager must exhibit excellent negotiation skills. These skills are important in helping a team arrive at decisions, gaining organizational support for a new plan, gaining the cooperation of another department or organization, and in many other facets of the manager's role.

The first rule of negotiation is to understand the positions of the stakeholders, including nurses, patients, interdisciplinary professionals, community members, families of patients, unlicensed assistive personnel, and administration. Communication is an important part of negotiation, and one of the vital attributes of a negotiator is to encourage discussion and trust among group members. Many times, negotiation surrounds a decision in which it is perceived that there will be "winners" and "losers." Negotiation focuses on understanding who the perceived winners and losers are; the best negotiations result in win-win solutions. Ask the question, "Under what circumstances do you think this goal can be accomplished?" This question frequently moves participants from a defensive position to one of creativity and innovation, and it uses the concept of establishing an attractor, which causes people to come together to discuss possibilities.

DELEGATOR

Delegation is no longer a "top-down" activity. Instead, the leader will recognize the wisdom of members of the health-care team, support the interconnectedness of team members in the health-care delivery system, and embrace a more fluid, innovative system. The manager will foster an environment that supports the notion of associates (1) being partners in the delivery of health care, (2) being accountable for evaluating the outcomes of their interventions, (3) having the equity in the organization to make "point of service delivery" decisions, and (4) feeling a sense of ownership in the organization (Wilson & Porter-O'Grady, 1999).

TABLE 2-5	Roles and Competencies of Nurse Managers

ROLES AND COMPETENCIES OF THE MANAGER		ACTIVITIES RELATED TO COMPETENCIES
Personal	Self-management	Values clarification; lifestyle management; goal setting; alignment with organizational mission, goals, and objectives.
	Collaborator	Nurtures relationships with organizational leadership and other key personnel within the organization.
	Networking	Develops strong liaisons with health-care leaders in the community.
Client	Advocate	Recognizes needs of clients in area of responsibility.
	Provider of care	Maintains evidence-based practice behaviors.
	Coordinator of care	Assesses and recognizes the needs of the client population and applies appropriate principles of delegation, interdisciplinary team care, education, and evaluation of outcomes.
Organizational	Member of the profession	Represents the organization to the community, serves as a mentor to new nurses, encourages professional behavior in others, role-models professional nursing, holds membership in professional organizations, and supports continuing education.
	Communicator	Communicates the organization's mission, goals, and objectives to the staff and community; facilitates communication and negotiation among members of the organization.

MENTOR

It is often said that effective managers are always in the business of replacing themselves so their professional development and advancement can continue. Mentorship is the process to accomplish this. The identification of potential protégés can occur through a variety of methods. Team members who express an interest in leadership, individuals who have recently taken on new leadership roles, and professionals who show promise in the area of leadership through their interactions with others are all likely candidates. Mentoring relationships can be formal (assigned through an organization) or informal (simply a handshake agreement between a seasoned leader and an aspiring one). Sigma Theta Tau International, the nursing honor society, is an example of an organization that seeks to foster formal mentoring relationships, as does the American Association of Colleges of Nursing.

Whether a mentoring relationship is formal or informal, there are a few guidelines for success. Mutual respect, goal setting, accountability to each other, and open dialogue are hallmarks of an effective mentoring relationship. The mentoring relationship must be mutually rewarding; it must involve the opportunity for real work and stimulating challenges; there must be agreement on ownership of any projects created through the partnership; and the relationship must remain on professional grounds at all times. The mentor has the responsibility to create opportunities for professional growth and involvement, whereas the protégé is responsible for responding to these opportunities. The mentor has the responsibility to provide opportunities for the protégé to gain recognition for the work accomplished; the protégé is accountable for being responsible and reliable with the work accepted. The mentor empowers, encourages, and challenges the protégé. All nurses have a professional responsibility to mentor new members of the profession. See Table 2-5.

All Good Things...

Management has evolved from its emphasis on control and measurement as conceptualized by Taylor, Fayol, and Weber. These strategies were helpful during the industrial revolution, but in the 21st century they are less useful for organizations that rely on the daily contributions of knowledge workers. The evolving management theories recognize the complexity of the work involved in professions such as nursing. "The uncertainty of healthcare flows from the quantum and chaotic nature of the world over time. Therefore, we should stop trying to plan every step and predict each happening. Indeed, we must realize that we can never come close to knowing all there is to know about a topic or planning every step. . . . Hence we have to accept that no matter how much we know about the world, there are far more questions than there are answers, and uncertainty is a natural part of our lives" (Grossman & Valiga, 2005, p. 125).

NCLEX Questions

1. Which of the following theorists represents a traditional management viewpoint?
   A. Fayol.
   B. Hock.
   C. Ouchi.
   D. Hawthorne.

2. The individual recognized as the "father of scientific management" is:
   A. Fayol.
   B. Weber.
   C. Taylor.
   D. Ouchi.

3. Traditional management theory was designed to provide control and structure to which types of organizations?
   A. Hospitals.
   B. Scientific laboratories.
   C. Manufacturing industry.
   D. Institutions of higher education.

4. Complexity science has developed from the field of:
   A. Health professions.
   B. Business.
   C. Industry.
   D. Quantum physics.

5. In complexity science, the movement of an organization as it changes from one attractor or mission statement to another is known as:
   A. Leverage.
   B. Bifurcation.

   C. Chaos.
   D. Order.

6. Japanese organizations are known for their:
   A. Short-term commitment to their employees.
   B. Individual approaches to decision making.
   C. Rapid promotion of employees.
   D. Development of consensus.

7. Fayol's principle of esprit de corps refers to:
   A. Subordination of individual interest to the common good.
   B. Development of a high level of employee morale.
   C. Encouragement of initiative and risk taking.
   D. Emphasis on goal setting.

8. Max Weber is known for the development of which management theory?
   A. Bureaucratic management.
   B. Scientific management.
   C. Humanistic management.
   D. Transformational leadership.

9. Which of the following management theorists conducted the famous experiment at the Hawthorne Electric Plant in which employee productivity increased regardless of the type of intervention implemented at the plant?
   A. Weber.
   B. Mayo.
   C. McGregor.
   D. Hock.

10. Dee Hock recommends that managers spend what percentage of their time managing the employees for whom they have direct responsibility?
    A. 0%.
    B. 50%.
    C. 75%.
    D. 100%.

REFERENCES

Bennis, W. (1994). *On becoming a leader*. New York: Addison-Wesley.
Bodek, N. (2002). Kaizen: Kazam! *T+D, 56*(1), 60–62.
Drucker, P.F. (2001). *The essential Drucker*. New York: HarperCollins Publishers, Inc.
Fayol, H. (1925). *General and industrial management*. London, England: Pittman & Sons.
Flynn, J. (1998). Taylor to TQM. *IIE Solutions, 30*(10), 22–29.
Gosling, J., & Mintzberg, H. (2003). The five minds of a manager. *Harvard Business Review*, (November), 1–10.

Grossman, S.C., & Valiga, T.M. (2005) *The new leadership challenge: Creating the future of nursing*. Philadelphia: F.A. Davis.

Hock, D. (2000). The art of chaordic leadership. *Leader to Leader, 15*(Winter):20–26. Retrieved January 15, 2005, from http://leadertoleader.org/leaderbooks/L2L/winter2000/hock.html

Huber, D. (2000). *Leadership and nursing care management*. Philadelphia: W.B. Saunders.

Inman, M.L. (2000). The relevance of traditional management theories to the 21st century. *ACCA News for Students.* Retrieved from http://www.accaglobal.com/publications/studentaccountant/32495

Marquis, B., & Huston, C. (2006). *Leadership roles and management functions in nursing, theory, and application*. Philadelphia: Lippincott Williams & Wilkins.

Mayo, E. (1953). *The human problems of an industrialized civilization*. New York: Macmillan.

McGregor, D. (1960). *The human side of enterprise*. New York: McGraw-Hill.

Mintzberg, H. (1999). Managing quietly. *Leader to Leader. 12*(Spring): 24–30. Retrieved January 15, 2005, from http://leadertoleader.org/leaderbooks/L2L/spring99/mintzberg.html

Morgan, D.A., Johnson, J.G., & Garrison, D.R. (2005) Reflective journaling: Bridging the theory-practice gap. In H. Feldman & M. Greenberg (Eds.), *Educating nurses for leadership* (pp. 110–118). New York: Springer.

Nixon, L. (2003) Management theories: An historical perspective. *Businessdate, 11*(4), 5–8.

Ouchi, W.G. (1981). *Theory Z: How American business can meet the Japanese challenge*. New York: Avon Books.

Rowland, H.S., & Rowland, B.L. (1997). *Nursing administration handbook* (4th ed.). Gaithersburg, MD: Aspen Publications, Inc.

Taylor, F. (1911). *The principles of scientific management*. New York: Harper & Row.

Weber, M. (1947). *The theory of social and economic organization*. (A.M. Henderson & T. Parsons, Trans.). New York: Free Press.

Wheatley, M.J. (1994). *Leadership and the new science*. San Francisco: Berrett-Koehler Publishers, Inc.

Wheatley, M.J. (2001). Innovation means relying on everyone's creativity. *Leader to Leader, 20*(Spring):14–20.

Whittemore, R. (1999). Natural science and nursing science: Where do the horizons fuse? *Journal of Advanced Nursing, 30*(5), 1027–1033.

Wilson, C.K., & Porter-O'Grady, T. (1999). *Leading the revolution in health care* (2nd ed.). Gaithersburg, MD: Aspen Publishers, Inc.

Zimmerman, B. (1999). Complexity science: A route through hard times and uncertainty. *Health Forum Journal, 42*(2), 42–48.

Motivating Yourself and Others for a Satisfying Career

BETSY FRANK, RN, PHD

CHAPTER MOTIVATION

"How does one motivate employees when so many are being asked to do more with less? The answer is, in a large part, to make the employee feel secure, needed and appreciated."

Benson & Dundis, 2003

CHAPTER MOTIVES

- Describe the various theories of employee motivation.
- Discuss the relationship between motivation and job satisfaction.
- Explore the effect job satisfaction has on organizational effectiveness.

Is motivation as simple as Benson implies? Perhaps not, but the heart of motivation is for employees to believe that their work is meaningful and that it offers them a reasonable standard of living. Mosley, Megginson, and Pietri (2005) said it well when they defined motivation "as the willingness of individuals and groups, as influenced by various needs and perceptions, to strive toward a goal" (p. 191).

Why is it important to understand motivation? When health-care workers are motivated and subsequently satisfied with their jobs, motivation leads to patient satisfaction and, ultimately, organizational effectiveness. Employee motivation holds a critical key to organizational success. If leaders and managers understand and take action to motivate their employees, the organization will increase its bottom line. This chapter will discuss theories of motivation and explore the links between motivation, job satisfaction, and patient outcomes.

Theories of Employee Motivation

Many theoretical perspectives have been used to explain worker motivation.

MASLOW

One theory, well known to nurses and other professionals, is Maslow's Hierarchy of Needs. Maslow (1970) stated that lower order needs, such as physiological and safety needs, must be met before higher order needs, such as love and belonging, esteem, and self-actualization, can be fulfilled. The physiological needs include such things as the need for food and sleep. Safety needs involve the need to be free from fear and to feel secure. Love, self-esteem, and self-actualization are the higher order psychological needs. Maslow's theory views individuals as holistic beings. This theory has been quite popular in managerial literature, despite the fact it was developed from observations of psychotherapists and not for the workplace environment. It does provide a framework to help managers understand the complexities of human behavior. A manager might use this theory, for instance, to help understand why an employee with financial difficulties may not have the motivation to undertake a complex work project that might bring some personal acclaim. While the

theory can help explain human behavior, research findings have not clearly supported the theoretical model's utility in the job environment (Porter, Bigley, & Steers, 2003).

ALDERFER

Alderfer (1972) revised Maslow's theory and applied it specifically to the organizational context (Porter, et al., 2003). His ERG theory (existence, relatedness, growth) classifies worker needs into three categories: existence needs, which are similar to Maslow's physiological needs; relatedness needs, which are similar to Maslow's belonging needs; and growth needs, which encompass Maslow's esteem and self-actualization needs. There are two important differences, however, between the theories of Alderfer and Maslow. An employee does not have to move through the need levels sequentially in Alderfer's theory. Unlike Maslow, Alderfer states that an employee can be motivated by more than one need category at the same time and not necessarily in a sequential fashion. For example, a nurse can have multiple motivations for working, including salary and self-esteem. If fulfillment of self-esteem needs is thwarted because staffing negatively affects the quality of care given, the nurse may focus on a lower order need, such as belongingness, and ignore the need to deliver high-quality care. For the manager, this change in motivation may help to retain the nurse for the time being, but quality care will continue to suffer until the staffing issues are addressed.

HERZBERG

Another well-known theory is Frederick Herzberg's Two-Factor, or Motivation-Hygiene, Theory (1966). Although his theory has been criticized for not taking into consideration an employee's individual needs, Herzberg's work has fostered much research on work motivation and is used widely by managers to foster a motivating work environment (Porter et al., 2003). Herzberg's theory is built on the proposition that workers have two sets of needs: intrinsic and extrinsic. The intrinsic needs (or motivators) are growth, advancement, responsibility, the work itself, recognition, and achievement. The extrinsic needs (or hygiene factors) are security, status, relationship with subordinates, personal life, relationship with peers, salary, work conditions, and

Practice Proof 3-1

Timmreck, T.C. Managing motivation and developing job satisfaction in the health care work environment. (2001). *Health Care Manager,* 2001, 20(1), 42-58. Copyright: Aspen Publishers, Inc.

[Note: Article is available as a full-text article via libraries that have subscriptions to Health Business Full Text through the EBSCO database.]

Using Herzberg's Motivation-Hygiene Theory as a framework for his questionnaire, the author surveyed 99 midlevel managers, including nurses and others in managerial positions. He asked the managers to what extent they believed certain factors served to motivate people; he also asked to what extent they used these factors to motivate employees. Each factor was rated on a Likert Scale of 1 to 5. He explored to what extent the managers used "negative motivators" such as guilt, threats, power, rebellion, and control. These factors could be identified as elements of hygiene deprivation according to Herzberg. Results showed that 37% believed that guilt should never be used as a motivator, and 42% never used guilt as a motivator. Four percent believed that guilt was a motivator, and one participant used guilt to motivate employees. Fifty-three percent believed rebellion should never be used as a motivator, and 65% never used it. Threats were never used by 55% of the managers, and 51% believed they should never be used. Power was believed effective by 23%, and 8% actually used power as a motivator. Timmreck used his findings to point out that managers often mistakenly believe that fear of hygiene deprivation can be used to motivate employees effectively. He reinforced the idea that promoting the use of motivators results in a high level of job satisfaction.

1. What negative motivators did the managers use in the study?
2. What were the findings related to hygiene factors and motivation?

points out that many human resource consultants focus on facts that satisfy extrinsic needs, such as compensation and human relations. Job enrichment, on the other hand, should not be overlooked. It promotes motivation and thus job satisfaction. For example, a nurse manager could send a staff nurse for training in a new procedure, thereby enhancing the staff nurse's knowledge and enabling her to grow in her position.

VROOM

Maslow, Alderfer, and Herzberg assume that motivational factors—whatever they may be—are global in scope or the same for all employees. Vroom (1964), on the other hand, recognized that motivation is more individualized and tailored to what individual employees expect from the job itself. According to Vroom, workers weigh their options and engage in behaviors that will bring about desired rewards or outcomes termed positive valences. If the worker sees that a certain behavior might bring about a negative outcome, Vroom called this negative valence. Behaviors, negative or positive, are reinforced if the expected outcome is achieved. In essence, if an expected outcome occurs, then the workplace behavior will continue. For example, Nurse Jones is late for work at least 2 days each week. The nurse manager counsels Nurse Jones and states the next time she is late a formal disciplinary notice will be placed in her personnel file. Nurse Jones is not late again because she knows what the negative outcome will be.

McCLELLAND

David McClelland (1971) also recognized that individual employees have different motivational needs and that managers could use information about individual employees to create a motivating work environment. McClelland stated that the three need categories are achievement, power, and affiliation. Those who have high achievement needs are motivated by task accomplishment. For many, the tasks need to be challenging, not routine (Porter, et al., 2003). Those that have a need for power might be more fulfilled in supervisory roles, and those that have a high need for affiliation have a strong need to be liked and to work in an environment that is friendly towards them and that involves team work. See Box 3-1 to learn about additional motivational theories.

relationship with supervisor, supervision, company policy, and administration. It is possible for an employee to be satisfied intrinsically but dissatisfied extrinsically. For example, a nurse may find herself enjoying her responsibilities and a recent promotion while at the same time bemoaning her coworker's unwillingness to be part of a team. What this means is that the nurse is satisfied with the work itself but is dissatisfied with her interpersonal relationships within the workplace environment. In order to be motivated, employees should be satisfied both extrinsically and intrinsically. Herzberg (2003)

Box 3-1

Additional Theorists*

The Porter-Lawler Model: Porter and Lawler (Porter, Bigley, & Steers, 2003) built upon Vroom's (1964) Expectancy Model. One key difference in their approach is that they assume that the link between effort toward anticipated job performance outcomes and employee behavior is not direct. Rather, this link is influenced by employee skill level and the task to be accomplished. If the tasks provide intrinsic rewards, such as a sense of a job well done, the employee may be more motivated than if the task provides just extrinsic rewards such as paid time off.

Equity Theory: The main assumption of Equity Theory (Adams, 1963; Mowaday & Colwell, 2003) is that employees are motivated by a sense of fairness of rewards and punishment in the workplace. For example, if the same work brings about lower pay than when done by a fellow worker, then the worker receiving the lower pay might not be motivated to perform at a high level.

Self-Efficacy Theory: Self-Efficacy Theory is grounded in social-cognitive theory (Bandura, 1997). Self-efficacy is shown in the employee's belief that a job can be performed at a certain level. If employees have faith they can perform at a high level, they will be motivated, then, to perform. Self-efficacy is influenced by the difficulty of the task and the strength of the belief in one's abilities to perform the task. A task may be difficult, but if an employee has a strong belief that the task can be accomplished, then the employee will be motivated to complete the task.

Control Theory: Control Theory (Carver & Scheier, 1981) demonstrates that an employee will be motivated if what needs to be accomplished helps to reach the goal the employee wishes to achieve. For instance, if an employee wants to learn more about critical care, the employee will be motivated by an assignment to take care of critically ill patients.

*Adapted from Porter, Bigley, and Steers, 2003.

GENERATION AFFECTS MOTIVATION

Generational differences can also account for variability in worker motivation (Atkinson, 2003; Billings & Kowalski, 2004; Cordeniz, 2002; Hill, 2004; Izzo & Klein, 1998). Baby Boomers are interested, for the most part, in job security. If an employee from this generation knows that performance will lead to long-term employment, the employee will work to maintain that employment.

Unfortunately, recent layoffs at major corporations, including health-care corporations, have challenged the notion that good performance leads to job security. Baby Boomers, born largely between the post–World War II era and 1964, grew up in era in which they learned to challenge those in power and authority (Cordeniz, 2002). Thus, Baby Boomers often question what others tell them to do and want to know the reasons why decisions have been made. Rules are not motivators for behavior for Baby Boomers.

Generation X'ers, born between 1965 and about 1977, grew up in an era when technology became paramount. This group works primarily for personal satisfaction and growth (Cordeniz, 2002). Balancing work and personal life is an important goal for this group. Whereas their parents valued organizational loyalty, members of this group change jobs when the work environment no longer challenges or satisfies them (Cordeniz, 2002; Hill, 2004). Money is more of a motivator for this group than for earlier generations.

The Net Generation is just now coming into the workforce. These workers were born in the 1980s. In McClelland's terms, these workers are motivated by affiliation. They prefer to work in groups and teams and are hands-on learners (Billings & Kowalski, 2004). Unlike earlier generations, they grew up in a very diverse society (Hill, 2004). The Net Generation is more motivated and satisfied when working within diverse group settings. This group is also most comfortable with technology; cell phones and e-mail have always existed for them. Exposed to a wide array of technology, the Net Generation is motivated by settings where the technology is advanced and current.

Motivation can be complex, and it differs by the individual. In order to maximize organizational effectiveness, the task for leaders and managers is to discover what motivates individual workers and to create a work environment that capitalizes on these motivations.

Motivation Yields Job Satisfaction Yields More Successful Organizations

Job satisfaction occurs when a nurse's motivational needs are met. Nurses and other employees work in

Chapter star

(The following is based on interviews with real people, but names have been changed.)

"Marilyn Jones is the unit manager on a general surgical unit. Her unit is noted for delivering high-quality care. Surgeons seek to have their patients on her unit, and the unit has been rewarded by being designated the Unit of the Quarter. Another measure of her success is the fact that voluntary turnover on her unit is lower than 7%. When asked how she creates a climate that promotes high-quality care and low nurse turnover, she states: "As for motivation, I think involvement is the driving force. Staff DO NOT buy into the process unless they have input of ideas and decision making. I have a unit team of three licensed nurses from days and nights and one unlicensed staff member. We meet monthly to discuss our scores and what we are doing right and wrong. These team members are my cheerleaders as well as my messengers. When I post new survey scores, I expect them to draw attention to these scores so the other staff see how we are doing. I am always talking survey scores. The staff also knows that when I make patient rounds—another very important component—I ask the patients if the staff is checking armbands, answering questions they have about their care, and showing concern about patient privacy. I also ask the patients and their families if they are having a VERY GOOD stay. If they say a good stay, I ask what we can do to make it a VERY GOOD stay. With the 1600 vital signs, staff members ask all patients to rate their care today on a scale of 1 to 5. When I come in the next day and find any 4 or below, I go see that patient right away to see how we can make it a 5. ...I'm always giving awards, pats on the back, hugs, and verbal public recognition to my employees. I keep a ledger of who I recognize; I wouldn't want to go overboard on one and not on another. ... I always ask what THEIR SOLUTION is when they come to me with a problem. This keeps them on their toes."

order to have certain needs met, such as finan-cial and growth needs. When those needs are met, employees express satisfaction with their jobs. This crucial link between motivation and job satisfaction has far-reaching consequences for an organization. In short, if nurses and other health-care employees are satisfied, personnel turnover decreases, the quality of patient care increases, and the organiza-tion's financial outlook improves.

JOB SATISFACTION FOR NURSES

What leads to job satisfaction for nurses and other health-care workers? Herzberg (2003) and Timmreck (2001) suggest that money is not the primary motivation for job satisfaction for nurses. Of course, nurses and others need to make a decent living, but other factors masy play a more important role in job satisfaction. McNeese-Smith (1999) found that while nurses did derive some satisfaction from salary, benefits, and the ability to balance work and family life, the most satisfying part of the job was patient care itself. Factors that inhibited job sat-isfaction were those that hindered the ability to accomplish patient care, including lack of supplies, feeling overloaded, and difficulties in communicat-ing with physicians. Relationships with coworkers could cause satisfaction or dissatisfaction as well.

Control over work environment and autonomy in decision making also contribute to job satisfac-tion (Freeman & O'Brien-Pallas, 1998). Allowing nurses to decide how patient care is to be delivered and the opportunity to use their skills promotes a satisfying work climate.

Hackman and Oldham's (1980) Job Characteris-tics Model of Work hypothesizes that the combina-tion of core job dimensions, such as skill variety, task identity, task significance, autonomy, feedback on job performance, perceived meaningfulness of work, and knowledge of and responsibility for outcomes, leads to job satisfaction. Edgar (1999) used this model to confirm that autonomy, mean-ingful work, and opportunity to use a variety of skills promote job satisfaction for nurses who work in hospitals.

Autonomy and work enrichment are also impor-tant for nurses who work in community-based set-tings. Laamanen, Broms, Happola, and Brommels (1999) found that work motivation and job satis-faction did increase when home health nurses had autonomy and variability in tasks. They became dis-satisfied when the workload became unmanageable. Likewise, school nurses have ranked autonomy as the most important job satisfier (Foley, et al., 2004). School nurses ranked the other following factors as important to job satisfaction: interaction with coworkers, professional status, pay, organizational policies, and task requirements. A study of hospice nurses also revealed that autonomy was positively linked to job satisfaction, as was positive supervi-sory support (DeLoach, 2003).

ORGANIZATIONAL AND PATIENT OUTCOMES

Knowing what promotes job satisfaction for nurses is significant because the level of job satisfaction has been connected to patient outcomes (Scott, Sochalski, & Aiken, 1999). In a series of studies of magnet hospitals, Aiken and her colleagues discovered a clear link between organizational characteristics, including nurse job satisfaction, and patient outcomes. According to Scott et al., magnet hospitals are characterized by lower nurse turnover, more nursing autonomy and control over practice, and better nursing relationships with physicians. Scott et al. noted that magnet hospitals also have lower patient mortality and higher patient satisfaction. More recently, Aiken, et al., (2002) reported that organizational characteristics such as high patient to nurse ratios contributed to nurse burnout, job dissatisfaction, and higher patient morbidity and mortality rates. Aiken and colleagues' work demonstrates that attending to job satisfaction is a necessity in order to achieve positive patient outcomes.

On an international scale, Tzeng and Ketefian (2002) demonstrated in an exploratory study conducted in Taiwan that nurse job satisfaction was related in part to some measure of patient satisfaction, such as satisfaction with pain management and arrangement for follow-up care post-discharge. This study confirms that nurse satisfaction does influence customer satisfaction, which is critical because if customers are not satisfied with care they receive, they will go elsewhere, and that health-care organization will suffer financially.

Nurse satisfaction also affects the bottom line of health-care organizations. If nurses become dissatisfied and subsequently leave their jobs, the organizations suffer. According to Atencio, Cohen, and Gorenberg (2003), the cost of turnover is up to two times the nurse's salary. For example, if the average nurse's salary in an organization is $46,000 and 10 nurses leave in a year's time, the cost to the organization is close to a million dollars.

As Herzberg's theory suggests, nurses will leave organizations if the dissatisfiers outweigh the motivators (Herzberg, 1966). Davidson, Folcarelli, Crawford, Duprat, and Clifford (1997) report that intent to leave was predicted by poor communication within the organization and heavy workload (Hinshaw & Atwood, 1983; Pearlin & Schooler, 1978; Price & Mueller, 1981). Additionally, Cline, Reilly, and Moore (2003) confirm that nurses will leave when management is nonsupportive, the pay is unsatisfactory, and staffing ratios are poor. They point out that nurses will tolerate understaffed and perceptually unsafe settings for only a limited amount of time. If nurses cannot get their concerns addressed, they will leave the organization.

Leadership Makes a Difference

One of the critical determinants of job satisfaction for nurses is relationships with supervisors. Being able to communicate effectively with supervisors can, in and of itself, serve as a motivating factor for nurses. Early on, McGregor (1960) described the relationship between leadership style and worker motivation. According to McGregor, a Theory X management style presupposes that humans inherently dislike work, do not want to be accountable and responsible for their actions, and need to be prodded to do work. Managers who espouse Theory X use such strategies as rewards, threats, and punishment to get workers to do their jobs. A Theory Y leadership style, on the other hand, assumes that workers can achieve their personal goals by integrating their goals with those of the organization. The Theory Y manager's job, then, is to foster this integration by using a variety of human relations approaches. For example, a nurse who wants to work for a master's degree in nursing may choose an organization that promotes educational mobility. The nurse's supervisor might work with the nurse to develop a schedule that will facilitate this goal. A manager who espouses the Theory Y approach is more likely to attract employees than a Theory X manager who rules with an iron fist.

One particular human relations approach was tested in research conducted by Mayfield, Mayfield, and Kopf (1998). They demonstrated that if a leader used motivating language in giving direction and sharing feelings, nurses expressed a higher level of job satisfaction and job performance. One such example of motivating communication could be telling a nurse in front of peers that he did a good job with a particular patient. They caution, however, that communication is not enough to sustain job satisfaction. Rather, communication plus organizational behavior, such as providing meaningful rewards, help to improve employee performance and job satisfaction.

Leadership style can also be characterized by whether leaders are transformational or transactional. Transformational leaders direct by role modeling, promoting employee development, providing a stimulating work environment, and inspiring optimism. Transactional leaders lead by being task-focused, focusing on the daily work of the organization, setting employee goals for them, and focusing on the reward system (Marriner-Tomey, 2004). Morrison, Jones, and Fuller (1997) found that

---

Practice to Strive For 3-1

The link between motivation, job satisfaction, and positive organizational outcomes is clear, but how to promote that link as a leader/manager is not as clear. Quint Studer (2003), a management consultant, provides some direction in this regard. He says that leaders must become "Fire Starters," or people who have the passion to keep an organization going. Fire Starters are those who use specific strategies (some focusing on employee satisfaction) to promote organizational success. One such strategy Studer names "Rounding for Outcomes." As a leader/manager, instead of going on patient rounds, go on employee rounds. Ask your coworkers what they need in order to do their jobs well. Show nurses, unlicensed personnel, and physicians that you are approachable and will work hard to provide the tools necessary to do a good job. On employee rounds, build relationships with employees; ask about families, school, and other items of interest to them. Ask what is going well for them in the job and what they need to do the job better. Focus on the positive to help structure a climate that is focused on improvement, not negativity. Show appreciation, and thank people when they do a good job.

Studer (2003) suggests that after rounding for outcomes with employees, leaders should round for patient outcomes. Bring employees into the process, and ask them for patient updates before entering patient rooms. In addition to asking patients if they have any concerns, Studer suggests asking patients, "Is there anyone you would like to recognize for a job well done?" Effective communication is one key to job satisfaction for nurses. Managers should discuss openly with staff both positive and negative findings from rounds.

Studer's recommendations are aimed at inpatient organizations, yet his template could be used in ambulatory settings as well. Managers could survey clients via telephone or when clients present for services.

---

job satisfaction was higher when leaders were perceived as both transformational and transactional but that the relationship between nurses and transformational-style managers was stronger. Only transformational leadership was positively related to empowerment (intrinsic task motivation). An interesting finding was that the relationship between job satisfaction and transformational leadership style was more powerful for unlicensed personnel. These findings may suggest that different categories of employees are motivated by different leadership styles.

Leaders who maintain a positive work environment also have more success in keeping employees satisfied. Spence-Laschinger, Finegan, and Shamian (2001) suggest that work environments that empower nurses to use their expert decision making promote trust within the organization and lead to job satisfaction. Nurse leaders/managers are crucial in promoting trusting work environments. Aside from staff nurse perceptions of the importance of leadership, nurse leaders, by their own admission, know that being accessible and fostering a professional practice environment that promotes teamwork are crucial to nurse job satisfaction (Upenieks, 2003). Like Frank, Eckrick, and Rohr (1997), Upenieks also noted that leaders play a critical role in obtaining resources for the delivery of optimal patient care, which in turn promotes job satisfaction. If leaders fail to promote teamwork and acquire the needed resources for quality patient care, job satisfaction and quality of patient care decrease.

All Good Things...

In this chapter, we have explored ways that nurse leaders/managers can motivate employees to deliver high-quality care. Motivating employees, while not a simple task, has significant payoffs both for the employees and the organization as a whole. A variety of theories can be used by leaders/managers to guide them in promoting a climate that fosters job satisfaction and subsequent quality patient care. Leaders/managers need to be cognizant of the fact that what motivates one employee may not motivate another. Therefore, they may need to use a variety of motivational strategies in order to achieve positive patient and organizational outcomes.

Let's Talk

1. Think of a time when you have been very satisfied with a job you have held. What made that job satisfying? Also think of a time when you have been dissatisfied with a job you have held. What made that job dissatisfying?

2. Think of a manager for whom you have worked. What did the manager do to promote job satisfaction among the employees in the organization?

3. Identify a nursing unit where you know good patient care is given. Discuss what factors in the environment promote the delivery of high-quality patient care. Pay particular attention to how the leader motivates the employees on the unit.

NCLEX Questions

1. According to Herzberg's theory, which job factor would be considered a motivator?
   A. Money.
   B. Vacation policies.
   C. Quarterly parties.
   D. Recognition of achievement through a clinical ladder.

2. Which theorist helps a manager understand why an employee who does not feel safe on the job cannot perform his or her job duties well?
   A. Maslow.
   B. Herzberg.
   C. Vroom.
   D. Alderfer.

3. Joe, the nurse manager for CCU, counsels Registered Nurse Bob about his errors in charting and tells Bob that the next time an error is made, a formal warning will be put in his personnel file. Bob does not make any more errors. Which theorist helped Joe to frame his disciplinary action?
   A. Maslow.
   B. Herzberg.
   C. McClelland.
   D. Vroom.

4. Which employee is most likely to be a representative of Generation X?
   A. Mary, who has worked at the hospital for 10 years and would not think of quitting.
   B. Sue, who is motivated by money and will change jobs when she is no longer challenged.
   C. Bill, who is a hands-on learner and likes teamwork.
   D. Jeff, who always wants to know why an action is being taken.

5. Which core job characteristic promotes job satisfaction for nurses?
   A. Rigid rules.
   B. Autonomy in decision making.
   C. Hierarchical decision making.
   D. Lack of communication with physicians.

6. According to Herzberg, a nurse is apt to leave a job if:
   A. Interpersonal relationships with coworkers are bad.
   B. Opportunities for promotion are rare.
   C. Achievements are not recognized.
   D. No clinical ladder is available.

7. Research by Aiken et al. on magnet hospitals shows:
   A. Job satisfaction has no impact on an organization's effectiveness.
   B. Magnet hospitals have high turnover rates.
   C. Job satisfaction is positively related to positive patient outcomes.
   D. Job satisfaction is not related to turnover rates.

8. Which statement might have been made by a manager who espouses the Theory X approach to management?
   A. "Employees on my unit are very goal-directed and need little supervision to get the job done."
   B. "Susie is a great worker, and I like to give her challenging things to do."
   C. "Most of my employees only work for the money and will do what is right only if I discipline them."
   D. "I work hard to get employees to go back to school."

9. Which manager uses a transformational leadership style to motivate employees?
   A. Dick, who works daily to get the task done and gives "to do" lists to employees.
   B. Martin, who is known for seeing that a thorough job is done and done correctly.
   C. Emily, who focuses on goal setting and rewards goal achievement.
   D. Jeanette, who is optimistic and makes a conscious effort to be a good role model.

10. Which statement best describes which theoretical perspective nurse managers should use to motivate their employees?
   A. Each employee has individual needs, so no one theory applies to all employees.
   B. Each employee has individual needs, but providing for autonomy and growth is supported by a number of theories.
   C. If a manager uses Herzberg's theory, most employees will be satisfied.
   D. A manager should use the theory that makes the most sense and fits his or her personal style.

REFERENCES

Adams, J.S. (1963). Toward an understanding of inequity. *Journal of Abnormal and Social Psychology 67*, 422–436.

Aiken, L.H., Clarke, S.P., Sloane, D.M., Sochalski, J., & Silber, J.H. (2002). Hospital nurse staffing and patient mortality, nurse burnout, and job dissatisfaction. *JAMA 288*, 1987–1993.

Alderfer, C.P. (1972). *Existence, relatedness, and growth.* New York: Free Press.

Atencio, B.L., Cohen, J., & Gorenberg, B. (2003). Nurse retention: Is it worth it? *Nursing Economic, 21*, 262–268, 299.

Atkinson, W. (2003). Managing the generation gap poses many challenges. *Hotel and Restaurant Management, 218*(19), 72–73.

Bandura, A. (1997). *Self-efficacy: The exercise of control.* New York: W.H. Freeman.

Benson, S.G., & Dundis, S.P. (2003). Understanding and motivating health care employees: Integrating Maslow's hierarchy of needs, training and technology. *Journal of Nursing Management, 11*, 315–320.

Billings, D., & Kowalski, K. (2004). Teaching tips: Teaching learners from varied generations. *The Journal of Continuing Education in Nursing, 35*(3), 104–105.

Carver, C.S., & Scheier, M.F. (1981). *Attention and self-regulation: A control-theory approach to human behavior.* New York: Springer-Verlag.

Cline, D., Reilly, R., & Moore, J.F. (2003). What's behind RN turnover? *Nursing Management, 34*(10), 50–53.

Cordeniz, J. (2002). Recruitment, retention, and management of Generation X: A focus on nursing professionals. *Journal of Healthcare Management, 47*, 237–249.

Davidson, H., Folcarelli, P.H., Crawford, S., Duprat, L.J., & Clifford, J. (1997). The effects of health care reforms on job satisfaction and voluntary turnover among hospital-based nurses. *Medical Care, 35*, 634–645.

DeLoach, R. (2003). Satisfaction among hospice interdisciplinary team members. *American Journal of Hospice and Palliative Care, 20*, 434–440.

Edgar, L. (1999). Nurses' motivation and its relationship to the characteristics of nursing care delivery systems: A test of the job characteristics model. *Canadian Journal of Nursing Leadership, 12*(1), 14–22.

Foley, M., Lee, J., Wilson, L., Cureton, V.Y., & Canham, D. (2004). A multi-factor analysis of job satisfaction among school nurses. *The Journal of School Nursing, 20*(2), 94–100.

Frank, B., Eckrick, H., & Rohr, J. (1997). Quality nursing care: Leadership makes the difference. *Journal of Nursing Administration, 27*(5), 13–14.

Freeman, T., & O'Brien-Pallas L.L. (1998). Factors influencing job satisfaction on specialty units. *Canadian Journal of Nursing Administration, 11*(3), 25–51.

Hackman, J.R., & Oldham, G.R. (1980). *Work redesign.* Reading, MA: Addison-Wesley.

Herzberg, F. (2003). Best of HBR: One more time: How do you motivate employees? *Harvard Business Review, 81*(1), 87–96.

Herzberg, F. (1966). *Work and the nature of man.* Cleveland: World Publishing.

Hill, K.S. (2004). Defy the decades with multigenerational teams. *Nursing Management, 35*(1), 32–35.

Hinshaw, A.S., & Atwood, J.R. (1983). Nursing staff turnover, stress and satisfaction: Models, measures and management. In J.J. Fitzpatrick & H.H. Werley (Eds.), *Annual Review of Nursing Research, Vol. 1* (pp. 133–153). New York: Springer.

Izzo, J., & Klein, E. (1998). The changing values of workers: Organizations must respond. *Healthcare Forum Journal, 41*(3), 62–65.

Laamanen, R., Broms, U., Happola, A., & Brommels, M. (1999). Changes in the work and motivation of staff delivering home care services in Finland. *Public Health Nursing, 16*(1), 60–71.

Marriner-Tomey, A. (2004). *Guide to nursing management and leadership* (7th ed.). St Louis: Mosby.

Maslow, A.H. (1970). *Motivation and personality* (2nd ed.). New York: Harper and Row.

Mayfield, J.R., Mayfield, M.R., & Kopf, J. (1998). The effects of leader motivating language on subordinate performance and satisfaction. *Human Resource Management, 37*, 235–248.

McClelland, D.C. (1971). *Assessing human motivation.* New York: General Learning Press.

McGregor, D. (1960). *The human side of enterprise.* New York: McGraw-Hill Book Company.

McNeese-Smith, D.K. (1999). A content analysis of staff nurse descriptions of job satisfaction and dissatisfaction. *Journal of Advanced Nursing, 29*, 1332–1341.

Morrison, R.S., Jones, L., & Fuller, B. (1997). The relation between leadership style and empowerment on job satisfaction of nurses. *Journal of Nursing Administration, 27*(5), 27–34.

Mosley, D.C., Megginson, L.C., & Pietri, P.H. (2005). *Supervisory management: The art of inspiring, empowering and developing people* (6th ed.). Mason, OH: Thomson South-Western.

Mowaday, R.T, & Colwell, K.A. (2003). Employee reactions to unfair outcomes in the workplace: The contributions of Adams's equity theory to understanding work motivation. In L.W. Porter, G.A. Bigley, & R.M. Steers (Eds.), *Motivation and work behavior* (7th ed.) New York: McGraw-Hill Higher Education.

Newman, K., & Maylor, U. (2002). Empirical evidence for "the nurse satisfaction, "quality of care and patient satisfaction chain." *International Journal of Health Care Quality Assurance, 15*(2/3), 80–88.

Pearlin, L., & Schooler, C. (1978). The structure of coping. *Journal of Health and Social Behavior, 19*(1), 2–22.

Porter, L.W., Bigley, G.A., & Steers, R.M. (2003). *Motivation and work behavior* (7th ed.). New York: McGraw-Hill Higher Education.

Price, J.L., & Mueller, C.W. (1981). *Academy of Management Journal, 24,* 543–565.

Scott, J.G., Sochalski, J., & Aiken, L. (1999). Review of magnet hospital research: Findings and implications for professional nursing practice. *Journal of Nursing Administration, 29*(1), 9–19.

Spence-Laschinger, H.K., Finegan, J., & Shamian, J. (2001). The impact of workplace empowerment, organizational trust on staff nurses' work satisfaction and organizational commitment. *Health Care Management Review, 26*(3), 7–23.

Studer, Q. (2003). *Hardwiring excellence: Purpose, worthwhile work, making a difference.* Gulf Breeze, FL.: Fire Starter Publishing.

Timmreck, T.C. (2001). Managing motivation and developing job satisfaction in the health care work environment. *Health Care Manager, 20*(1), 42–58.

Tzeng, H.M. & Ketefian, S. (2002). The relationship between nurses' job satisfaction and inpatient satisfaction: An exploratory study in a Taiwan teaching hospital. *Journal of Nursing Care Quality, 16*(2), 39–49.

Upenieks, V.V. (2003). The interrelationship of organizational characteristics of magnet hospitals, nursing leadership, and job satisfaction. *Health Care Manager, 22*(2), 83–98.

Vroom, V. (1964). *Work and motivation.* New York: John Wiley and Sons.

BIBLIOGRAPHY

Hiam, A. (2003). *Motivational management: Inspiring your people for maximum performance.* New York: American Management Association.

Hodgetts, R.M., & Hegar, K.W. (2005). *Modern human relations at work* (9th ed.). Mason, OH: Thomson South-Western.

Noe, R.A., Hollenbeck, J.R., Gerhart, B., & Wright, P.M. (2004). *Fundamentals of human resource management.* New York: McGraw-Hill.

Whetton, D.A., & Cameron, K.S. (2005). *Developing managements skills* (6th ed.). Upper Saddle River, NJ: Pearson Prentice Hall.

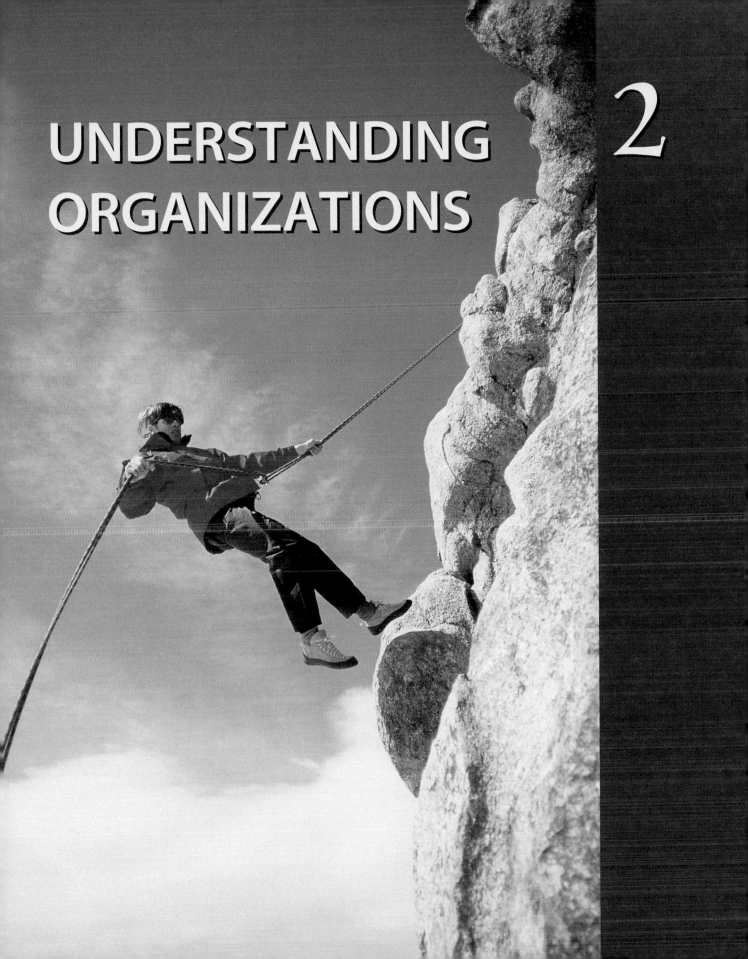

UNDERSTANDING
ORGANIZATIONS

2

Understanding Organizational Structures

CONNIE J. BOERST, MSN, RN, BC

CHAPTER MOTIVATION

*"The goal of most organizations—certainly of philanthropic organizations—
is not just to deliver services, but also to foster change and improve lives."*

Peter Drucker

CHAPTER MOTIVES

- Compare and contrast the different theories of organizations.
- Describe the purpose of an organization chart.
- Define the components included in an organization chart.
- Differentiate between organizational culture and climate.

Organizational mergers and health-care changes are rampant in the 21st century. In health care today, organizational structures are affected by the economic, political, social, and technological pressures in society (Marriner Tomey, 2000, p. 231). The structure identifies the authority, the responsibility, and the decision-making processes. Today's structures are no longer simple and hierarchical; they are complex systems with cross-functional teams and communications and interactions occurring at many levels. The structure of the organization is representative of its mission, vision, and values and how it functions.

Nursing is an integral and major component of the health-care organization, with nursing being the largest group of employees within the health-care setting. As a result, it is essential that nurses know their organization, the structures within which they function, and be able to relate this to their individual clinical unit. As health-care delivery expands, organizations will continuously take on a new look and approach to structure. By studying and learning the organizational structure, nurses will better understand their role within it. The nurse is the key person at the bedside, coordinating the care for the patient. Registered nurses work within a matrix of systems within the health-care organization, being a gatekeeper of information that can improve outcomes for the organization.

In this chapter, the reader will learn about organizational theory and its role; review the characteristics and the different types of health-care organizations; and understand how the corporate vision, mission, values, and philosophy guide the organization. The chapter also presents information on governance models, the different types of health-care delivery settings, and the importance of continuity of care for the health of the organization. The chapter concludes with predictive future trends related to organizations.

Organizational Theory

Organizations consist of groups of people coming together for a common purpose. An **organization** can be defined as "a group of persons with specific responsibilities who are acting together for the achievement of a specific purpose determined by the organization" (Huber, 2000, p. 454). It is "the structure that supports the organizational processes," according to Yoder-Wise (2003). Organizations comprise people who are given specific tasks to complete within their defined job role.

Organizational "theory," technically, dates back to biblical times, when thought was given to how groups were organized. Pharaoh utilized theories to build the pyramids of Egypt. Workers were organized into specific groups with specific tasks to be completed for the success of the structure. Modern organizational theory began during the Industrial Revolution. Many theories have been reviewed to demonstrate the how and the what of organizational structure. Today's view of the structure emphasizes the relationships of the groups within the organization, the people, and how work is accomplished in a self-organized system (Crowell, 1998).

It is important to understand the different theories of how organizations have come to be because the theory serves as the foundational component and the driving force for how groups are formed and function in today's health-care arena. As we discuss the theories, it will reveal the transitions and variations that shape organizational functions today. By studying organizational theories, the reader will understand the functionality of organizational structures.

CLASSICAL THEORY

The **Classical Theory,** dating to the 1890s, is one of the oldest theories regarding organizational structure. The focus of this theory was on the structure of the formal organization: it examined the efficiency of the organization as a by-product of the design of the system. The concept was that the people of an organization will be productive if they are given a well-defined task to complete. By dividing work into tasks and requesting employees to complete the same task every day, the theory proposed that productivity would increase because of the repetition of the task. This worked from an industrial perspective.

Results of this theory have come to be known as the classical principles of organizational design. These principles examine how members are divided into work teams, who reports to whom, the number of people for whom the managers are responsible, and the shape of the structure. From classical principles, Max Weber, called the Father of

Organizational Theory, created the bureaucratic model of organizational structure. Weber's model consists of the following components:

- Organizational structure
- Division and specialization of labor
- Chain of command
- Span of control

The **organizational structure** concerns the arrangement of the work groups within the organization and is intended to support the organization's survival and success. The structure determines accountability and responsibility. It dictates who makes the decisions and who has authority and oversight of workers. The structure shows who reports to whom and gives a pictorial view of the organization. In the Classical Theory, workers were placed into departments in relation to the work they were assigned to complete.

Specialization of labor dictates that the work of the organization be divided into tasks and employees be assigned a specific task to complete. Limiting the number of tasks assigned to each individual increases the efficiency and improves the organization's product. Just as in an assembly line, the worker who puts steering wheels on a car every day will become very proficient at the task. The risk of error is reduced, and efficiency is increased.

Chain of command refers to the formal line of authority and responsibility within the organization. Authority is the power to guide and direct workers within their specific area. This authority is usually depicted by vertical lines on an organization chart. This linkage is from the key position on top to the positions directly below. Responsibility refers to the obligation to produce or to complete the task. Each worker is responsible to finish the task assigned by a superior.

Span of control refers to the number of employees who report to a manager or a supervisor. A wide span of control indicates that many employees report to a supervisor; a narrow span means that few employees report to one. The number of people reporting determines the organizational structure (Altaffer, 1998). A narrow span of control is indicative of a tall structure because each manager has only a few people in the reporting structure. There are many managers responsible for a limited number of people, which results in many layers to get to the top of the organizational structure. There are often many layers for the change of command, and the span of control is narrow. A wide span of control is indicative of fewer managers and more reporting workers, resulting in a flat organizational structure.

Many organizations still base their structure on the Classical Theory principles, utilizing some of the components to make up their structure. As organizations begin to function leaner with limited resources, other approaches and options to organize the employees are being implemented. The Classical Theory is based on the concept that the employee does one job and will learn it well. In health-care organizations today, multiple tasks are being managed and completed by fewer employees.

NEOCLASSICAL THEORY (HUMANISTIC THEORY)

The **Neoclassical Theory** became popular in the 1930s. It placed emphasis on cooperation and participation in the workplace (Sullivan & Decker, 2001). The key factor in this theory is motivation. A motivated employee will produce better output in the job setting (see Chapter 3 on motivation in this book). If employees are given satisfactory working conditions and have opportunities to socialize with other employees, job satisfaction will improve, and the employee will be more motivated.

The Neoclassical Theory links with a democratic style of leadership because the employees are encouraged and allowed to participate in the functions of the organization and the decision-making process. For example, employees may participate on committees related to patient education and care outcomes. Nurses and other members of the health-care team have a voice in the decision-making process. The Neoclassical Theory relates to a flat organizational structure. Processes are decentralized, and member involvement is encouraged.

SYSTEMS THEORY

Systems Theory is based on the work of Von Bertalanffy (1968). This theory asserts that systems are a whole and that organizations should be viewed as a whole, considering the relationships within the structure of the organization. A system is a complex mix of intertwined elements, including inputs, throughputs, and outputs. Inputs are the

hot topic:
Nurses and the Public

Nurses today have many opportunities to expand their services to the public domain. In the past, private duty nursing was common; nurses provided services for a fee or in exchange for room and board. Essentially, the nurse was considered a free agent and could take her services just about anywhere. Today, nurses have many more chances to incorporate their services and provide care for a fee. The nurse can still function as a free agent. One example is the nurse anesthetist. This nurse can work for a variety of hospitals and free-standing surgical centers at the same time. The nurse can incorporate the services provided and have contracts with many agencies at the same time.

Another example is the consultation nurse. The nurse may have expertise in the area of technology and sign contracts with a variety of health-care institutions to assist them with their technology development. Forensic nursing is still another example. The forensic nurse possesses expertise in investigating crime, evidence gathering, and providing health-care services to victims of crime. A nurse with this type of background can contract with prison systems, emergency rooms, lawyers, and the legal system.

Free agency for nursing is not a forgotten topic. In the 21st century, it is an opportunity to expand services to the public as well as to gain independence within the selected specialty. Nurses today have many opportunities to become autonomous within their practice and to develop and expand their potential.

items being put into the organization to create the product. The throughputs are the processes put into place to assist with the creation of the outputs. These elements work together to accomplish specific goals within the organization. Changes in one part of the system affect the other parts of the system, creating a ripple effect. The resources are inputs, such as the employees, patients, materials, money, and equipment imported from the environment. The work is considered the throughput. This is the work within the organization, transforming energy and resources to yield a product. The product (the output) is then exported to the environment. The organization is a constant recurring cycle of inputs, throughputs, and outputs.

CHAOS THEORY

The **Chaos Theory** stresses the importance of change within organizations. Change is the stimulation of the organization, and it is constant in health care today. Change can create stress or relief for organizations, depending on how it is perceived and interpreted (see Chapter 11 on leading change). Leaders must constantly assess the organizational environment and determine whether there is consistency within the structure. Organizational leaders working under the Chaos Theory will excel with change and creativity (McGuire, 1999). Management is flexible and will reward those organizational members who thrive on adaptive behaviors and innovation. The overall goal of the organization is to be successful in an environment of constant change. This theory works well with health-care organizations today. Change is inevitable, and employees must learn to adapt and excel to remain employable in health care.

CONTINGENCY THEORY

The concept within the **Contingency Theory** is that the organization's structure must match the working of the environment. The most common aspect of the Contingency Theory recognizes the style of the leader and how this influences the situation. How the leader leads will determine how the organizational structure is established. There is variation in leadership style to gain expected outcomes. There is no one leadership style that fits every situation; a good leader will learn how to adapt to each situation to support the desired outcomes. The organizational structure based on this theory is flexible and varies based on the needs of the organization and the leader.

LEARNING ORGANIZATIONS

In a **learning organization,** the people and the systems respond and expand their capabilities to obtain the results that are desired. The basic concept is that in situations of change, the organization that is adaptive to the change will thrive. Learning organizations are becoming more popular in businesses today. Members of organizations have the ability to create and manage the changes (Senge, 1999). Particular people are employed because of their commitment to the organization, and this commitment serves as a resource for the success of the organization. Peter Senge (1990) identifies five disciplines for a learning organization to be successful: systems thinking, personal mastery, mental models, building a shared vision, and team learning.

Systems thinking is the ability to examine an organization as a whole entity, not separate units, and to see the interrelationships between the units. Successful organizations explore systems as a whole and as very dynamic processes. Personal mastery refers to a continuous learning process by each individual. It is based on self-discipline and the idea that individuals never stop learning. Mental models refer to an individual's ability to see things differently and work with pictures within the mind to influence how a given situation is seen and interpreted. This means taking a situation and being able to view all sides of it to discover the objectivity of it. Building a shared vision is the ability of the organization to create a shared idea of the future goals and dreams. This vision creates energy for the members of the organization to work together as a team and meet the goals of the organization. The final component, team learning, refers to the organizational members' ability to unite as a whole for the betterment of the organization. This will improve organizational results. When members work together, processes improve, and outcomes are enhanced.

Organizational theory plays an important role in the productivity and success of the organization. The theory helps determine the type of organizational structure and how the organization will function. It is important for managers and leaders to understand the theories, how they relate to their organizations, and how they can influence the members of their organization.

Organizational Components and Planning

Health-care organizations have been transformed by the many changes in social, structural, political, and human resource allocations (Bolman & Deal, 2003). Some specific factors that have contributed to these changes include quality care issues, increasing health-care costs, and the focus on patient satisfaction. These factors affect how the organization is run and contribute to changes within the structure. Organizations with a strong value set, mission, vision, and philosophy will be more prepared to successfully meet these ever-changing events. Goals and objectives, policies and procedures, and strategic planning are also key components of facile organizational operation.

ORGANIZATIONAL VALUES

The stated values of an organization give meaning to its existence and help its members act in concert with its motives. The values clarify what is important to the organization in regard to its customers, products, and/or services. Values set the standards for behavior within the organization and support the mission and the strategic plan. Organizational leaders determine a set of values that align with the mission and the vision of the organization.

The values for the organization serve as the foundational cornerstone for the events and activities of the facility. Organizational values are related to the success of the organization and determine how it will function when working with its customers. For example, if a hospital as an organization values service, the members will work hard on methods to improve their patient satisfaction surveys. A client who returns for future care at the hospital is usually one who is pleased with the type of service given. Leaders of the organization express these values on a daily basis within their work and responsibilities to the system. Values can be an implicit or explicit part of the mission statement and are incorporated implicitly into the organization's culture. See Box 4-1 for some examples of organizational values.

MISSION STATEMENTS

The purpose or the mission statement encapsulates the intent and goal of the organization. It explains, in a short statement, the core reasons behind the organization's existence and a primary focus on a single strategic thrust for the organization. The purpose of each area of the organization is to pursue the stated mission of the organization. The mission statement sets standards for the organization's philosophy and its goals and objectives; it is the baseline for decisions of the organization. The mission statement drives the organization's existence and is

BOX 4-1

Organizational Values

Integrity	Caring
Quality	Respect
Service	Competence

BOX 4-3

Sample Vision Statement

To be the premier leader in quality health-care education and service.

a reflection of the culture. See Box 4-2 for an example of a mission statement.

VISION STATEMENTS

The vision statement incorporates an organization's mission and values. It serves as the future-oriented plan for the organization, the wish list of future development ideas, and the plan to set this wish list into motion. The vision statement serves as the dream of the organization and provides guidance on where an organization wants to be 10–15 years into the future. See Box 4-3 for an example of a vision statement.

ORGANIZATIONAL PHILOSOPHY

The philosophy of an organization is derived from its mission and incorporates the organizational values that direct the behavior of the organization. The information provided in the philosophy—the values and principles of the organization—provides the framework for the decision-making process of the organization and shapes the social and professional development of the organization. The philosophy serves to allow employees to achieve common goals (Wendenhof & Strahley, 1995). The philosophy underlies the goals and objectives of the organization, so it is imperative that nurses understand and know their organization's philosophy. See Box 4-4 for a sample philosophy.

ORGANIZATIONAL GOALS AND OBJECTIVES

The specific goals and objectives of the organization provide more concrete information on what and how the organization plans to provide/act, under the guiding hands of its established mission and philosophy. The organizational goals are the broad statements of intent, and the objectives are the specific ways to accomplish the goals. Goals are a part of the planning process, which is one of the functions of management. Generally, the goals and the objectives explain the services offered, the resource allocation, the future plans, and the responsibility to the customer (Box 4-5).

ORGANIZATIONAL POLICIES AND PROCEDURES

Each organization also has established policies and procedures. A policy is a written plan stating how the organization will function and work together. Policies help the organization to accomplish the established goals and directives and provide cohesive guidance for the members of the organization. The procedures are the methods and direction on how the policy will be implemented. Procedures

BOX 4-2

Sample Mission Statement

Provide a personal approach to the services offered by demonstrating a commitment to quality health care and offering services that promote well-being of the community through education and advanced technology.

BOX 4-4

Sample Philosophy

Hospital and Health-Care Organization, in conjunction with the Board of Trustees and entire health-care staff, believe that human beings are unique and holistic, having value and worth as individuals with individualized health-care needs. The health-care team at Hospital believes in providing the best possible care and education (using enhanced technology) to the community it serves. Each client has diverse learning needs and individualized goals to meet health-care needs. The focus of care is on wellness, caring, and the highest standards of customer service and quality.

Sample List of Goals

- An environment will be established that is conducive to patient teaching and learning.
- Nursing staff will identify the patient's need for independence and foster relationships to develop this.
- Quality nursing care will be provided within all levels of the organization.
- Annual development and assessment plans will be implemented with all employees of Hospital.

offer step-by-step guidance as to how to implement and carry out the policy. Policies and procedures are used during employee orientation, daily routines, and decision making. Both establish interdepartmental consistency within the organization. The policies and procedures familiarize employees with the rules and also serve to provide guidance and organizational direction.

ORGANIZATIONAL STRATEGIC PLANNING

Many organizations do strategic planning 3–5 years (see Chapter 14) out for the purpose of preparing to reach future goals. Strategic planning begins with analysis of where the organization stands currently and where it wants to be in the future.

The strategic plan has to have value for the members of the organization, and it needs to fit with the vision and mission of the organization. The strategic plan may include new services for patients, building opportunities, and other growth for the organization. It serves as the blueprint for the future. The strategic plan maps out ideas from the vision while focusing on the mission of the organization.

Implementation of the strategic plan requires strong leadership and managerial skills, support from the board of directors, administrative acceptance, and an understanding by all employees. It is critical that members of the organization understand what the strategic plan contains and where it will guide them for the future. Many organizations hold informational sessions to obtain employee input and feedback. Informed employees are happy employees, and there will be greater acceptance when all understand and participate in creating the goals for the organization's future.

The Organization Chart

The organization chart outlines the formal working relationships and the way people interact within the given structure. The organization chart establishes the following:

- Formal lines of authority—the official power to act
- Responsibility—the duty or assignment
- Accountability—the moral responsibility

The chart displays the decision-making authority within the organization, illustrating who has the power to make and enforce decisions for the organization. Organizational leadership has the unique ability to implement and follow the values, mission, vision, philosophy, and strategic plan in order to ensure the organization's future. The leadership of the organization is identified and described in the organization chart.

The formal channels of communication are identified as well as how members fit within the given structure. The chart demonstrates the formal relationships within the organization but does not demonstrate the informal communication and relationships that often develop as a result of working within the organization. The chart shows how the organization is supposed to run and how departments support one another in this process. Charts change frequently and require updating at least annually so that they represent what is really happening within the organization. Organization charts generally reflect the components displayed in Figure 4-1.

CHAIN OF COMMAND

Chain of command demonstrates who formally reports to whom within the organization. The vertical lines in the chart represent chain of command. It is a formal line of authority and communication within the organization and the structure. Authority and responsibility are delegated down through the chain of command. This philosophy works well, as organizations are attempting to decrease the number of layers within their structures in order to decrease the number of management positions and save money.

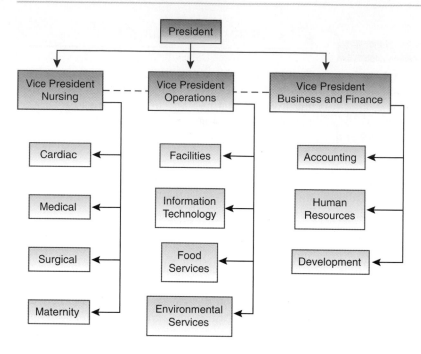

FIGURE 4-1 Organizational components.

Line Positions

Line positions are depicted by the solid vertical lines within the organization chart. These lines demonstrate who is responsible to whom within the organization. The positions with the most decision-making power are near the top of the organization chart. An example of a line position would be the Nurse Manager of the Pediatric unit, who has power and authority over the staff nurses on the unit. Another example would be the vice president of the organization who reports directly to the president.

Staff Positions

Staff positions are broken horizontal lines or dashes within the organization chart, showing the relationship between two people who work together to support objectives within the organization. These positions are primarily advisory in nature, with no direct authority over the people they are working with. The staff positions support each other within the organization by consultation, education, role modeling, and development. An example would be the vice presidents of the organization with respect to one another. These members advise and consult with each other but report to a person in a higher position, through the vertical line connection.

Organizations would be hard-pressed to function without staff positions. Managers usually work closely with people in staff positions to support a specific cause or opportunity for the unit. For example, the manager works closely with the nursing educator to support the educational needs of the nursing unit. The manager would find it difficult to do this task without the educator's assistance and expertise. The educator does not necessarily report to the manager, nor do the staff nurses directly report to the educator. This is an example of the advisory nature of the staff position.

Unity of Command

The concept of unity of command is central to the hierarchy of the organization. The overall thought is that each person on the organization chart has one manager or one boss. This is observed on the chart by the vertical solid lines that connect positions on the chart. As health-care organizations continue to grow and increase in complexity, there may be more than one person to whom an employee must report.

Span of Control

Span of control is denoted on the chart as the number of people reporting to each manager. The span of control determines how the organizational structure will appear on paper (Altaffer, 1998). A wide span of control indicates that many people are reporting to a manager, and a narrow span of control indicates that only a few people are reporting to the manager. In the 1990s, many managers were let go, and their positions were combined to cover many different units in an effort to reduce management costs. Due to the hierarchical nature of the chart, the higher a leader resides within the organizational structure, the fewer the people who report, but the greater the overall responsibility that leader has within the organization. As health-care organizations change and consolidate, upper-level managers are taking on a greater span of control (Altaffer, 1998).

DECISION MAKING

Organization charts also depict how decisions are made within an organization. **Centralized** decision making occurs when a few people at the top levels of the organizational structure make decisions. Such a chart will appear tall and hierarchical on

paper. **Decentralized** decision making occurs when decisions are made throughout the organization, at the lowest level possible within the organization. Such an organization chart takes on a flattened appearance. In decentralized decision making, authority, responsibility, and accountability are given to the person closest to the problem to resolve the issue. This method increases employee morale and job satisfaction. Employees given such authority tend to be more motivated and feel valued as members of the organization (Huber, 2000; Marquis & Huston, 2003).

The management and the leadership of the organization have to be comfortable with the type of decision making that will evolve with the organization. The method used to make decisions is influenced by the mission, the vision, the values, and the philosophy. The size of the organization may also influence what method is used.

Type of Organizational Structures

Health-care providers should be familiar with the type of structure used within their organization. The structure affects communication patterns, relationships, and authority within the health-care setting (Marquis & Huston, 2006). The structure provides stability for the mission, the vision, the values, and the goals of the organization. The structure aligns itself with the goals of the organization and provides efficiency for the organization.

The structure provides stability for decision making within the organization. The structure determines how the decision will be made. The organization chart depicts the lines of authority and chain of command and identifies communication patterns and relationships for the employees of the organization.

TALL/CENTRALIZED/BUREAUCRACY

The centralized structure, a tall structure, also known as the bureaucracy, is a hierarchical structure (Fig. 4-2). Decision making and power are held by a few people within the top level. Each person who has some power and authority is responsible for only a few people. There are many layers of

---

Practice to Strive For 4-1

Today's organizations face many challenges with changes in health-care technology, reimbursement, and practice. The organizational leader's jobs are to formulate an organizational culture and climate that is supportive of the vision, mission, and values of the organization. One main point to strive for is autonomy for the nursing staff. The culture should provide the members opportunities to grow and develop within their profession, such as with shared governance practice models and magnet status. Both affect nurses and how they will function within the organizational structure. The culture surrounding magnet status is one of care centers, with leaders who work with the staff to plan and evaluate the organization's services to meet the needs of the community.

Magnet status allows the nursing staff to participate and share in the development of policies and procedures through committees detailing research, practice, and education. Quality care and indicators are a part of all performance appraisal processes and patient satisfaction surveys. The overall nursing structure includes autonomy, collaboration, and delegation as key processes within the nursing philosophy. Nurses participate in all levels of decision making within the shared governance model. Organizations strive for excellence and ensure this within all of the services and activities offered. This philosophy is threaded throughout within the vision, mission, and values.

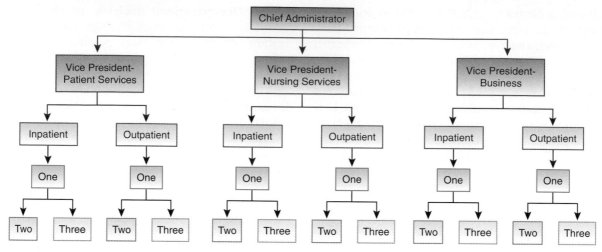

FIGURE 4-2 Bureaucracy.

departments, and communication tends to be slow as it travels through this type of a system. This type of structure is noted for its subdivision and specialization of labor. Advantages to this type of structure are that managers have a narrow span of control and can maintain close supervision of their employees. A disadvantage is that there may be a delay in decision making due to the many layers of people that the decision must pass through to get to the top administrative level. It predisposes leaders to an autocratic style of leadership because many decisions must go to the top of the organization or the higher-level supervisor for an answer.

FLAT/DECENTRALIZED STRUCTURE

The decentralized structure is flat in nature, and organizational power is spread out throughout the structure (Fig. 4-3). There are few layers in the reporting structure, and managers have a broad span

of control. Communication patterns are simplified, and problems tend to be addressed with ease and efficiency at the level at which they occur. Employees have autonomy and increased job satisfaction within this type of structure. A disadvantage is the broad span of control, which may make it hard for management to process information quickly and efficiently for the employees. This is especially true for decisions that need to span the whole structure. Management at all levels takes on a greater sense of responsibility within this structure, so education across teams is important. Managers may be supervising areas with which they are not familiar or have limited working experience.

AD HOC/ADHOCRACY STRUCTURE

The organic or **adhocracy structure** of organization is an open, free-form system. This system has resulted from behavioral research based on job

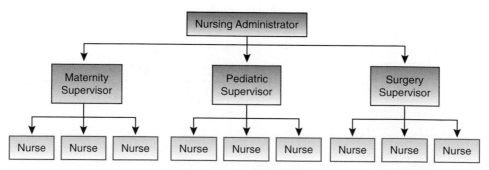

FIGURE 4-3 Decentralized structure.

satisfaction and efficiency. This type of structure is used with specialized teams to complete a specific task. From an organizational perspective, the entire organization consists of specialized teams, each assigned to complete a specific task. The major disadvantage of this type of structure is the lack of a formal chain of command. The teams work together, but when problems are encountered there is no assigned person within the structure on whom they can rely for resolution.

MATRIX STRUCTURE

The matrix structure is a combination of two structures, consisting of the product (output) and the function, linked into one structure. The function consists of all of the activities and duties needed to produce an end product, and the product is the result of the function. The structure works to balance the function and service of the organization into one operational outcome. The functions are the tasks required to complete the product. The manager of the product division works with the manager of the function division, creating two lines of authority, accountability, and communication. The team approach is incorporated, and there is a decrease in the number of formal rules for this type of structure. Issues with the matrix structure include the vague chain of command and goal variation between the two structures. This type of structure implements the use of resources efficiently.

STRUCTURES SPECIFIC TO HEALTH CARE

As health-care organizations continue to change and reorganize services to meet the needs of the customer, so will the look of the structure. Many services are changing and becoming more accessible for the patient entering the complex health-care arena.

Integrated Health-Care System

Integrated health-care systems can be defined as innovative, patient-centered hospital delivery systems that continuously improve quality and use resources cost-effectively (Effken & Stetler, 1997). This type of system evolved as a result of changes in reimbursement and managed care. An integrated health-care system is a **network** of structures combined into one to provide better continuity of care

for patients in the most applicable setting. The networks share the risks associated with the cost to provide care to the patients (McCarthy, 1997). By providing services in the most appropriate setting, the costs can be contained, which allows for a better patient outcome.

The push for an integrated system stems from the need to improve the quality of care within organizations, to reduce costs associated with health care, and to ensure patient/customer satisfaction (Wolf, Hayden, & Bradle, 2004). The single hospital of yesterday is now a component of a much larger system, offering a wide range of services for the consumer. Integrated health-care systems attempt to keep costs down and keep dollars for care within their own systems. This type of consolidation also assists and prepares for managed competition. One example of a cost control measure includes redesigning practice to serve the organizational and patient needs better. Management systems look collaboratively at patient care and outcomes of care. It is important for nurses to know and understand how these systems work and what can be done to enhance them.

The services offered can include a combination of any of the following: hospital, clinics, home health, community health, school nursing, long-term care, and rehabilitation services. When services vary like this, it is known as vertical integration, which provides a range of health-care services across the life span (Newhouse & Mills, 1999). When the integrated system consists of a chain of similar services, such as all hospitals or clinics, this is known as horizontal integration.

TYPES OF HEALTH-CARE SERVICES

There are three types of health-care services on the health-care continuum. Integrated systems often provide all three types. The shift to managed care has also changed the focus from secondary and tertiary care to primary health care. **Primary health care** prioritizes the importance of health promotion and illness prevention. This is the first line of defense for health care. Examples of health-care services provided in primary care include physician visits, immunization clinics, mammography, and teaching and education for clients. Primary health care covers services that prevent illness. **Secondary health-care** services focus on treating disease through intervention. The patient has a health alteration and seeks treatment to improve the current state of health. Secondary health-care settings include the acute care setting, such as inpatient hospitals, surgical centers, and birthing centers. **Tertiary health-care** services focus on the restoration and rehabilitation services for patients with chronic health-care needs. The goal is to maintain the current state at the best possible level of health. Health-care settings include long-term care facilities, hospice, and rehabilitation centers.

Managed care is the umbrella term that is used to address the financing and risk management for services provided in integrated health-care systems. Managed care unites the financing groups with the providers of care. The goal of managed care is to establish programs that benefit all key participants, including the insurance companies and the physicians. The push for managed care was evident as the health-care industry continued to become more complex and difficult for patients to maneuver and understand. Intensifying these concerns was the increase in cultural diversity served by the private sector (Valanis, 2000). The managed care model is the only health-care delivery model formulated from market and customer response, as compared with government and legislative initiatives (Kelly-Heidenthal, 2003; Liberman & Rotarius, 2001).

Managed care involves a prepaid mechanism, which means that a predetermined dollar amount is established to cover the cost of the health-care service. Care that is rendered is selective and requires prior authorization. There are many types of managed care products in use currently. The most common is the health maintenance organization (HMO). The HMO plan offers health care for its members for a fixed prepaid amount. An enrolled group of patients participates in the plan, and the provider is considered an employee. The provider receives a fixed payment for the services from the subscriber and assumes the financial risk. The advantage of a managed care program is cost reduction. There is a gatekeeper for the patient, usually the primary care physician. The gatekeeper's role is to oversee and coordinate services for the patient in the mix of the system. A disadvantage to managed care includes limitations to specialized care needs; some organizations are profit-driven and limit their services. Patients in health care today are discharged quicker and sicker, with only limited services available outside of the acute care setting.

Professional Practice Models

In organizations where nurses are employed and valued, management has developed and implemented opportunities for professional, autonomous nursing practice. Shared governance is defined as "structures... based on a set of principles about the relationship between the worker and the workplace" (Porter-O'Grady, 2003, p. 251). The push was for decentralized nursing leadership and decision making for professional nurses. Such a structure is based on the values of interdependence and accountability for nursing practice. The objective is to empower the nursing staff through involvement in decisions that affect their specific work areas (Erickson, Hamilton, Jones, & Ditomassi, 2003). The outcome from implementation of a professional practice model is that nurses have control of their nursing practice. Nursing staff participates in nursing committees that cover topics such as education, community involvement, research, quality control, and staffing, scheduling, and hiring practices.

The uniqueness of this structure is that nurses gain control and autonomy over their professional nursing practice. Governance models are designed to link values and nursing practice beliefs to achieve quality care (Anthony, 2004). There are more opportunities to be involved in decision making and have a voice within the organizational structure. As the nursing staff members serve on the various committees, they plan and organize the care of the patients and establish standards for nursing care based on research and evidenced-based practice.

MAGNET STATUS

The American Academy of Nursing (AAN) began to review and identify as magnet hospitals those hospitals that had solid organizational structures and a decentralized, open management style. This concept became popular in the 1980s in relation to professional practice model concepts. The goal of the magnet organization was to demonstrate autonomous nursing practice through self-governance, appropriate staffing, clinical expertise, and clinical ladder career opportunities (Upenieks, 2003).

To obtain magnet status, hospitals demonstrate that the structure in place is exemplified through a professional practice model that promotes excellence in nursing. Compliance with the identified standards must be demonstrated at all levels of nursing care within the organization (McClure, Poulin, Sovie, & Wandelt, 1983). Multiple days of onsite evaluations to assess organizational magnetism are conducted by the accrediting organization, American Nurses Credentialing Center, to determine if magnet status can be awarded. Status is awarded for 4 years. To achieve magnet status, there must organizational and nursing leadership linkages. There are 14 criteria necessary to obtain magnet status:

1. Quality of nursing leadership
2. Organizational structure
3. Management style
4. Personnel policies and programs
5. Professional models of care
6. Quality of care
7. Quality improvement
8. Consultation and resources
9. Autonomy
10. Community and the hospital
11. Nurses as teachers
12. Image of nursing
13. Interdisciplinary relationships
14. Professional development

Organizational Culture and Climate

All organizations have an informal structure that is not identified on the organization chart. It comprises the social networks and relationships that develop in the work setting. It provides a sense of belonging within the organization, also known as the culture and climate of the organization. These concepts provide insight into the organization and help influence change.

ORGANIZATIONAL CULTURE

Culture can be defined as the assumptions and beliefs that organizational members have in common. It is the "shared values and beliefs within the organization" (Huber, 2000, p. 437). The culture of the organization contains the norms that characterize the environment (Sleutel, 2000). The culture gives a sense of identity to its members and their commitment to the organization, and it helps to determine the behavior of the organization. It drives the work and the quality of the care within the organization (Gershon, Stone, Bakken, & Larson, 2004).

Culture also means that there are things in the environment that are constant, unspoken, and rarely subject to change. The culture consists of things that are not written down but are known by all members. The organizational culture affects the outcomes of quality for the organization. The culture is learned through the relationship between behaviors and the consequences (Jones & Redman, 2000).

ORGANIZATIONAL CLIMATE

The climate of the organization is the "perception of how it feels to work in a particular environment" (Snow, 2002, p. 393). Components of the climate are specific and easy to measure. Some characteristics of climate include amount of involvement members can have, supervisor support given, amount of responsibility given, commitment of the members, flexibility of the work setting, and standards set for improving practice. The key assessment question to ask regarding the climate of an organization is "Would I want to work here? Why or why not?" The climate comprises the social aspects of the organization that make the members feel like they are a part of the team.

All Good Things...

Health-care organizations face many changes in today's world. Nurses are a major component of a health-care organization, and it is imperative they understand the structure in which they provide nursing care. The structure of the organization is defined by the organization chart. This chart indicates who reports to whom and who is responsible and accountable for the functions of the organization. The organizational structure defines the arrangement of the work groups. Organizations today that have a strong value set, mission, vision, and philosophy are better prepared to meet ever-changing events and the needs of their customers. This chapter defines organizational theories, different types of structures, lines of authority and accountability, and the components of the organization chart. These are all elements that help members understand their work environment. Nurses need to be knowledgeable and comfortable within the culture and the climate of the organization. Many organizations are improving their work environment through shared governance and magnet status for the nurses. This provides autonomy and demonstrates the importance of a professional practice environment for the registered nurse.

Let's Talk

1. *Determine what your personal values are, and compare them with those of a local health-care setting. Do you see a fit with your values and those of the organization?*

2. *Think of the last position you had or the current job you are in. What type of organizational structure was in place? Was it working for the organization? Did you feel comfortable within the structure?*

3. *Describe the type of culture and climate you believe will best serve your needs as a practicing registered nurse.*

NCLEX Questions

1. Which theory emphasizes the importance of cooperation and participation in the workplace?
   A. Chaos Theory.
   B. Systems Theory.
   C. Classical Theory.
   D. Neoclassical Theory.

2. When reviewing an organizational chart, what represents the formal line of authority and responsibility within the organization?
   A. Specialization of labor.
   B. Chain of command.
   C. Span of control.
   D. Organizational structure.

3. The basic concept behind a learning organization is:
   A. The popularity to change.
   B. The people change.
   C. The adaptation to change.
   D. The resources of change.

4. Which one of the following sets the standards for behavior within the organization?
   A. The mission.
   B. The values.
   C. The philosophy.
   D. The vision.

5. Line and staff positions are identified on the organization chart. What does the line position denote?
   A. Who is responsible to whom within the organization.
   B. Advisory relationships between employees.
   C. The number of people reporting to each manager.
   D. How the decisions are made by the employer.

6. Which type of structure has decision making and power being led by a few people?
   A. Flat.
   B. Integrated.
   C. Matrix.
   D. Tall.

7. What is characteristic of a flat structure?
   A. Narrow span of control.
   B. Fewer layers in the reporting structure.
   C. Combines two structures into one.
   D. Is cost-effective with use of resources.

8. A patient was admitted to the hospital for an outpatient surgical procedure. Discharge was on the same day, and recovery continued at home. This is an example of what type of health care?
   A. Primary.
   B. Secondary.
   C. Tertiary.
   D. Quarterly.

9. Professional practice models allow for autonomous nursing practice. This concept is based on the relationship between the worker and the workplace. An example of a professional practice model is:
   A. Matrix.
   B. Integrated health care.
   C. Shared governance.
   D. Nursing care delivery.

10. Organizational culture and climate are important aspects of the organization. Which of the following are characteristic of the culture of the organization?
    A. Supervisor support given.
    B. Flexibility of the work setting.
    C. Responsibility given.
    D. Determines the behavior of the organization.

REFERENCES

Altaffer, A. (1998, July). First line managers: Measuring their span of control. *Nursing Management, 36–40.*

Anthony, M. (2004). Shared governance models: The theory, practice, and evidence. *Online Journal of Issues in Nursing, 9*(1)1–10.

Bolman, L., & Deal, T. (2003). *Reframing organizations: Artistry, choice, and leadership.* San Francisco: Jossey-Bass.

Crowell, D. (1998, May). Organizations are relationships, a new view of management. *Nursing Management,* 28–29.

Effken, J., & Stetler, C. (1997). Impact of organizational redesign. *Journal of Nursing Administration. 27*(7/8), 23–32.

Erickson, J., Hamilton, G., Jones, D., & Ditomassi, M. (2003). The value of governance/staff empowerment. *Journal of Nursing Administration, 33*(2), 96–104.

Gershon, R., Stone, P., Bakken. S., & Larson, E. (2004). Measurement of organizational culture and climate in healthcare. *Journal of Nursing Administration, 34*(1), 33–39.

Huber, D. (2000). *Leadership and nursing care management* (2nd ed.). Philadelphia: W.B. Saunders.

Jones, K., & Redman, R. (2000). Organizational culture and work redesign. *Journal of Nursing Administration, 30*(12), 604–610.

Liberman, A., & Rotarius, T. (2001). Managed care evolution—where did it come from and where is it going? In Kelly-Heidenthal, P. *Nursing leadership and management.* Australia: Thomson-Delmar Learning.

Marquis, B., & Huston, C. (2003). Leadership roles and management functions in nursing. Theory & application (4th ed.). Philadelphia: Lippincott Williams & Wilkins.

Marriner-Tomey, A. (2000). Guide to nursing management and leadership (6th ed.). St. Louis: Mosby.

McCarthy, R. (1997, September). Do integrated delivery systems do it better? *Business & Health,* 39–43.

McGuire, E. (1999). Chaos theory: Learning a new science. *Journal of Nursing Administration, 29*(2), 8–9.

McClure, M., Poulin, M., Sovie, M., & Wandelt, M. (1983). *Magnet hospitals: Attraction and retention of professional nurses.* Washington, D.C.: American Nurses Association.

Newhouse, R., & Mills, M. (1999). Vertical systems integration. *Journal of Nursing Administration, 29*(10), 22–29.

Porter-O'Grady, T. (2003). Researching shared governance. *Journal of Nursing Administration, 33*(4), 251–252.

Senge, P. (1990). *The fifth discipline: The art & practice of the learning organization.* New York: Currency Doubleday.

Senge, P. (1999). The practice of innovation. In Hesselbein, F., & Cohen, P. (Eds.), *Leader to leader* (pp. 57–68). San Francisco: Jossey-Bass.

Sleutel, M. (2000). Climate culture, context or work environment? Organization factors that influence nursing practice. *Journal of Nursing Administration, 30*(2), 53–58.

Snow, J. (2002). Enhancing work climate to improve performance and retain valued employees. *Journal of Nursing Administration, 32*(7/8), 393–397.

Sullivan, E, & Decker, P. (2001). *Effective leadership and management in nursing.* Upper Saddle River, NJ: Prentice Hall.

Upenieks, V. (2003). What's the attraction to magnet hospitals? *Nursing Management, 34*(2), 43–44.

Valanis, B. (2000). Professional nursing practice in an HMO: The future is now. *Journal of Nursing Education, 39*(1), 13–20.

Wendenhof, J., & Strahley, J. (1995). Realizing a corporate philosophy. *Organizational Dynamics, 23,* 4–19.

Wolf, G., Hayden, M., & Bradle, J. (2004). The transformational model for professional practice. A system integration focus. *Journal of Nursing Administration, 34*(4), 180–187.

Yoder-Wise, P. (2003). *Leading and managing in nursing* (3rd ed.). St. Louis: Mosby.

BIBLIOGRAPHY

Aikman, P., Andress, I., Goodfellow, C., LaBelle, N., & Porter-O'Grady, T. (1998). System integration: A necessity. *Journal of Nursing Administration, 28*(2), 28–34.

Belcher, J., & Alexy, B. (1999). High-resource hospital users in an integrated delivery system. *Journal of Nursing Administration, 29*(10), 30–36.

Drucker, P. (1980). *Management in turbulent times.* New York: Harper & Row Publishers.

Hudson, K. (2005). From research to practice on the magnet pathway. *Nursing Management, 36*(3), 33–37.

Ingersoll, G., Kirsch, J., Ehrlich-Merk, S., & Lightfoot, J. Relationship of organizational culture and readiness for change to employee commitment to the organization. *Journal of Nursing Administration, 30*(1), 11–20.

Osland, J., Kolb, D., & Rubin, I. (2001). *The organizational behavior reader* (7th ed.). Upper Saddle River, N.J.: Prentice Hall.

Tappen, R., Weiss, S., & Whitehead, D. (1998). *Essentials of nursing leadership and management.* Philadelphia: F.A. Davis Company.

Taylor, N. (2003). The magnetic pull. *Nursing Management, 34*(7), 48–56.

Von Bertalanffy, L. (1968). *General systems theory.* New York: George Braziller.

Walton, M. (1986). *The Deming management method.* New York: Perigee Books.

Additional Bibliography

Jones, L.B. (1998). *The path: Creating your mission statement for work and life.* New York: Hyperion.

Mitzberg, H. (1983). *Structures in fives: Designing effective organizations.* Englewood Cliffs, NJ: Prentice-Hall.

Norton, D., & Kaplan, R. (2000). *The strategy-focused organization.* Boston: Harvard Business School.

Porter-O'Grady, T. (1992). *Implementing shared governance: Creating a professional organization.* St. Louis: Mosby–Year Book.

Legal and Ethical Knowledge for Nurses

SHIRLEY GARICK, PHD, RN, MSN, ABQARP Diplomate, Legal Nurse Consultant (LNC)

CHAPTER MOTIVATION

"Mercy and Justice balance the scales of Justice; if mercy fails then justice must prevail."

Anonymous

CHAPTER MOTIVES

- Discuss foundations of the law.
- Describe general areas of the law.
- Explain the difference between civil and criminal law.
- Define ethics.
- Describe ethical principles and theories.
- Discuss the interrelationship between law and ethics.

Understanding the legal and ethical issues involved in nursing practice is critical for all nurses, especially managers and leaders. Legal and ethical issues are intertwined in many ways, but the two entities are distinct bodies of thought and practice. Ethics and laws both derive from societal values. Ethics is a branch of philosophy that involves clarification of the "shoulds" and "oughts" of individuals and society. Ethical decision making entails a distinctive choice between undesirable options. Ethical algorithms help to guide decisions by looking at multiple dimensions of the situation under review. Laws, on the other hand, are set down by the state or federal governments, administrative agencies, or courts, to establish boundaries of behaviors for society. The legal process constantly questions and debates the law on both legal and ethical planes.

To clear some of the confusion that often surrounds ethics and law, it is important to point out that ethics deals with the "should and should nots" that are related to behavior or actions taken by an individual. Ethics also deals with the questions of why an action is reprehensible or not reprehensible (Fry & Veatch, 1992). The legality of these choices is always a strong consideration when attempting to resolve ethical dilemmas. Ethical dilemmas in health care come up frequently, and they often address life and death issues. Nurse leaders must be prepared to address these issues in order to guide the members of their nursing staff. This chapter considers the aspects of the legal system with which the nurse leader must become familiar and then explores the foundations of ethics and ethical decision making.

The Legal System

The American legal system is based on the early English system of common law. **Common law** refers to case law that is directed and made by a judge rather than by a governmental legislative body. This type of law is set by precedent or the principles of *stare decisis,* along with the factual scenario of a given case. These laws build from one case to the next, as each judge's decision sets the precedent for future cases. In addition to federal law, Pohlman points out that each state court system has it own "**case law** [emphasis added] based

on the interpretation of its respective statutes" (Pohlman, 1990, p. 296). State and federal legislative bodies create statutes according to societal need. Administrative agencies detail the implementation of these statutes, and the courts interpret confusion over the meaning of the statutes.

FEDERAL LEGISLATION

Federal laws affect nursing practice by setting minimum standards of care for all agencies receiving federal funding. Nurses must become familiar with federal legislation, such as the Health Insurance Portability and Accountability Act, which guarantees the privacy of a patient's personal health information; the Emergency Medical Treatment and Active Labor Law (EMTALA), and the Americans With Disabilities Act (ADA). According to Moy (2003), EMTALA prohibits refusal of care for indigent and uninsured patients seeking emergency care in the emergency department. It prevents hospitals from "dumping" indigent individuals on other hospitals. The ADA also affects nursing intimately. This law proscribes any discrimination against individuals with disabilities by offering them the same opportunities as individuals without disabilities. For instance, if an individual with disabilities is the most qualified individual for a job but requires reasonable accommodations by the employer in order to take the job, the employer must make these accommodations. See Box 5-1 for others federal laws affecting nurses.

STATE LEGISLATION

State laws also regulate nurses. **Nurse practice acts (NPAs)** are created by state legislatures to define, limit, and oversee nursing practice. Nurses must be familiar with the NPA in the state in which they are practicing. NPAs set the requirements for becoming licensed as a nurse in a given state, for renewing one's license, and for continuing education. They define the duties and responsibilities of nurses in the state and limit the scope of practice. Many NPAs include safe harbor laws, which limit nurses to practicing only in their area of expertise. For example, they prevent a rehabilitation nurse from being pulled into intensive care because of a staff shortage. Other NPAs include good samaritan provisions, which protect nurses from liability for volunteering to help in an emergency situation. These provisions apply, for example, if a nurse stops at the scene of a car accident to assist victims. If something goes wrong, the victims of the car accident could not sue the nurse for malpractice. NPAs also address charting and physician orders. They specify that nurses must be skillful, correct, timely, and thorough in their charting. With respect to physician orders, most NPAs make nurses responsible for ensuring that orders are clear and accurate. If the nurse needs clarification, she must seek it from the physician giving the orders. The nurse is obligated to follow the physician order, but if she believes that doing so would be dangerous to the health of the patient, she is responsible for contacting her supervisor and following through with the institution's policy regarding physician orders.

COMMON LAW

Along with federal and state statutes, common law guides nursing practice. In order to understand how common law works in practice, consider the precedent-setting case of *Utter v. United Hospital Center, Inc.* (Giordano, 2003). This case involved a patient developing compartment syndrome after his arm was put in a cast. The nurse caring for this patient failed to acknowledge and recognize the signs and symptoms of compartment syndrome and did not request medical intervention. This case set a legal precedent that is still followed by other courts: nurses are required to exercise independent judgment to ensure patient safety and to prevent harm. Case law touches on a range of issues that involve nursing practice, including nursing malpractice, practicing medicine without a license, wrongful termination, legal challenges to a nurse's license, and questions regarding collective bargaining and labor laws. Nurse managers must work in collaboration with risk managers to make staff nurses aware of and educated about relevant case law.

There are two major categories of common law that nurses must understand: civil and criminal law. Civil law involves violations between people regarding everyday matters. Criminal law regulates offenses against individuals and society, violations made with criminal intent. Tort law is one of the major branches of civil law. Contracts is the other major branch. According to Hall (1990), a tort is a wrongdoing or injury that is committed against a person's property or person. The basis of this type of action is the liability by one individual against another. Contracts law revolves around an offer and acceptance of terms between two or more individuals or organizations. The law specifies when these agreements should be upheld and when they should not be upheld.

Torts

There are two types of torts: unintentional and **intentional**.

Unintentional Torts

Unintentional **torts** include the two types of tort that most frequently affect nurses, negligence and malpractice. Negligence is the failure to act as a reasonable or prudent person would act in the same or similar circumstances. Malpractice is a form of negligence committed by a professional, such as a nurse, by which professional misconduct, unreasonable lack of professional skills, and/or noncompliance with accepted standards of care causes injury to the client (Creighton, 1986).

There are a number of elements involved in both negligence and malpractice (Box 5-2). In order to establish liability for negligence, the existence of a duty must first be established. This duty and/or

Box 5-2

Elements of Malpractice

Duty to client	Owed to the client by nature of employment and standards of care by which the nurse must practice.
Breach of duty	A failure to meet the standard of care owed to the client.
Causation	A direct relationship between the failure to meet the standard of care and the client's harm.
Damages	It must be proved that the client/patient has incurred harm through the unsafe nursing practice.
Forseeability	The nurse must recognize or have prior knowledge that failing to meet a standard of care may cause this type of harm to the client/patient.

obligation from the nurse to the patient is created by law, standards of practice, or contract (Creighton, 1986). For instance, if a nurse is late to shift change, the nurse waiting for the nurse running late may not leave or abandon the clients in their care until the other nurse arrives because that nurse has a legal duty to the clients. If there is an urgent reason that the nurse on duty must leave, then the manager or supervisor must be notified so that another nurse may fill the position until the late nurse arrives. This leads to the second element needed to establish negligence, a **breach of duty** by the nurse. If the nurse breaches a duty (i.e., left the clients without waiting for the late nurse to arrive and without finding a replacement), there is evidence of the second element of negligence (Fry & Johnstone, 2002).

The third element needed to establish liability for malpractice is **causation,** or proximate cause. Causation means that the nurse's breach of duty is reasonably close to or causally connected to the injury or damage to the client. Damage or actual harm is the fourth element needed to prove malpractice. Without harm or injury, no cause of action exists. This harm may be physical, emotional, and/or financial (Furrow, et al., 1991). There must be proof of a direct relationship between not meeting a standard and the injury sustained by the client.

The fifth and final element of malpractice is the **forseeability** of an event. Foreseeability in this context means that the damages must be a reasonably expected result from the breach of duty.

Nurse executives/managers need to be aware of the current trend toward the criminalization of professional nurses' negligence. A nurse-attorney shares a personal communication of May 14, 1997, reported by Burkhardt and Nathaniel (1998). The communication is as follows:

"Until recently, the risk of criminal prosecution for nursing practice was non-existent unless nursing action arose to the level of criminal intent, such as the case of euthanasia leading to murder charges. However, in April, 1997, three nurses were indicted by a Colorado grand jury for criminally negligent homicide in the death of a newborn. Public records show that one nurse was assigned to care for the baby. A second nurse offered to assist her colleague in caring for the baby. A third nurse was a nurse practitioner working in the hospital nursery. Because the baby was at risk for congenital syphilis, the physician ordered that the nurse give 150,000 units of intramuscular penicillin, which would have required five separate injections. In relation to other problems the same day, the baby was subjected to a lumbar puncture, which required six painful attempts. To avoid inflicting further pain, Nurse Two asked the nurse practitioner if there was another route available for administration of the penicillin. Nurse Two and the nurse practitioner searched recognized pharmacology references and determined that IV administration would be acceptable. The nurse practitioner had the authority to change the route and directed Nurse Two to administer the medication intravenously rather than intramuscularly. Unrecognized by the nurses, the pharmacy erroneously delivered the medication prepared and ready to administer in a dose ten times greater than was ordered—1.5 million units. As Nurse Two was administering the medication IV, the baby died. The Colorado Board of Nursing initiated disciplinary proceedings against Nurse Two and the Nurse Practitioner, but not against Nurse One. The grand jury indicted all three nurses on charges of criminally negligent homicide, but did not indict the pharmacist" (Burkhardt & Nathaniel, 1998, p. 124). This is a very disturbing example of the criminalization of negligence. The case should be made that the nurses should have double-checked the medication, but there really does not seem to be criminal intent involved. However, recklessness can rise to the level of criminal negligence, and in this case recklessness, not intent, became the issue. Extreme cases of negligence that rise to the level of recklessness, however, can sometimes replace the need for criminal intent.

Vicarious liability arises when other parties are held responsible for causes of negligence. In these cases, employers become responsible for employees' actions. Most employees are supervised, so employers, by virtue of their oversight responsibilities, are held accountable for negligent acts employees commit in the course of employment. Employers also tend to have "deeper pockets" than individual employees, so the doctrine of vicarious liability affords injured clients a greater pool of resources from which to draw. There is often the temptation by nurses to believe they are protected by their employer, but they need to keep in mind the principle of **indemnification** when practicing. Under this doctrine, the institution may in turn sue the nurses for damages paid out for substandard care. Nurse managers play an important role in avoiding corporate liability problems by ensuring that employees are delivering high-quality care to their consumers. They must recognize the significance of information gathered, reports, implementation of plans, and evaluation of care on an ongoing basis. This includes client satisfaction surveys and/or other tools, which give information on the consumers' perception of the care they have received in the institution.

Intentional Torts

Intentional torts are "willful or intentional acts that violate another person's rights or property" (Berzweig, 1996). There are basically three components to intentional torts:

- The acts are intended to interfere with the plaintiff and/or the plaintiff's property.
- The acts are intentional by the defendant.
- The acts cause the consequences.

There is no legal requirement for the act causing injury or damage, only proof of intention is sufficient for the courts (Fiesta, 1988). Intentional torts include fraud, assault, battery, informed consent, false imprisonment, invasion of privacy, and defamation, which includes slander and libel. This section briefly describes each in turn.

Fraud is deliberate deception to gain unfair or unlawful advantage of a situation. Fraud may occur if a nurse falsifies her employment record or any records at her disposal. According to Guido (2001), civil assault is a threat to touch an individual without consent and causing an immediate fear of harm.

The touch does not have to take place; the individual just has to be fearful that it will take place. Battery, on the other hand, is the actual and unlawful touching of the individual's body or clothes or anything attached to the individual without the individual's consent. The nurse manager must make sure that their employees understand these two intentional torts and the differences. Fiesta (1988) presents an interesting case in which a Christian Scientist client refused medication and treatment. This client was nonetheless forced to take medication, which the courts ultimately ruled was a battery and awarded remuneration.

Interestingly, one of the most common examples of battery in a hospital setting is surgery being performed without informed consent. Informed consent is the process whereby a client is informed of all possible outcomes, risks of treatments, and alternatives in order to be able to consent freely to the recommended procedure. This means the client has the opportunity and the freedom to make choices in health-care treatment. Confusion arises when the patient is not mentally competent to make decisions about treatment, when there is a language or cultural barrier to understanding the explanation of the treatment and risks, when the patient has not reached legal age to consent but is an emancipated minor, in emergency situations, and when patients refuse to consent despite expected dire consequences for refusal. State laws vary on these subjects. Informed consent is an active and complex area of litigation. Nurses should ensure that valid informed consent exists before performing or assisting with any procedure or treatment. Otherwise, nurses risk possible cause of action for battery.

According to Creighton (1986, p. 197), false imprisonment is the unjustifiable and unlawful detention of a client within fixed boundaries or an act with the intention to keep the individual in such a confinement. There are many cases involving false imprisonment. In *Big Town Nursing Home, Inc. v. Newman* (1970), a 67-year-old man was brought to the nursing home by a nephew, and when he tried to leave, the staff restrained him and denied him use of the telephone or his clothes. The court found the reckless actions of the nursing home willful and malicious in detaining him.

Invasion of privacy is the right to be left alone or free from unwanted publicity. Fiesta (1988) describes four types of privacy invasion: the intrusion of the client's physical and mental solitude, public disclosure of private facts, any type of publicity that puts the client in the public eye under false pretenses, and any type of appropriation that is a benefit due to the client's name or likeness (p. 160). The case of *Bethiaume v. Pratt* involved a dying client who had cancer of the larynx and was repeatedly photographed for use by the physician. The client asked not to be photographed, but these wishes were ignored, and the court found the physician liable for invasion of privacy (Fiesta, 1988, p. 160). Nurse leaders and managers must make sure that a client's privacy is not invaded during their care. This includes ethical as well as legal overtones in client care delivery. Confidentiality is one of the ethical principles that nursing practice upholds via the American Nurses Association Code of Ethics with Interpretative Statements (2001). Nurse managers must make certain that the privileged information regarding clients in their care is kept confidential. Nurses are privy to highly confidential information regarding client care. Information should be disseminated exclusively on a need-to-know basis. Nurse managers should also caution their staff not to discuss interesting client cases in open areas. Nurse managers are charged with the maintenance of nursing standards within the ranks of their nursing staff.

Contract Law

The area of contract law most relevant to nurse managers is employment. Most employment relationships between nurses and employers are "at will," which allows the employees to quit "at will" and the employer to terminate "at will," for no reason. An actual employment contract between employee and employer is more binding, however. The nurse promises to provide specific nursing services in exchange for financial reimbursement. If either side violates its promises under the contract, the contract has been breached, and the other part may seek damages.

Contracts also come into play in the labor law arena. Many nurses work under the auspices of a union. The Massachusetts Nurses Association (2003) points out that 35% of nurses with union affiliation make a higher wage and work less mandatory overtime than nonunion nurses. This brings into play collective bargaining agreements, which protect the nurse and will not allow the discharge of a nurse without "good cause." Nurse

---

Practice to Strive For 5-1

Catalano (1991); Guido (1997); and Mitchell & Grippando (1993) all point out Best Practices for Reducing the Risk of Malpractice Litigation:

I. Maintain good communication with the clients in your care. This means being courteous and respectful; listening carefully; not making value judgments; assessing the ability of your client to follow and understand and then explaining treatments, orders, and medications at the level of understanding and in the language the client understands. Always verify and clarify telephone orders; optimally, do not take any telephone orders or give instructions or advice over the phone.

II. Always keep your knowledge and skills up to date. Do not administer any medication with which you are not familiar, and always practice within the professional standards and statutory span of your practice.

III. Follow and know your institution's policies and procedures, and always pay close attention to your clients' changing health status. Keep close attention to all details surrounding your clients, and document thoroughly, accurately, objectively, and in a timely manner.

IV. Always seek attention for a client's changing health status, and question physician orders if they are unclear or not in keeping with the client's condition. Remember to challenge policies or bureaucratic structures that may threaten your client's welfare.

---

supervisors are not allowed to participate in collective bargaining.

Ethical Foundations

Ethics is a philosophy based on moral values and reasoning. It contains distinct conduct rules that

Administrative Law

Administrative law includes the regulatory and adjudicatory power that is placed in the hands of agencies like the state boards of nursing. For example, state boards of nursing are given authority to further define state-legislated nursing practice acts by setting out the needed preparation for nursing practice and disciplinary actions for nurses who fail to follow the rules governing the practice of nursing.

hot topic:
Advance Directives

Advance directives include living wills, do not resuscitate (DNR) orders, and durable power of attorney for health care. Patients and their families as well as nurse managers and leaders must be conversant in these topics. Advance directives allow the individual who is of sound mind to make decisions regarding end-of-life or emergency treatment before situations arise. Advance directives may be executed through a living will, which designates the type of care the individual would like to receive in circumstances in which the individual is no longer able to decide.

Because living wills sometimes do not hold legal validity, many individuals execute a durable power of attorney for health care, which names a person who will be responsible for end-of-life decision making and care. Nurses are obligated to ask patients about advance directives, living wills, and durable power of attorney. The Patient Self-Determination Act directs all healthcare institutions receiving Medicare/Medicaid funds to inform adult patients of their right to determine their care. This includes informing them of advance directives and their right to have an advance directive. Health practitioners have a duty to follow medical directives, out of respect for patients' wishes. The physician must adhere to state statutes when writing these orders, and the nurse must follow these orders. In fact, nurses have been sued for not observing these orders (Tammelleo, 1997). Claims that may be lodged against the nurse for violating DNR orders include battery and negligence.

regulate particular choices of actions or decisions (Mappes & DeGrazia, 2001). These rules are based on philosophical theories. Ethics and ethical decision making stem from works of major philosophers, such as Immanuel Kant, Rawls, and Mill (Brannigan & DeGrazia, 2001). Deontology, or formalism, is a theory that focuses on an individual's motives rather than on the consequences of actions. Deontology encompasses natural law and incorporates dutiful actions of the individual (Hill & Zweig, 2003). Kant further recognized that reasoning is sufficient in leading an individual to moral actions and that these actions should be commenced as ends in themselves rather than as means to an end (Raphael, 1994). For example, a physician asks a

nurse to monitor a depressed 40-year-old patient who has been placed on a new, experimental antidepressant medication. The nurse monitors the patient and tells the physician that the patient said, "The medication makes me feel nauseated all of the time," but the depression has lifted. The physician makes the decision to maintain the patient on the medication because of the need to continue testing on this new medication. The physician is using the patient as a means to an end rather than demonstrating concerns for the patient's needs and feelings. Kant insisted that moral actions be placed within the boundaries of reason. He further pointed out that an action is not right unless it has the capability of becoming a binding law for everyone. For instance, in truth telling, if the caveat of telling a lie to please a patient exists, then to tell the truth is not a categorical imperative for everyone.

The other major ethical theory is teleology, or consequentialism. Utilitarianism, which is part of teleology and supports the "the greatest good for the greatest number of people," considers consequences of actions (Beauchamp & Childress, 2001). For instance, if there were to be a flu epidemic and flu vaccine was limited, the decision would be to allow the greatest number of individuals who would be affected to receive the vaccine first. If after their vaccinations, more vaccine became available, then the remainder of the population could be vaccinated. Utilitarianism truly considers real-life and commonsense approaches. John Stuart Mill expressed the view that pleasure and happiness have different qualities. This followed with the distinction that applying the golden rule in one's conduct takes precedence over immediate gratifications. Mill thought that the greatest happiness must involve everyone concerned, not just an individual. Therefore, the emphasis of this principle is based on groups aimed at producing the most happiness, focusing on utility, consequences, and means to an end (Raphael, 1994).

Another ethical theory is the more contemporary ethics of care. Mappes and DeGrazia (2001) point to the history of this ethical theory as being based on the moral experiences of women, with a focus on personal relationships and responsibilities of the relationship. Munson (2004) determines that individuals who prescribe to the care ethic think in terms of specific circumstances by using individual context rather than universal rules and principles. Furthermore, in resolving ethical dilemmas and accepting complex circumstances, the people involved must utilize critical thinking within the context of solving or coming to a resolution of the ethical situation.

Mappes and DeGrazia (2001) also considered virtue ethics as part of the ethical picture. Virtue ethics, according to these authors, originated with Aristotle and is based on the character of the individual. Virtue ethics deals with the good or virtuous character traits that may be engendered within the individual. Aristotle named courage as a virtue, striking a balance between excess courage (rashness) and appropriate courage within a situation. The Greek philosophers always strove for balance between two ends of excesses. Balance was always considered the best approach in dealing with virtues. Aristotle also believed that virtues were attained and developed through training and routine practice. In understanding virtue ethics, it would be reasonable to believe that virtuous individuals facing complex ethical dilemmas would make the right decisions due to their virtuous character.

Beauchamp and Childress (2001) laid the foundation for ethical dilemma resolution in their first edition of *Principles of Biomedical Ethics*. This book is now into its fifth edition and continues to act as a guide for ethical decision making. Nurse leaders/managers need to consider the following ethical principles in their decision-making process or if they are participating on an ethical committee.

ETHICAL PRINCIPLES

The principles listed in Box 5-3 act as a basic foundation for ethical decision making. The first principle is autonomy, which involves the right to self-determination and to make independent personal decisions regarding care. Beauchamp and Childress (2001) imply that the principle of autonomy is sometimes described as respect for autonomy. An example in health care is the patient's right to refuse treatment. The only restriction on autonomy that may preclude this right would be a com-

municable disease, in which case the patient's autonomy would be restricted. Devettere (2000) points to the Patient Self-Determination Act of 1990 as the first federal initiative that was introduced and designed to educate patients on the use of advance directives. Currently, hospitals and other institutions provide education and paperwork for patients being admitted who have not implemented an advance directive.

Beneficence is a principle that speaks to deeds of charity, mercy, and kindness toward the individual. It also means promoting the welfare of others (Beauchamp & Childress, 2001) or doing good. Nurses, by the nature of nursing practice, perform beneficent acts.

Nonmaleficence literally means to not harm the patient. Munson (2004) believes this is the overriding principle in the care of patients. Aiken and Catalano (1994) declares that nonmaleficence is the other side of beneficence but that the two cannot be considered independent of each other. Nurses may sometimes violate this principle in the short term in order to give a positive long-term result. An example is chest compressions in the event of heart stoppage in an elderly patient; ribs may be broken, and/or sternal fractures may occur that are harmful, but recovering the patient's life takes precedence over the harm.

The principle of justice is actually the deontological ethical theory. According to Beauchamp and Childress (2001), it encompasses the entire field of ethics and refers to the right to be treated justly, fairly, and equally. Munson (2004) points out that justice in health care often refers to distributive justice and/or the distribution of scarce health-care resources. Social justice becomes a part of this; Munson continues that it implies fairness in the treatment of individuals. Nurses should be aware that when indigent patients arrive in the emergency department, they must be treated in an equitable way and that if persons require emergency service due to trauma, nurses must proceed to deliver the service as deemed appropriate. This goes along with Rawls' concept of a *Theory of Justice* (1971). Brannigan and DeGrazia (2001) cited Rawls' two principles of equality and justice: (1) that everyone should be given equal liberty no matter what adversities exist; and (2) that differences among people ought to be recognized by being inclusive of the least advantaged and given their share of improvements. Others have explored this concept in health care, according to Brannigan and Boss, by proposing

---

Box 5-3

Ethical Principles

Autonomy	Fidelity
Beneficence	Veracity
Nonmaleficence	Sanctity of human life
Justice	

equitable health-care systems, benchmarks, and accessible points of entry.

Fidelity focuses more on the delivery of health care and literally means keeping one's promises or obligations to an individual. Munson (2004) suggests that keeping these commitments becomes of paramount importance when considering patient care standards that are to be met by the nurse. Likewise, nurse managers are bound by their commitments to their employees. In particular, a verbal commitment involving a shift change is a contract with the employee and should be considered as such by the manager.

Veracity involves truth telling by all concerned in patient care. The nurse certainly has an obligation to tell the truth, for instance, when a patient asks about his or her condition. This, however, can take on tones of nonmaleficence when, for example, a cancer patient asks the nurse how long he might live. In this instance, it may be the duty of the nurse not to take hope away from the patient and to provide a positive answer to this question. The answer might include the idea that no one is able to predict death and that there is always hope in life. Here again the balancing of beneficence and nonmalfeasance within the boundaries of veracity is important in the nurse's actions (Munson, 2004).

The sanctity of life principle is a part of ethical decisions when it comes to withholding or withdrawing life-sustaining treatments or assisting suicide. Sanctity of human life is defined as the obligation not to take human life (Fry & Veatch, 2000). The American Nurses Association (ANA) implies that nurses caring for patients should direct their care toward the relief and prevention of the suffering that is often associated with the process of dying (ANA, 1985, p. 4). This brings into focus the ANA's position statement (1994) on active euthanasia and its position statement on withholding nutrition and hydration for the patient (ANA, 2001). The latter position should be made by the client or surrogate with the health-care team. The ANA carefully considered the benefit-and-harm relationship of withholding nutrition, recognizing that, sometimes, living causes more harm to the individual than dying. The ANA differentiates between artificial nutrition and the individual being able to consume food and water by mouth. The ANA states that only artificial nutrition may or may not be justified. If the individual is unable to make decisions, then the surrogate must be relied upon. Nurses must continue to give good care and

educate client family members about the dying process and provision of comfort measures (ANA Ethics and Human Rights Position Statements, April 2, 1992).

ETHICAL DECISION MAKING

Nurses must learn how to make ethical decisions, and nurse managers/leaders must direct and guide nurses in making such decisions. Nurses, in increasing numbers, are being invited to participate on ethical committees. These committees are structured with members of the health-care team, administrators, risk managers, attorneys for the institution, and others. A popular ethical decision model called MORAL was put forward by Thiroux (1977) and Halloran (1982). This model offers a very concise and systematic way of making ethical decisions (Box 5-4). It is most important that

---

Box 5-4

MORAL Model of Ethical Decision Making

M—Massage the dilemma. Identify and define the issues in the dilemma. Consider the options of all the major players in the dilemma and their value systems. This includes patients, family members, nurses, physicians, clergy, and any other interdisciplinary health-care members.

O—Outline the options. Examine all of the options, including those that are less realistic and conflicting. This stage is designed only for considering options and not for making a final decision.

R—Resolve the dilemma. Review the issues and options, applying basic principles of ethics to each option. Decide the best option, based on the views of all those concerned in the dilemma.

A—Act by applying the chosen option. This step is usually the most difficult because it requires actual implementation, whereas the previous steps require only dialogue and discussion.

L—Look back and evaluate the entire process, including the implementation. No process is complete without a thorough evaluation. Ensure that those involved are able to follow through on the final option. If not, a second decision may be required, and the process must start again at the initial step.

Modified from Thiroux, J. (1977). *Ethics: Theory and practice*. Philadelphia: Macmillan; and Halloran, M.C. (1982). Rational ethical judgments utilizing a decision making tool. *Heart and Lung 11*, 566–570.

Box 5-5
Essential Values and Behaviors

Altruism is a concern for the welfare and well-being of others. In professional practice, altruism is reflected by the nurse's concern for the welfare of patients, other nurses, and other health-care providers. The professional behaviors involved with this essential value include: *understanding* of cultures, beliefs, and perspectives of others; *advocacy* for patients, particularly the most vulnerable; *risk taking* on behalf of patients and colleagues; and *mentoring* other professionals.

Autonomy is the right to self-determination. Professional practice reflects autonomy when it respects patients' rights to make decisions about their health. The professional behaviors involved with this essential value include: *planning* care in partnership with patients; *honoring* the right of patients and families to make decisions about health care; and *providing* information so patients can make informed choices.

Human dignity is respect for the inherent worth and uniqueness of individuals and populations. In professional practice, human dignity is reflected when the nurse values and respects all patients and colleagues. The professional behaviors involved with this essential value include: *providing* culturally competent and sensitive care;

protecting patients' privacy; *preserving* the confidentiality of patients and health-care providers; and *designing* care with sensitivity to individual patient needs.

Integrity is acting in accordance with an appropriate code of ethics and accepted standards of practice. Integrity is reflected in professional practice when the nurse is honest and provides care based on an ethical framework that is accepted within the profession. The professional behaviors involved with this essential value include: *providing* honest information to patients and the public; *documenting* care accurately and honestly; *seeking* to remedy errors made by self or other; and *demonstrating* accountability for own actions.

Social justice is upholding moral, legal, and humanistic principles. This value is reflected in professional practice when the nurse works to ensure equal treatment under the law and equal access to quality health care. The professional behaviors involved with this essential value include: *supporting* fairness and nondiscrimination in the delivery of care; *promoting* universal access to health care; and *encouraging* legislation and policy consistent with the advancement of nursing care and health care.

American Association of Colleges of Nursing, 1998.

ethical decisions be reached in a timely manner. and the use of this model certainly facilitates the process.

Ethics and ethical decision making have become a thread that is followed throughout the nursing curriculum. The American Association of Colleges of Nursing (AACN) has presented a set of nursing values for nursing students to internalize into their nursing education (Box 5-5). These essential values follow closely the aforementioned ethical principles as a guide for the profession and provide a foundation for future nursing leaders and managers to build upon.

All Good Things...

Legal and ethical issues are moving to the forefront of professional nursing practice. The current socie-

tal values are changing, and there is an increasing abundance of litigation in the health-care arena. Along with this, the rapid changes in technological advancement keep health professionals in a constant state of training. Nurse executives and managers must know the law and ethics as well as understand the ramifications of making sure their employees are also knowledgeable of the law and ethical dilemmas. The laws that affect nurses are critical for nurse executives to understand and follow by making their employees knowledgeable about the pitfalls that may arise due to not meeting standards of care in their units and what may happen to them legally due to this failure to meet standards of care. Along with the legalities of practice and care go the ethical issues involved in practice. Understanding ethical foundations, ethical decision making, and ethical committees is an important part of the nurse executive/managerial role.

Let's Talk

1. *Discuss the interrelationship of law and ethics.*

2. *Discuss federal laws affecting nursing and their impact on the profession.*

3. *Describe the difference between the two types of common law.*

4. *Discuss the elements of malpractice, and give an example of each.*

5. *Give an example of the criminalization of negligence.*

6. *What are the three components of intentional torts?*

7. *Give an example of an intentional tort of battery.*

8. *Give one example of a best practice for reducing the risk of malpractice litigation.*

9. *Discuss advance directives and claims that may be lodged for not following them.*

10. *Give an example of each of the seven ethical principles.*

11. *Discuss the five steps of ethical decision making in the MORAL model.*

NCLEX Questions

1. Legal and ethical issues are intertwined but:
   A. They are not distinct bodies of thought or practice.
   B. They are individual and distinct bodies of thought and practice.
   C. Have no effect on each other.
   D. Are not of great influence on each other.

2. Ethics is a body of knowledge that deals with:
   A. Primarily legal aspects of health care.
   B. Trying to get individuals to behave correctly.
   C. The "shoulds" and "should nots" of individual behavior or actions.
   D. Religion only.

3. Common law refers to:
   A. Laws that societies have in common.
   B. Ethical ideas only.
   C. Statutes.
   D. Case law.

4. Some of the federal laws affecting nurses are:
   A. Not important because only state laws impact nursing.
   B. Age discrimination act and equal pay act.
   C. Very important but not relevant to practice.
   D. The nurse practice acts.

5. It is important for nurses to know the Nurse Practice Act in their state because:
   A. It affects their practice.
   B. It authorizes their licensure.
   C. Neither a nor b.
   D. Both a and b.

6. Nonmaleficence actually means:
   A. For the nurse to take care of the client.
   B. There is negligence.
   C. To not harm the patient.
   D. Malpractice.

7. Deontology encompasses:
   A. Duty.
   B. Natural law.
   C. Utilitarianism.
   D. All of the above.

8. Ethic of care is:
   A. Part of all health-care philosophy.
   B. Consequentialism.
   C. Formulated by John Mill.
   D. Based on the moral experiences of women.

9. Ethics is:
   A. Based on moral values and reasoning.
   B. Only part of the legal system.
   C. Not as important as the legal system.
   D. Important to philosophical studies.

10. Ethical principles are:
    A. Autonomy, fidelity, veracity.
    B. Only abstract ideas.
    C. Not used in practice.
    D. Not applicable to legal situations.

REFERENCES

Aiken, T.D., & Catalano, J.I. (1994). *Legal, ethical and political issues in nursing.* Philadelphia: FA Davis.

American Nurses Association. (1998). *Standards for nurse administrators.* Kansas City, MO: Author.

American Nurses Association (1988). *Standards for nurse administrators.* Kansas City, MO: Author.

American Nurses Association Committee on Ethics (2001). *Code for nurse with interpretative statements,* Washington, DC: American Nurses Association.

Beauchamp, T.L., & Childress, J.F. (2001). *Principles in biomedical ethics* (5th ed.). New York: Oxford University.

Berzweig, P. (1996). *The nurse's liability for malpractice* (6th ed.). New York: Mosby.

Black's law dictionary (6th ed.) (1996). St. Paul: West.

Brannigan, M.C., & DeGrazia, D. (2001). *Health care ethics in a diverse society.* Mountain View, CA: Mayfield.

Burkhardt, M., & Nathaniel, A. (1998). *Ethics & issues in contemporary nursing.* Albany, NY: Delmar Publishers.

Chambliss, D.R. (1996). *Beyond caring: Hospitals, nurses, and the social organization of ethics.* Chicago: University of Chicago Press.

Cofer, M.J. (1998). How to avoid age bias. *Nursing Management, 29*(11), 34–36.

Creighton, H. (1986). *Law every nurse should know* (5th ed.). Philadelphia: W.B. Saunders.

Curtin, L. (2001). The first 10 principles for the ethical administration of nursing services. *Nursing Administration Quarterly, 25*(1), 7–13.

DeMello, A. (1985). *One-minute wisdom.* New York: Doubleday.

Devettede, R.J. *Pretrial decision making for health care ethics: Cases of concepts* (2nd ed.). Washington, DC: Georgetown University Press.

Edwards, P.A., & Roemer, L. (1996) Are nurse managers ready for the current challenges of health care? *Journal of Nursing Administration, 26*(9), 11–17.

Fiesta, J. (1999a). Do no harm: When caregivers violate our golden rule, part I. *Nursing Management, 30*(8), 10–11.

Fiesta, J. (1999b). Informed consent: What health care professionals need to know, part 2. *Nursing Management, 30*(7), 6–7.

Fiesta, J. (1999c). Know your boundaries in sexual assault litigation. *Nursing Management, 31*(1), 10.

Fiesta, J. (1988). *The law and liability: A guide for nurses* (2nd ed.) New York: John Wiley & Sons.

Fowler, M.D., & Benner, P. (2001). Implementing the new code of ethics for nurses: An interview with Marsha Fowler. *American Journal of Critical Care, 10*(6), 434–437.

Fry, S., & Johnstone, M.J. (2002). *Ethics in nursing practice: A guide to ethical decision making* (2nd ed.). Oxford, UK: Blackwell Science.

Fry, S.T., & Veatch, R.M. (1992). *Case studies in nursing ethics* (2nd ed.). Boston: Jones and Barlett Publishers.

Furrow, B.R., Johnson, S.H., Jost, T.S., & Schwartz, R.L. (1991). *Liability and quality issues in health care.* St. Paul: West.

Giordano, K. (2003). Examining nursing malpractice: A defense attorney's perspective. *Critical Care Nurse, Apr*(23).

Guido, G.W. (2001). *Legal and ethical issues in nursing* (3rd ed.). Upper Saddle River, NJ: Prentice Hall.

Hall, J.K. (1990). Understanding the fine line between law and ethics. *Nursing 90*(10), 37.

Hellinghausen, M.A. (1996). Providers face more liability as duties grow. *Nursing & Allied Health Week, 1*(15), 1.

Hill, T.C., & Zweig, R.M. (2003). *Immanuel Kant: Groundwork for the metaphysics of morals,* New York: Oxford University Press.

Iowa Hospital Association (1991). *The patient self-determination act of 1990: Implementation in Iowa hospitals.* Author.

Kelly, C. (2000). *Nurses' moral practice: Investing and discounting self.* Indianapolis: Sigma Theta Tau, International Center Nursing Press.

LaDuke, S. (2000). What to expect from your attorney. *Nursing Management, 31*(1), 10.

Mappes, T.A., & DeGrazia, D. (2002). *Biomedical ethics* (5th ed). Boston: McGraw Hill.

Massachusetts Nursing Association (2003). *MNA Publication, May,* 11.

Moy, M.M. (2005). A year later: EMTALA final rule clarifies obligations. *ED Legal Letter, 16*(4), 37–48.

Moy, M.S. (2003). EMTALA revisions provide clearer explanation of critical terms. *ED Legal Letter, 15*(2), 13–24.

Munson, R. (2004). *Intervention and prediction: Basic issues in medical ethics* (7th ed.). Victoria, Australia: Thomas Wadsworth.

Nguyen, B.Q. (2000a). ADA coverage: Defining who is "qualified individual with a disability." *American Journal of Nursing, 100*(3), 87.

Nguyen, B.Q. (2000b). If you're replaced by a younger nurse. *American Journal of Nursing, 100*(3), 82.

Olson-Chavarriaga, D. (2000). Informed consent: Do you know your role? *Nursing 2000, 30*(5), 60–61.

Patient Self-Determination Act/Omnibus Budget Reconciliation Act of 1990, Pub L No. 101–508, Sec. 4206; 42 U.S.C. Sec. 1395cc(a)(1).

Pohlman, K.J. (1989a). Legal issues in nursing: DNR? CPR? *Focus on Critical Care, 16*(3), 224–225.

Pohlman, K.J. (1989b). Legal issues in nursing: Nursing negligence. *Focus on Critical Care, 16*(4), 296–298.

Pohlman, K.J. (1990). Against nursing advice? *Focus on Critical Care, 17*(1), 57–58.

Pozgar, G.D. (1999). *Legal aspects of health care administration* (7th ed.). Gaithersburg, MD: Aspen Press.

Raphael, D.D. (1994). *Moral philosophy* (2nd ed.). New York: Oxford University Press.

Rawls, J. (1971). *A theory of justice.* Cambridge, MA: Harvard University Press.

Steckler, S.L. (2000). Nursing case law update. *Journal of Nursing Law, 7*(1), 55–64.

Yoder-Wise, P. (2003). *Leading and managing in nursing* (3rd ed.). St. Louis: Mosby.

chapter 6

Regulating Nursing

MARY O'KEEFE, RN, PHD, JD

CHAPTER MOTIVATION

"The nurse promotes, advocates for, and strives to protect the health, safety, and rights of the patient."[1]

Disclaimer[2]

CHAPTER MOTIVES

- Explore nursing regulation through nursing practice acts.
- Define nursing standards and competencies.
- Identify nursing standards specific to advanced practice, management, and informatics.
- Analyze evidence-based nursing practice as the standard of care.
- Analyze nursing research as the mechanism to provide evidence-based nursing and best practice.
- Explore accreditation as nursing regulation.
- Explore policies and procedures as nursing regulation.
- Explore regulations of staffing to provide standardized patient care.
- Discuss state and federal legislative and administrative regulation of nursing.

[1]American Nurses Association. (2001 June). Code of Ethics for Nurses. Retrieved December 14, 2004, from http://www.nursingworld.org/ethics/chcode.htm

[2]The information contained in this chapter is not intended to be legal advice. Further, this information related to regulating nursing is dynamic, and may have changed or be changing at any point. Therefore, when seeking legal advice regarding any of the information contained in this chapter, retain the legal counsel of an attorney.

Nursing practice is regulated on the state and federal level. Nursing regulation "began as a simple registry process to protect the nursing title and the public" (Flook, 2003, p. 160). The primary purpose of nursing regulation today is not only protecting the public through a defined nursing practice but also regulating nursing education and "overseeing the competence of nurses through licensing and disciplinary rules and regulations" (Flook, 2003, p. 160). The authority to license and discipline the nursing profession is granted to each state's board of nursing, often called the board of nurse examiners (BNE) through state legislation creating a nursing practice act and mechanisms for licensure.

The Nursing Practice Act

At the state level, nursing is regulated by the **nursing practice act,** which provides for licensure as a registered nurse. A state's act defines nursing and the standards of care. The nurse is licensed to practice under the state's act. The act defines specifically what the reasonable nurse is licensed to do to meet the standards of patient care.

STANDARD OF CARE FOR THE REGISTERED NURSE

The **standard of care** (Box 6-1) is "that degree of care, expertise and judgment exercised by a reasonable and prudent nurse under the same or similar circumstances [through] use of nursing process" (O'Keefe, 2001, pp. 552–553).

Licensure is the "mechanism by which a state establishes and verifies compliance with [nursing] standards" (O'Keefe, 2001, p. 542). The act regulates nursing through the BNE, which oversees the nurse's compliance with the nursing standards and grants licensure.

Certification acknowledges nursing competence at an advanced level of practice. Gunn (1999, p. 135) believed that society and patients in general have grown skeptical of the willingness of the nursing profession to police itself. In the 1970s, skepticism coupled with a malpractice crisis forced regulators of nursing practice to move beyond "one-time testing for a lifelong credential, to other alternatives for assuring competency in nursing

---

Box 6-1

BNE Rule 217.11: Standards of Nursing Practice for the Registered Nurse (22 Tex. Admin. Code 217, Part 11, 2004)

The Texas Board of Nurse Examiners is responsible for regulating the practice of nursing within the State of Texas for Vocational Nurses, Registered Nurses, and Registered Nurses with advanced practice authorization. The standards of practice establish a minimum acceptable level of nursing practice in any setting for each level of nursing licensure or advanced practice authorization. Failure to meet these standards may result in action against the nurse's license even if no actual patient injury resulted.

(3) Standards Specific to Registered Nurses. The registered nurse shall assist in the determination of healthcare needs of clients and shall:

(c) Utilize a systematic approach to provide individualized, goal-directed, nursing care by:

(d) performing comprehensive nursing assessments regarding the health status of the client;

(ii) making nursing diagnoses that serve as the basis for the strategy of care;

(iii) developing a plan of care based on the assessment and nursing diagnosis;

(iv) implementing nursing care; and

(v) evaluating the client's responses to nursing interventions;

(B) Delegate tasks to unlicensed personnel in compliance with 22 Tex. Admin. Code chapter 224, relating to clients with acute conditions or in acute care environments, and chapter 225, relating to independent living environments for clients with stable and predictable conditions.

---

practice." Currently, the focus varies on a state-by-state basis, from voluntary to mandatory requirements for continuing education as a mechanism for either continuing certification or recredentialing. Certification involves "examinations developed by professional organizations which provide certification of a claim to competence at a certain level of practice" (O'Keefe, 2001, p. 532). The graduate nurse must possess the competence to practice independently, a declaration that must be demonstrated and supported by documentation (Texas Board of Nurse Examiners, 2004). A **nursing competency** is the skill and behavior required to perform the role of a nurse.

STANDARDS OF CARE FOR ADVANCED NURSING PRACTICE

By definition, an **advanced practice nurse** (APN) is "a registered professional nurse who is prepared for advanced nursing practice by virtue of knowledge and skills obtained through a post-basic or advanced educational program of study, [and] acts independently and/or in collaboration with other health care professionals in the delivery of health care services" (O'Keefe, 2001, p. 529).

Regulating Advanced Practice

Advanced nursing practice is regulated by and built upon standards of care for the registered nurse, identified within each state's nursing practice act. See Box 6-2 for the definition of an APN in Texas.

Prior to 1971, most states made it illegal for any nurse to perform diagnosis or prescribe treatment. Regulation of APNs and programs for their preparation by boards of nursing vary from state to state. Fenton and Thomas (1998) reported that boards have authority only to regulate advanced practice through: (1) the recognition of the APN and (2) the setting of standards and scope of practice. Fenton (1998, p. 78) noted the "lack of consistent APN educational program standards and experiences and criteria for recognition of APNs was problematic at the levels of accreditation, certification, and regulation." As a consequence, the Texas Board of Nurse

Examiners developed a model designed to ensure the education and recognition of the APN, emphasizing both professionalism and public safety (Fenton & Thomas, 1998).

For example, APNs practice via protocols or other written authorizations. See Box 6-3 for a definition of these protocols and other written authorizations under the Texas Nursing Practice Act.

Roemer (1977) reported that states have been increasingly liberalizing the scope of nursing functions, making it possible for the APN to assume functions formerly not within the nurse's scope of clinical practice. In some states, some of these advanced practice functions are allowed under doctor's supervision. In other states, especially in rural areas, the APN may function independently. The independent action, however, such as dispensing medications, may be limited to a single course of treatment.

Midwives tend to function independently. According to Roemer (1977), nurse-midwives have been accepted as extensions of scarce medical facilities, generally authorized to provide prenatal and postpartum care, handle normal deliveries, and do family planning work, including fitting diaphragms and inserting and removing IUDs. Moreover, courses for family planning nurse practitioners have been set up across the United States. Graduates may, with medical direction: (1) perform bimanual pelvic examinations and breast examinations; (2) prescribe contraception; (3) fit diaphragms, insert IUDs, and examine vaginal secretions microscopically; and (4) refer patients with problems to physicians.

Roemer (1977) also reported a California program of both registered and nonregistered nurses trained as women's health specialists, who make routine examinations in both pregnant and nonpregnant women, to give family planning advice. Non-RN family planning specialists being trained included (1) licensed vocational nurses, (2) baccalaureate degree holders in non-nursing fields, and (3) qualified persons with less formal education. This 24-week course was authorized under the California State Department of Health. According to Roemer, the use of the APN would (1) help make family planning and well-baby services more generally available and (2) conserve valuable physician time for those cases that need greater skill and training.

As standards of nursing care vary from state to state, so does the regulation of the APN. Ponto,

---

Box 6-2

BNE Rule 221.1(3): Definition of an Advanced Practice Nurse (22 Tex. Admin. Code 221.1(3), 2001)

(3) Advanced practice nurse—A registered nurse approved by the board to practice as an advanced practice nurse based on completing an advanced educational program acceptable to the board. The term includes a nurse practitioner, nurse-midwife, nurse anesthetist, and clinical nurse specialist. The advanced practice nurse is prepared to practice in an expanded role to provide health care to individuals, families, and/or groups in a variety of settings including but not limited to homes, hospitals, institutions, offices, industry, schools, community agencies, public and private clinics, and private practice. The advanced practice nurse acts independently and/or in collaboration with other health care professionals in the delivery of health care services.

Box 6-3

BNE Rule 221.13: Core Standards for Advanced Practice (22 Tex. Admin. Code 221.1(3), 2001)

(a) The advanced practice nurse shall know and conform to the Texas Nursing Practice Act; current board rules, regulations, and standards of professional nursing; and all federal, state, and local laws, rules, and regulations affecting the advanced role and specialty area. When collaborating with other health care providers, the advanced practice nurse shall be accountable for knowledge of the statutes and rules relating to advanced practice nursing and function within the boundaries of the appropriate advanced practice category.

(b) The advanced practice nurse shall practice within the advanced specialty and role appropriate to his/her advanced educational preparation.

(c) The advanced practice nurse acts independently and/or in collaboration with the health team in the observation, assessment, diagnosis, intervention, evaluation, rehabilitation, care and counsel, and health teachings of persons who are ill, injured or infirm or experiencing changes in normal health processes; and in the promotion and maintenance of health or prevention of illness.

(d) When providing medical aspects of care, advanced practice nurses shall utilize mechanisms which provide authority for that care. These mechanisms may include, but are not limited to, Protocols or other written

authorization. This shall not be construed as requiring authority for nursing aspects of care.

(1) Protocols or other written authorization shall promote the exercise of professional judgment by the advanced practice nurse commensurate with his/her education and experience. The degree of detail within protocols/policies/practice guidelines/clinical practice privileges may vary in relation to the complexity of the situations covered by such Protocols, the advanced specialty area of practice, the advanced educational preparation of the individual, and the experience level of the individual advanced practice nurse.

(2) Protocols or other written authorization:
   (A) should be jointly developed by the advanced practice nurse and the appropriate physician(s),
   (B) shall be signed by both the advanced practice nurse and the physician(s),
   (C) shall be reviewed and re-signed at least annually,
   (D) shall be maintained in the practice setting of the advanced practice nurse, and
   (E) shall be made available as necessary to verify authority to provide medical aspects of care.

(e) The advanced practice nurse shall retain professional accountability for advanced practice nursing care.

Sabo, Fitzgerald, and Wilson (2002) report that many other state boards of nursing are examining advanced nursing practice to determine a process to recognize and regulate such practice for the purpose of eventual uniformity of the nursing law. For example, in 1999, Minnesota state law was redesigned to define and provide protection for advanced practice registered nurses. The Minnesota Board of Nursing convened to develop (1) recommendations regarding issues of certification, (2) criteria for determining acceptable certifying organizations, (3) procedures in the event of examination failure, and (4) a process for communicating this information to the nursing community (Ponto et al., 2002).

Scope of Practice for Clinical Nurse Specialists

A **clinical nurse specialist** (CNS) is an APN who has specialized education and training in one clinical area. For example, the psychiatric CNS focuses on treating the patient in the clinical area through patient or staff education, consultation with psychiatric nursing or other staff, and structuring patient therapies. See Box 6-4 for the scope of practice for the APN.

Heitkemper and Bond (2004) believed that the CNS is critical to providing leadership to improve patient care, advancing nursing practice, and strengthening health-care delivery systems.

The scope of nursing practice has been expanded to encompass nursing via various technologies. For example, with the advent of telenursing, states must now extend the scope of practice across state boundaries.

The Effects of Telenursing Upon Expansion of Nursing Practice Acts

Nursing practice acts—developed by the individual states—traditionally have regulated the nurses that practice within the state. Telenursing challenges this boundary-driven regulation. **Telenursing** is

Box 6-4

BNE Rule 221.12: Scope of Practice for the Advanced Practice Nurse (22 Tex. Admin. Code 221.12, 2001)

The advanced practice nurse provides a broad range of health services, the scope of which shall be based upon educational preparation, continued advanced practice experience and the accepted scope of professional practice of the particular specialty area. Advanced practice nurses practice in a variety of settings, and according to their practice specialty and role they provide a broad range of health care services to a variety of patient populations.

(1) The scope of practice of particular specialty areas shall be defined by national professional specialty organizations or advanced practice nursing organizations recognized by the Board. The advanced practice nurse may perform only those functions which are within that scope of practice and which are consistent with the Nursing Practice Act, Board rules, and other laws and regulations of the State of Texas.

(2) The advanced practice nurse's scope of practice shall be in addition to the scope of practice permitted a registered nurse and does not prohibit the advanced practice nurse from practicing in those areas deemed to be within the scope of practice of a registered nurse.

 hot topic:

National Health Care: Is Nursing Ready?

Health care and nursing have been transformed, by technology and other external forces, into a national and international system that has (1) reshaped professional nursing practice to cross state boundaries, (2) facilitated nursing regulation on a multistate level, (3) enabled the implementation of the national interstate practice model, and (4) placed nursing within the global health-care marketplace (Fernandez & Herbert, 2004).

The National Health Care Program (NHCP) is often referred to as "socialized medicine," as the government will administer, regulate, and control health care by providing for health and hospital care for the public. Other terms for NHCP are "universal health care" and "single payer health care."

Currently, only those older than 65 years are the beneficiaries of government-paid medical benefits through Medicare. Through NHCP, payment for all public health care will be subsidized by public funds. Health-care providers will be subject to salaries, as all providers will work for and receive their salaries from the government.

National and international health care exists in the geographic sense for nursing, through federal and state government regulations, such as the Nursing Licensure Compact (NLC). Has the NLC created the structure for nurses to participate in a national health care program? Are levels of nursing practice and competencies clearly identified in preparation for an NHCP? Can levels of competencies be standardized across state boundaries to nationalize basic nursing competencies in preparation for an NHCP?

the "electronic transfer of nursing data, nursing information, and nursing expertise between two points" (O'Keefe, 2001, p. 552). Because nurses are now able to practice outside of their state without actually traveling, telenursing has had a considerable impact on the expansion of nursing practice acts. Hutcherson (2001, p. 4) opined: "During the last century the world has become increasingly reliant on a variety of technologies to manage information needs. Escalation in deployment of remote technology to enhance health care, accompanied by expanded public and private reimbursement for distant care, indicates increasing acceptance of these technologies. Yet many legal and regulatory questions regarding the provision of health care using these technologies remain."

The age of informatics has opened a new era for nursing practice, taking advantage of advances in telecommunications technology that has allowed nurses to provide patient care in different geographic locations throughout the country (Hardin & Langford, 2001). The state-based system of nurs-

ing practice acts is being challenged by this new practice environment.

The Nurse Licensure Compact

To accommodate new technology, states have created the **interstate compact** (Hardin & Langford, 2001). An interstate compact "is an agreement between two or more states established for the purpose of remedying a particular problem of multi-state concern" (National Council of State Boards of Nursing, 2005, citing *Black's Law Dictionary*). In this instance, the compact, developed by the National Council of State Boards of

Nursing, "allows nurses to practice outside their state of licensure, as long as the nurse adheres to the nurse practice act in the state in which he/she practices" (O'Keefe, 2001, p. 541).

The compact utilizes the **mutual recognition model,** which is a model of nursing licensure that "allows a nurse to have one license (in the nurse's state of residency) and to practice in other states, as long as that individual acknowledges that he or she is subject to each state's practice laws and discipline. Under mutual recognition, practice across state lines is allowed, whether physical or electronic, unless the nurse is under discipline or a monitoring agreement that restricts practice across state lines. In order to achieve mutual recognition, each state must enter into an interstate compact, called the Nurse Licensure Compact (NLC or Compact)" (National Council of State Boards of Nursing, 2005).

The NLC grants the nurse a **multistate licensure privilege,** meaning "the authority to practice nursing in any compact state that is not the state of residency," without the need of an additional license. See Box 6-5 for a listing of states currently participating and/or pending participation in the NLC.

But the NLC also provides that the nurse is accountable for complying with the nursing practice laws, regulations, standards of care, and competencies in the state where the patient is located at the time care is provided (National Council of State Boards of Nursing, 2005). This is a daunting task because the terminology within the nursing practice acts varies from state to state.

NURSING PRACTICE ACTS LACK UNIFORMITY FROM STATE TO STATE

The terminology used within the acts differs and varies from state to state. For example, Lavin, Meyer, and Carlson (1999) reviewed the use of the term "nursing diagnosis" in the nursing practice acts in the United States. They divided the nursing practice acts of the 50 states and the District of Columbia into those that did or did not include within a nursing context: (1) the term "nursing diagnosis" or (2) the word "diagnosis." The findings revealed that 33 of the 51 nursing practice acts used the term "diagnosis" within the nursing context. They concluded (p. 57): "The majority of practice acts now define the practice of professional

---

Box 6-5

Nurse Licensure Compact Implementation (National Council of State Boards of Nursing, 2005)

The following list shows which states have enacted the **RN and LPN/VN Nurse Licensure Compact.** Please note that although New Jersey, New Hampshire, and South Carolina have enacted the Nurse Licensure Compact, these states have not yet implemented (passed into law) the compact. On April 25, 2005, the states of Iowa and Utah agreed to mutually recognize APRN licenses. No date has been set for the implementation of the APRN Compact.

COMPACT STATES	IMPLEMENTATION DATE
Arizona	7/1/2002
Arkansas	7/1/2000
Delaware	7/1/2000
Idaho	7/1/2001
Iowa	7/1/2000
Maine	7/1/2001
Maryland	7/1/1999
Mississippi	7/1/2001
Nebraska	1/1/2001
New Mexico	1/1/2004
North Carolina	7/1/2000
North Dakota	1/1/2004
South Dakota	1/1/2001
Tennessee	7/1/2003
Texas	1/1/2000
Utah	1/1/2000
Virginia	1/1/2005
Wisconsin	1/1/2000

If you are seeking Compact licensure, please contact your state board of nursing for primary state of residence requirements.

Compact States Pending Implementation

PENDING COMPACT STATES	STATUS
New Jersey	Signed by Governor
New Hampshire	Signed by Governor
South Carolina	Signed by Governor

---

nursing as including the diagnostic act, although the manner in which they use the term varies."

Marrs and Alley (2004) conducted a descriptive study to explore related regulatory terminology used in nurse practice acts from the 50 states and Washington, DC. They discovered, for example, that although terms such as moral turpitude, moral character, and morality were used by approximately half of the states, the terms typically were not defined. They suggested (p. 54): "Agreement among states on uniform definitions and standards of nursing practice can be a step toward aligning practice acts, bringing consistency to disciplinary actions, and informing the public about the profession's standards for practice."

DISCIPLINE AND REHABILITATION UNDER THE TERMS OF THE NURSING PRACTICE ACT

Nursing regulatory boards have the power to take disciplinary action against licensees who have violated the state's act. Typically, license suspension is a common penalty. For examples of violations of an act and grounds for disciplinary action, see Box 6-6.

Disciplinary action in most states is a function of the state board of nursing. But boards also promote rehabilitation for nurses while they regain competence. Lewallen and McMullan (2001) reported that as part of the disciplinary process, the state board of nursing may require licensees to take courses in legal-ethical decision making and/or pharmacology. They indicate that this form of rehabilitative discipline redevelops nursing competence in the following manner: (1) during the courses, the licensees must acknowledge their specific violation and explore the reasons for occurrence and strategies for prevention and (2) on completion of the courses, instructors submit required course materials that are used for consideration of relicensure decisions. These rehabilitation courses, designed to return the nurse to competence, are developed based on nursing standards and required competencies identified in the state's nursing practice act.

Nursing Competencies

The graduate nurse must possess the competence to practice independently, a declaration that must be demonstrated and supported by documentation (Texas Board of Nurse Examiners, 2004). A **nursing competency** is the skill and behavior required to perform the role of a nurse.

Carlson, Kotze, and van Rooyen (2003, p. 30) have noted "the clinical learning environment creates many opportunities for student learning and the development of critical competencies in the

Box 6-6

Texas Nursing Practice Act: Grounds for Disciplinary Action (301 Tex. Occ. Code 452, 2005) Sec. 301.452. Grounds for Disciplinary Action

(a) In this section, "intemperate use" includes practicing nursing or being on duty or on call while under the influence of alcohol or drugs.

(b) A person is subject to denial of a license or to disciplinary action under this subchapter for:

(1) a violation of this chapter, a rule or regulation not inconsistent with this chapter, or an order issued under this chapter;

(2) fraud or deceit in procuring or attempting to procure a license to practice professional nursing or vocational nursing;

(3) a conviction for, or placement on deferred adjudication community supervision or deferred disposition for, a felony or for a misdemeanor involving moral turpitude;

(4) conduct that results in the revocation of probation imposed because of conviction for a felony or for a misdemeanor involving moral turpitude;

(5) use of a nursing license, diploma, or permit, or the transcript of such a document, that has been fraudulently purchased, issued, counterfeited, or materially altered;

(6) impersonating or acting as a proxy for another person in the licensing examination required under Section 301.253 or 301.255;

(7) directly or indirectly aiding or abetting an unlicensed person in connection with the unauthorized practice of nursing.

nursing profession." They conducted a study that "revealed that the students experience uncertainty due to the lack of opportunities to develop competence in providing nursing care." Four factors these researchers identified as contributing to the students' ability to develop essential nursing competencies included (1) availability and accessibility of competent staff; (2) sufficient equipment to fulfill nursing duties and meet the needs of patients; (3) consensus in the expectations of nursing school and clinical nursing personnel in hospitals on the patient standard of care; and (4) awareness among faculty of the needs and problems of first-year nursing students in the clinical health-care environment in meeting standards of care. Unfortunately, students often find that the very nature of the clinical learning experience may interfere with their ability to develop nursing competencies, as the guidance and support by nursing personnel in the clinical learning environment are often inadequate due to the current critical nursing shortage.

The development, measurement, and documentation of essential nursing competencies will be discussed through exploration of (1) essential nursing competencies, (2) measurement of competencies in clinical practice, (3) competencies critical to nursing management, (4) competencies critical to advanced nursing practice, and (5) competencies in nursing informatics.

ESSENTIAL NURSING COMPETENCIES

Nursing competencies to be developed, documented, and validated in the student's clinical setting include (1) the core competency of caring, (2) competencies essential to patient care, and (3) competencies in specialty practice.

The Core Competency of Caring

Care is a competency often elusive of measurement and/or validation. But caring in professional nursing has been described as the essence of nursing (Sadler 2003). Woodward (2003, p. 215) postulated: "Human caring, while instinctive, can also be taught, learned, and measured through the nursing education system … suggest[ing] people enter nursing because they value interpersonal relationships, altruism, and a desire to help others."

This "caring ethic" can be built upon. Woodward (2003) believes that nursing students can be professionally trained to develop the competency of caring through the concepts of modeling and role modeling. Modeling is "the process used by the nurse to develop an image and understanding of the client's world—an image and understanding developed within the client's framework and from the client's perspective." This simply means to "walk a mile" in the patient's shoes. "Role modeling" was defined as utilizing "the facilitation and nurturance of the individual in attaining, maintaining and/or promoting health through purposeful interventions" (Woodward, 2003, p. 215; citing Erickson, Tomlin, & Swain, 1983, p. 95).

But Sadler (2003) measured the self-reported competency of caring in baccalaureate nursing students, using the Coates Caring Efficacy Scale (CES)

(2003). Sadler found that "final semester seniors identified their families as making the greatest contribution to their development of caring; only a few reported the influence of the nursing curriculum" (Sadler, 2003, p. 295). Regardless of its origin, the competency of caring appears to be the basis and framework for the development of other essential nursing competencies.

Competencies Essential to Patient Care

Part of the challenge of preparing new graduates for practice is ensuring skill in providing a broad continuum of patient care. Utley-Smith (2004, pp. 166–170) identified six categories of competencies for new baccalaureate graduates in today's health-care environment:

1. Health Promotion Competency: involves interventions initiated by the nurse to promote and improve health in individuals, families, and communities. The focus of the intervention "is on assisting clients to maximize their health potential and enhance their well-being." Therefore, client assessment and intervention are equally important parts of this competency.
2. Supervision Competency: involves the graduate nurse's ability to coordinate the implementation of a nursing care plan, by ancillary or subordinate members of the health-care team who are responsible for carrying out specific aspects of the health plan.
3. Interpersonal Communication Competency: "encompasses relationship skills that enable the nurse to work effectively on a team … such as communication, negotiating, problem-solving, and collaboration."
4. Direct Care Competency: encompasses the psychomotor skills necessary to deliver patient care including, for example, medication administration, wound care, and injections. Essentially, these competencies are those skills that "require the nurse to use hands or body to manipulate equipment and the client."
5. Computer Competency: "refers to the ability of the nurse to use electronic and technological equipment to access, retrieve, and store information that assists in the delivery of effective nursing care."

6. Caseload Management Competency: concerns the nurse's ability to coordinate care for a specific number of clients. This may involve direct care as well as time and resource management over a particular period.

These findings identify and encompass critical outcome competencies that define the standards of care for the graduate nurse in both the classroom and clinical settings (Utley-Smith, 2004). Graduate nurse will also have the opportunity to develop specialty competencies within their traditional coursework.

Competencies in Specialty Practice

RN-to-BSN specialty courses often move from a traditional model to a competency-based model, according to Foss, Janken, Langford, and Patton (2004). For example, within a psychiatric nursing program, a student may be assigned to work with a probate court as the court's visitor, assessing the ward's psychiatric status and need for continuing guardianship. Specialty competencies as a court visitor are then used to measure the student's course learning outcomes, such as the student's ability to determine if the psychiatric ward meets the standard of care for the psychiatric patient. Faculty can then document not only student learning outcomes but also mastery of competencies within this specialty area of practice.

MEASUREMENT OF COMPETENCIES IN CLINICAL PRACTICE

Staff development professionals and continuing education instructors have always been concerned with maintaining continued competency of the clinical practitioner in nursing practice. Waddell (2001) reported that the issue of competence reached new levels of significance because of proposals made by the Pew Commission Taskforce on Health Care Workforce Regulation and the National Council of State Boards of Nursing.

Waddell (2001, p. 2) believed that these two powerful organizations have forced the nursing profession to re-examine the question, "How do we promote and assure continued competence?" Waddell believed competence should be assessed via (1) mandatory continuing education, (2) peer

---

Box 6-7

Pew Commission Taskforce on Health Care Workforce Regulation: Ten Recommendations for Reform (Gragnola & Stone, 1997)

1. "States should use standardized and understandable language for health professions regulation and its functions to clearly describe them for consumers, provider organizations, businesses, and the professions."
2. "States should standardize entry-to-practice requirements and limit them to competence assessments for health professions to facilitate the physical and professional mobility of the health professions."
3. "States should base practice acts on demonstrated initial and continuing competence. This process must allow and expect different professions to share overlapping scopes of practice. States should explore pathways to allow all professionals to provide services to the full extent of their current knowledge, training, experience and skills."
4. "States should redesign health professional boards and their functions to reflect the interdisciplinary and public accountability demands of the changing health care delivery system."
5. "Boards should educate consumers to assist them in obtaining the information necessary to make decisions about practitioners and to improve the board's public accountability."
6. "Boards should cooperate with other public and private organizations in collecting data on regulated health professions to support effective workforce planning."
7. "States should require each board to develop, implement and evaluate continuing competency requirements to assure the continuing competence of regulated health care professionals."
8. "States should maintain a fair, cost-effective and uniform disciplinary process to exclude incompetent practitioners to protect and promote the public's health."
9. "States should develop evaluation tools that assess the objectives, successes and shortcomings of their regulatory systems ad bodies to best protect and promote the public's health."
10. "States should understand the links, overlaps and conficts between their health care workforce regulatory systems and other systems which affect the education, regulation and practice of health care practitioners and work to develop partnerships to streamline regulatory structures and processes."

review, and (3) practice or process audits used to assess continued competence. But Waddell suggested that the actual measurement involved in the assessment and verification of nursing competence should be established by (1) utilization of appropriate measurement scales; (2) selection of accurate measurement instruments, i.e., a reliable, validated competency scale; and (3) interpretation of the measurement data by nurses qualified in informatics.

Nursing competence may be measured and validated by utilizing a variety of mechanisms to document compliance, including the (1) videotaping, (2) preceptors' record of competency-based orientation, (3) development of a portfolio of competence in clinical practice, (4) nurse's self-assessment of competence, and (5) utilization of the hospital intranet.

Videotaping to Assess and Document Competencies and Course Outcomes

The challenge in nursing education, according to Winters et al. (2003, p. 472), is how to develop a mechanism for "effectively teaching competencies and allowing students to safely practice essential nursing skills." They suggested videotaping, as this medium "offers a safe way ... to practice skills and develop confidence prior to actual performance ... [it] is a teaching-learning strategy used to help...develop effective communication, physical assessment, and selected psychomotor skills ... [and] also provides ... a mechanism for detailed instructor feedback to improve performance." For example, the graduate nurse or registered nurse, both required to attend annual cardiopulmonary resuscitation training exercises, may provide videotaped documentation of either attainment or updating of this competence.

The Preceptors' Record of Competency-Based Orientation

According to Harper (2002, p. 198, quoting Alspach, 1995): "Competency-based orientation is [a program that is] learner focused ... based on the attainment of core [nursing] competencies ... that are necessary for new employees to function in their [health care] role at the completion of the orientation period."

Harper (2002) conducted a research study designed to describe preceptors' perceptions of a competency-based orientation. The results of a 26-item questionnaire indicated that the majority of preceptors agreed on the following components as necessary to meet standards for a basic nursing orientation: (1) attainment of core competencies that are role- and unit-specific, (2) sufficient time for attainment and completion of core competencies, and (3) a preceptor to ensure that competencies are in fact attained and validated, e.g., via an orientation checklist.

Development of Portfolios of Competence in Clinical Practice

A **portfolio** is a set of documents that "captures learning from experience, enables an assessor to measure student learning, acts as a tool for reflective thinking, illustrates critical analytical skills and evidence of self-directed learning and provides a collection of detailed evidence of a person's competence" (Scholes, et al., 2004, p. 595).

The purpose of a portfolio is to document and verify achievement of the clinical competencies required to meet the standard of patient care in the area of practice to which the nurse is assigned. They concluded (p. 595): "To achieve maximum benefit from the portfolio as a learning tool to link theory and practice, there needs to be a clear fit between the model of portfolio and the professional practice that is to be assessed."

When designing a portfolio, nurses, faculty, and/or nursing students must match learning outcomes and/or competencies to their practice, reconstructing those clinical experiences into the format required for portfolio documentation, such as a skills checklist. Through this process, nursing faculty and students undergo a process of deconstructing learning outcomes/competencies, then fitting this information into their unique practice. Competencies are then reconstructed to fit the structure of the portfolio.

According to the University of Michigan School of Nursing (2005), when comparing a résumé with a portfolio: "A career portfolio ... is a much more in-depth document, and supplements—not replaces—your résumé ... a key feature is the inclusion of artifacts ... [or] tangible objects that demonstrate your work ... [such as] care plans, brochures, outlines of training sessions, manuals, spreadsheets, memos, etc., that you created by yourself or as part of a group effort."

These portfolios can be in many formats, including paper or electronic, Web pages, PDF documents, and even PowerPoint. Included within the portfolio may also be documents addressing the nurse's good faith self-assessment of competency.

A Nurse's Self-Assessment of Competence

Self-assessment tools can also be utilized to document and measure competence in clinical practice. Meretoja, Isoaho, and Leino-Kilpi (2004, p. 124) reported that "self-assessment assists nurses to maintain and improve their practice by identifying their strengths and areas that may need to be further developed ... encourag[ing] them to take an active part in the learning process of continuing education."

Meretoja, Eriksson, and Leino-Kilpi (2002, p. 95) collected descriptive data addressing competent nursing practice in a variety of settings. The data came from staff nurses, head nurses, and nursing directors in an acute 1000-bed university hospital. The descriptive data obtained were then analyzed to identify a set of clinical indicators for generic competencies that could be applied to all clinical practice environments.

The Nurse Competence Scale, an instrument utilized to measure the level of nurse competence, was then designed and developed by Meretoja et al. (2004). The 73 competencies were categorized into the following seven roles and functions: (1) helping role, (2) teaching-coaching role, (3) diagnostic functions, (4) managing situations, (5) therapeutic interventions, (6) ensuring quality, and (7) work role.

Categories of the scale were derived from Benner's *From Novice to Expert* competency framework. The results revealed that the higher the frequency of using competencies, the higher the nurse's self-assessed level of competence. Age and length of work experience had a weak positive correlation with level of competence (Meretoja et al., 2004). See Box 6-8.

The nurses' self-evaluation of competence in their own job performance may be conceptualized as an indicator of the standards for the quality of nursing care. Tzeng (2004) clustered nursing competencies into the following three general groups: (1) basic-level patient care skills, (2) intermediate-level patient care and fundamental management skills, and (3) advanced-level patient care and supervision skills. The results of the study revealed "that nurses' self-assessment of intermediate

---

Box 6-8

Nurse Competence Scale: Helping Role

1. Planning patient care according to individual needs.
2. Supporting patient's coping strategies.
3. Critically evaluating own philosophy in nursing.
4. Modifying the care plan according to individual needs.
5. Utilizing nursing research findings in relationships with patients.
6. Developing the treatment culture of own unit.
7. Decision making by ethical values.

Adapted from Meretoja et al., 2002.

---

patient care skills, the difference between nurses' self-assessment and job demands for basic patient care skills, and nurses' overall satisfaction with their own nursing competencies were three significant predictors of overall satisfaction with nurses' own job performance. Nurses' self-assessment on basic patient care skills and advanced patient care skills contributed to nurses' levels of overall satisfaction with their own nursing competencies. These results suggest a relationship between competency and performance" (Tzeng, 2004, p. 487).

Based on these findings, academic nursing courses and on-the-job training programs may be amended to place emphasis on these competencies required to provide high-quality patient care (Tzeng, 2004). Further, self-assessments demonstrate to nursing regulatory bodies good faith in the nurse's efforts to either achieve or maintain competencies essential to meet the standard of practice.

Utilization of the Hospital Intranet to Validate and Document Compliance With State Competency Standards

Currently, regulatory agencies require hospitals to provide evidence that employees are in compliance with state-mandated competencies. Wolford and Hughes (2001, pp. 188–189) identified "Intranet-delivered computer-based training as an effective and efficient method of providing and documenting training to meet regulatory requirements."

For example, regulatory agencies require competency in adapting nursing care standards to the developmental needs of patients. Although Welton, Nieves-Khouw, Schreiber, and McElreath (2000) suggested that training programs on age-specific care competencies vary widely in format, content, and method, these authors developed computer-based training (CBT) programs on age-specific care competencies, using traditional self-paced learning modules. The authors converted printed modules to CBT and pilot-tested experiences of using CBT with clinical staff, ultimately implementing an organization-wide CBT deployment for age-specific care competency and other mandatory training.

COMPETENCIES CRITICAL TO NURSING MANAGEMENT

Nursing management has its own set of unique competence functions. Connelly, Yoder, and Miner-Williams (2003) categorized a total of 54 charge nurse competencies within the following four categories: (1) clinical/technical competencies, (2) critical thinking competencies, (3) organizational competencies, and (4) human relations skills. These researchers believe that these competencies define the standard for leadership and management skills required to function as effective, front-line charge nurses. See Box 6-9.

Kleinman (2003) noted, "nurse managers are often less well prepared to manage the business activities than the clinical activities." The nurse managers and nurse executives who were subjects of this research identified staffing and scheduling, management, and human resources as the three most important competencies for nurse managers.

Box 6-9

Categories of Generalist Versus Specialist Nursing Competencies

1. Decision-making competencies
2. Developing practice competencies
3. Health education competencies
4. Interpersonal competencies
5. Knowledge "how to" competencies
6. Knowledge "about" competencies
7. Organizing competencies
8. Practice/intervention competencies
9. Professional responsibilities competencies
10. Personal qualities competencies
11. Teaching competencies
12. Values competencies

Adapted from Gibson et al., 2003

Based on the results of Kleinman's research (p. 451), and in an effort to develop and validate knowledge of the regulations and standards of practice for a nurse manager that encompass not only the organizational but also the clinical/technical competencies, the subjects of this research suggested: "Strategies nurse executives may employ to develop nurse manager business knowledge include traditional undergraduate and graduate degree programs, online programs, certificate programs, continuing education, in-service education offerings, seminars, and mentoring activities."

COMPETENCIES CRITICAL TO ADVANCED NURSING PRACTICE

The level and type of competence and education required in advanced nursing practice depend on the area of specialty practice and vary from state to state. The following section discusses (1) generalist versus specialist nursing competencies and (2) competencies required in critical care.

Generalist Versus Specialist Nursing Competencies

A generalist nurse is one who has a duty to comply with the standards of nursing practice as identified in the nursing practice act of the state of licensure. A specialist nurse has a duty to comply with the state's standards of nursing practice and a duty to comply with the standards of practice as identified in the specialty area, e.g., psychiatric nursing.

This distinction between the standards of practice for generalist versus specialist nursing requires analysis of the "characteristics of knowledge, skills, abilities, values and qualities displayed in the context of professional work for both groups of nurses" (Gibson, Fletcher, & Casey, 2003, p. 591). These authors conducted a research study to determine if there was a difference between the basic competencies of a generalist versus those of a specialist nurse. They ordered 198 competencies into 26 subcategories that were then classified into 12 categories. See Box 6-10.

In conclusion, the researchers noted: "There is a significant common element in these two areas of nursing practice, and generalist preparation in ... nursing is the foundation of specialist ... nursing practice. Generalist knowledge and skills are

Box 6-10

Charge Nurse Competencies: Clinical/Technical Competencies

Responsibilities directly related to patient care or some technical aspect of working on a clinical unit:

1. Calculate patient acuities and enter them in the computer (or ensure these are done).
2. Complete administrative duties (examples: complete 24-hour report, pre-op charts, up-date census/assignment board).
3. Assist staff in completing their work.
4. Act as a clinical resource, sharing knowledge.
5. Use computer skills to chart and complete reports.
6. Delegate workload appropriately and fairly.
7. Check emergency equipment, handle unit emergencies.
8. Conduct initial unit-wide patient assessments.
9. Use knowledge of medical equipment to provide care.
10. Use knowledge of available clinical resources when needed.
11. Use knowledge of unit, type of patients, procedures, etc., to plan work.
12. Maintain a safe, clean physical unit environment.
13. Provide direct patient care as needed, balancing patient care with charge nurse duties.
14. Provide for patient safety.

Adapted from Connelly, et al., 2003.

expanded in specialist practice and there is also evidence of specialist practice that is beyond the scope of general nursing practice" (Gibson et al., 2003, p. 591).

Competencies Required in Critical Care

Nationally accepted critical care competencies have not been formulated. Therefore, critical care programs in each educational institution tend to redefine the essential competencies necessary to meet the standards of practice in the area of critical care, resulting in variations in accepted practice from state by state basis and within practice.

But core critical care competencies can be identified on a national basis. Jones (2002) conducted a research study designed to elicit core critical care competency statements from a sample of nurses working in London, England, in critical care. According to Jones, a core critical care competency framework can be developed by expert nurses draw-

ing on their own experience and knowledge of critical care nursing. The author suggested that this process would be useful to (1) educationalists designing competency-based curricula, (2) critical care managers as a tool for recruitment and retention and for education and training of staff, and (3) individual critical care nurses to facilitate continuous professional development.

Competencies Required in Nursing Informatics

Informatics is the "application of computer and statistical techniques to the management of information" (University of New Castle upon Tyne, 2004). The standards on which nursing informatics competencies are based are still evolving. Some of the essential nursing informatics competencies will be categorized according to their relevancy to (1) national nursing education strategies designed to develop nursing informatics competencies, (2) nurses at four levels of practice, (3) risk assessment, and (4) computerization of records

National Education Strategies Designed to Develop Nursing Informatics Competencies

Herbert (2000) proposed that advances in the sophistication of information and communication technologies offer the nurse practitioner opportunities for (1) better information management, (2) more complete documentation of work, and (3) knowledge development to support evidence-based nursing practice. Herbert suggested a shift in emphasis from specialists in nursing informatics (NI) to NI being integrated into all domains of nursing clinical practice, pointing to the need for nursing informatics education strategies on a national level.

According to Herbert (2000), steps in developing a plan to implement an education program on informatics competencies and standards must include (1) recognizing the role and history of the NI specialists, (2) defining NI and the required NI competencies, and (3) adapting the educational infrastructure required to support this initiative. A national committee, the National Nursing Informatics Project, was working on a plan to address these competencies in nursing informatics (Herbert, 2000). This project ultimately demonstrated, however, that informatics does not seem to be as successful in providing evidence-based research for establishing standards and competencies for practice as individual nursing researchers, such as Staggers, Gassert, and Curran (2002).

Informatics Competencies for Nurses at Four Levels of Practice

Bickford (2002) noted that, although nurses have always dealt with data, information, and knowledge, the standard for nursing now requires core competencies not only in computer skills but also in data and information management. Informatics competencies differ according to the nurse's level of skill.

Staggers, Gassert, and Curran (2002, p. 383) conducted a research study designed "to produce a research-based master list of informatics competencies for nurses and differentiate these competencies by level of nursing practice." The four levels of practice were identified as the beginning nurse, the experienced nurse, the informatics specialist, and the informatics innovator. Based on a comprehensive literature review and item consolidation, an expert panel of informatics nurse specialists defined initial competencies for the beginning informatics nurse. See Box 6-11 for a master list of valid computer competencies for the Level 1 Beginning Nurse.

The results of the research of Staggers, et al. (2002) indicated that: (1) computer skills are only one set of competencies within the larger category of informatics standards, and (2) programming skills or competencies of the third-level informatics specialist nurse are generally not a necessary standard for the first-level beginning and/or second-level experienced nurse.

Thus, Staggers, et al. (2002) agreed with Herbert's (2000) conclusion that general, not specialized, informatics should be the standard for integration into all areas of clinical nursing practice.

Informatics Utilized in Regulating Safety Standards

Nursing informatics may be utilized to design or redesign computerized risk assessment programs that monitor whether patient safety standards have been met. Browne, Covington, and Davila (2004) reported that such computerized tools provide (1) an accurate assessment of the safety risk to each patient; (2) indicators that are embedded into routine assessment documentation, eliminating added charting time and ensuring safety; (3) tailored interventions for specific patient safety risks; (4) an integration of fall-risk information into the care

---

Box 6-11

Level 1 Beginning Nurse: Master List of Valid Computer Competencies

Computer Skills—Administration: applications for structured patient data entry
Computer Skills—Communication (e-mail, Internet, telecommunications)
Informatics Knowledge—Data access: for patient care
Informatics Knowledge—Documentation of patient care
Computer Skills—Education of patient, instruction of staff
Computer Skills—Monitoring patient systems
Computer Skills—Basic desktop software: uses word processing
Computer Skills—Systems: use of peripheral devices, e.g., CD-ROM; knows basic components of the current computer system
Computer Skills—Data to improve nursing practice
Computer Skills—Impact: requires time, persistent effort, and skill for computers to become an effective tool
Computer Skills—Privacy/security: describes patients' rights as they pertain to computerized information management

Adapted from Staggers, et al., 2002

---

plan, report sheets, and care conferences; and (5) an interdisciplinary communication network regarding the standards of care for safety.

Informatics Utilized in Establishing the Standard of Care

A descriptive study, designed by Scott and Elstein (2004) using the Nursing Home Quality Initiative, found that the standard of nursing care may be achieved, regulated, and maintained through nursing informatics by (1) utilizing quality measurement methods and tools in monitoring patient care, (2) utilizing quality data to ensure desired patient care outcomes, (3) monitoring organizational and cultural factors affecting utilization of quality data in the clinical setting, (4) utilizing informatics systems to gather and implement quality data, and (5) documenting and measuring impact evaluation and research outcomes. The findings of this study may be generalized to establish the standard of care, ensuring quality nursing care. Thus, the nursing standard becomes regulated through evidence-based research.

Box 6-12

Level 3 Nursing Informatics Specialist: Master List of Valid Computer Competencies

Computer Skills-Basic Desktop Software: develops/writes spreadsheets used for complex problems

Computer Skills-Project Management

Computer Skills-Quality Improvement: determines data indicators, quality and effectiveness of nursing informatics practice

Computer Skills-Systems: integrate different applications or programs

Informatics Knowledge-Data: demonstrates fluency in informatics and nursing terminologies

Informatics Knowledge-Education: plans and develops application/system training programs for users, clients

Informatics Knowledge-Impact: interprets current legislation, research, and economics affecting computerized information management in health scope of user passwords, devises strategies to protect the confidentiality of computerized information

Informatics Knowledge-Regulations: incorporates relevant law and regulations into informatics practice

Informatics Knowledge-Systems: applies theories that influence computerization in health care; evaluates applications/systems available in health care

Informatics Knowledge-Usability: applies human factors and ergonomics to the design of the computer screen, location and design of devices, and design of software

Informatics Skills-Analysis: applies principles and techniques of systems analysis; interprets information flow within the organization

Informatics Skills-Data/Data Structures: constructs data structures and maintains data sets; integrates nursing taxonomies, unified nomenclatures and other data needed by nurses within database design

Informatics Skills-Design, Development: develops screen layouts, report formats, and custom views of clinical data by working directly with clinical departments and

individual users; coordinates the development of integrated computer-based patient record technologies; maintains database (e.g., adding, deleting fields, structuring input for others, relational database)

Informatics Skills-Evaluation: existing technologies for cost-effectiveness; evaluates hardware, software, and vendor support

Informatics Skills-Fiscal Management: uses strategies to optimize application use after implementation (benefits realization)

Informatics Skills-Implementation: devises strategies for installing applications/systems

Informatics Skills-Management: determines project scope, objectives, and resources for each proposed application, system or enhancement; functions as a project manager

Informatics Skills-Privacy/Security: develops policies related to privacy, confidentiality, and security of patient and client data

Informatics Skills-Programming: applies principles of computer programming to communicate with software developers

Informatics Skills-Requirements: modifies information technologies to meet changing data requirements/needs

Informatics Skills-Role: consults about informatics with clinical, managerial, educational, and/or research entities

Informatics Skills-Systems Maintenance: assists in the resolution of basic software problems

Informatics Skills-System Selection: designs evaluation criteria and strategies for selecting applications and systems

Informatics Skills-Testing: conducts tests of information management applications, systems.

Informatics Skills-Training: produces short-term and long-term training plans, materials, and operating manuals tailored to the organization.

Adapted from Staggers, et al., 2002

Evidence-Based Practice: The Standard of Care

Evidence-based nursing practice is an expected part of the nursing standard of care. Evidence-based nursing practice utilizes the best current clinical evidence or research when implementing the nursing process. Evidence-based practice is the basis upon which nursing standards are developed. Thus, evidence-based nursing practice is a clinical

decision-making process that is integrated into the nursing process. This scientific, step-by-step process combines (1) the best available research evidence, (2) the nurses' clinical expertise, and (3) the patient's preferences for patient care.

Nurses integrate evidence-based nursing into the nursing process by doing the following:

1. Identifying the patient's care need by assessment, based on analysis using current nursing knowledge, expertise, and clinical practice.

2. Researching the literature for best evidence relevant to meeting the patient care need.
3. Evaluating the research, or best evidence, for interventions specific to the patient care need.
4. Choosing the best intervention designed to meet the patient care need, justifying the selection based on valid, reliable research (University of Minnesota, 2004).

Evidence-based practice challenges nurses to develop patient care interventions and expand the relevant knowledge, based on the best research. But van Meijel, Gamel, van Swieten-Duijfjes, and Grypdonck (2004) reported limited literature on the development of evidence-based nursing interventions. They presented a model for developing evidence-based nursing interventions, designed to guide the process of developing and testing complex nursing interventions while incorporating the experience of the client.

The model consisted of four stages: (1) problem definition, (2) accumulation of building blocks for intervention design, (3) intervention design, and (4) intervention validation.

The model allowed for the accumulation of empirical evidence and theory development during the formulation of the evidence-based intervention. The authors suggested (p. 84) that the "use of the model could facilitate effective communication among nurses, researchers and educators when discussing the development and testing of nursing interventions."

Plouffe and Seniuk (2004) promoted evidence-based clinical practice as the goal of professional nursing. Unfortunately, they reported (p. 14) that "linking research to the clinical realm appears logical and sounds simplistic, yet frequently our preconceived thoughts and ideas of ease of change do not equate with the reality of the situation." Although relevant research may exist, and the patient care need may be there, the question remains of "how shall the two meet?"

For example, a study was designed by Olade (2004), whose purpose was: (1) to identify the extent to which rural nurses utilize evidence-based practice guidelines from scientific research in their practice, (2) to describe previous and current research utilization activities, and (3) to identify the specific barriers they face in their practice settings. The results of the study revealed that only 20.8% of the participants, nurses with bachelor's degrees, were involved in research utilization. The two most common areas of research were pain management and pressure ulcer prevention and management. Barriers to research identified by Olade included rural isolation and lack of nursing research consultants.

But Winch, Creedy, and Chaboyer (2002, p. 56) commented that evidence-based nursing practice either will or does direct nursing practice, arguing: "It is possible to identify the governance of nursing practice and hence nurses across two distinct axes; that of the political (governance through political and economic means) and the personal (governance of the self through the cultivation of the practices required by nurses to put evidence into practice.) ... Evidence-based nursing is an emerging technology of government that judges nursing research and knowledge and has the capacity to direct nursing practice at both the political and personal level."

EVIDENCE-BASED PRACTICE THROUGH NURSING RESEARCH: THE ROAD TO BEST PRACTICE

Best practice is the process through which competence and evidence-based practice lead to the desired health-care outcome. Nursing research is the mechanism to provide evidence-based practice. Thus, for desired patient outcomes and to ensure cost-efficient and effective best practice, application of nursing research findings is essential to the establishment and regulation of the standard of nursing practice.

Many variables affect regulations and standards that are the subject and/or outcome of nursing research. Olsen (2003) identified Health Insurance Portability and Accountability Act (HIPAA) privacy regulations, which became effective April 14, 2003, as having had the most significant current impact on nursing research. The privacy requirements of the regulations have affected nursing research in (1) the research process, (2) accessing data (including recruitment and using medical records), (3) creating data (including intervention studies, survey, and interview research), and (4) disclosing data to others, such as nursing colleagues at other health-care institutions.

Hodge, Kochie, Larsen, and Santiago (2003) identified a "research-practice gap," a situation in which research findings that should become best nursing practice are not implemented. In an attempt to diminish the research-practice gap via evidence-based nursing practice, the authors studied ways to implement best practice. A patient care research utilization committee was formed to review and revise each patient care policy and procedure, based on best research evidence. The impetus for the project was a belief that current patient care policies and procedures were (1) based on tradition rather than on science and (2) did not provide best practice in patient care, missing skills required for new equipment, treatments, and research findings. The beneficial outcomes of this research project included (1) a revision of patient care policies and procedures, based on scientific evidence; (2) generation of new research questions, based on gaps in the nursing literature; and (3) an increase in the number of clinical nurses involved in using research to provide best practice.

Staff education is another important component of best practice. A research utilization project was designed by Cruz, Abdul-Hamid, and Heater (1997) for the purpose of (1) selecting and implementing a research-based restraint education program, (2) reducing the use of restraints in an acute care setting, and (3) changing the perception about restraints in the direction of decreased importance. The existing restraint policy and procedure and new restraint products and alternative restraint methods were reviewed by a multidisciplinary team. Based on the evidence provided by a review of the literature on restraint education programs, the multidisciplinary team concluded that education was the key component in promoting best practice. Education programs could be monitored by risk management and quality assurance to ensure best practice in accordance with nursing regulations.

Accreditation as Nursing Regulation

Accreditation is a voluntary process of compliance with a set of standards established by a nongovernmental organization (University of New Castle upon Tyne, 2004). Accreditation is the process utilized by an organization, such as a school of nursing or health-care facility, to verify a competent educational or health-care program, respectively. For example, the state's governing board for nursing typically provides accreditation for schools of nurs-

ing, providing validation that the educational program is in compliance with the state's standards of instruction for teaching qualified students how to provide standardized nursing care. Private accrediting agencies like the Joint Commission on Accreditation of Healthcare Organizations **(JCAHO)** monitor compliance with state and federal standards, but utilization of these private accrediting agencies is voluntary, not mandatory.

JOINT COMMISSION ON ACCREDITATION OF HEALTHCARE ORGANIZATIONS (JCAHO)

Established over 50 years ago, JCAHO is an independent, not-for-profit accreditation organization. Governed by a board that includes physicians, nurses, and consumers, JCAHO sets the standards by which quality of health care provided in hospitals is measured in the United States and around the world (JCAHO, 2004).

Hospitals and ambulatory surgery centers may voluntarily choose to apply for accreditation through JCAHO or other such organizations. According to Saufl and Fieldus (2003), before accrediting a hospital, JCAHO requires compliance with its standards regarding the environment of care, provision of care, and quality of care. Quality of care is ensured by JCAHO conducting regular surveys of each agency's performance. The value of the accreditation, according to the authors (p. 152), is that this process "… certifies to the health care community and the community-at-large that the facilities meet nationally accepted standards through a recognized accreditation program."

JCAHO is committed to improving and regulating safety in patient care by providing (1) standards of patient care, (2) survey evaluations on the healthcare provider's status in meeting standards of care, and (3) professional consultative and educational services on mechanisms for meeting the standard of patient care (Saufl & Fieldus, 2003). To meet JCAHO standards, nursing standards and operating strategies of health-care organizations must be in a continual state of readiness, including performance improvement practices. Gantz, Sorenson, and Howard (2003) believe that nurses have a unique role in identifying and guiding the nursing process, central to quality care, and the commitment to establishing and maintaining quality care, as identified by JCAHO. They believe that the paradigm of health care must be shifted from just meeting the standards to continual readiness and performance improvement throughout the organization.

COMPLIANCE WITH POLICIES AND PROCEDURES

A **policy** is a stated system by which health care is administered. A **procedure** is a step-by-step process by which a health-care outcome is achieved.

The American Nurses Association (ANA) plays a significant role in the development of model policies and procedures on both the state and national levels. Standards of care also affect the development of policies and procedures regulating nursing practice. Policies and procedures must meet or exceed minimum standards of care as set by nurse practice acts and other sources.

For example, the ANA provides a foundation for policies and procedures related to patient safety by (1) developing and disseminating policies and procedures to meet the standard for patient safety, (2) lobbying for legislation and regulations that protect and serve users of nursing services, and (3) advocating for patients and issues that affect a nurse's ability to meet the standards for safe care.

Policies and procedures are designed to regulate, standardize, and drive nursing practice (Zeitz & McCutcheon 2002). Evidence-based nursing practice is essential in developing policies and procedures. Zeitz and McCutcheon (2003) reported that although evidence-based nursing is the mechanism for achieving best practice in the clinical setting, in reality it has had very little impact on the clinical practice that nurses deliver on a daily basis. For example, the authors noted that although the collection of vital signs is a ubiquitous component of practice in the postoperative general surgical setting, there is little evidence, in the form of evidence-based policies and procedures, to support this practice.

Further, they indicated that nursing policies and textbooks, in general, present traditional, routine-regulated clinical practice without an evidence base. Traditional policies and procedures are being used to (1) control rather than support evidence-based practice and (2) limit opportunities for clinicians to make patient-specific decisions. They suggested that evidence-based practice, and ultimately best practice, may be achieved through creation of policies and procedures based on (1) rigorous relevant

evidence that supports standardized nursing interventions, (2) the nurse's clinical expertise, and (3) the changing and expanding environment in which nurses develop and practice. One of the most important environmental factors affecting nursing practice is the level of staffing.

Compliance With Staffing Requirements

Regulation of staffing affects productivity, the delivery of patient care, and thus the standard of nursing care. Bednar, Haight and Street (2003, p. 47) reported that: "… state-mandated staffing ratios, coupled with restrictive nurse practice acts, may be impacting the delivery of care to … patients." They found that patient-to-staff ratios vary state by state.

Mark, Harless, McCue, and Xu (2004) conducted a study designed to evaluate previous research findings exploring the relationship between nurse staffing and quality of care. In evaluating this relationship, they examined the effects of change in registered nurse staffing on change in quality of patient care from 1990 to 1995 They found (p. 279) that "improving registered nurse (RN) staffing unconditionally improves quality of care." Levels of registered nurse staffing must also comply with state and federal legislative and administrative regulations.

Legislative and Administrative Regulation of Nursing

Nursing practice is regulated through state and federal legislative and administrative laws and agencies. The state and federal legislatures develop and pass laws. Federal administrative agencies, such as the Veterans Administration, oversee compliance with regulations by their agencies. Some examples of federal administrative regulatory agencies include the Centers for Medicare and Medicaid Services (CMS), the Occupational Safety and Health Administration (OSHA), and the Centers for Disease Control and Prevention (CDC). State administrative agencies, such as state boards of nursing, create regulations to accompany, detail, and implement state laws.

CENTERS FOR MEDICARE AND MEDICAID SERVICES (CMS)

The CMS administers the Medicare program and collaborate with states to administer Medicaid, the

State Children's Insurance Health Care Program, and HIPAA. CMS is specifically responsible for simplification of standards for implementation of and HIPAA and maintenance of quality standards for health care through its surveys and certification functions (CMS, 2004).

HEALTH INFORMATION PORTABILITY AND ACCOUNTABILITY ACT (HIPAA)

CMS oversees implementation of HIPAA standards and regulations. Title I of HIPAA is designed to protect health insurance coverage for workers and their families when they change or lose their jobs. Title II of HIPAA, The Administrative Simplification provisions, "requires strict security measures to protect the electronic health data of patients" (Follansbee, 2002, p. 42). Consequently, nursing policies and procedures associated with the management of health-care information have changed dramatically (Follansbee, 2002).

Requirements under HIPAA require nursing service to comply with privacy standards by (1) developing appropriate policies and procedures, (2) providing notice of privacy practices and other forms, (3) implementing measures to secure privacy, (4) contracting with business associates to secure privacy, and (5) training all nursing staff involved in patient care (Lucas, Adams, & Wachs, 2004). According to these authors (pp. 178–179): "HIPAA's privacy regulations are considered 'the floor' or minimum standard for the protection of PHI [protected health information]. As such, it is likely that these privacy regulations will become the 'industry standard' to which all health care professionals will be held."

Research in Long-Term Care: Issues, Dilemmas, and Challenges

Scott and Elstein (2004) reported that as the American population ages, already sizable long-term care expenditures are likely to increase. The CMS, as the largest purchaser of health care for the aging population, is continuously working to improve the standard of long-term patient care through (1) quality monitoring and enforcing of patient care standards, (2) providing information to beneficiaries about the standard of patient care, and (3) enhancing resources to improve standardized patient care.

Medicare and Medicaid also establish program requirements in long-term care facilities. For example, according to regulations created by CMS (CMS, 2003, September), long-term care facilities may, in specific circumstances, utilize paid feeding assistants to supplement the services of certified nurse aides. The training and certification of the feeding assistants must have occurred under standardized guidelines, established by CMS.

OCCUPATIONAL SAFETY AND HEALTH ADMINISTRATION

The Occupational Safety and Health Administration (OSHA, 2004) is a federal agency whose mission is designed to: "assure the safety and health of America's workers by setting and enforcing standards; providing training, outreach, and education; establishing partnerships; and encouraging continual improvement in workplace safety and health."

OSHA provides a foundation for understanding workplace health and safety by producing publications, pamphlets, audiovisual programs, computer access programs, and other documents designed to promote compliance with safety standards (Nester, 1996). OSHA works to build partnerships between occupational safety and health-care administration, according to Nester (1996). For example, the Office of Occupational Health Nursing within OSHA is an active advocate for health-care workers, such as nurses, assisting with the establishment of standards that protect and provide for the safety of patients and all health-care providers.

The OSHA Pathogens Standard

In 1991 the OSHA standard designed to protect health-care providers from exposure to blood and other potentially infectious materials became mandatory. According to Goldstein and Johnson (1991), health-care employers were required to institute an infection control plan based upon this OSHA standard, which included universal precautions, engineering and work practice controls, personal protective equipment, and housekeeping. Occupational health nurses (1) coordinated the development, maintenance, and revision of this infection control program, in compliance with the OSHA regulations, (2) educated management about the hazards of blood-borne pathogens, and (3) provided assistance to ensure compliance with the

OSHA standard, resulting in a safe and healthy work environment for the health-care provider.

Nursing plays an active role in OSHA's functions. Nurses are not only regulated/protected by OSHA standards but also play an important role in their implementation to meet standards for patient safety.

CENTERS FOR DISEASE CONTROL (CDC)

The Centers for Disease Control and Prevention (CDC, 2004) is the leading federal agency for protecting the patient's health and safety both at home and abroad. The CDC is responsible for (1) developing and applying disease prevention and control, (2) maintaining environmental health, and (3) promoting health and education activities designed to improve the well-being of the people of the United States. But research has demonstrated that more nursing expertise is needed in the area of disease control, as this environmental concern is a "front line" patient care safety issue in nursing practice.

Disease Control: A Safety Issue in Nursing Practice

According to Larson and Butterfield (2002), clients often use nurses as their primary contact for expressing concerns about health problems related to environmental disease control. In response to this need, core competencies for nursing expertise in the field of environmental disease control were developed by the Institute of Medicine, Agency for Toxic Substances and Disease Registry, and National Institute of Nursing Research. These core disease control competencies comprise a baseline of knowledge and awareness as well as a standard by which nurses intervene to prevent and minimize environmental disease. Nursing standards for disease control focused on the following four competencies:

1. Basic knowledge and disease control concepts: "Understanding scientific principles [of] ... basic mechanisms of exposure...prevention and control strategies ... applied research, and the interdisciplinary nature of environmental health."
2. Assessment and referral: "Completing a comprehensive environmental exposure history and making appropriate referrals ... locating

and providing appropriate scientific information for individual patients and communities."
3. Advocacy, ethics, and risk communication: "Understanding the role of advocacy, principles of environmental justice, and risk communication in addressing environmental health issues."
4. Legislation and regulation: "Understanding ... environmental health policy as well as state and national regulations" (Larson & Butterfield, 2002, pp. 301–308; quoting Pope, Snyder, & Mood, 1995).

Establishing Safety Protocols Based Upon CDC and OSHA Recommendations

In 1987 OSHA was petitioned by the ANA and labor unions to issue an emergency infection control standard, subsequent to the first documented reports of occupationally acquired human immunodeficiency virus (HIV) in health-care providers (Miramontes, 1990). OSHA responded by enforcing voluntary guidelines developed by the CDC 4 years earlier. Subsequently, OSHA drafted regulations containing the final set of HIV safety protocols in1991.

According to Miramontes (1990), OSHA established HIV safety standards and protocols to be utilized by all health-care providers, addressing (1) types of protective clothing and equipment, (2) housekeeping and laundry areas, (3) infectious waste disposal, and (4) tracking employees, pre- and postexposure. In enforcing these standards, hospitals stress continued education and training in order to increase compliance. Miramontes (pp. 561–562) cited a research study that found "after a two-year training/evaluation period, physician compliance with infection control procedures increased from 20% to 80%, and nurse compliance rose from 50% to 86%."

All Good Things...

Nursing practice is regulated on the state and federal levels. On the state level, nursing is regulated via the state's nursing practice act, which provides for licensure as a registered nurse. Subsequently, certification acknowledges nursing competence at an advanced level of practice.

The nursing practice act establishes the standard of care and scope of practice, which are monitored by the state's governing board, usually the board of nursing examiners. The nursing practice act also regulates advanced practice; for example, the clinical nurse specialist. The scope of nursing practice has been expanded by telenursing, requiring the development of the Nurse Licensure Compact (NLC). The NLC creates standardization within nurse practice acts that vary and lack uniformity from state to state, providing more standard methods of compliance, discipline, and rehabilitation.

Nursing has been developed upon the core competence of caring, a concept difficult to measure, document, or legislate. Other essential competencies, which appear to be measurable behaviors, include health promotion, supervision, interpersonal communication, direct care, computer, and case load competencies. Competencies may be documented with videotaping, orientation records, portfolios, self-assessment tools, records of mandatory intranet training courses, and continuing education records. Advanced areas of nursing practice have more specialized sets of competencies.

Specific competencies are required in nursing informatics at four levels, consisting of the beginning, experienced, informatics specialist, and informatics innovator nurse. Informatics may be integrated into the nursing standards.

Evidence-based nursing practice is the expected standard of care. Nursing research is the mechanism to provide evidence-based practice. The nurse may integrate evidence-based practice into the nursing process, for example, by following a four-step clinical decision-making process. Policies and procedures also establish the standard of care and thus regulate nursing practice.

Independent organizations, such as JCAHO, monitor a health-care provider's compliance with state and federal laws and regulations. Accreditation is the process utilized by an organization, such as a school of nursing or health-care facility, to verify competency of its educational or health-care program, respectively. Staffing and productivity must also be regulated under these accreditation guidelines to meet the standard of care.

Legislative and administrative regulation of nursing occurs on the federal level; for example, through CMS. CMS oversees the administration of HIPAA, a federal law that regulates confidentiality issues related to patient care. OSHA is a federal agency that promotes standards for patient safety in the health-care environment. The CDC is the federal agency that develops and promotes disease prevention and control.

Let's Talk

1. What is the nursing standard for advanced practice, management, and informatics?

2. Do you believe that nurses should seek certification? If so, why?

3. In what areas can a nurse specialize that are considered advanced practice?

4. How has telenursing expanded nurse practice acts?

5. Does an interstate compact have to exist for a nurse to practice telenursing in those states?

6. How does lack of uniformity in state nurse practice acts affect interstate compacts and telenursing?

7. What can influence student nurse learning of competencies in the clinical area?

NCLEX Questions

1. A nursing competency:
   A. Is a skill that the nurse has to perform.
   B. Is a specific behavior that a nurse must demonstrate.
   C. A and B.
   D. Is the proficiency level that the nurse must obtain.

2. A standard of care:
   A. Requires use of the nursing process.
   B. Is the degree of care, expertise, and judgment exercised by nurses under similar circumstances.
   C. A and B.
   D. Is the number of patients that a competent nurse can care for on any given shift.

3. What affects nursing regulation?
   A. A state nurse practice act.
   B. Accreditation by an official body.
   C. Policies and procedures.
   D. All of the above.

4. The goal of state and federal legislation is to:
   A. Protect the public.
   B. Regulate nursing education.

   C. Oversee nurse competency via licensure and discipline.
   D. All of the above.

5. A nurse practice act:
   A. Governs the role of the nurse.
   B. Governs nursing education.
   C. A and B.
   D. Prescribes the competencies for the nursing role.

6. Certification is:
   A. An examination.
   B. Developed by a professional organization.
   C. Aids a nurse in demonstrating competency.
   D. All of the above.

7. What types of disciplinary action can a board of nursing take?
   A. License suspension.
   B. Licensure denial.
   C. Mandate that the offender take courses in legal ethical decision making or pharmacology.
   D. All of the above.

8. An advanced practice nurse:
   A. Is a registered nurse.
   B. Has studied in a post-basic or advanced educational program of study.
   C. Acts independently of other health-care professionals in the delivery of health-care services.
   D. All of the above.

9. Portfolios:
   A. Can be used to demonstrate to state boards of nursing that one is qualified to be a registered nurse.
   B. Can be designed to demonstrate one's competence.
   C. Consist of documentation that captures learning from experience.
   D. B and C.

10. Modeling:
    A. Is the facilitation and nurturance of an individual.
    B. Assists one in attaining, maintaining, and promoting health.
    C. Is a purposeful nursing intervention.
    D. Is a process used by nurses to develop an understanding of the client's world.

REFERENCES

Alspach, J. (1995). *The educational process in nursing staff development.* St.Louis: Mosby.

American Nurses Association. (2001 June). *Code of ethics for nurses.* Retrieved December 14, 2004, from http://www.nursingworld.org/ethics/chcode.htm

Bednar, B., Haight, D., & Street, J. (2003). State-mandated staffing ratios within ESRD: Benefits and costs. *Nephrology News Issues, 17*(5):47, 51–55, 56.

Bickford, C.J. (2002). Informatics competencies for nurse managers and their staffs. *Seminar in Nurse Management, 10*(2): 110–113.

Browne, J.A., Covington, B.G., & Davila, Y. (2004). Using information technology to assist in redesign of a fall prevention program. *Journal of Nursing Care Quality, 19*(3): 218–225.

Carlson, S., Kotze, W.J., & van Rooyen, D. (2003). Accompaniment needs of first year nursing students in the clinical learning environment. *Curationis, 26*(2):30–39.

Centers for Disease Control and Prevention. (2004). *About the CDC.* Retrieved November 22, 2004, from http:// www.governmentguide.com/govsite.adp?bread=*Main& url=http%3A//www.governmentguide.com/ams/clickThruRedirect.adp%3F55076483%2C16920155%2Chttp%3A//www.cdc.gov/

Centers for Medicare and Medicaid Services. (2004).*Facts about the Center for Medicare and Medicaid Services.* Retrieved November 22, 2004, from http://www.cms.hhs.gov/researchers/projects/APR/2003/facts.pdf

Centers for Medicare and Medicaid Services, HHS. (2003 August). Medicare and Medicaid programs: Changes to the hospital inpatient prospective payment systems and fiscal year 2004 rates. Final rule. *Federal Register, 68*(148): 45345–4672.

Centers for Medicare & Medicaid Services, HHS. (2003 September). Medicare and Medicaid programs: Requirements for paid feeding assistants in long term care facilities. Final rule. *Federal Register, 68*(187): 55528–55539.

Centers for Medicare and Medicaid Services. (2004). *The Health Insurance Portability and Accountability Act of 1996.* Retrieved November 22, 2004, from http://www.cms.hhs.gov/hipaa/

Connelly, L.M., Yoder, L.H., & Miner-Williams, D. (2003). A qualitative study of charge nurse competencies. *Medical Surgical Nursing, 12*(5):298–306.

Cruz, V., Abdul-Hamid, M., & Heater, B. (1997). Research-based practice: Reducing restraints in an acute care setting Phase I. *Journal of Gerontological Nursing, 23*(2): 31–40.

Erickson, H., Tomlin, E., & Swain, M.A. (1983). *Modeling and role modeling: A theory and paradigm for nursing.* Englewood Cliffs, NJ: Prentice Hall.

Fenton, M.V., & Thomas, K.A. (1998) Advanced practice nursing in Texas: The interface of accreditation, regulation, and certification. *Advanced Practice Nursing Quarterly, 4*(3): 78–85.

Fernandez, R.D., & Herbert, G.J. (2004). New modalities of treatment and care require the development of new structures and systems to access care. *Nursing Administration Quarterly, 28*(2):129–132.

Flook, D.M. (2003). The professional nurse and regulation. *Journal of Perianesthetic Nursing, 18*(3):160–167.

Follansbee, N.M. (2002). Implications of the Health Information Portability and Accountability Act. *Journal of Nursing Administration, 32*(1):42–47.

Foss, G.F., Janken, J.K., Langford, D.R., & Patton, M.M. (2004). Using professional specialty competencies to guide course development. *Journal of Nursing Education, 43*(8):368–375.

Gantz, N.R., Sorenson, L., & Howard, R.L. (2003). A collaborative perspective on nursing leadership in quality improvement: The foundation for outcomes management and patient/staff safety in health care environments. *Nursing Administration Quarterly, 27*(4):324–329.

Gibson, F., Fletcher, M., & Casey, A. (2003). Classifying general and specialist children's nursing competencies. *Journal of Advanced Nursing, 44*(6):591–602.

Goldstein, L., & Johnson, S. (1991). OSHA blood-borne pathogens standard: Implications for the occupational health nurse. *American Association of Hospital Nursing Journal, 39*(4):182–188.

Gragnola, C.M., & Stone, E.S. (1997). *Responses from the field to the Pew Health Professions Commission's December 1995 report: Reforming health care workforce regulation: Policy considerations for the 21st Century.* UCSF Center for the Health Professions. Retrieved January 1, 2006, from http://www.futurehealth.ucsf.edu/pdf_files/futwkreg.pdf

Gunn, I.P. (1999). Regulation of health care professionals, Part 2: Validation of continued competence. *Certified Registered Nurse Anesthetist, 10*(3):135–141.

Hardin, S., & Langford, D. (2001). Telehealth's impact on nursing and the development of the interstate compact. *Journal of Professional Nursing, 17*(5):243–247.

Harper, J.P. (2002). Preceptors' perceptions of a competency based orientation. *Journal of Nurses Staff Development, 18*(4):198–202.

Heitkemper, M.M., & Bond, E.F. (2004). Clinical nurse specialists: State of the profession and challenges ahead. *Clinical Nurse Specialist, 18*(3):135–140.

Herbert, M. (2000). A national education strategy to develop nursing informatics competencies. *Canadian Journal of Nursing Leadership, 13*(2):11–14.

Hodge. M., Kochie. L.D., Larsen. L., & Santiago. M. (2003). Clinician-implemented research utilization in critical care. *American Journal of Critical Care, 12*(4):361–366.

Hutcherson, C.M. (2001). Legal considerations for nurses practicing in a telehealth setting. *Online Journal of Issues in Nursing, 6*(3):4.

Joint Commission on Hospital Accreditation. (2004). *What is the Joint Commission on Hospital Accreditation.* Retrieved on November 22, 2004, from http://www.jcaho.org/general+public/who+jc/index.htm

Jones, M. (2002). Critical care competencies. *Nursing Critical Care, 7*(3):111–120.

Kleinman, C.S. (2003). Leadership roles, competencies, and education: How prepared are our nurse managers? *Journal of Nursing Administration, 33*(9):451–455.

Larson L.S., & Butterfield P. (2002). Mapping the future of environmental health and nursing: Strategies for integrating national competencies into nursing practice. *Public Health Nursing, 19*(4):301–308.

Lavin, M.A., Meyer, G., & Carlson J.H. (1999). A review of the use of nursing diagnosis in U.S. nurse practice acts. *Nursing Diagnosis, 10*(2):57–64.

Lewallen, L.P., & McMullan, K.G. (2001). Returning to competence after discipline. *JONAS Health Law Ethics Regulations, 3*(3):88–91.

Lucas, B., Adams, S., & Wachs, J.E. (2004). Roadmap to HIPAA: Keeping occupational health nurses on track. *American Association of Hospital Nursing Journal, 52*(4):169–179.

Mark, B.A., Harless, D.W., McCue, M., & Xu, Y. (2004). A longitudinal examination of hospital registered nurse staffing and quality of care. *Health Service Research, 39*(2):279–300.

Marrs J.A., & Alley, N.M. (2004). Moral turpitude: A benchmark toward eligibility for registered nurse licensure? *JONAS Health Law Ethics Regulations, 6*(2):54–59.

Meretoja, R., Eriksson, E., & Leino-Kilpi, H. (2002). Indicators for competent nursing practice. *Journal of Nursing Management, 10*(2):95–102.

Meretoja, R., Isoaho, H., & Leino-Kilpi, H. (2004). Nurse competence scale: Development and psychometric testing. *Journal of Advanced Nursing, 47*(2):124–133.

Miramontes, H. (1990). Progress in establishing safety protocols based on CDC and OSHA recommendations. *Infection Control in Hospital Epidemiology, 11*(10 Supp):561–562.

National Council of State Boards of Nursing. *Nurse Licensure Compact: Nurse licensure compact implementation.* Retrieved December 26, 2005, from http://www.ncsbn.org/nlc/rnlpvncompact_mutual_recognition_state.asp

Nester, R.M. (1996). Occupational Safety & Health Administration: Building partnerships. *American Association of Hospital Nursing Journal, 44*(10):493–499.

Occupational Safety and Health Administration. (2004). *OSHA's mission.* Retrieved November 22, 2004, from http://www.osha.gov/oshinfo/mission.html

Olade, R,A. (2004). Evidence-based practice and research utilization activities among rural nurses. *Journal of Nursing Scholarship, 36*(3):220–225.

Olsen, D.P. (2003). HIPAA privacy regulations and nursing research. *Nursing Research, 52*(5):344–348.

Plouffe, J., & Seniuk, C. (2004). Walking the walk: Living evidence-based practice. *Dynamics, 15*(1):14–17.

Ponto, J., Sabo, J., Fitzgerald, M.A., & Wilson, D.E. (2002). Operationalizing advanced practice registered nurse legislation: Perspectives from a clinical nurse specialist task force. *Clinical Nurse Specialist, 16*(5):263–269.

Pope, A.M., Snyder, M.A., & Mood, L.H. (Eds.). (1995). *Nursing, health and the environment: Strengthening the relationship to improve the public's health.* Washington, DC: National Academy Press.

Roemer, R. (1977). The nurse practitioner in family planning services: Law and practice. *JOICFP Review, 6*(3):28–34.

Sadler, J. (2003). A pilot study to measure the caring efficacy of baccalaureate nursing students. *Nursing Education Perspective, 24*(6):295–299.

Saufl, N.M., & Fieldus, M.H. (2003). Accreditation: A "voluntary" regulatory requirement. *Journal of Perianesthia Nursing, 18*(3):152–159.

Scholes, J., et al. (2004). Making portfolios work in practice. *Journal of Advanced Nursing, 46*(6):595–603.

Scott, J.C., & Elstein, P. (2004). Research in long-term care: Issues, dilemmas, and challenges from the public purchaser's perspective. *Medical Care, 42*(4 Supp):11–18.

Staggers, N., Gassert, C.A., & Curran, C. (2002). A Delphi study to determine informatics competencies for nurses at four levels of practice. *Nursing Research, 51*(6):383–390.

Texas Board of Nurse Examiners. (2001). *Advanced practice nurse.* 22 Texas Administrative Code 221.1(3). Retrived December 31, 2005, from http://info.sos.state.tx.us/pls/pub/readtacext.TacPage?sl=R&app=9&p_dir=&p_rloc=&p_tloc=&p_ploc=&pg=1&p_tac=&ti=22&pt=11&ch=221&rl=1

Texas Board of Nurse Examiners. (2001). *Approval for prescriptive authority.* 22 Texas Administrative Code 222.2. Retrieved January 2, 2006, from http://info.sos.state.tx.us/pls/pub/readtacext.TacPage?sl=R&app=9&p_dir=&p_rloc=&p_tloc=&p_ploc=&pg=1&p_tac=&ti=22&pt=11&ch=222&rl=2

Texas Board of Nurse Examiners. (2001). *Core standards for advanced practice.* 22 Texas Administrative Code 221.13. Retrieved December 31, 2005, from http://info.sos.state.tx.us/pls/pub/readtacext.TacPage?sl=R&app=9&p_dir=&p_rloc=&p_tloc=&p_ploc=&pg=1&p_tac=&ti=22&pt=11&ch=221&rl=13

Texas Board of Nurse Examiners. (2001). *Minimum requirements for carrying out or signing prescriptions.* 22 Texas Administrative Code 222.4. Retrieved January 2, 2006, from http://info.sos.state.tx.us/pls/pub/readtacext.TacPage?sl=R&app=9&p_dir=&p_rloc=&p_tloc=&p_ploc=&pg=1&p_tac=&ti=22&pt=11&ch=222&rl=4

Texas Board of Nurse Examiners. (2001). *Protocols or other written authorizations.* 22 Texas Administrative Code 221.1(12). Retrieved December 31, 2005, from http://info.sos.state.tx.us/pls/pub/readtacext.TacPage?sl=R&app=9&p_dir=&p_rloc=&p_tloc=&p_ploc=&pg=1&p_tac=&ti=22&pt=11&ch=221&rl=1

Texas Board of Nurse Examiners. (2001). *Scope of Practice.* 22 Texas Administrative Code 221.12. Retrieved December 31, 2005, from http://info.sos.state.tx.us/pls/pub/ readtacext.TacPage?sl=R&app=9&p_dir=&p_rloc=&p_tloc=&p_ploc=&pg=1&p_tac=&ti=22&pt=11&ch=221&rl=12

Texas Board of Nurse Examiners. (2004). *Standards of Nursing Practice.* 22 Texas Administrative Code 217, Part 11. Retrieved December 26, 2005, from http://info.sos.state.tx. us/pls/pub/readtac ext.TacPage?sl=R&app=9&p_dir=&p_rloc=&p_tloc=&p_ploc=&pg=1&p_tac=&ti=22&pt=11&ch=217&rl=11

Texas Board of Nurse Examiners. (2004). *Temporary Authorization to Practice.* 22 Texas Administrative Code 217, Part 3(a)(1). Retricved December 27, 2005, from http://www.bne.state.tx.us/grads.htm

Texas Nursing Practice Act. (2005). *Grounds for disciplinary action.* 301 Texas Occupational Code 452. Retrieved December 26, 2005, from http://www.bne.state.tx.us/npa1.htm#452

Thalman, J.J., & Ford, R.M. (2004). Labor and productivity measures. *Respiratory Care Clinics of North America, 10*(2):211–221.

Tzeng, H.M. (2004). Nurses' self-assessment of their nursing competencies, job demands and job performance in the Taiwan hospital system. *International Journal of Nursing Studies, 41*(5):487–496.

University of Michigan.(2005). *Resume vs. portfolio.* Retrieved December 29, 2005, from http://www.nursing. umich.edu/ studentresources/resumes/resumeVsPfolio.html

University of New Castle upon Tyne. (2004). *Online medical dictionary.* Online at http://cancerweb.ncl.ac.uk/cgibin/ omd?action=Home&query=

Utley-Smith, Q. (2004). Competencies needed by new baccalaureate graduates. *Nursing Education Perspectives, 25*(4): 166–170.

van Meijel, B., Gamel, C., van Swieten-Duijfjes, B., & Grypdonck, M.H. (2004). The development of evidence-based nursing interventions: Methodological considerations. *Journal of Advanced Nursing, 48*(1):84–92.

Waddell, D.L. (2001). Measurement issues in promoting continued competence. *Journal of Continuing Education Nursing, 32*(3):102–106; 138–139.

Welton, R., Nieves-Khouw, F., Schreiber, D.A., & McElreath, M.P. (2000). Developing computer-based training for age related competencies. *Journal Nurses Staff Development, 16*(5):195–201.

Winch, S., Creedy, D., & Chaboyer, W. (2002). Governing nursing conduct: The rise of evidence-based practice. *Nursing Inquiry, 9*:156–161.

Winters, J., et al. (2003). Use of videotaping to assess competencies and course outcomes. *Journal of Nursing Education, 42*(10):472–476.

Wolford, R.A., & Hughes, L.K. (2001). Using the hospital Intranet to meet competency standards for nurses. *Journal of Nurses Staff Development, 17*(4):182–189.

Woodward, W. (2003). Preparing a new workforce. *Nursing Administration Quarterly, 27*(3):215–222.

Zeitz, K., & McCutcheon H. (2003). Evidence-based practice: To be or not to be, this is the question! *International Journal of Nursing Practice, 9*(5):272–279.

Zeitz, K., & McCutcheon, H. (2002). Policies that drive the nursing practice of postoperative observations. *International Journal of Nursing Studies, 39*(8):831–839.

BIBLIOGRAPHY

Aroskar, M.A., Moldow, D.G., & Good, C.M. (2004). Nurses' voices: Policy, practice and ethics. *Nursing Ethics, 11*(3): 266–76.

Bell, D., Bowen, T., & Dilling, D. (1991). Computerizing records for continuing education. *Journal of Nursing Staff Development, 7*(1):36–39.

Bergren, M.D. (2004). HIPAA-FERPA revisited. *Journal of Scholastic Nursing, 20*(2):107–112.

Drenkard, K.N. (2004). The clinical nurse leader: A response from practice. *Journal of Professional Nursing, 20*(2):89–96.

Editorial. (2000). Recognizing nursing's independent license: Prescriptive authority for APNs. *Michigan Nurse, 73*(3): 11–12.

Laine, G.A, et al. (1994). Hospital-wide medication policies and standards. *American Journal of Hospital* Pharmacy, *51*(23): 2949–2951.

Lewis, M.A., & Tamparo, C.D. (2002). *Medical law, ethics and bioethics for ambulatory care* (5th ed.). Philadelphia: FA Davis.

Lorimer, K. (2004). Continuity through best practice: Design and implementation of a nurse-led community leg-ulcer service. *Canadian Journal of Nursing Research, 36*(2):105–112.

Lyon, B.L., & Minarik, P.A. (2001). Statutory and regulatory issues for clinical nurse specialist (CNS) practice: Ensuring the public's access to CNS services. *Clinical Nurse Specialist, 5*(3):108–114.

MacEachern, L. (2003). Providers issue brief: Scope of practice and prescriptive authority: Year-end report 2003. *Issue Brief Health Policy Track Service,* 1–29.

Menenberg, S.R. (1995). Standards of care in documentation of psychiatric nursing care. *Clinical Nurse Specialist, 9*(3)· 140–142, 148.

Meretoja, R., & Leino-Kilpi, H. (2003). Comparison of competence assessments made by nurse managers and practicing nurses. *Journal of Nursing Management, 11*(6):404–409.

Merriam Webster. (2004). Medical dictionary. Online at http://www2.merriam-webster.com.

Mikos, C.A. (2004). Inside the nurse practice act. *Nursing Management, 35*(9):20–22, 91.

Oermann, M.H. (2002). Developing a professional portfolio in nursing. *Orthopedic Nursing, 21*(2):73–78.

O'Keefe, M. (Ed.) (2001). *Nursing practice and the law: Avoiding malpractice and other legal risks.* Philadelphia: F.A. Davis.

Rowell, P.A. (2003). The Professional Nursing Association's role in patient safety. *Online Journal of Issues in Nursing, 8*(3):3.

Sattler, B. (1996). Occupational and environmental health: From the back roads to the highways. *American Association of Hospital Nursing Journal, 44*(5):233–237.

Schwab, N.C., & Pohlman, K.J. (2004). Records—the Achilles' heel of school nursing: Answers to bothersome questions. *Journal of School Nursing, 4*:236–241

Slimmer, L., & Andersen, B. (2004). Designing a data and safety monitoring plan. *Western Journal of Nursing Research, 26*(7):797–803.

Tanner, A., Pierce, S., & Pravikoff, D. (2004). Readiness for evidence-based practice: Information literacy needs of nurses in the United States. *Medinformatics 2004,* 936–940.

University of Minnesota.(2004). *Evidence-based health care project: Evidence-based nursing.* Retrieved October 23, 2004, from http://evidence.ahc.umn.edu/ebn.htm

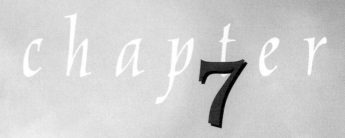

Economic Influences

MICHELLE B. HAGADORN, MA, CPA
NANCY HOWELL AGEE, RN, MN

CHAPTER MOTIVES

- Describe economic changes in the health-care industry and the resulting challenges to managers.
- Discuss who pays for health-care services and the unique complexities of payment methods to health care organizations.
- Explore the challenges of balancing supply and demand for health-care services and understand what factors managers can influence.
- Review the two primary forms of business organizations and focus on their different goals and objectives.
- Discuss the current forms of health-care rationing.

*L*eadership is a challenging job as described by De Pree above. Leaders are asked to be stewards for their organizations' assets, which range from financial resources and human resources to the overall reputation of the organization. Leaders keep the organization continually moving forward by looking for ways to improve while managing the delicate balance between the goals of the customer and those of the organization. This chapter describes why health economics is important to managers within the health-care industry and some of the unique challenges facing those managers. Health economics has received increased focus in recent years due to the increase in technological innovations, the greater availability of data, and the surge in health-care spending. The need for managers to be effective stewards has never been greater.

Current Status of Health Care in the United States

In order to understand the current turmoil in the U.S. health-care system, a brief review of several dramatic changes that have occurred over the last 40 years is warranted. The emphasis of medical care shifted from diagnosis of the illness to intervention and, now, has shifted to prevention of the illness. New technologies have revolutionized the ways in which health care is practiced. A few examples of these innovations include organ transplants, radiation and chemotherapy treatment plans for cancer, in vitro fertilization, and vast enhancements in drug treatments. The role of health insurance coverage has risen dramatically from less than 10% of the U.S. population in 1940 to more than 84% today (Weisbrod, 1991). In addition, in 1935 when Social Security was enacted as a benefit for older citizens, only 5% of the population lived past the age of 65 years. Social Security did not anticipate life expectancy increases and the resulting need for longer-term use (Cypher, 2003). Finally, health-care expenditures continue to grow in proportion to the gross domestic product, making up 15.3% of total spending in the U.S. economy in 2003, or $1.7 trillion annually, up from 5.3% in the 1960s. Health-care spending is outpacing growth in the overall economy by 3 percentage points (Highlights—National Health Expenditures, 2003). See Figure 7-1.

Why is there so much focus on the increase in health-care spending? One reason is that the United States spends more on health care per person than any other major industrialized country but fares worse on key health indicators such as life expectancy and infant mortality rates. (Anderson, 1997). In addition, the continuing growth in health-care spending leaves a smaller proportion of national income for other purposes, such as education or defense. This has prompted the federal government and employers to question whether the benefits of this increased spending are warranted, which has spurred the current discussions of how to reform the health-care system. Central to the reform debate is how much to pay for health care. In order to understand the issues fully, an overview of the current payment systems is necessary.

OVERVIEW OF HEALTH-CARE PAYMENT SYSTEMS

Who pays for medical care? In most industries, the process of obtaining payment for services or products is fairly straightforward. A customer will purchase a product or service and be presented with a bill that represents the quantity of goods or services received, multiplied by an appropriate price. Discounts may encourage sales of slow-moving inventory; however, the basic method is a fixed price per unit set by the business. But health care does not follow this simple process. In the United States, there is a complex structure in place for obtaining payment for health-care services, due to various contractual relationships with third parties (Cleverley & Cameron, 2003). As seen in Figure 7-2, 83% of all payments come from third parties. Nevertheless, it is important that managers remember that the consumer is the ultimate payer for health-care services. Although most consumer payments are indirect in the form of insurance premiums or taxes, increases in health-care costs will force consumers to spend less on other goods and services and more on items like insurance benefits. Reactions to increases in health-care costs can vary, such as consumers dropping their health insurance coverage, employers reducing the health insurance benefits offered to employees, or insurance companies reducing payments for services. Even insured consumers are required to make some direct payments for health-care services, often referred to as

National Health Expenditures									
		Total			Private Funds			Public Funds		
Calendar Year	GDP in billions	Amount in billions	Per Capita	Percent of GDP	Amount in billions	Per Capita	Percent of Total	Amount in billions	Per Capita	Percent of Total
1965	$720	$41.0	$205	5.7	$30.6	$154	75.1	$10.2	$51	24.9
1966	759	45.1	324	5.7	31.6	156	69.9	13.5	67	30.1
1967	834	50.7	249	6.1	31.8	156	62.8	18.9	93	37.2
1970	1,040	73.1	348	7.0	45.4	216	62.2	27.5	131	37.8
1975	1,635	129.6	590	7.9	74.8	340	57.6	55.0	250	42.4
1980	2,795	245.8	1,067	8.8	140.9	512	57.3	104.8	455	42.7
1981	3,131	255.1	1,225	9.1	153.9	704	57.5	121.2	521	42.5
1982	3,259	321.0	1,366	9.8	186.7	794	55.2	134.3	571	41.8
1000	3,535	353.5	1,489	10.0	206.1	868	55.3	147.5	621	41.7
1984	3,933	390.1	1,628	9.9	229.3	957	55.6	160.6	671	41.2
1985	4,213	425.8	1,765	10.1	252.2	1,043	59.1	174.6	722	40.9
1986	4,453	457.2	1,672	10.3	256.9	1,093	55.4	190.4	760	41.6
1987	4,742	496.0	2,020	10.5	259.3	1,174	55.1	208.8	847	41.9
1988	5,106	558.1	2,243	10.9	331.7	1,333	59.4	225.4	910	40.5
1989	5,449	622.7	2,477	11.3	370.9	1,476	59.6	251.8	1,002	40.4
1990	5,803	696.0	2,738	12.0	413.5	1,627	59.4	262.5	1,111	40.6
1991	5,956	761.8	2,966	12.7	441.3	1,718	57.9	320.6	1,248	42.1
1992	6,319	827.0	3,184	13.1	458.5	1,503	56.6	358.5	1,380	43.4
1993	6,642	888.1	3,381	13.4	497.7	1,895	55.0	390.4	1,486	44.0
1994	7,054	937.2	3,534	13.3	509.8	1,922	54.4	427.3	1,611	45.6
1995	7,400	990.1	3,967	13.4	532.5	1,968	53.8	457.7	1,709	46.2
1996	7,813	1,039.4	3,647	13.3	557.5	2,063	53.6	481.9	1,784	46.4
1997	8,318	1092.7	4,007	13.1	589.2	2,160	53.9	503.5	1,845	46.1
1998	8,781	1,150.0	4,178	13.1	626.4	2,283	54.6	521.6	1,895	45.4
1999	9,274	1,219.7	4,392	13.2	659.7	2,411	54.9	550.0	1,960	45.1
2000	9,825	1,310.0	4,672	13.3	718.7	2,563	54.9	591.3	2,109	45.1
2001	10,082	1,425.5	5,035	14.1	777.9	2,749	54.6	646.7	2,265	45.4

NOTES: These data reflect Bureau of Economic Analysis Gross Domestic Product as of October 2001. Per capita is calculated using Census resident based population estimates.
November 2003

FIGURE 7-1 National health-care trends in public versus private funding in selected years. (Source: U.S. Bureau of the Census, U.S. Department of Commerce, Bureau of Economic Analysis)

out-of-pocket payments, co-pays, or deductibles. Some out-of-pocket payments are for services that are not covered by the policy or for services in excess of the policy's coverage limits.

Most health-care organizations have a master price list referred to as the **charge description master** (CDM). The CDM has the specific charges for a defined unit of service, such as an x-ray, specific laboratory test, or 1 hour of surgery time. The unique aspect of pricing in the health-care industry is that often the payment for a specific unit of service in no way relates to the charge that actually appears on the patient's bill from the CDM. This

dilemma is discussed in more detail in the review of reimbursement methods.

Uninsured Consumers

Currently, about 16% of the population (45 million people) does not have health insurance (Centers for Medicare and Medicaid Services, 2005). These consumers must pay for their health-care needs from their own resources. Customers without insurance are expected to pay the total billed charges, based on the health-care organization's price list, while insured customers receive dis

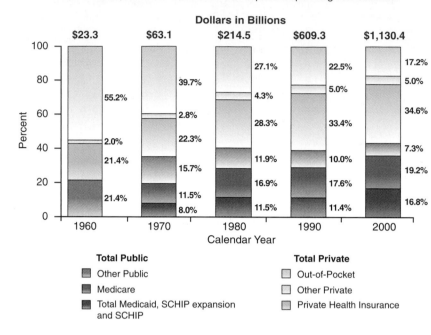

Personal Health Care Expenditures by Source of Funds: Selected Years 1960–2000

Over the last several decades, the public sector share of health spending has increased, while the share from out-of-pocket spending has declined.

Dollars in Billions

FIGURE 7-2 Personal health-care expenditures by source of funds. (Source: CMS Office of Actuary, National Health Statistics Group)

counts for services based on contracts their insurance companies have negotiated with the providers. When personal resources are not adequate, often the uninsured consumer must rely on charity care or do without the service. The rising share of the population without medical insurance is seen as a major problem in the United States and one of the key issues driving the need for health-care reform. See Figure 7-3.

Reimbursement Models

Health-care managers need to understand the basic payment methods for customers with insurance. There are two main categories of payment methods: fee-for-service and capitation.

Fee for Service

In **fee-for-service payment methods**, reimbursement increases based on the number of services provided. There are three primary methods of reimbursement: cost-based reimbursement, charge-based reimbursement, and the prospective payment system

Cost-based reimbursement is not frequently encountered in practice today; Medicare reimbursed

health-care providers in this manner from 1966 to 1983. Under cost-based reimbursement, the payer agrees to reimburse the provider for the costs incurred in providing services to the insured populations. The payment is limited to allowable costs, which is defined as costs directly related to the provision of health-care services (Gapenski, 2003). For example, if the hospital's cost to care for a patient delivering a baby included 2 days in the hospital at a nursing cost of $480 per day, medical supplies of $200, drugs of $125, and equipment use of $250, the hospital would be reimbursed the sum of all these costs, $1,535.

Charge-based reimbursement was common in the early days of health insurance, when payers reimbursed providers on the basis of billed charges. The current trend is away from paying on billed charges; however, some payers now reimburse based on a discount of billed charges ranging 20 % to 40 % (Gapenski, 2003). For example, if the patient bill for the same 2-day maternity stay included charges that totaled $3,500, the hospital would be paid some percentage of this amount under charge-based reimbursement.

In the **prospective payment system** (PPS) a predetermined rate is paid for services. Reimburse-

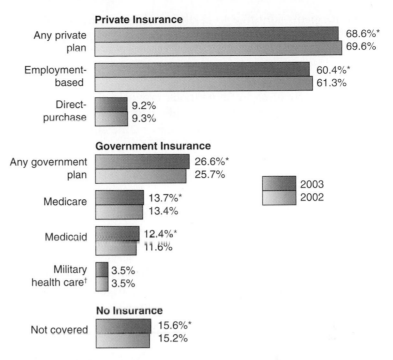

FIGURE 7-3 Coverage by type of health insurance: 2002 and 2003. (Source: U.S. Census Bureau, Current Population Survey 2003 and 2004, annual social and economic supplements)

* Statistically different at the 90-percent confidence level.

† Military health care includes: CHAMPUS (Comprehensive Health and Medical Plan for Uniformed Services)/Tricare and CHAMPVA (Civilian Health and Medical Program of the Department of Veterans Affairs), as well as care provided by the Department of Veterans Affairs and the military.

Note. The estimates by type of coverage are not mutually exclusive; people can be covered by more than one type of health insurance during the year.

ment of services is based on a per-unit payment, such as diagnosis, procedure, day, or episode. Several common PPS examples follow:

1. Per-procedure reimbursement, which is commonly used in outpatient settings.
2. Per-diagnosis reimbursement, in which diagnoses that require a higher resource utilization have higher reimbursement rates. "Medicare pioneered this basis of payment in its diagnosis related group system, which was first used for hospital reimbursement in 1983" (Gapenski, 2003). For further discussion, see the Medicare section below.
3. Per-day reimbursement, in which the healthcare provider is paid a fixed amount for each day that service is provided, regardless of the nature of the services.
4. Global pricing, which is a single payment that covers all services delivered in a single episode of care. For example, one payment is made for maternity services, covering physi-

cian visits prior to and following delivery and hospital care for the delivery.

Capitation

The second major category of reimbursement is **capitation,** in which the provider is paid a fixed number per covered life per period (usually a month), regardless of the number and type of services provided. Although similar to the prospective payment system, a capitated payment system pays a fixed number per month for all services provided to an individual versus per procedure or episode under the PPS. Initially, everyone believed that capitation would become the dominant method of payment; however, the popularity of capitation plans has declined and became popular only in certain geographic locations. The administrative skills and data demands required to manage risks appropriately are quite substantial. In addition, the financial risks to the insurer are greater under capitation due to the importance of accurately projecting the appropriate payment per member. Currently, fee-for-service plans continue to be the most common form of reimbursement (Gapenski, 2003).

Financial Incentives and Risk

Each of the reimbursement methods provides different financial incentives to providers of health-care services. In cost-based reimbursement, for example, providers are paid more if their costs are higher; therefore, no incentive exists to contain costs. In charge-based reimbursement, on the other hand, providers have an incentive to increase their prices because that results in higher payments. Generally, in a competitive marketplace, consumers will only be willing to pay so much for a service, but because most payments for health-care services come from third parties, providers have limited ability to pass on higher charges. As third-party payers transition to a discount charge-based methodology, providers have an incentive to manage costs to maintain the same level of profit. Additional costs are no longer able to be recouped through increasing charges for services, as only a portion of the charges will be reimbursed.

In all of the prospective payment methods, regardless of the unit of payment (procedure, diagnosis), an incentive exists to reduce costs because the payment is fixed. The overall incentive under the PPS is to work more effectively by managing costs and increasing the utilization of the most profitable services. Under global pricing, for example, one payment is made for an entire episode of services, so a strong incentive exists for the physicians and hospitals to work together to offer the most effective treatment. Finally, under capitation, the key to profitability is to increase efficiency and decrease utilization. In a capitation setting, providers have the incentive to practice preventive medicine rather than just treating the illness so they can limit unnecessary utilization of services.

Health-care providers also face several financial risks created by the reimbursement methods in place. The risks create some uncertainty regarding the profitability of the organization. First, providers now bear the risk that costs will exceed revenues. Due to reimbursement for services being somewhat fixed under current payment methods, providers can no longer increase revenues to offset additional costs. Revenues can be increased, but the reimbursement will be the same, regardless of the charge. A key difference among the reimbursement methods is the ability of the provider to influence the profit of each service by setting the prices above the costs. In the PPS, risk is increased due to the payment being fixed regardless of the charge to the patient. The PPS payment is based on the resource utilization necessary for the average patient, and because some patients need more intensive treatments than others, the health-care provider is at greater risk to manage costs to maintain profitability. It is important to realize that the recent trends in reimbursement represent a shift in risk from the insurers to the providers. By implementing a fixed payment for services regardless of patient charges, the providers are now responsible for managing costs to ensure a profit is made on services.

Major Third-Party Payers

There are two broad categories of third-party payers, which provide insurance coverage to the populations: private insurers and public programs. Currently, approximately 54% of all hospital payments come from private sources, with the remaining 46% coming from governmental programs such as Medicare and Medicaid. Over the last several decades, the trend has been toward an increase in public sector funding of health-care spending, with public funding projected to be 49% of total funding by 2014 (*USA Today,* 2005).

PRIVATE INSURERS

The major private insurers include Blue Cross/Blue Shield, commercial insurers, and self-insurers.

During the Depression, the Blue Cross/Blue Shield concept emerged as a way for patients to afford care at hospitals and from local physicians. Blue Cross was created by Justin Ford Kimball; 1300 school teachers were allowed to finance 21 days of hospital care by making small monthly payments to the Baylor University Hospital (Flanagan & Kjesbo, 2004). Blue Shield was emerging in the Pacific Northwest as a result of serious injuries and chronic illness in the lumber and mining camps. "Employers who wanted to provide medical care for their workers made arrangements with physicians who were paid a monthly fee for their services" (History of Blue Cross/Blue Shield, 2006). These organizations developed across the country as independent not-for-profit corporations. Today, the various Blue Cross/Blue Shield plans continue to operate as independent organizations and are members of a single national association that sets standards. In 1986 Congress eliminated their tax-exemption status because the organizations were offering commercial insurance. As a result, several plans have converted to for-profit status; due to the complexities involved in converting from not-for-profit to for-profit status, others maintain their not-for-profit status (Gapenski, 2003). Because all Blue Cross/Blue Shield corporations operate independently, reimbursement methods vary by state. Just as with Medicare, the trend has been toward a prospective payment methodology. Many private insurers have adopted Medicare's **diagnosis-related group** (DRG) system and developed their own payment rates based on specific diagnoses.

Several types of organizations, most often for-profit insurance companies, offer commercial health insurance. Traditionally, **commercial insurers** have reimbursed providers for health-care services on the basis of billed charges. As health-care costs continue to grow, and as these organizations have begun charging higher insurance premiums, a trend has started toward more cost-effective reimburse-

ment methods. As for-profits, these organizations have an incentive to maximize their owners' profits.

Another form of private insurance is where companies set aside funds to pay for future health costs of their own employees rather than using an outside organization to provide their health insurance. This form of insurance is referred to as self-insurance and is very popular among organizations with a large number of employees. The next section of the chapter focuses on the two major government insurance programs, Medicare and Medicaid.

Medicare

The Medicare and Medicaid programs were established through the Social Security Act in the mid-1960s. These programs were administered by the Department of Health, Education, and Welfare (HEW). "In 1977, the Health Care Financing Administration (HCFA) was created under HEW to effectively coordinate Medicare and Medicaid. In 1980, HEW was divided into the Department of Education and the Department of Health and Human Services. In 2001, HCFA was renamed the Centers for Medicare & Medicaid Services (CMS)" (Medicare Information Resource, 2005).

CMS is the federal agency that administers the Medicare program. Currently, Medicare provides coverage to approximately 40 million Americans. Medicare is the national health insurance program for:

- People age 65 years or older
- Some people younger than age 65, with qualifying disabilities that have been recognized by the Social Security Administration
- People with end-stage renal disease, which is permanent kidney failure requiring dialysis or a kidney transplant

Medicare coverage is separated into two plans:

- Part A coverage provides hospital and some skilled nursing home coverage.
- Part B coverage provides outpatient, physician, ambulatory surgical, and several miscellaneous services.

Most people do not pay a monthly Part A premium because they or their spouses are eligible for Social Security, and it comes as a benefit of Social Security. The Part A premium in 2005 for individuals not eligible for Social Security benefits was $375

Common Types of Managed Care Plans

Many private insurers have moved to offering managed care plans. "Managed care plans are designed to control healthcare costs through monitoring, prescribing or proscribing the provision of healthcare to a patient" (Cleverley, 2003). The two most common plans are health maintenance organizations and preferred provider organizations. There is much variability in how these plans work; however, they both seek to change incentives in several ways:

   Limiting subscribers' choices to a provider within the network of providers.

   Relying on the primary care physician to serve as the gatekeeper for referral and approval of services.

   Encouraging preventive care services by offering lower co-pays.

Discouraging use of brand name drugs by higher co-pays.

Changing financial incentives for health-care providers to limit the number of services ordered for patients

Implementing utilization review processes prior to services being rendered.

per month. Part B coverage is optional to all individuals who have Part A coverage. In 2005, the monthly premium for Part B was $78.20 (HHS Announces, 2005).

Until 1983 Medicare reimbursed providers for health-care services based on provider costs. In 1983 the federal government implemented a new reimbursement system for Part A providers called the PPS, discussed earlier. The objective of the PPS was to curb Medicare spending and provide incentives for providers to manage costs. The ultimate goal was to curb growth in health-care spending and to free up funds in the national budget for other services. Unfortunately, over the years PPS payments have not kept pace with hospital costs. To make matters worse, the Balanced Budget Act (BBA) of 1997 placed significant restrictions on the growth in Medicare spending. The Balanced Budget Relief Act of 1999 restored some of the spending cuts from the BBA, but payment growth is still below the growth in operating costs (Gapenski, 2003).

In the PPS system, providers have an incentive to look for ways to contain costs and maintain profitability. From the early 1980s until 2000, outpatient services continued to be reimbursed at cost while inpatient services were reimbursed under the PPS, so providers shifted services from inpatient to outpatient. As a result, Medicare spending for outpatient services grew quickly and offset some of the expected savings from the PPS. As a result, in August 2000, Medicare implemented a fixed payment system for outpatient services as well.

Medigap Plans

A Medigap policy is a health insurance policy sold by private insurance companies that must follow state and federal laws. Many people choose to buy these policies because Medicare does not pay for all their health-care costs. For example, consumers must pay for coinsurance, co-pays, and deductibles, which are called gaps in coverage, and they often choose to buy a Medigap plan to cover these gaps. In addition, Medigap plans often cover benefits that the original plan does not offer, such as emergency health care while traveling. Monthly premiums are paid to the private insurance company for the Medigap coverage. There are 12 standardized plans from which to choose that vary in cost, based on the specific details of each plan, such as deductible and co-pay limits and restrictions on which facilities can be used (Medicare and You, 2006).

Inpatient Prospective Payment System

The foundation of Medicare's inpatient PPS is the DRG assigned to the patient at discharge from the hospital. The DRG provides a way to classify patients based on their primary diagnosis. The diagnosis is influenced by which medical diagnostic category a patient is in. There are approximately 543 DRGs. Each DRG is assigned a relative weight, which represents the average number of resources used in treating the average patient with a certain diagnosis. The average weight of all DRGs is assumed to be 1, so DRGs with a relative weight greater than 1 are more resource-intensive than DRGs with a relative weight of lower than 1. The Medicare case mix index of an institution is a weighted average of all the different diagnoses being treated at a particular organization. For example, a case mix index of 1.5 indicates that a facility's diagnoses are more complex and resource-intensive than a facility with a case mix index of 0.80. CMS reviews the relative weights of specific DRGs annually and makes adjustments based on changes in resource consumption, treatment patterns, and technology.

The DRG payment assigned by Medicare is based on standardized payment rates for labor and nonlabor costs and the relative weight of the DRG. The labor portion of the payment must be adjusted for the local area wage index, which attempts to reflect relative labor costs across the United States. Local wage indices and standardized payment rates are published annually by CMS. Table 7-1 contains an illustration of this calculation for DRG 106 Cardiac Bypass with a PTCA for a hospital in Atlanta, Georgia.

The inpatient PPS works fairly well when patient costs are distributed symmetrically for each DRG, and the payment should be sufficient to cover the costs of an average patient. For example, if within the DRG for pneumonia more patients have a severe rather than a mild case, the charges would be higher for the sicker patients yet the reimbursement will be the same regardless. In the event that certain hospitals treat sicker patients who require more resources for certain DRGs, the PPS payment will fall short in covering the costs of care. To provide some cushion for high-cost patients, the PPS provides an additional outlier payment for patients whose costs exceed certain thresholds.

The regular PPS payment covers only operating costs. Because hospitals have to bear the costs of financing assets necessary to provide services,

TABLE 7-1	Example of Inpatient PPS Reimbursement*
DRG 106 CORONARY BYPASS WITH PTCA	**HOSPITAL: ATLANTA, GA**
National unadjusted labor payment	$2,823.63
Wage index: Atlanta, GA	× .9960
Wage-adjusted labor payment	= $2,812.34
National nonlabor payment	+ 1,730.62
Total adjusted payment for a relative weight of 1	= $4,542.96
DRG 106 relative weight	× 7.3062
Total PPS payment for DRG 106	$33,191.74

*The current labor payment rate is $2,823.63, which is multiplied by the local wage index for Atlanta, Georgia, of .9960 to calculate the adjusted labor payment rate. This amount is added to the nonlabor payment amount to derive the adjusted hospital rate. The adjusted hospital rate is an attempt by CMS to account for differences in costs due to geographic location. Finally, the adjusted hospital rate is multiplied by the DRG relative weight to determine the hospital payment for DRG 106. Once the adjusted hospital rate has been determined, it is relatively simple to analyze the payment for any number of DRGs by multiplying the appropriate DRG weight by the adjusted hospital rate to determine the total payment.

Medicare provides additional dollars to assist in covering capital costs. Currently, the capital payment rate is $416.53, which is multiplied by the DRG relative weight, for each Medicare discharge during the year. So hospitals receive additional reimbursement equal to $416.53 × DRG weight × the number of Medicare patients.

Outpatient PPS

On August 1, 2000, CMS implemented an outpatient PPS based on ambulatory payment classifications (APCs). Services grouped under each APC are similar clinically and in terms of the resources required. A payment rate is established for each APC, and hospitals may be paid for more than one APC for an encounter. Currently, there are approximately 350 APCs that specify surgical and nonsurgical procedures, visits to clinics and emergency departments, and ancillary services.

The APC payment calculation is based on a standard national payment rate, the national Medicare payment percentage, and the patient's co-payment amount. The national payment rate is divided into labor and nonlabor components. Labor represents 60% of the payment rate and nonlabor the remaining 40%. As in the DRG calculations, the labor component of the payment rate is adjusted for the hospital's local wage index. The calculation of the payment for an individual APC is fairly straightforward. Complications arise, however, when multiple procedures are performed within the same visit for a patient. The procedure with the highest value is paid at 100% of the APC payment, and additional procedures are paid at 50%. Certain outpatient services are paid based on a fee schedule, such as physical, occupational and speech therapy, ambulance services, and diagnostic laboratory services.

In addition to inpatient and outpatient hospital services moving to a PPS of reimbursement, nursing homes and home health agency payment methods have also been revised to shift more risk to the health-care provider by capping payments for services.

Medicaid

Medicaid was created under Title XIX of the Social Security Act in 1965 as an entitlement program

Practice Proof 7-1

Popularity of new drug-coated stents exceed supply. *Cardiovascular Watch*, July 21, 2003, p. 15.

Stents have been used since 1987 in conjunction with angioplasties to help prevent arteries from reclosing from plaque buildup. In the spring of 2003, Cordis Corporation released a new stent that was coated with the drug sirolimus. Research indicates that the drug-coated stents prevent scar tissue from reclogging the artery, which often results in another angioplasty within a year of the first procedure. Demand for the new stents is outpacing supply. At the time of this article, Cordis Corporation had the only drug-coated stent on the market. It is anticipated that Boston Scientific will receive approval from the Federal Drug Administration (FDA) within the next year to offer its own drug-coated stent. In addition, the Cordis stents sell for approximately $2,100 more than the bare metal stents, which is creating financial losses for some hospitals on these procedures.

1. What are the factors driving the demand for the drug-coated stents?
2. What are the possible rationing issues as a result of the shortage? What are possible solutions to this dilemma?
3. Explain the potential reimbursement ramifications from the new stents.

jointly funded by the federal and state governments to provide medical assistance for qualified individuals and families with low income and resources. "Medicaid is the largest source of funding for medical and health-related services for America's poorest people" (Medicaid: A Brief Summary, 2005).

States have tremendous autonomy in how they structure their Medicaid programs. States decide on:

- Eligibility criteria
- Type, amount, duration, and scope of services
- Payment rates for services
- Administration

Due to the flexibility each state possesses in structuring its Medicaid programs, considerable variations occur. For example, an individual may be eligible for Medicaid in one state and not be eligible in another state.

The federal government pays a portion of expenditures under each state's Medicaid program. The percentage the federal government pays is updated annually by comparing the state's average per capita income level with the national income average. States with higher income levels are reimbursed a smaller percentage. By law, federal payment cannot be lower than 50% or higher than 83% of a state's Medicaid costs. In 2004, the overall average payment percentage was 60.2%, ranging from 50% in 12 states to a high of 77% in Mississippi (Medicaid: A Brief Summary, 2005). See Box 7-1 for an example.

Basic Economic Theories of Supply and Demand

Based on the current state of health-care spending, there is little argument that resources are limited and consumers (and professionals) are forced to make decisions on how to allocate these resources best. The study of economics helps managers analyze the allocation of scarce resources. **Resources** are anything useful in the consumption or production of a product or service, such as nursing care, new equipment, surgical supplies and, of course, money. For example, individuals must choose daily how to allocate their resources for food, gas, entertainment, and health care. Basic supply and demand theories help illustrate how this allocation of resources takes place. Managers can use these concepts to make both broad strategic decisions and detailed pricing decisions.

In a market system, price is used to ration goods and services. A price system is easy to operate because the price of a product or service self-corrects when the quantity supplied exceeds the quantity demanded. A price system allows individuals with different preferences to make their own choice. In the health-care industry, the market system may appear to work unfairly, as when low income consumers or individuals with preexisting medical conditions are unable to afford needed services (Lee, 2000).

DEMAND THEORY

Most organizations begin their annual strategic planning process by projecting demand for their products. In the health-care setting, the focus is on predicting demand for the appropriate level of services to provide, which also results in planning the required staffing levels to meet this demand. Managers routinely project revenues based on a certain volume of services at a given price. This type of demand forecasting is an essential part of management. It is very important to understand the relationship between price and quantity. The demand curve describes the quantity of goods or services that will be purchased at different prices when all other factors are held constant. Generally, the demand curve slopes downward, which means that a price decrease will reflect more sales of a product. See Figure 7-4. For example, in looking at Figure 7-4, a consumer is willing to buy 80 units at a price of $50 each; however, at a price of $100, consumers are only willing to buy 60 units. Other factors that may influence demand for health services include consumer income, insurance coverage, perceptions of health status, and changes in the prices of other products (Lee, 2000).

The demand for medical care is more complex than the demand for many products due to the:

1. Influence of insurance coverage on the price of care.
2. Complexity in understanding the relationship between the cost and value of a medical service compared with the likely outcome or benefit of the service. This is in part due to the

BOX 7-1

The Medicaid Program in the State of New York

Let's take a look at the state of New York's Medicaid plan to learn more about eligibility requirements and services covered. Citizens of New York may be eligible for Medicaid if they have high medical bills, receive Supplemental Security Income (SSI), or meet certain income, age, or disability requirements. The following table illustrates the 2006 income and resource limits to qualify for Medicaid in New York. Resources include property of all kinds, including real and intangible property: e.g., retirement accounts, life insurance policies, stocks, bonds, automobiles, and personal property. Individuals may still qualify for Medicaid even if they own a home, car, or personal property.

NUMBER IN FAMILY	MONTHLY NET INCOME	RESOURCES
1	$692	$4,150
2	$900	$5,400
3	$1,017	$6,100
4	$1,025	$6,150
5	$1,034	$6,200
6	$1,134	$6,800
7	$1,275	$7,650
8	$1,417	$8,500

The above income levels are expanded for pregnant women and children.

The following services are paid by Medicaid, but some services may not be covered because of age, financial circumstances, family situation, transfer of resource requirements, or living arrangements. Some services have small co-payments.

- Smoking cessation agents
- Treatment and preventive health and dental care (physicians and dentists)
- Hospital inpatient and outpatient services
- Laboratory and x-ray services
- Care in a nursing home
- Care through home health agencies and personal care
- Treatment in psychiatric hospitals (for persons under 21 or those 65 years and older), mental health facilities, and facilities for the developmentally disabled
- Family planning services
- Early periodic screening, diagnosis, and treatment for children under 21 years under the child/teen health program
- Medicine, supplies, medical equipment, and appliances (wheelchairs, etc.)
- Clinical services
- Transportation to medical appointments, including public transportation and car mileage
- Emergency ambulance transportation to a hospital
- Prenatal care
- Some insurance and Medicare premiums

Citizens of New York may apply for Medicaid by writing, phoning, or going by their local social services department (New York State Department of Health: Medicaid, 2006).

lack of information related to these costs and benefits.

3. Difficulty in making informed choices, which leads consumers to turn to health-care professionals for advice. These professionals have significant influence on demand and often make choices that reflect their own best interests.

SUPPLY CURVE AND EQUILIBRIUM PRICE

The supply of services offered is based on how much the producer is willing to sell at each price. This relationship is graphically illustrated in Figure 7-4 by an upward-sloping supply curve, demonstrating that producers are willing to sell more as the price increases. For example, at a price of $150 a provider would be willing to supply 80 units; the consumer is only willing to buy 80 units at a price of $50. Markets generally move toward an equilibrium price at which producers want to sell the amount that consumers are willing to buy. Movements along the demand curve describe the different quantities that consumers are willing to buy at various prices; however, certain circumstances can cause the entire demand curve to shift to the right or left. An example of a situation that would result in the entire demand curve shifting to the right would be the expansion of insurance coverage (i.e., insurance will pay a larger portion of the bill, more people are covered by insurance, or possibly a reduction in deductibles). The increased coverage of mammograms or colonoscopies for patients of a certain age has created a shift in demand for these services. See Figure 7-5.

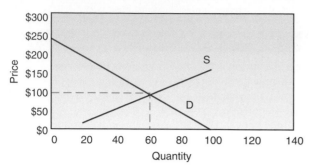

FIGURE 7-4 Supply and demand at equilibrium.

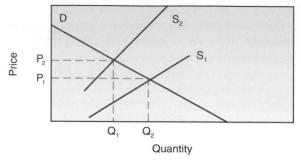

FIGURE 7-6 Shift in supply due to change in regulations allowing freestanding ambulatory surgery centers.

A shift in the supply curve to the right indicates that at every price a producer wants to supply a smaller quantity. A change in regulations might cause such a shift in the supply curve by making care more expensive. For example, recent changes in the approval process for freestanding ambulatory surgery centers in certain states have led to a major shift to provision of services outside the hospital (Lee, 2000). Hospitals saw a decrease in the demand for their services, which caused a reduction in the quantity of services offered. See Figure 7-6.

Health-care managers face many challenges in balancing the supply and demand for services. To illustrate some of the unique challenges, compare an automobile manufacturer with a health-care organization. Prices are set in the competitive marketplace for automotive manufacturers. Consumers have a choice among many suppliers of automobiles, and there is easy access to information to help distinguish between the qualities of competing models, such as Internet Web sites). The assumption is that consumers make a rational decision based on the price and quality of the product. In addition, consumers directly pay for the full price of the purchase. In contrast, health-care organizations often do not provide a wide array of serv-

ices; for example, limited organizations offer open heart surgery or organ transplant services. Historically, it has been difficult to obtain necessary information to compare services from one facility with those of another. In addition, the information is very complex, and consumers often seek the advice of health-care professionals, which allows the professionals to influence the choice of which service to purchase. Finally, the payment for the service, in the majority of cases, is made by a third party, such as the federal government or private insurance companies. Predicting supply and demand for services is difficult for health-care organizations because of the involvement of multiple third parties in the decision process of where to seek health-care services.

Health-care organizations are currently facing additional pressures because of resource shortages that do not meet demand. Services are constrained by, for example, the current shortage of nurses and the projected shortage of physicians. Consequently, the prices (hourly rates, salaries) to attract nurses and physicians are increasing, reducing profits even further. In addition, the cost of drugs and medical supplies has skyrocketed. Finally, a dramatic increase in demand for health-care services is expected over the next 20 years because of a projected 72% increase in the population over age 65, coupled with technological advances offering more treatment options and extending the life expectancy (U.S. Department of Health and Human Services, 2003).

Maximizing Profits

As evident in the previous discussion of supply and demand, producers of health-care services strive to

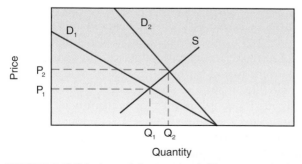

FIGURE 7-5 Shift in demand due to expanded insurance coverage of colonoscopies.

increase the demand for their services in hopes of maximizing profits. Even if one is employed in a not-for-profit organization, which does not explicitly seek profit maximization as a goal, it is important to realize that profits are necessary to carry out the mission of the organization.

Profits are dollars that are left over after total costs are subtracted from total revenue. Managers are able to influence profits by reducing costs and/or expanding the quantity of services offered and thereby increasing revenue. Reducing costs generally requires improvements in clinical management, which focuses on how clinical plans are designed and the associated resource usage. Reengineering and quality management are two strategies that some organizations have used to improve the performance of their organization and thereby reduce costs. Reengineering is generally a more radical approach, in which all business processes are reviewed and revised to improve the efficiency of key organizational processes while reducing costs. Quality management often focuses on improving clinical processes and how the delivery of care to the patient can be improved while saving costs. The impact of the changes on the organizational culture is a key factor that must be managed in order for the improvements to be successful.

The second option for maximizing profits is increasing the services offered in order to increase revenue. As a general rule, it is profitable to expand output as long as the additional revenue generated is greater than the additional costs incurred.

FOR-PROFIT VERSUS NOT-FOR-PROFIT HEALTH ORGANIZATIONS

Although all firms do not have maximizing profits as a primary goal, profits are necessary to maintain long-term financial viability in the increasingly competitive health-care environment. Traditionally, not-for-profit organizations have dominated the health-care industry. A closer examination of the differences between for profit and not-for-profit health-care organizations will provide a better understanding of the overall goals and objectives of these organizations.

For-profit organizations are often referred to as investor-owned, which means that investors buy shares of stock in the firm, representing ownership interests. A primary goal of for-profit entities is to maximize profits for their owners, keeping in mind

---

Practice to Strive For 7-1

Cost reduction is a hot topic in the health-care industry, and many articles have been written about how to redesign clinical processes to increase profits. A recent article in Healthcare Financial Management *describes a success story at Lucile Packard Children's Hospital (LPCH) in Stanford. This hospital improved patient flow, which thereby increased bed capacity, profits, and patient satisfaction. There are several strategies that managers can take from this example and apply to their own organizations.*

A critical first step in clinical reengineering projects entails an accurate assessment of the current environment. At LPCH, a comprehensive assessment included detailed observations, a review of historical data, and interviews with all stakeholders, including physicians, housekeeping, case managers, and many others. Actions that resulted from this assessment included a comprehensive implementation of strategies rather than a piecemeal approach.

Because many of the improvements to patient flow depended on changes to multiple processes in various departments, a comprehensive rollout allowed larger benefits to be achieved. The hospital created workflow and reporting tools to provide daily and weekly key performance measures for key stakeholders. In addition, communication with staff to explain the process and create consent was critical to the success of the project. LPCH saw significant improvements within 11 months, such as a 7% increase in capacity, increased operating income of $3.3 million, and improvements in several bed placement and turnover measures (Flanagan & Kjesbo, 2004).

Pricing Services

The manager of an outpatient cancer center was approached by the local Veterans Administration (VA) hospital to provide certain treatment unavailable at the VA for $250 per treatment. The manager agreed to this proposal because there was extra time in the schedule that was already being covered by staff. This allowed the manager to increase the department's revenue without adding any additional costs. Had the demand from the VA grown beyond what could be fit into the existing schedule, the manager would have had to reevaluate the situation based on the projected revenue compared with the additional staffing costs that would have been required.

that investors have many choices regarding how to invest their money in today's competitive marketplace. The investors in the firm are referred to as stockholders and have several basic rights:

1. The right to vote for the firm's board of directors and on other relevant issues.
2. A claim to the earnings of the firm, primarily through cash or stock dividends.
3. In the case of bankruptcy or liquidation, the stockholders are entitled to any proceeds that remain after all other obligations have been satisfied.

There are two basic types of for-profit organizations: publicly held firms and privately held firms. **Publicly held firms** are owned by a large number of investors, and the shares of stock in the firm are traded through various mechanisms, such as the New York Stock Exchange, American Stock Exchange, or over-the-counter market. Examples of publicly held health-care organizations include Healthcare Corporation of America and Beverly Enterprises. In contrast, **privately held firms** are owned by just a few investors and are not publicly traded. In general, for-profits are thought to be more efficient because of the scrutiny by shareholders on financial performance. In addition, for-profits can readily access large amounts of capital by issuing additional shares of stock to modernize their facilities and compete for customers (Marsteller, Bovbjerg, & Nichols, 1998).

An alternative form of ownership is the **not-for-profit organization,** which is also referred to as a tax-exempt or nonprofit corporation. Unlike the for-profit entities, not-for-profit organizations traditionally had serving the community as their primary goal. The IRS Tax Code Section 501C (3) sets forth the criteria that a firm must meet to qualify for tax exemption as a charitable organization: if it is formed for some defined public good and if none of the net earnings will be disbursed to any shareholder or individual as a "dividend" or share of the net. There are several key characteristics of not-for-profit organizations:

1. Historically, not-for-profit organizations received **significant revenues from charitable sources and other donations.** Nonprofits today receive a small portion of total income from donations; they are being challenged to increase efficiency to gain access to capital and remain competitive (Harrison & Sexton, 2004).
2. Not-for-profit organizations have no shareholders; therefore, a board of trustees, often residents from the local community who are not owners of the firm, exercise control over the organization's operations (Josephson, 1997).
3. Not-for-profit organizations have **limited access to capital** because they cannot issue shares of stock. Tax-exempt bond issues are their primary source of funding for capital needs.
4. In the event of **liquidation or sale,** proceeds must be used for a charitable purpose.
5. **Tax subsidies** are often provided to not-for-profit organizations through exemptions on local, state, and federal taxes.
6. Not-for-profit organizations are expected to provide free care for poor people, regardless of their ability to pay.
7. Not-for-profit organizations are expected to **provide benefits to the community,** such as access to services that are not profitable, medical education and research, community education, and health screening (Josephson, 1997; Marsteller, Bovbjerg, & Nichols, 1998). Patients expect that not-for-profit organizations will not reduce quality to increase profits and that earnings above costs will be used for beneficial services or other worthy investments (Marsteller, Bovbjerg, & Nichols, 1998).
8. In many **small communities**, the very existence of a hospital may be owed to its not-for-profit status as substantial donations of money and time from the community often support the hospital. Local hospitals are a valuable part of the community infrastructure and have fostered community development and civic pride (Marstellar, Bovbjerg, & Nichols, 1998).

Not-for-profit hospitals represent 58% of total hospitals in the United States, according to a recent American Hospital Association Survey (Fast Facts, 2005). Although not-for-profits clearly play a dominant role in the health-care industry, many federal and state policy makers are starting to question the validity of the true differences between for-profits and not-for-profits. With health-care costs growing at the state and federal levels, policy makers, looking for additional sources of revenue as a way to balance their budgets, are scrutinizing the current tax subsidies that not-for-profits receive. Several states, such as Texas and Utah, are now requiring health-care organizations to meet minimum levels of indigent care to maintain their tax-exempt status.

All Good Things...

This chapter has provided a broad overview of the unique challenges facing managers in the health-care industry today. It is of vital importance for managers to understand the economic pressures facing health-care organizations and why their role is so important in effectively managing their organizations' scarce resources. Even with the additional complexities of health care, however, there are several factors that managers can influence. Accurately forecasting demand for services is a very important management task, as is managing the costs of meeting the demand for services. Cost management can be as focused as staffing and supply utilization within a particular unit or as broad as a clinical reengineering project for a certain patient diagnosis. An understanding of the patients who utilize the services is crucial to understanding how the organization will ultimately be paid for the services provided.

 hot topic:

Health-Care Rationing

Rationing is one method that society uses to balance demands with limited resources. Even though the United States is viewed as a world leader in both scientific and technological aspects of medical care, not all citizens have access to basic health-care services. Current issues providing the context for rationing of health care are as follows:

1. Health-care services are restricted to individuals with sufficient financial resources (Cypher, 2003).

2. Health-care providers can choose not to accept certain forms of insurance, such as Medicaid or HMO plans, due to low payment (Cypher, 2003).

3. High deductibles and increasing insurance premiums are forcing many middle-income families to forego health-care coverage. In addition, small businesses are unable to supplement the cost of premiums for employees or even offer health-care coverage (Cypher, 2003).

4. Individuals with preexisting medical conditions are restricted in their access to health care coverage.

5. Public policy covers only Medicare recipients.

The reality is that millions of Americans' access to care is limited either because they are unable to afford or qualify for insurance coverage or the coverage they have does not cover the services needed. Private insurance compa-

nies using a managed care system ration services through such methods as primary care gatekeeping, financial incentives to physicians, utilization review of services, and capitation. Primary care physicians serve as the point of access, or gatekeeper, to specialists, hospitalization, and other services. Limiting services or having consumers choose less costly treatments or simply no treatment at all is a primary objective of the managed care system. Physicians receive incentives that encourage them to ration health-care services. In addition, most managed care systems have a utilization review process in place, which requires prior authorization before a nonroutine service can be provided to a patient. Traditional insurance programs also attempt to ration services by not covering certain services in their policies. Often customers will avoid these procedures because they have to pay for them from their personal finances. Patients likewise self-ration their use of services when they do not have insurance coverage. This is often referred to as price-based rationing, because the patient has to evaluate the cost of receiving the services versus the perceived benefits of care (Baur, Wang, & Fitzgerald, 1996).

The potential legal and ethical issues surrounding the ability of citizens to receive needed health-care services is a controversial topic without an easy solution. It is clear that the current system is in need of a dramatic reform to correct these inequalities.

Let's Talk

1. What impact have recent trends in legislation had on the health-care industry?

2. What is the key difference in prospective reimbursement methods? How would hospital management policies differ for PPS methodologies of reimbursement?

3. Think of a time in your work experience when services for a certain patient were limited. What were the circumstances surrounding this situation and details of how the decision was made? How did you feel about it?

4. Give an example of a time when your organization or department experienced a shift in supply or a shift in demand for certain services.

5. Using Table 7-1 as a guide, calculate the hospital payment rate for DRG 371 Cesarean without CC with a relative weight of .6221 for a hospital in New York City with a local wage index of 1.3595.

NCLEX Questions

1. In the United States, the majority of health-care services are paid by:
   A. Consumers.
   B. Employers.
   C. Insurance companies.
   D. Financial institutions.

2. Increases in health-care costs often lead to:
   A. Consumers dropping insurance coverage.
   B. Employers reducing health insurance benefits.
   C. Insurance companies reducing payments for services.
   D. All of the above.

3. The primary reimbursement methods under the fee-for-service category are:
   A. Cost-based reimbursement.
   B. Charge-based reimbursement.
   C. Capitation.
   D. A and B only.

4. The advantages of a price-based market system are:
   A. Easy to operate because the price is self-correcting.
   B. Individual choice is limited.
   C. Goods and services are allocated in a fair manner.
   D. All of the above.

5. Predicting demand for medical care is more complex due to:
   A. Third parties paying for the majority of services.
   B. Difficulty in comparing cost and quality of services.
   C. Need for professional advice to make an informed decision.
   D. All of the above.

6. Which of the following is NOT a characteristic of a not-for-profit organization?
   A. Unlimited access to capital.
   B. Proceeds from liquidation must be used for a charitable purpose.
   C. Exemption from local, state, and federal taxes.
   D. Free care for poor citizens.

7. Current health-care rationing issues include:
   A. Restriction of services to individuals with sufficient resources.
   B. Providers choosing to accept only certain forms of insurance.
   C. Difficulty for individuals with preexisting conditions to obtain insurance coverage.
   D. All of the above.

8. Which reimbursement method demonstrates a shift in the financial risk from the insurer to the provider?
   A. Cost-based reimbursement.
   B. Percentage of charges.
   C. Prospective payment.
   D. All of the above.

9. Under the Medicare inpatient system a DRG with a relative weight of 2.0 compared with a DRG with a relative weight of .80 is:
   A. More complex and resource-intensive.
   B. Less complex and resource-intensive.
   C. The same in complexity and resource usage.
   D. None of the above.

10. Characteristics of the Medicaid program are as follows:
    A. Federally and state-funded program for low-income individuals and families.
    B. Federal government has specific guidelines how the program is structured.
    C. Eligibility for Medicaid is the same regardless of the state of residence.
    D. The federal government's share of the Medicaid program's cost has not changed over the last several years.

REFERENCES

Anderson, G.F. (1997). In search of value: An international comparison of cost, access and outcomes. *Health Affairs, 16*(6): 163–171.

Baur, M., Wang, J., and Fitzgerald, J. (1996). Insurance rationing versus public political rationing: The care of the Oregon health plan. *Public Budgeting and Finance, 16*(1): 60–74.

Centers for Medicare and Medicaid services. Retrieved March 17, 2005, from http://www.cms.hhs.gov/charts/healthcare system/chapter1.pdf

Cleverley, W., and Cameron, A. (2003). *Essentials of health care finance.* Sudbury, MA: Jones & Bartlett.

Cypher, D. (2003) Healthcare rationing: Issues and implications. *Nursing Forum, 32*(4): 25–34.

Fast facts on U.S. hospitals from AHA hospital statistics. Retrieved February 11, 2005, from www.aha.org//aha/resource_center/fastfacts/fast_facts_US_hospitals.html

Flanagan, S., and Kjesbo, A. (2004). Conquering capacity: By improving its patient flow, one hospital has been able to admit an additional 400 patients since January 2003 and expects to maintain that potential. *Healthcare Financial Management, 58*(7): 92–97.

Gapenski, L. (2003) *Understanding healthcare financial management.* Chicago: Health Administration Press.

Harrison, J., and Sexton C. (2004). The paradox of the not-for-profit hospital. *The Health Care Manager, 23*(3):192–205.

Healthcare Tab Ready to Explode. (2005, February 24). *USA Today* p. 1A.

HHS Announces Medicare Premium, Deductibles for 2005. United States Department of Health and Human Services. Retrieved March 23, 2005, from http://www.hhs.gov/news/press/2004pres/20040903a.html

History of Blue Cross Blue Shield. Retrieved February 6, 2006, from http://www.bcbs.com/history/index.html/

Lee, R. (2000). *Economics for healthcare managers.* Chicago: Health Administration Press.

Marsteller, J., Bovbjerg, R., and Nichols, L. (1998). Non-profit conversion: Theory, evidence, and state policy options. *Health Services Research, 33*(5): 1495–1500.

Medicaid: A Brief Summary. Centers for Medicare and Medicaid Services. Retrieved March 23, 2005, from http://www.cms.hhs.gov/publications/overview-medicare-medicaid/default4.asp

Medicare and You. Retrieved February 4, 2006, from http://www.medicare.gov/publications/pubs/pdf/10050.pdf

Medicare Information Resource. Centers for Medicare and Medicaid Services. Retrieved March 23, 2005, from http://www.cmc.hhs.gov/medicare/

New York State Department of Health: Medicaid. Retrieved February 5, 2006, from http://www.health.state.ny.us/health_care/medicaid/#income

U.S. Department of Health and Human Services. Centers for Medicare and Medicaid Services. Office of Research, Development and Information. *CMS Publication No. 03445.* June 2003

Weisbrod, B.A. (1991). The health care quadrilemma: An essay on technological change, insurance, quality of care, and cost. *The Journal of Economic Literature 29*: 523–552.

BIBLIOGRAPHY

Barr, D. (2002) *Where do we go from here? An introduction to U.S. health policy: The organization, financing and delivery of healthcare in America* (pp. 223-237). San Francisco: Benjamin Cummings.

Health care costs. Agency for Healthcare Research and Quality. Retrieved February 9, 2005, from www.ahrg.gov

Highlights—National Health Expenditures, 2003. *Centers for Medicare and Medicaid Services.* Retrieved February 9, 2005, from http://www.cms.hhs.gov/statistics/nhe/historical/highlights.asp

Josephson, G. (1997). Private hospital care for profit? A reappraisal. *Health Care Management Review, 22*(3): 64–74.

Random House Webster's college dictionary. (1996). New York: Random House.

Scott, J.S. (2004). Dare we use the word (gasp)—rationing? *Healthcare Financial Management 58*(5): 32–34.

Organizational Communication

CARLA G. PHILLIPS, PHD, RN

CHAPTER MOTIVATION

*"The greatest problem in communication is the illusion
that it has taken place."*

George Bernard Shaw

CHAPTER MOTIVES

- Identify the communication process.
- Describe perspectives of communication as they relate to organizational communication.
- Explore the relationship of organizational structure to organizational communication.
- Discuss the importance of organizational communication to patient safety and quality care.
- Distinguish between formal and informal channels of communication.

*E*ffective **communication** is essential to the well-being of an organization. Communication is critical to the strategic planning process of any organization, and it is crucial for attainment of short- and long-term organizational goals. Likewise, good communication is pivotal to the day-to-day operation of any organization, affecting patient safety and quality care, employee satisfaction, and customer relations and satisfaction. Adamson, Emswiller, and Ollier (1991) recognize the importance of **organizational communication** and point out that if something cannot be communicated in a consistent and inspiring way, it cannot be done, no matter how well it is planned and financed.

Communication can be considered as occurring along a continuum, from interpersonal communication to small-group communication to organizational communication. Interpersonal communication occurs when the participants are face to face. Although there is disagreement in the literature as to how many people can be involved in interpersonal communication, it is generally agreed that it involves only two or three people. According to Trenhom (1991), because the interaction is face to face, there is spontaneity to the communication, and although the communication is focused, there is no need for messages to be "prepackaged." Small-group communication becomes more complex than interpersonal communication primarily because the number of participants increases. Again, although the exact number of participants in small-group communication is not definite, the literature suggests that it may range from two to seven or so participants. Whereas small-group communication can provide the same sensory impact and immediacy of feedback as interpersonal communication, with participants knowing and reacting to one another, the possible combinations of relationships increase dramatically, and messages may be sent via a variety of networks (Trenholm, 1991). Organizational communication is different from the other two in that the number of participants is greater, and the communication occurs within the context of an organizational hierarchy. Trenholm notes that organizational communication is usually highly structured and goal-oriented and that roles in the communication process may correspond to roles within the organizational hierarchy. Therefore, because messages may be sent by a variety of people in a variety of formats, the immediate feedback of interpersonal and small-group communication is not possible. In organizational communication, messages are, by necessity, carefully planned and structured. Trenholm states that "communication within the organization involves a higher degree of strategic planning than it does with a dyad or small group" (p. 24).

This chapter focuses on organizational communication, although interpersonal and small-group communication may also be used as part of the overall communication strategy. This chapter presents an overview of the communication process, a discussion of three theoretical perspectives relevant to organizational communication, and other information relevant to the understanding of effective communication in organizations.

Communication Theories

Communication between humans is of critical importance whether occurring between two individuals or between multiple people in an organization, but communication is often difficult. Communication is usually taken for granted; that is, someone sends a message to another person, either verbally or in writing, and assumes that the person receiving the message understood the message exactly as it was intended. When communicating with a few people, it is fairly easy to validate whether the message was understood as intended. When communicating with many people in organizations, it becomes more difficult to ascertain whether a message was understood correctly.

Because communication is basic and constant in the lives of humans, it has been studied for centuries. If communication within organizations is to be effective, it is important to have an understanding of the underlying precepts of communication. For example, in order for nurse managers to be effective communicators, they should practice communication founded on sound theoretical perspectives. The following theories are summarized here: the mechanistic perspective, the psychological perspective, and the interactionist perspective.

MECHANISTIC PERSPECTIVE

According to Trenholm (1991), the mechanistic perspective of communication is a linear, one-directional, sequential model of communication. Trenholm explains the model by applying it to a face-to-face spoken communication between two people: "The two people become sender and receiver. The sender encodes the message into units of spoken language that are conveyed by sound waves to the receiver, who decodes the message. Any feature not intended by the sender but inadvertently included in the message is called noise" (p. 33). Noise may interfere with the message so that it is not received as intended. Whether communicating between two people or between groups of people, it is important to consider the factors that may hinder the clear transmission of a message: environmental noise, the emotional content of the message, and tone of voice as well as the **nonverbal** behavior of the sender.

PSYCHOLOGICAL PERSPECTIVE

The psychological perspective builds on the mechanistic perspective, acknowledging the sender, receiver, and the message, but goes beyond the linear approach. The psychological perspective is based, in large part, on learned behavior. It suggests that when a message is received, it serves as a stimulus to the receiver to respond to the message. This process of give and take, in which (1) a message is sent, (2) it stimulates the receiver to respond, (3) a response is sent, which then (4) stimulates the receiver to respond, is a learned behavior. Children learn from an early age, as they develop their ability to communicate, that when they are spoken to, they are expected to respond either behaviorally or verbally. This perspective recognizes that people constantly receive and respond to stimuli. "All responses are elicited by stimuli, and all stimuli lead to responses. Human beings are both senders and receivers because we simultaneously react to and produce stimuli" (Trenholm, p. 34). Trenholm further theorizes that humans both seek out and process stimuli according to learned responses. As children are socialized, for example, they learn which behaviors and actions are met with approval, including their communication. Trenholm asserts, "As communicators, we actively choose to attend to certain stimuli, interpret them by means of our own unique mental structures, and respond by emitting certain behaviors capable of stimulating others" (p. 37). According to this perspective, a message is sent by some means, and the potential for noise exists,

but the sender and receiver become joint senders and receivers. For example, a person sends a message to a receiver either verbally or by some other means. When the message is received, it stimulates the receiver to respond, and the receiver then becomes the sender of a message, and so on.

INTERACTIONIST PERSPECTIVE

The interactionist perspective is based on the body of work known as symbolic interactionism. This perspective developed as a way to understand the development of self as learned through a process of interaction within the larger society/environment. According to symbolic interaction, the self emerges during interaction between an individual and the environment beginning in infancy. The self emerges as that which makes each person unique and comprises a set of ideas, values, and experiences, all arrived at through social interaction. Trenholm (1991) notes that the concept of symbols is foundational to this perspective and that symbols are generally agreed upon by members of a group and become socially significant because of this agreement. She summarizes by stating, "Humans exist in and through communication; human action can be understood through the shared symbol systems that make action possible" (p. 39). Given that people have different experiences, ideas, and values, they are likely to interpret messages differently based on their own unique socialization. This theoretical perspective has provided the basis for continuing research in the field of communication and other disciplines. It provides the basis for managers and others involved in organizational communication to understand that people will engage in the communication process based, in part at least, on their own experiences.

Symbols in Communication

Trenholm (1991) believes that "words are symbols, and human language is a symbolic code, just as the Morse Code, sign language, semaphore codes and traffic lights are symbolic systems. The meanings of these codes are established through convention; their use is generally intentional" (p. 12). Dahnke and Clatterbuck (1990) state that "one common view of communication holds that it is a process in which a message producer puts thoughts or feelings into words and transmits those words to a hearer who then gets the information from them" (p. 24). They further state that the notion of a code is essential to this viewpoint, with language being representative of a code. Barnum and Kerfoot (1995) state, "The act of putting meaning into symbolic form is called encoding, and the act of extracting meaning from symbols is termed decoding. The degree of agreement between the message sent and the message received will depend on the degree to which the symbols have the same meaning for the two parties" (pp. 296–297).

It is clear that in organizations messages are sent through a variety of means to many categories of workers, using words as symbols. Words and other symbols often bear many different meanings. In order for people to derive a common meaning from a message, they must have a common understanding of the symbols, in this case the words. For example, assume a top governing body of a health-care system is composed of both health-care professionals and a mix of lay people. When the administration of the health-care system brings proposals to the group seeking approval for programs or equipment, the proposals must not be filled with technical jargon that the lay members of the group cannot understand. The administrative team presenting the reports or proposals should present them in easily understandable terms or at least interpret the technical language for the audience. This holds true for messages sent throughout the organization. Many people who work in health-care settings do not have a clinical background and therefore cannot interpret messages about clinical issues accurately. By the same token, clinical people often lack a background in business or finance, so issues of budget may pose difficulty if not presented in easily understandable terms. But executives and clinicians who live with technical terms on a daily basis often forget that the audience does not share that same language. Therefore, messages must be worded appropriately for varied audiences and categories of workers throughout an organization.

Organizational Structure as It Influences Communication

In order to understand how communication can occur in organizations, it is necessary to understand what constitutes an organization and the impact of the chain of command on communication in organizations. (See Chapter 4 for a complete discussion of organizations and their characteristics.) "An organization is a systematic arrangement of two or more people or entities who fulfill formal roles and share a common purpose" (Wolper, 2004 p. 653). All health-care systems fulfill this definition of an organization, regardless of their size or purpose. Even though a public health agency has a different purpose than a long-term care facility, each has its own purpose and people who fulfill the roles necessary to achieve the goals of the organization. Wolper observes that hospitals usually have pyramidal, or hierarchical, forms of structure in which people at the top levels have a span of control and authority that is passed down to other employees in the chain of command. In such a structure, a manager may delegate to two or three supervisors, who delegate to several charge nurses, and so on. This hierarchical structure is common in most health-care organizations and becomes more pronounced in larger organizations. This structure usually dictates how communication flows within an organization. For example, the nurse administrator may communicate with nurse managers, who then pass the message along to staff nurses.

The notion of the chain of command has to do with the lines of authority throughout the organization. Employees are expected to respect the chain of command; a break in the chain suggests a violation of authority, according to Wolper (2004). For example, if an employee has an issue or concern, the employee is expected to communicate the concern to his or her immediate supervisor, who then takes the message through the organizational hierarchy. The manager should return to the employee with an answer to the employee's concern. Employees often get frustrated as it takes time for an issue to be taken up through the hierarchy and then back down through the channels to the employee. The larger the organization, the more time required for communication to travel through the levels.

Because of the complexities of health-care organizations, it is necessary that all functions are well coordinated. Much of the coordination in hospitals occurs at the level of middle managers. Effective communication between people, units, and departments facilitates coordination of decision making and the quality of the day-to-day operations.

Ruthman (Kelly-Heidenthal, 2003) states, "Avenues of communication are often defined by an organization's formal structure. The formal structure of the organization establishes who is in charge and identifies how different levels of personnel and various departments relate within the organization" (p. 126). For example, nurses on a unit may have concerns about the transportation of clients to surgery. They tell their concerns to the nurse manager, who in turn discusses the issue with the nurse manager of the surgery department or others within the organization who could solve the problem. The formal structure of the organization dictates who has the authority to deal with certain issues and to speak to others within the organization to resolve problems. Marquis and Huston (2003) note the impact the formal organizational structure has on communication and observe that people in lower levels are more likely to have inadequate communication from higher levels. They state, "This occurs because of the number of levels communication must filter through in large organizations. As the number of employees increases (particularly more than 1000 employees), the quantity of communication generally increases; however, employees may perceive it as increasingly closed" (p. 337).

Often, employees see a great deal of communication coming down through the levels of the hierarchy and perceive that there is very little opportunity for them to respond or to initiate communication from their level. They are bound by the formal lines of the organizational structure and must rely on their immediate supervisor to relay their concerns or input upward. Much communication in organizations is designed to inform employees, but little communication invites employee input. This may be especially true in larger organizations where there are many layers in the hierarchy.

Communication within organizations has become more challenging as health systems have grown in size and complexity. Advances in technology, greater acuity of patients, managed care, diagnosis-related groups, and regulatory requirements have changed the way health-care organizations function. The pace of most health-care organizations is faster than in the past, with many regulatory requirements dictating organizational performance. Effective communication is required for the coordination, cooperation, and collabora-

Interpersonal and Group Communication in Organizations

Although interpersonal and group-level communications are at lower levels of organizational communication, they are major forms of communication. People exchange vital information as they meet one on one or in group meetings. For instance, a group of nurse managers may meet with the nurse executive to work through solutions to staffing problems, or the nurse executive may meet with the chief of the medical staff to address a clinical issue. Staff nurses may meet to solve a problem on a nursing unit. Organizational communication requires nurse executives, managers, and employees to have the necessary skills to communicate at all levels within the organization to accomplish goals.

tion necessary to achieve unit and organizational goals. The complexities of the health-care environment require effective communication for keeping employees informed of the status and challenges of the unit and organization, the organizational goals, and the unit expectations and responsibilities in meeting those goals. Communication serves to give employees the knowledge and guidance necessary to do their jobs, build commitment to unit and organizational goals, and make them feel that they are an integral part of the organization.

Nurse executives and managers must be able to ascertain what and how many details need to be provided to employees and make considered judgments about the best means by which to provide that information. Nurse executives in particular may need to deliver the messages on the same topic to several audiences and will need to tailor the message to the audience. If seeking approval for funding for a program from the governing board of the agency, the nurse executive would provide enough information for the board to make an informed decision, usually in a formal presentation. When presenting the program to employees who will be responsible for implementing the program, the level of specificity would increase and might be communicated personally, through nurse managers, in educational session, or by memo. Employees must also understand their responsibility to be proactive in bringing nursing issues—including problems and solution suggestions—to the attention of management, using the proper chain of command.

Types of Organizational Communication

Organizational communication includes **verbal** and **nonverbal** means of communication throughout the organization. Large, complex organizations use a variety of channels of communication, including **vertical, horizontal, diagonal**, and the grapevine (Marquis and Huston, 2003).

Managers have to determine the best mode of communication to be used to convey a particular message. For example, layoffs or some other change in the organization with strong, potentially negative consequences for employees warrant a face-to-face meeting so that management can provide immediate clarification and can receive feedback. The immediate feedback and clarification may prevent misunderstandings and rumors that misconstrue the intent of the message. Other more routine information may be communicated successfully by memo or e-mail. Marquis and Huston (2003) note that "a message's clarity is greatly affected by the mode of communication used" (p. 341).

VERBAL COMMUNICATION

Both face-to-face and written messages constitute verbal communication. Written messages, including e-mail, provide documentation of the message but may be misinterpreted by the recipients and are time-consuming for managers. People will likely interpret written messages from their own perspectives, experiences, and position in the organization, making unlikely a common understanding of written messages by all who receive them. Efficient and effective writing skills are important for nurse managers. Spears (1997) interviewed nurse managers concerning their feelings about writing business communications. Nurse managers reported that on average they spent between 12.4 and 16 hours of a 40-hour work week writing. They noted the need for good writing skills, and many expressed the need for more education in developing writing skills. They reported that often written requests

and recommendations garnered more attention from top managers than oral messages. Written requests, recommendations, and proposals also provide a record of the communication.

Marquis and Huston (2003) observe that face-to-face communication is rapid but that fewer people may receive the information. Common strategies used by managers and nurse executives are to have open meetings with staff on all shifts. However, it would be rare if 100% of the staff members were able to attend these meetings at the times scheduled. Therefore, other means of conveying information might be necessary, such as memos or written summaries of the content of the meetings. Nonetheless, nurse managers communicate face-to-face in a variety of formats, including formal meetings, presentations, and work groups. Top-level managers typically spend many hours in meetings. Barnum and Kerfoot (1995) state, "Person-to-person communication has advantages such as forcing the receiver's attention to the issue, providing immediate feedback and clarification, and allowing the message to be adapted to a specific audience" (p. 300). Crow (2002) suggests that personal interaction may build more trust than written communication, such as memos, and that it provides people the opportunity to question each other.

Whatever mode of verbal communication is used, several points are important. Messages should be checked carefully for accuracy, completeness of detail, and clarity. Some managers ask others to read a message to evaluate these points before the message is sent to the target audience. This review becomes more important in light of a survey of 1000 "average" workers in the United States (Schumann, 2004). The study found that employees want truthful information from their employer and that only about half were satisfied with the information they received. The researcher found that employees want plain talk that is easy to evaluate on items that are important to them. The tone of a message is also of utmost importance. The message should convey respect for the intended audience. Barnum and Kerfoot (1995) state that it is a mistake for a manager to write a message in anger. A communication written or spoken in an angry, confrontational tone almost always engenders a negative response from employees. A message that conveys respect and invites cooperation and collaboration is likely to be well received. The tone must be appropriate for the topic and the targeted audience, and both the short- and long-term effects of the message must be considered.

NONVERBAL COMMUNICATION

In face-to-face communication, the spoken word is accompanied by nonverbal behaviors. Sometimes the nonverbal behavior is planned and calculated, and other times it is unconscious on the part of all parties involved in the communication process. Communication is commonly considered a process, with words as symbols and language representing a code. When a person assumes a rigid posture and shakes a fist at someone else, words are not necessary to understand the meaning of the message. In a work setting, an angry, frowning face may convey a louder message than the words spoken or the tone of voice used. Gillies (1994) states, "To compensate for the inadequacy of verbal message information, people unconsciously use facial expression, gesture, touch, and vocal tone to amplify the meaning of spoken communication" (p. 184). Nonverbal communication includes appearance, tone of voice, gestures, body movements, glances, facial expressions, dress, smell, proximity, and gait (Dahnke and Clatterbuck, 1990; Ruthman in Kelly-Heidenthal, 2003). Tone may be more important than the words in a message, and facial expression may be more important than either. Even if the content of a message is fairly neutral and informative, if it is delivered by someone with an angry facial expression using a sharp tone of voice, the content of the message will most likely be overshadowed by the nonverbal behavior of the sender. Because nonverbal communication is usually unconscious, it is hard to control. It is important for the nonverbal message to be consistent with the verbal message. For example, it would be inappropriate to deliver a serious message of a planned layoff while smiling. Managers and employees should be aware of their nonverbal behavior and recognize its impact on all communication. Both managers and employees should monitor their nonverbal behaviors. They may also find it useful to seek feedback from others to determine if their nonverbal behaviors are consistent with their verbal messages and to determine the impact of their nonverbal behavior on the overall impression generated by their communication.

Nonverbal Cues

- Posture
- Gait
- Facial expression
- Gestures
- Body language
- Tone, pitch, and volume of voice

Note: There may be gender and cultural differences in communication that may impact/influence nonverbal behavior

VERTICAL, HORIZONTAL, AND DIAGONAL COMMUNICATION

In complex organizations, it is necessary for communication to flow in a variety of directions in order to attain organizational goals. Vertical, horizontal, and diagonal communications are used to communicate effectively.

Vertical Communication

Vertical communication is communication that occurs between superiors and subordinates. Vertical communication includes downward communication, in which information and other types of communication are sent by superiors to subordinates. Downward communication reflects the hierarchical structure of the organization. Downward communication can occur in a variety of ways depending, in part, on the content of the message. For example, news that will please subordinates, such as a bonus, would be delivered differently than news that might be distressing to them, such as upcoming layoffs (Barnum and Kerfoot, 1995). Some messages may need to be delivered by a variety of modes, such as face-to-face, mediated forms like video or audio, and written. For example, if a procedure is being changed, it may be announced in a unit meeting, reinforced by a memo to all employees affected by the change, and shown in a video detailing the proposed change. The revised procedure would then be written and placed on the nursing unit. The mediated and written messages also serve to provide a record of the communication. If employees do not adhere to the new procedure, they cannot say they were not informed of the changes if it is clear that they received a written notification or were present for a video detailing the procedure. Mantone (2004) reports the case of a chief executive officer (CEO) who was nearly removed from office because of great unrest in the medical staff due to poor communication. Although the organization was providing information to and communicating with the elected leaders of the medical staff, the information was not reaching the actual medical staff. The CEO learned that reinforcing the message is as important as delivering it initially. It is clear that the CEO should have communicated not only with the leadership of the medical staff but also with the medical staff as a whole, either in face-to-face meetings or in written format.

Upward communication occurs when employees or managers who are subordinate to top level management send messages up through the chain of command (Marquis and Huston, 2003). Each employee is expected to respect the chain of command and submit the communication to an immediate manager. Organizations should establish a culture that supports upward communication from employees. Subordinates should be educated as to how to use the chain of command to elicit information, provide input, and express concerns. If the immediate manager is unable to address the issue, it must be clear how that manager should move the message through the organization in order to respond to the person who submitted the message. Employees often feel that their input and questions are not welcomed and complain that they do not receive satisfactory responses, which may have a negative impact on employee satisfaction and productivity. It is generally easier to filter information down through the layers than to filter information upward (Keefe, 2004). For example, nursing staff members may be concerned about inadequate staffing on a unit. They bring their concerns to their nurse manager, who listens to them and assures them that their concerns are viable and will be addressed. Several weeks pass, and the staff nurses have had no further communication regarding staffing from the nurse manager. They again pose their concerns to the nurse manager, who assures them again that the administration is aware of the staffing difficulties and is working toward a solution. Nurses are likely to become increasingly frustrated when more time elapses with no definitive communication from the nurse manager and with no changes in the staffing patterns.

Horizontal Communication

Horizontal communication occurs when managers and others communicate with people on the same level in the organizational structure. Staff nurses communicate with other staff nurses, or nurse managers communicate with other managers. Communicating with others at the same level in the hierarchy is often more efficient than moving a communication up and down through the chain. Effective horizontal communication can facilitate coordination between departments as well as problem solving and decision making. Horizontal communication provides a direct, often expedient, way of solving problems and addressing issues critical to the effective functioning of the organization.

Diagonal Communication

In diagonal communication, managers interact with managers, physicians, and groups of people in other departments in the organization who are not on the same level in the hierarchy (Marquis and Huston, 2003). This type of interaction is important to the functioning of the organization and usually does not occur through formal means. Diagonal communication serves much the same function of being an expedient, direct route of decision making and problem solving as horizontal communication but encompasses a wider range of people throughout the organization. Diagonal communication allows managers to go directly to a person at a different level in the bureaucratic structure to resolve issues. For example, a nurse executive might work with the leadership of the medical staff to address a clinical issue.

FORMAL VERSUS INFORMAL COMMUNICATION

Organizations have both formal and informal communication networks. "Formal communication networks follow the formal line of authority in the organization's hierarchy. Informal communication networks occur between people at the same or different levels of the organizational hierarchy but do not represent formal lines of authority or responsibility" (Marquis & Huston, 2003, p. 339). Formal communication occurs when a nurse manager takes a unit problem to an immediate superior. Much communication occurs informally between employees who are not formally connected within the hierarchy. For example, nurses may have lunch with employees from the laboratory and discuss a process or procedure. Informal communication can occur in chance encounters within the organization but may be useful in accomplishing goals. Duemer and Mendez-Morse (2002) believe that people who hold higher positions in the organization have access to more formal communication, and those lower in the organization participate more easily in informal communication. The higher positions in the organizational hierarchy provide more access to key people in the organization, so formal communication can occur fairly easily. Further, managerial and administrative people often conduct business in regularly scheduled meetings. People who hold lower positions in the organization do not have the same access to key people. Given the difficulty in upward communication, employees may find it more expedient and convenient to engage in informal communication networks. Informal communication may be facilitated by proximity of employees to one another, making communication convenient. Baker (2002) observes that, traditionally, formal communication was considered to be the more effective type of communication in large bureaucratic organizations. Informal communication, traditionally considered as interpersonal or horizontal, was thought to hinder effective communication. Today, however, both formal and informal communication may be necessary for effectively conducting the work of modern organizations. Astute nurse executives recognize the need to incorporate informal communication into the communication network. The nurse executive may use informal communication, however, to clarify a formal communication, to provide or seek additional information on an issue, or as a vehicle for negotiation and persuasion.

GRAPEVINE

A common vehicle for informal communication in organizations is the grapevine. "The grapevine is the informal and unsanctioned information network within every organization" (Mishra, 1990, p. 213). The grapevine is essentially the rumor mill in an organization. Word is spread from one person to another outside the formal communication network. The grapevine is the spread of information without regard for the traditional networks of communication. Because management does not control the grapevine, it moves in every direction within the organization. Dowd, Davidhizar, and Dowd (1997) believe that in the absence of factual information, employees will fill in the lack of information with rumors. Grapevines carry both positive and negative messages. Rosnow (1983) suggests that productivity and morale are decreased when the grapevine consistently carries negative messages. In those situations, Crampton, Hodge, and Mishra (1998) believe management should focus more on the conditions in the organization that lead to the rumor rather than on the rumor itself. They observe that rumors usually develop when formal communication has been absent or unclear. Rosnow suggests that the more anxious people are, the more likely they are to participate in rumors. When focusing on the conditions that lead to rumors, managers should be aware of employee satisfaction and employee concerns. When employees believe they are being kept well informed of issues important to them, they may decrease the use of the grapevine. However, the grapevine is not all negative. Rosnow uses the example that if an employee is disciplined by a manager for tardiness, word will spread rapidly, and tardiness across the organization or department is likely to decrease. The grapevine is faster than memos or distributing policy or other more formal means of communication because the rumors are spread without regard for the conventional networks of communication dictated by the organizational structure.

Dowd, Davidhizar, and Dowd (1997) also believe that rumors may have the positive effect of relieving tension and helping employees adapt to change. If employees are concerned about a proposed change in policy or procedure, hearing others talk about the change may provide employees the opportunity to become accustomed to the idea. Further, if employees are worried about an issue or do not have complete official information about an impending change, listening to and passing along what others are saying or believing about the situation may relieve some stress and tension.

It is clear that managers need both to monitor and manage the grapevine as appropriate. If misinformation is rampant and is causing unrest, managers must intervene and provide factual information quickly. The most astute managers not only manage the grapevine but use it advantageously. Leftridge et al. (1999) report a technique used for managing the grapevine at one hospital. Members of management hung a grapevine wreath in the corridor of the nursing service and announced their plan at a staff meeting. They encouraged staff to write down any questions or rumors they wanted addressed and post them anonymously to the "grapevine." Managers' answers were written on purple paper, posted by e-mail, answered in staff meetings. and posted on the grapevine. This method allowed employees to ask questions they might not have asked in a formal setting. This exchange of ideas and information between employees and managers can be highly advantageous to the organization. It serves as a means of providing factual information and may serve to build trust between employees and management. The grapevine is a fact of life in every organization. The challenge becomes finding the best ways to use it to the organization's advantage.

Gender and Generational Differences in Communication

Many factors can affect communication in organizations where many people are involved in the communication process. Two such variables include gender and generational differences.

GENDER

It has long been recognized that men and women differ in their communication styles and prefer-

 chapter star

Nurse Manager M plans a staff meeting in order to share *organizational information* with the staff of Medical Surgical Unit 4 North. The information she received is *vertical information* as it came from the Director of Nursing for all medical-surgical areas, and there was no more opportunity to provide feedback into the decision-making process. This occurred during the budget preparation process. She chooses the staff meeting because this is a *formal* monthly meeting for her unit, and she has bad news about the next year's budget for the unit. Nurse Manger M wants to provide the information to her staff in a *face-to-face meeting* in order to provide an opportunity for questions. Three meetings are planned, one from 8 to 9 a.m. for the night shift, one from 2 to 3 p.m. for the evening shift, and one from 3 to 4 p.m. for the day shift. Evening staff members are on a weekday schedule at the time the monthly staff meetings are planned. Thus, everyone who works on the unit receives the same information in 1 day. Refreshments, drinks, and a nutritious snack are available at the beginning of each meeting. Nurse Manager M begins each of the three meetings in the same manner. She invites the employees into the meeting room and encourages them to have some refreshments. She is aware of her nonverbal behavior to assure that she appears formal, cordial, and open to staff members beginning casual conversation. She begins the meeting with an announcement about upcoming continuing education (CE) offerings. Then she proceeds to the budget information for next year's budget. She explains that, due to a projected lower census and change in Medicare reimbursement, the merit pool for the unit will only be 3%. She explains this means that if people are eligible for a merit raise, they can receive a maximum of only 3% of their base salary, and there will be no bonuses. She also informs staff that the education budget for the unit has been decreased. Therefore, they will be funded to attend only CE offerings hosted by the hospital CE Department. There will be no funds for anyone to attend any external conferences. Staff Nurse B asks her to explain the merit pool again. She repeats the same information. Staff Nurse B asks if employees will still be permitted administrative leave to attend an external conference if they pay their own way. Nurse Manager M responds that if staffing is covered and they do not have to use overtime or agency nurses to cover a vacancy, that could be a possibility. The meeting ends. She sends every staff member a *written memo* containing the key points that were covered at the meeting. The memo closes with information about how to reach her via e-mail if questions arise and the address of the hospital intranet, where members may read an electronic copy of the memo and have an opportunity to share ideas or ask questions. Nurse Aide C e-mails a question about changes in the paid time off accrual plan. Nurse Manager M responds by *e-mail* that there will be no changes for the next budget year and proofs and spellchecks the message before pressing the send button. Staff members post ideas for saving money for next year's budget in order to replace the lost travel and merit pool dollars.

ences. Tripp (2002) cites research by Nicotera and Rancer in 1994, which suggests that males are expected to and actually do exhibit more verbal aggressiveness and are more argumentative than females, which may place men in more credible positions in the hierarchy. Vanfosson (1996) reviewed the research on gender and communication and observed that men are more likely than women to initiate interaction and are more likely to interrupt other people than women. She ascertained that in meetings men obtain the "floor" more often and hold it longer than women. Vanfossen notes that the significance of the findings is that those who talk more in decision-making groups tend to become leaders. People in more powerful positions spend more time talking than people in less powerful positions. Tripp suggests that socialization and acculturation account for the vast majority of the differences in male and female communication behavior. He further notes that these findings in basic research are important to those involved in organizational communication. It is important for nurse administrators and managers to be aware of the general differences in communication patterns between males and females. This is particularly important because nursing is a discipline consisting primarily of females functioning in bureaucratic organizations potentially led by males. Nurses need to be aware of their own and others' communication styles so they can be equally effective within the organization as others. For example, female nurses may be less willing to speak out in meetings than their male counterparts but may find it necessary to do so in order to have equal input into important issues. When males are interacting within groups composed primarily of females, they may find it advantageous to modify their communication style to foster input from all members of the group.

GENERATIONAL

An organization comprises people of many ages, which can pose challenges for communicating throughout the organization. People across generations have different socialization and experiences that necessarily affect communication styles and preferences. Generalizations about younger people and older people and their attitudes about communication should be made cautiously, but some broad generalizations may apply. Many older people com-

plain that younger people are too casual, do not value face-to-face communication, and are too technology-dependent. Many younger people complain that older people are set in their ways and are not computer-savvy (Lieberman and Berardo, 2005). Even though all members of a generation may not share the same values and traits, most people are shaped by the important events in their early to middle years (Executive Update, 2000).

People of different generations prefer different methods of communicating and have different comfort levels with technology (Burke, 2004). According to this author, providing important information in a variety of formats increases the likelihood of people receiving the information in a format that they prefer.

Because people of different generations hold different goals, beliefs, and experiential backgrounds, misunderstandings occur in the workplace. These intergenerational misunderstandings can create tensions and strife, which results in unproductive use of time and energy (Executive Update, 2000). To decrease such tensions, managers may engage employees in team-building activities that draw on the strengths of each generation and provide learning opportunities for all members of the team. Having employees of several generations in an organization can bring a richness of experience and perspectives to the organization. Managers should strive to create a positive, empowering work environment that is valued by all generations in the workforce. Such a work environment can be created by using team- and camaraderie-building strategies and emphasizing communication. Management should provide information to employees in a variety of formats and facilitate interaction between people of all ages to foster mutual understanding and collaboration.

Information Technology and Electronic Communication

Technology has transformed clinical practice and has changed organizational communication itself. Clinical information systems allow nurses to chart at the bedside, eliminating duplicate documentation. Wireless technology allows nurses, for example, to access patient records, answer call lights from remote locations, and access databases for clinical practice. Technology also allows caregivers to have access to data when needed (Newbold, 2003).

As new clinical or administrative technology is being introduced, communication concerning resulting changes may be an important determinant of success. Simpson (1996) observes that when implementing an information technology system, organizational communication about the technology must be tailored to the specific audience. Employees should be kept well informed of the new systems throughout the change process. If employees believe they have been a part of the change process, they are more likely to accept the proposed change.

ELECTRONIC HEALTH RECORDS

It has been widely recognized that information technology systems have the potential to improve safety and quality of patient care. Electronic health record (EHRs) are an integral part of the information technology system that can positively affect patient care. Kauka (2005) recognizes several benefits of EHRs, including facilitating faster and better communication among providers, allowing for faster and simultaneous access to patient data by authorized providers, reducing errors resulting in better outcomes and lower costs, and improving patient confidentiality.

The Institute of Medicine of the National Academies has identified a set of core functions that EHRs should fulfill in order to promote patient safety and increase quality and efficiency in health-care delivery (The National Academies, 2003). The eight functions fall into the categories of: (1) health information and data, (2) results management, (3) order entry/management, (4) decision support, (5) electronic communication and connectivity, (6) patient support, (7) administrative processes, and (8) reporting and population health management (Institute of Medicine, 2003). The National Academies (2003) note that immediate access to health information and data regarding patients' diagnoses, allergies, medications, laboratory test results, etc., is useful in timely decision making. Results management speaks to the ability of providers of care in multiple settings to have quick access to new and past data, such as laboratory test results, thereby increasing patient safety and quality of care. Decision support includes computerized decision support systems to facilitate compliance with best practices. It uses reminders, prompts, and alerts; identifies possible drug interactions; facilitates screenings and preventive practices; and facilitates diagnoses and treatments. The National Academies go on to observe that electronic communication and connectivity include readily accessible communication among providers and patients that is secure, efficient, and readily accessible, which reduces the frequency of adverse events through timely diagnoses and treatment. Patient support includes tools that assist patients in controlling chronic conditions through home monitoring and self-testing, having access to their health records, and providing interactive patient education. Administrative processes include computerized tools that improve provider efficiency. Reporting includes data storage using uniform data standards, which help health-care organizations fulfill reporting requirements. These functional categories will serve as a basis for development of industry standards for EHRs and will guide the development of software that includes those functional areas (The National Academies, 2003). Ideal EHRs are still in development, and health systems and vendors alike continue to work toward refining them.

EHRs have the potential to alter the way patient information is managed throughout the system with positive effects on patient safety and quality of care. Patients may view their medical records through secure access using the Internet. Ross, Moore, Earnest, Wittenvrongel, and Lin (2004) state that such access to their medical records may help patients in the management of chronic diseases. They conducted a study to ascertain the effects on patient care and clinic operations of patient-accessible online medical records concerning patients with congestive heart failure. They used software that included an educational guide and messaging system between patients and staff. The sample included 107 patients, 54 of whom were in the intervention group and 53 in the control group. The researchers found that providing these patients with an online medical record was not only feasible but also improved treatment adherence (Ross, et al., 2004).

The use of computerized systems has altered not only methods of patient care delivery but also the way people communicate in organizations. Norton and Lester (1996) observed that electronic communication breaks down rigid organizational structure and actually circumvents hierarchy because infor-

Practice Proof 8-1

Hassol et al. (2004) conducted a study to ascertain patients' attitudes toward access to their EHRs and Web-based communication with providers. Most respondents indicated that they found the system easy to use and that their medical records were complete, accurate, and understandable. The researchers found that only a minority of the respondents were concerned about confidentiality of their records or about seeing abnormal test results after they had received an electronic explanation of the results from their health-care provider. The respondents preferred e-mail communication for general medical information and prescription renewals but preferred personal communication for getting treatment instructions. They did not indicate a preference for telephone or written communication for any of their needs. However, the physicians were more likely to prefer telephone communication to e-mail communication.

1. Why might patients prefer personal communication for treatment instructions as opposed to general medical information and prescription renewals?
2. Identify at least one reason physicians may prefer telephone communication to e-mail.
3. From the study, it is clear that EHRs must be complete, understandable, and accurate if patients are to find them useful. What other component is essential to patients' use of EHRs?

mation flows around rather than through the traditional organizational hierarchy. They note that organizational culture and common sense can control such communication fairly well and that there should be rules and procedures to govern use of information technology. For example, if a communication is sent to staff from the chief nurse executive, it should be made clear whether the staff members can respond to the communication directly or if they should go through their supervisor. In health care, there is always the overriding issue of privacy, so each organization will have policies governing what information is accessible to categories of staff and under what circumstances.

INTRANETS

One way that organization-wide communication has changed through technology is the establishment of intranets using Web technology. Intranets are private, in-house systems that allow people to communicate and share information easily and efficiently (Cupito, 1997). Use of intranets varies, but the commonality is that they improve communication. Notices that keep employees informed on a given topic can be posted; information that is specific to the organization becomes accessible to staff, such as policies, announcements, events, and so on. White (2004) believes that in order to get the most from an intranet, the intranet has to be a part of the overall communication strategy of the organization. He stresses the importance of people being able to trust the information they obtain and being able to find current and correct information on the system. Sinickas (2004) reports on research from 20 organizations over 4 years. Of the employees surveyed, only about 33% said they would like to rely on the intranet exclusively for communication in the workplace, and about 50% said they would like it to be a component of the communication system in the organization. Only about 10% of the employees stated that they did not wish to receive any information through the intranet. These findings point out the necessity for managers to use a variety of techniques when communicating to a diverse population.

E-MAIL AS COMMUNICATION

Electronic mail (e-mail) is a widely accepted communication technique. Organizations have come to rely on e-mail as a fast, efficient means of communicating with large numbers of people or a single person. Although e-mail allows the recipient to answer when time allows, it is expected that e-mail will be answered in a timely manner. A recent cartoon depicted a manager standing at the desk of an employee, stating that the employee should have checked his e-mail more often as he was fired weeks ago. This exemplifies two important points. E-mail would be an inappropriate means of informing an employee of something as serious as termination of employment. It also points out the need for employees to read e-mails in a timely manner to stay informed and receive current information.

E-mail allows large numbers of employees to receive the same message at the same time. However, e-mail is not a perfect way to communicate and should only be part of an overall communication strategy. Simpson (1996) notes that an e-mail cannot be sent to 100 people with an expectation that the message will be commonly understood and interpreted correctly by all of the recipients. Managers must understand that employees may not all interpret an e-mail in exactly the same way. Interpretation will vary, depending on the topic, complexity of the message, position of the employee in the organization, and personal perception. Sinickas (2004) notes that electronic communication seems to reduce employees' need for or expectation of face-to-face communication more than it decreases their desire for printed communication. With the use of e-mail, employees seem to have fewer expectations that communications in the organization will occur face-to-face. Many people may still wish to have notices written and posted or provided to them by some means other than e-mail, however.

E-mail is an expedient way to communicate within organizations but less confidential and secure than some other forms of communication. When using this mode of communication, there is need for security to avoid unauthorized disclosure of patient information or other privileged information. Because the very nature of e-mail encourages spontaneous communication, and because much information in a health-care organization warrants confidentiality, organizations should have an e-mail usage policy. The policy should be designed to protect confidential information, ensure that the organization is in compliance with all relevant national and state laws, and inform employees of the rules that apply to their appropriate use of e-mail. Organizations may establish rules that deal with personal use of e-mail, including the kinds of messages and material that are suitable for transmission in the workplace. Van Doren (1996) notes that while employers consider monitoring of e-mail as their responsibility to protect confidential information, employees may view the monitoring as an invasion of their privacy. Van Doren further observes that e-mail communication of employees in hospitals and long-term care facilities is being obtained by the legal system and used as evidence against them in lawsuits. The issue of liability points out the importance of policies to govern use of e-mail within an organization.

One major advantage of e-mail is that managers can provide immediate information to many people within the organization, for example, to counter the rumors spread through the grapevine. Managers should proofread their messages before they are sent to be sure they are accurate and carry the intended message. E-mail is a convenient way for managers to keep employees feeling that they are well informed of issues of importance to them.

Importance of Organizational Communication

Effective communication is an essential component of organizational functioning. It is generally accepted that communication directly affects patient safety and quality of care. "According to findings from a study released in a national briefing of healthcare stakeholders, the prevalent culture of poor communication and collaboration among health professionals relates significantly to continued medical errors and staff turnovers" (Kohn & Henderson, 2005). Adubato (2004) observes that many thousands of people die each year from medical errors during their hospital stay. He states, "These are not caused by high-tech medical equipment breakdown, but by sloppy, downright poor communication by health-care professionals who should know better" (p. 33). Amatayakul and Cohen (2004) believe that optimal communication is as important in reducing medication errors as computerized physician order entry and other efforts to improve patient safety.

Hanlon (1996) says that poor communication is often cited as a source of stress for nurses. He believes that when nurses have repeated unsatisfactory communication experiences, there is a cumulative effect that creates stress. This stress, according to Hanlon, may contribute to burnout, job dissatisfaction, and increased turnover, all of which serve to decrease the quality of care received by patients. Similarly, Breisch (1999) believes that effective communication, as well as accountability and recognition, is necessary for motivating employees. She explains that nurses' responsibilities have become more complex with greater patient acuity, more rigorous documentation requirements, and technological advances. These factors support the need for nurse managers to create a work environment that supports the needs of the work group. In fact, the importance of effective communication in the organization is reflected in The Scope and Standards for Nurse Administrators, which states that the nurse administrator "creates a climate of effective communication" (American Nurses Association, p. 26).

PRACTICE TO STRIVE FOR

Adena Health System in Chillicothe, Ohio, developed an innovative way to meet the accreditation requirements of the Joint Commission on Accreditation of Healthcare Organizations (JCAHO). Effective organizational communication was key to Adena's innovative approach to the accreditation process.

JCAHO instituted a new process whereby surveyors selected approximately 11 active patients and retraced their care through different departments. The surveyors observed care given, reviewed policies and procedures, and questioned staff and patients in different areas of the hospital. Because of the uniqueness of each patient and the differences in each area of the hospital, preparing the facility for a survey was challenging. The unpredictable nature of tracer activities proved to be difficult for even the most experienced managers and survey coordinators. Historically, Adena had used mock surveys and electronic communication to prepare the staff for the JCAHO visit, but these methodologies had failed to generate any enthusiasm among the staff. Further, following the accreditation visit, most practices returned to the way they had been prior to the visit.

The "Survivor Adena" concept was developed based on the popular *Survivor* television series. The objectives of Survivor Adena were to provide a framework to motivate and engage the organization in survey readiness to sustain the results of the preparation. A tribal council was developed to lay the groundwork for Survivor Adena, which focused on innovative ways to communicate effectively with staff to engage them in the accreditation process, empower staff to make changes, and provide ongoing education needed to make the required organizational changes. Adena's staff was given the task of developing over 120 "tribes." Each tribe had the challenge of picking an area of focus that combined the concepts of JCAHO's "Shared Visions" tracer methodology and any "hot button" areas such as patient safety, medication management, and infection control. Tribes were encouraged to collaborate with other departments and collaborate on a common goal.

Weekly, mini-challenges were electronically mailed to Adena's staff. The mini-challenges were quizzes that focused on specific topics or standards of care. It was mandatory for staff to complete the weekly quizzes. A Survivor Adena Fair was held to bring various departments together to provide educational booths and fun activities to promote sustained excitement and motivation concerning the upcoming survey. Complete participation was expected from the staff, and 99% indicated on a survey that the fair was beneficial and provided a good learning opportunity. Incentives were built into the plan, with people and tribes earning tickets that were cashed for various prizes at the end of the 18-month Survivor Adena project.

Adena had a successful survey and received very few requirements for improvement. Dawn Allen, Director of Quality Management and Medical Staff Services at Adena, stated that the participation, enthusiasm, and activity from the staff in preparing for the JCAHO survey were unprecedented in this system. She further noted that traditional methods of a unilaterally driven project will no longer meet the expectations of JCAHO's Shared Vision framework and that creating a culture of continuous survey readiness is crucial. The system believes that the shared vision at Adena of communicating effectively with employees and encouraging communication between departments was instrumental in developing ownership of the concept of continuous survey readiness. The outcome of their efforts is a system with a culture of safety and quality that is imbedded within the organization.

All Good Things...

Communication is essential to the goal attainment and overall success of an organization. Effective organizational communication is challenging in many ways, given the complexity of health-care systems. Because good communication is such an important component of successful operation, it is well worth the time and effort it takes to develop effective communication strategies. Nurse administrators and managers responsible for internal communication must recognize that people interpret messages differently, depending on several factors, including their experiential background and position in the organization. Further, there are gender and generational differences that must be recognized and accommodated when communicating with many people in an organization. Managers must choose the correct mode of communicating messages depending on the intent of the message. Some messages may need to be delivered face to face, and others may be sent by memo, e-mail, in a group setting in meetings, or some combination of modes. Managers also have the obligation to ascertain whether important information has been understood correctly by diverse employee groups. Employees must understand their responsibility in the communication process and how the flow of information is to occur from the level of the employee to those at higher levels of the hierarchy. Management is then obligated to address employee concerns in a timely and effective manner.

Communication has been shown to require a time commitment by managers in order for it to be effective throughout the organization. This commitment is well worth the effort as effective communication influences employee satisfaction, quality care, and customer satisfaction. Effective communication within an organization improves the coordination of decision making and may decrease the use of the grapevine. Excellent organizational communication facilitates the attainment of organizational goals and is necessary for almost every aspect of operations. Effective communication within the organization should be a priority of every nurse manager and is an essential component of effective leadership.

Let's Talk

1. *Name at least two benefits of effective organizational communication.*

2. *Think of an example of how interpersonal communication, small-group communication, and organizational communication can be used in the organization.*

3. *Identify at least three factors that might cause employees to interpret a message differently.*

4. *Provide an example of vertical, horizontal, and diagonal communication in a health-care organization.*

NCLEX Questions

1. A chief nurse executive sends a memorandum to the nursing staff announcing a change in the policy concerning absenteeism. This represents an example of:
   A. Horizontal communication.
   B. Diagonal communication.
   C. Upward communication.
   D. Vertical communication.

2. Organizational communication involves relaying information to many people in order to accomplish organizational goals. Organizational communication includes small-group communication and:
   A. Interpersonal communication.
   B. Repetition.
   C. Discipline of employees.
   D. Role development.

3. The act of extracting meaning from symbols is termed:
   A. Encoding.
   B. Symbolic code.
   C. Transmission.
   D. Decoding.

4. When communicating within an organization, employees are expected to respect the:
   A. Use of technology.
   B. Chain of command.
   C. Decision-making method.
   D. Time factor in the communication process.

5. From an employee perspective, the most difficult communication mode is often:
   A. Horizontal communication.
   B. Diagonal communication.
   C. Verbal communication.
   D. Upward communication.

6. If a nurse manager finds it necessary to terminate an employee, the most appropriate means of delivering this message would be by:
   A. E-mail.
   B. Written letter.
   C. Face-to-face discussion.
   D. Memorandum.

7. Which type of communication is most likely to be misinterpreted by employees?
   A. Written messages.
   B. Face-to-face communication.

C. Nonverbal communication.
D. Diagonal communication.

8. Nonverbal communication includes:
A. Facial expression.
B. Vocal tone.
C. Gestures.
D. All of the above.

9. Factors that may cause different interpretation of messages by employees include personal experiences, socialization, educational background, age, and _____.
A. Years of service as an employee.
B. Gender.
C. Department in which employed.
D. Selective hearing.

10. Research has shown that e-mail seems to decrease employees' need for face-to face communication but does not necessarily reduce their desire for:
A. Group meetings.
B. More confidential means of communication.
C. Written communication.
D. Phone messages.

REFERENCES

Adamson, G., Emswiller, T., and Olliver, C. (1991). Communicating the vision; visions communicated. *The Healthcare Forum Journal, 34*(12).

Adubato, S. (2004). Making the communication connection. *Nursing Management, 35*(9), 33–35.

Amatayakul, M., & Cohen, M.R. (2004). First communication, then automation. *Healthcare Financial Management, 58*(5), 102–104. Retrieved March 14, 2005, from http://proquest.umi.commmmmmm/pqdweb?did=639202301&Fmt=3&clientID=52052&RQT=309&VName=PQD

Baker, K. (2002). Organizational communication Chapter 13. *Organizational Communication,* June 8, 2002. Retrieved March 8, 2005, from www.sc.doe.gov/sc-5/benchmark/Ch%2013%20Organizational%20Communication%202006.08.02.pdf

Barnum, B.S., & Kerfoot, K.M. (1995). The nurse as executive. (4th ed.). Gaithersburg, MD: Aspen.

Breisch, L. (1999). Motivate. *Nursing Management, 30*(3), 27–30

Burke, M.E. (2004). Generational differences survey report. *Society of Human Resource Management.* Retrieved June 30, 2005, from www.shrm.org/hrresources/surveys_published/Generational%20Differences%20Survery%20

Crampton, S.M., Hodge, J.W., & Mishra, J.M. (1998). The informal communication network: Factors influencing grapevine activity. *Public Personnel Management, 27*(4), 569–584.

Crow, G. (2002). The relationship between trust, social capital, and organizational success. *Nursing Administration Quarterly, 29*(3), 1–11.

Cupito, M. (1997). Intranets: Communication for the internal universe. *Health Management Technology, 18*(7), 20–24. Retrieved March 14, 2005, from http://proquest.umi.com/pqdweb?did=12566403&Fmt=4&clientId=52052&RQT=309&VName=PQD

Dahnke, G.L., & Clatterbuck, G.W. (1990). *Human communication: Theory and research.* Belmont, CA: Wadsworth.

Dowd, S.B., Davidhizar, R., & Dowd, L. (1997). Rumors and gossip: A guide for the health care supervisor. *The Health Care Supervisor, 16*(1), 65–71.

Duemer, L.S., & Mendez-Morse, S. (2002). Recovering policy implementation: Understanding implementation through informal communication. *Education Policy Analysis Archives, 10*(39). Retrieved March 14, 2005, from http://epaa.asu.edu/epaa/10n39.html

Executive Update. (July 2000). *Uncommon threads: Mending the generation gap at work.* Retrieved June 30, 2005, from http://www.centeronline.org/knowledge/article.cfm?ID=841&ContentProfileID=122864&...

Gillies, D.A. (1994). *Nursing management* (3rd ed.). Philadelphia: W.B. Saunders.

Hanlon, J.M. (1996). Teaching effective communication skills. *Nursing Management, 27*(4), 48–49.

Hassol, A., et al. (2004). Patient experiences and attitudes about access to a patient electronic health care record and linked web messaging. *Journal of the American Medical Informatics Association, 11*:505–513.

Institute of Medicine of the National Academies. (2003). *Key capabilities of an electronic heath record system.* The National Academies Press.

jamia.org/cgi/content/abstract/11/6/505

Kauka, M. (2005). Computerized patient record, electronic medical record and electronic record: A comparison in differences. (2005) Retrieved November 30, 2005, from: http://www.avazmd.com/resoures/emr_cpr_ehr.html

Keefe, L. (2004). Generating quality interaction. *Occupational Health and Safety, 73*(5), 30–32.

Kelly-Heidenthal, P. (2003). *Nursing leadership and management.* Canada: Thomson-Delmar Learning.

Kohn, K., & Henderson, C.W. (2005). *Managed Care Weekly,* 5.

Leftridge, D.W., et al. (1999). Improved communication in a shared governance system. *Nursing Management, 30*(3), 50–51.

Lieberman, S., & Berardo, K. (2005). Simma Lieberman Associates. Retrieved June 30, 2005, from http://www.simmalieberman.com/articles/archived_news/april_2005.html

Mantone, J. (2004). Communication is key. *Modern Healthcare, 34*(45), S12–13.

Marquis, B.L., & Huston, C.J. (2003). *Leadership roles and management functions in nursing.* Philadelphia: Lippincott Williams & Wilkins.

Mishra, J. (1990). Managing the grapevine. *Public Personnel Management, 19*(2), 213–228.

National Academies. (2003). Institute of medicine report identifies core capabilities that should be part of an electronic health record system. Retrieved November 22, 2005, from: http://www4.nationalacademies.org/news.nsf/isbn/N1000427?

Newbold, S.K. (2003). New uses for wireless technology. *Nursing Management: IT Solutions.* Retrieved March 6, 2005, from http://proquest.umi.com/pqdweb?did=44288665& Fmt=3&clientid=52052&RQT=309&VName=PQD

Norton, M., & Lester, J. (1996). Digital accessibility: Information value in changing hierarchies. American Society for Information Science. *Bulletin of the American Society for Information Science, 22*(6), 21–25. Retrieved March 7, 2005, from http://proquest.umi.com/pqdweb? did=10220417& FMT=3&clientId=52052&RQT=309& VName=PQD

Rosnow, R.D. (1983). Corporate rumors: How they start and how to stop them. *Management Review, 72*(4), 44–50.

Ross, S., Moore, L., Earnest, M., Wittenvrongel, L., & Lin, C. (2004). Providing a Web-based online medical record with electronic communication capabilities to patients with congestive heart failure: A randomized trial. *Journal of Medical Internet Research, 6*(2), e12.

Schumann, M. (2004). Enhancing corporate credibility. *Communication World,* 28–32.

Scope and standards for nurse administrators. (2004). (2nd ed.). American Nurses Association.

Simpson, R. (1996). What we have is a failure to communicate. *Nursing Management, 27*(10), 18–20.

Sinickas, A.D. (2004). Intranet anyone? Take the guesswork out of using electronic channels. *Communication World,* January–February.

Spears, L.A. (1997). Writing business communications: Are nurse managers prepared? *Nursing Management, 28*(12), 43–45.

Trenholm, S. (1991). *Human communication theory* (2nd ed.). Englewood Cliffs, NJ: Prentice Hall.

Tripp, M.A. Gender differences in communication. Retrieved April 7, 2005, from http://www.umm.maine.edu/resources/beharchive/bexstudents/MarkTripp/mt320.html

Van Doren, J.A. (1996). If you monitor e-mail, have a policy. *The Health Care Supervisor, 15*(1), 12.

Vanfossen, B. (1996). Gender differences in communication. Institute for Teaching and Research on Women, Towson University, Towson, MD. Retrieved April 7, 2005, from http://pages.towson.edu/itrow/wmcomm.htm

White, M. (2004). Does your intranet have a win-win strategy? *EContent Wilton, 27*(3), 41. Retrieved March 14, 2005, from http://proquest.umi.com/pqdweb?did=589394&Fmt=3& clientId=52052&RQT=309&VName=PQD

Wolper, L.F. (2004). *Health care administration* (4th ed.). Boston: Jones and Bartlett.

BIBLIOGRAPHY

Adams, D.A., Nelson, R.R., and Todd, P.A. (1993). A comparative evaluation of the impact of electronic and voice mail on organizational communication. *Information and Management, 22*(1), 9–21.

Allen, D.G., & Griffith, R.W. (1997). Vertical and lateral information processing: The effects of gender, employee classification level, and media richness on communication and work outcomes. *Human Relations, 50*(10), 1230–1260.

Herring, S. (2000). Gender differences in CMC: findings and implications. *The CPSR Newsletter 18*(1). http://www.cpsr.org/prevsite/publications/newsletters/issues/2000/Winter 2000/herring.html

Ngwenyama, O.K., & Lee, A.S. (1997). Communication richness in electronic mail: Critical social theory and the contextuality of meaning. *MIS Quarterly, 21*(2), 145–167.

Rothenberg, R.L. (1995). Using information networks for competitive advantage. *Healthcare Financial Management 49*(1), 73.

Weening, M.W.H. (1999). Communication networks in the diffusion of an innovation in an organization. *Journal of Applied Social Psychology, 29*(5), 1072–1092.

Yazici, H.J. (2002). The role of communication in organizational change: An empirical investigation. *Information and Management 39*, 539–552.

Informatics

SHARON MCLANE, MBA, RN, BC

"Without continual growth and progress, such words as improvement, achievement, and success have no meaning."

Benjamin Franklin (1706–1790)

CHAPTER MOTIVES

- Define nursing informatics.
- Compare and contrast the nursing process and standards of informatics practice.
- Describe the role of information system standards in supporting communication between practitioners.
- Discuss the implications of nursing terminology to future nursing practice.
- Identify the six goals of information systems in the 21st century.
- Identify ways in which nursing informatics influences clinical practice.
- Identify personal accountabilities with regard to informatics.

Nursing informatics is a relatively new specialty, which has been marked by rapid growth in terms of numbers of practitioners as well in the explosion of domain knowledge. Beginning with the Social Security Act amendment of 1965, which established Medicare and Medicaid, the growth in the use of computers in health care was assured. This act required documentation of care, most notably nursing care, and the progression of nursing documentation in the medical record received a significant boost (Thede, 2003).

The first nursing informatics specialists emerged in 1981, when approximately 15 nurses identified nursing informaticists as their practice specialty (Saba & McCormick, 2006). Nursing informatics was recognized as a specialty by the American Nurses Association (ANA) in 1992, thereby denoting it as a distinct nursing practice specialty with a unique scope of practice. In 1994, ANA published the first Scope of Practice for Nursing Informatics, followed by the Standards of Practice for Nursing Informatics in 1995. Once the scope and standards of practice were clearly articulated, the American Nurses Credentialing Center (ANCC) offered the first certification examination in December 1995. As of December 31, 2005, 566 nurses were certified across the United States as Nurse Informaticists (T. Norris, ANCC, personal communication, April 20, 2006).

Throughout the last two decades of the 20th century, informatics grew as a specialty in health care as well as within the nursing profession. As the use of electronic documentation systems grew from small, isolated demonstration projects to a mainstream reality, it became clear to nursing leaders that the profession needed to define taxonomies and classification models and minimum data sets that could be coded for documentation, storage, and retrieval in electronic medical record systems. Additionally, demand was growing for nursing protocols, innovative methods to support nursing and patient education, and expert systems incorporating knowledge representation and decision support and evidence-based practice. With these compelling objectives, nursing informatics has a practice agenda on which to focus for the foreseeable future (Saba, 2001).

Definition of Nursing Informatics

Graves and Corcoran provided the first definition of nursing informatics in 1989: "A combination of computer science, information science, and nursing science designed to assist in the management and processing of nursing data, information, and knowledge to support the practice of nursing and the delivery of nursing care" (Graves & Corcoran, 1989, p. 227). These two scholars also clarified that professional information systems serve as a foundation for the dimensions of supporting decisions and advancing the knowledge of the discipline. The Graves and Corcoran definition has been expanded by the ANA: "Nursing informatics is a specialty that integrates nursing science, computer science, and information science to manage and communicate data, information, and knowledge in nursing practice. Nursing informatics facilitates the integration of data, information, and knowledge to support patients, nurses, and other providers in their decision making in all roles and settings. This support is accomplished through the use of information structures, information processes, and information technology" (American Nurses Association, 2001, p. 17).

Several important factors are inherent in these definitions. First, the definitions illustrate that nursing informatics is a multidisciplinary science practice. Second, the definitions clarify that nursing informatics is not to be equated with the generic term informatics; it is specific to nursing and nursing practice because of the inclusion of the nursing science domain. Nurses specializing in nursing informatics employ their nursing science knowledge to mold, provide direction to, and influence the design of nursing information systems. Another core component is computer science. Nursing informatics is not about computers but rather the core elements derived from computers—data, information, and knowledge—and how best to structure nursing documentation systems to ensure that the output will meet the needs of patient care and nursing science. We will discuss these three concepts later, but it is important to note that computer technology is the tool by which the outputs of information science are derived and which are an important facet of nursing informatics.

Dr. James Turley suggested the addition of cognitive science to the definition of nursing informatics. Understanding the processes employed in structuring knowledge; representing knowledge; and employing knowledge in decision making, recall, and perception are important dimensions in the practice and application of informatics. Ongoing research in the cognitive domain provides important understanding to guide the design of information system software, helping to create systems that are increasingly more useful and more effective in supporting decision making by clinicians.

Turley suggests a model that incorporates the elements of Graves and Corcoran's model—nursing, information, and computer science—and adds the domain of cognitive science. Furthermore, Turley suggests that the nursing science is the foundation on which the other three sciences rest. Turley's model also suggests that it is the *intersection* of the cognitive, information, and computer sciences that constitutes nursing informatics (Turley, 1996). Nursing science is the raison d'être of nursing informatics, and without the needs and context of nursing science nursing informatics would have no purpose. Turley's model has the further advantage of flexibility: the model can be translated to other health-care science disciplines by changing the foundational domain.

Nursing informatics has the purpose and the potential to support and improve the care of patients and communities through the collection, management, and communication of information about and for the patient. As well, nursing informatics can assist in making the contributions of nursing visible in the medical record and assist the nurse by providing decision support tools. Nurses are presented with an increasing array and complexity of information that they are expected to synthesize and incorporate into their patient care decisions. More information does not necessarily result in better care unless it is thoughtfully analyzed, organized, and presented in ways that are meaningful to nurses and their practice. The timing, content, and format of the information can vary with the recipient; the information needs of clinicians at the point of care are different from the needs of the manager or administrator, and those needs differ from the needs of the policy maker.

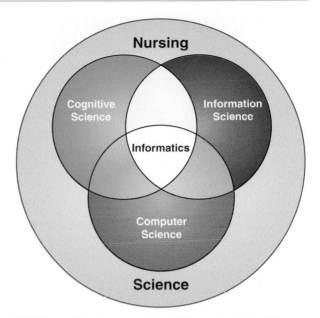

FIGURE 9-1 Turley's suggested model for nursing informatics.

Consequently, a pivotal role of the informaticist is to collaborate with those individuals and groups to discover their information needs and the decisions that will result and translate those needs into creation of appropriate data collection, analysis, and presentation formats.

Nursing Informatics Standards of Practice

The standards of nursing informatics practice carefully parallel the nursing process (see Table 9-1). The clinical nurse focuses on assessing the needs of a patient and the individuals in the patient's support system. The nurse then develops a plan of care based on careful prioritizing of the nursing diagnoses. Then the plan is implemented and assessed and evaluated according to the patient's responses to the plan. Data collected during evaluation are thoughtfully analyzed, and appropriate modifications are made to the plan of care.

The focus of the nurse informaticist is assessment of systems problems as identified by a group of clinical practitioners; identification of the problems,

TABLE 9-1	Comparing the Nursing Process and Nursing Informatics Standards of Practice

NURSING PROCESS	STANDARDS OF INFORMATICS PRACTICE
Assessment: ■ Collect data from physical examination of patient ■ Collect data from listening to patient and family ■ Analyze data ■ Identify patient's problems related to health status	Identify the issue or problem: ■ Prepare a project charter and initial project plan based on assessed problems, opportunities, and directives of the project ■ Define business requirements for a new system ■ Define the desired functional requirements, or activities and services, of the new system
Diagnoses ■ Formulate a nursing diagnosis related to each health problem ■ Prioritize the problems and diagnoses in collaboration with patient and/or family	Identify alternatives: ■ Analyze requirements in terms of data, processes, interfaces, etc., the system will require ■ Analyze possible solutions in terms of technical, operational, economic, and timeline feasibility ■ Prepare solution recommendation(s) for discussion with the users
Plan: ■ Discuss patient's expectations ■ Establish outcome goals for patient in collaboration with patient and/or family Implement: ■ Set plan of care in action, delegating responsibilities as appropriate ■ Communicate plan of care to other team members	Choose and develop a solution: ■ Select a solution in collaboration with users ■ Create a project plan, which include timelines, dependencies, evaluation milestones, and evaluation metrics Implement the solution: ■ Implement programming of the solution ■ At defined intervals, evaluate the developing solution in collaboration with users ■ Implement the fully completed solution
Evaluate: ■ Evaluate plan and implementation as ongoing events ■ Adjust plan as appropriate in context of data collected ■ Return to assessment in context of changing needs and data collected	Evaluate and modify: ■ Evaluate solution with evaluation metrics ■ Implement programming and workflow modifications in response to feedback ■ Evaluate solution after completion of programming modifications to determine further needs or issues (Whitten, Bentley, & Dittman, 2000)

opportunities, and constraints; and description of the outcomes the group desires to achieve. Using the information gathered during the assessment phase, the nurse informaticist prioritizes the problems and constraints; carefully explores alternatives in the context of time, fiscal, and resource constraints; and prepares recommendations for the team to consider. Working closely with the clinicians, the nurse informaticist facilitates and supports the clinical team in selecting a solution from the options presented, ensuring that the advantages and limitations of each solution are explored carefully. Once the clinical team has chosen the most appropriate solution, the nurse informaticist works with the system programmers during design of the software solution, reviewing the progress of the plan with the clinical

team at key junctures. Upon completion of the programming process, the system is implemented, and the evaluation phase begins. Employing evaluation measures defined during the planning phase, the nurse informaticist gathers the evaluation data, analyzes them, and works with the programmers and the clinical team to define the nature of system modifications necessary to resolve identified system issues. The evaluation process and subsequent system modification are iterative.

It is important to recognize that the above summary is just that—a very high-level summary. Just as the brief description of the nursing process does not begin to describe the details of interventions and decisions a nurse makes during an episode of patient care, the same can be said for the processes, interventions, and decisions of the nursing informaticist. It is also important to point out that the process of identifying and implementing systems solutions necessitates development of detailed workflow information, and the solutions often include changes in workflow that are not related to the software solution. Nonetheless, there is value in identifying and comparing the parallels between the nursing processes of patient care and the analysis processes of information system design and informatics.

Health-Care Data Standards

Data standards are intended to minimize confusion and assure that data are collected, stored, transmitted, and retrieved in a manner that ensures that the original meaning is intact and that actions taken in response to the data are consistent with the original meaning of the data (Sensmeier, 2006, p. 218). A discussion of data standards should begin with a clear understanding of what constitutes a standard. A standard is an agreed-upon reference point, criterion, or value against which something can be measured. To be effective, data standards include discrete, precise definitions, adherence to which is not optional (Thede, 2003, p. 205). Dr. Thede used an apt analogy from the 19th century U.S. railroad industry in discussing her vision of standards. In the railroad's early days, standards for track width, or gauge, had not been established, and each railroad company was free to create its own gauge. The problems associated with multiple widths quickly became apparent when trains from different railroad companies could not travel beyond their own territory. The problems this created for passenger and product movement quickly became apparent and necessitated that the competing companies come to agreement on a standard gauge. In the health-care industry, much work is focused on standard development. Some standards are widely accepted, and others are evolving. The following discussion will briefly describe some of the collaborative work currently being conducted in the United States and globally.

Interoperability is another term that is frequently used in discussions regarding health-care information systems standards. Systems that can effectively exchange data and effectively and effi-

ciently use the data that have been exchanged have interoperability. Health-care data standards are designed to support and enable interoperability.

Data standards include "methods, protocols, terminologies, and specifications for the collection, exchange, storage, and retrieval of information associated with health care applications, including medical records, medications, radiological images, payment and reimbursement, medical devices and monitoring systems, and administrative processes" (Washington Publishing Company, 1998). Data standards encompass four primary areas:

1. Definition of data elements.
2. Determining data interchange formats to establish how data elements are to be encoded as well as to assure relationships between data elements through defining how documents and information models should be structured.
3. Terminologies, which identify and define the terms and concepts used to classify and code data elements and establish relationships between the concepts and terms.
4. Knowledge representation, as provided by electronic medical literature, guidelines, evidence-based practice protocols, and clinical decision support (Institute of Medicine, 2004, pp. 128-129).

Data Elements

Data elements are the most basic pieces of information collected, and in order to be able to use the collected data they must be defined clearly, discretely, and unambiguously. Definition includes determining how the data are to be collected, by what software application, by what hardware, and when they are to be collected. It is also important to establish how the data will be entered into the software system, e.g., as free text or by selection of predefined responses using coded values. Without clearly defined, consistently entered, unambiguous data, the ability to recover data with assurance of content is greatly diminished, as is the potential of the use of the data in future research.

The question of what data should be collected was answered in part through the development of minimum data sets, an example of which is the Nursing Minimum Data Set (NMDS) (Table 9-2).

| TABLE 9-2 | ANA-Approved Terminology Standards (February 24, 2006) |

DATA SET	PURPOSE
NMDS (Nursing Minimum Data Set)	The NMDS has 3 categories (nursing care, demographics, and service elements) with 16 data elements. This seminal work defined the minimum information that should be collected for every patient receiving nursing care and contributed to the foundation necessary for the development of nursing terminologies. http://www.nursing.uiowa.edu/NI/collabs_files/Synopsis%20NMDS%20Nov%202003.pdf
NMMDS (Nursing Management Minimum Data Set)	NMMDA was developed to meet the needs of nursing administrators. The NMMDS data set includes 17 data elements across the categories of nursing environment, nursing resources, and financial resources, and it is necessary to inform the strategic decisions of the nurse executive. (Huber D., Schumacher L., & Delaney C. [1997]. Nursing management minimum data set [NMMDS]. *Journal of Nursing Administration, 27*(4), 42–48.

TERMINOLOGIES	PURPOSE
CCC (Clinical Care Classification)	CCC emerged from a Medicare-funded nursing research study designed to assess and classify patients to determine the resources required to provide home health services. CCC comprises two interrelated taxonomies: ■ 182 nursing diagnoses and outcomes, modified by an expected outcome or actual outcome axis, each of which is modified by three possible conditions: improved, stabilized, or deteriorated. ■ 198 nursing interventions modified by four types of action: assess/monitor, care/perform, teach/instruct, and manage/refer. http://www.sabacare.com/
ICNP (International Classification for Nursing Practice)	International Council of Nurses (ICN) is a federation of national nurse associations representing nursing in more than 128 member nations. ICNP is a derivative of the ICN, with the goal of articulating the contribution of nurses around the world to health care and promoting international standardization of nursing. ICNP includes nursing diagnoses, nursing interventions, and outcomes. http://www.icn.ch/icnp.htm
NANDA (North American Nursing Diagnosis Association)	NANDA provides nurses at all levels and in all areas of practice with a standardized nursing terminology with which to: ■ Name client responses to actual or potential health problems, life processes, and wellness ■ Document care for reimbursement of nursing services ■ Contribute to the development of informatics and information standards, ensuring the inclusion of nursing terminology in electronic health-care records ■ Facilitate study of the phenomena of concern to nurses for the purpose of improving patient care. http://www.nanda.org/
NIC (Nursing Intervention Classification)	NIC includes the full range of nursing interventions from general practice to specialty areas. Interventions include physiological and psychosocial, illness treatment and prevention, and health promotion for individuals, families, and communities as well as indirect care. Both independent and collaborative interventions are included. http://www.nursing.uiowa.edu/centers/cncce/nic/index.htm
NOC (Nursing Outcome Classification)	NOC labels and provides measures for comprehensive patient-focused outcomes that respond to nursing intervention. The outcomes are intermediate to the achievement of longer-range outcomes and employ a scale that provides quantifiable information. NIC facilitates the identification of risk adjustment factors for population groups. http://www.nursing.uiowa.edu/centers/cncce/noc/index.htm

DATA SET	PURPOSE
OMAHA System	This is a comprehensive practice and documentation tool for multidisciplinary health-care practitioners in any setting. The three components of the system are problem classification, intervention scheme, and problem rating for outcome. http://www.omahasystem.org/
PCDS (Patient Care Data Set)	The PCDS was developed as a data dictionary of elements abstracted from clinical information systems. The PCDS is multiaxial and combinatorial (a system in which atomic terms are combined to create more complex concepts or problems or structures). http://www.duke.edu/~goodw010/vocab/PCDS.html
PNDS (Perioperative Nursing Data Set)	Developed by the Association of Perioperative Registered Nurses, the PNDS is a standardized nursing vocabulary that addresses the perioperative patient experience from preadmission through discharge. It is the first, and to date the only, nursing language developed by a specialty organization that has been recognized by the ANA as a data set useful for perioperative nursing practice. http://www.aorn.org/research/pnds.htm

MULTIDISCIPLINARY TERMINOLOGIES	PURPOSE
ABC (Alternative Billing Codes)	ABC defines 5-character alphabetic symbols to represent thousands of integrative health-care products and services. The codes reflect the care delivered by acupuncturists, behavioral health-care workers, chiropractors, medical doctors, massage therapists, mental health–care practitioners, midwives, nurses, nutritionists, etc. http://www.abccodes.com/ali/abc_codes/
LOINC (Logical Observation Identifiers Names and Codes)	The purpose of the LOINC database is to facilitate the exchange of laboratory and diagnostic results, generated by vendor systems, with other clinical information systems. LOINC creates the translation so that other systems can understand and file the data. LOINC data are used by practitioners for clinical care, outcomes management, and research. http://www.regenstrief.org/loinc/
SNOMED-CT (Systemic Nomenclature of Medicine Clinical Terms)	SNOMED-CT consists of health-care concepts, with unique meanings and formal logic-based definitions, that are organized into hierarchies. The number of terms and attributes presently enables approximately 1.5 million relationships to be defined in order to support a robust and discrete terminology system. SNOMED-CT can also be mapped to other medical terminologies and classification systems already in use. http://www.snomed.org/

The NMDS identifies a limited set of data elements that should be collected for every patient. These elements are clearly defined and serve as a foundation for further data collection. Fortunately, these data elements are generally collected by most electronic medical record systems.

Data elements are the most basic pieces of information to be collected, and each element must have a unique definition in order to ensure clear and consistent meaning. This process is not inconsequential. For example, "blood pressure" is a term often assumed to be understood. The term, taken alone, can have various meanings relative to the context of the user: a physical therapist may think of blood pressure in terms of pre- or postexercise; a neuroscience practitioner may think in terms of the position of the client at the time of measurement; the nurse clinician may evaluate blood pressure in the context of pre- or postprocedure. It becomes obvious just how critical it is to have a clear, discrete, nonambiguous definition of each data element: "Common data standards are essential to simplify and streamline data requirements and allow the information systems that carry the data to function as an integrated whole" (Institute of Medicine, 2004, p. 132).

Data can be appreciated best in the data-information-knowledge continuum. Data are fundamental building blocks; they combine into a clear, objective definition of a specific fact, without attached meaning. Data are transformed into information when they are interpreted or analyzed and when a structure or organization has been applied. Information becomes knowledge when it is incorporated into the creation of thoughtful relationships and used to support decision processes meaningfully (American Nurses Association, 2001). For example, assessment of pain at a specific moment in time provides data. The data gathered during that assessment gain meaning when placed in the context of previous pain assessments, and the pain data become information. Finally, when this pain assessment information is evaluated in the context of information regarding recent pain medication administration and other pain alleviation measures, the nurse develops knowledge regarding the effectiveness of the patient's pain management plan.

Knowledge work uses transformed information in the context of specialized knowledge and expertise (Mayes, 2001). Registered nurses are knowledge workers by the very nature of the work they do and the continual synthesis of information and knowledge they weave throughout the decision processes inherent in patient care. Clinical judgment implies that nurses use their knowledge to interpret information in the context of the individual patient and apply that knowledge to higher-level clinical plan development. The electronic medical record systems and knowledge representation systems support and enhance the ready access of the clinical nurse to such data, information, and knowledge.

DATA INTERCHANGE STANDARDS

Four types of data interchange standards have been developed in health care. These standards address:

1. Communication between medical devices and between devices and electronic medical records (EMRs)
2. Digital imaging communications
3. Administrative data exchange
4. Clinical data exchange (Mayes, 2001; Sensmeier, 2006)

Transfer of physiological data from a cardiac monitor to the EMR is an example of communication between devices and the EMR. Radiology departments employ digital imaging communication every day as they make x-ray films available to practitioners over the Internet. Administrative data exchange is an integral part of the billing systems of hospitals, enabling information to be shared with payers. Clinical data exchange is woven throughout an EMR system as, for example, data from the laboratory information system are sent to the EMR for integration in the patient record. The National Committee on Vital and Health Statistics, through its accountabilities under the Health Insurance Portability and Accountability Act of 1996, recommended adoption of several standards for data exchange. Table 9-3 is a sample of the more widely known data standards and includes a brief description of the purpose of the standards. Each standard addresses at least one type of data interchange. It is important to know why these standards have been created and that they are necessary for effective and safe patient care. The specifics of the standards will continue to evolve as a result of technological innovations.

Knowledge Representation

Effective data standards are fundamental to knowledge representation, and knowledge representation is a cornerstone of establishing and communicating best practices. As new knowledge is discovered, best practices evolve and change. At this point, the health-care industry does not have effective technological processes for quickly translating new knowledge into best practices. However, information systems, particularly the EMR, offer considerable promise. A major goal of information system developers is design of software systems that can translate up-to-the-moment evidence-based practice guidelines into clinical decision support and provide that information to practitioners when they work with the EMR (Institute of Medicine, 2004). The promise is there, but the timeline for realization is not clear at this juncture.

One means of knowledge representation currently available is electronic linkage to the biomedical literature and other medical knowledge bases. This level of functionality supports practitioner access at the point-of-care, providing information to support clinical decision making. Often the links to literature, formulary, and other knowledge bases

TABLE 9-3	Health-Care Data Standards Organizations

STANDARDS ORGANIZATION	PURPOSE
IEEE (Institute of Electrical and Electronic Engineers)	IEEE establishes international standards in a great number of fields, including medical information devices. The IEEE standards enable communication between medical devices and computer systems, providing real-time, automatic, comprehensive, and consistent data capture and storage in computer systems. Equipment that uses IEEE standards includes monitoring equipment, ECG devices, ventilators, infusion pumps, and wireless transmission devices. http://standards.ieee.org/announcements/pr_1073.html
DICOM (Digital Imaging and Communications in Medicine)	Collaborating with the American College of Radiologists, the National Electrical Manufacturers Association has created and maintains international standards for communication of biomedical diagnostic and therapeutic information in disciplines that use digital images and associated data. The goals of DICOM are to achieve compatibility and to improve workflow efficiency between imaging systems and other information systems in health-care environments worldwide. http://www.nema.org/prod/med/
ACS (Accredited Standards Committee)	ACS develops and maintains standards for electronic data interchange and document structure standards to support business transactions. Within health care, these X12N standards have been adopted nationally to facilitate administrative functions that support patient care, such as submission of claims, enrollment of participants, and similar functions (Accredited Standards Committee, 2003). Given the unique nature of the health-care environment in the United States, including the privacy provisions of HIPAA, these standards are generally not used outside of the United States. http://www.x12.org/
HL7 (Health Level Seven)	HL7 develops specifications for data transmission. The most widely used specification is a standard that enables disparate health-care applications to exchange key sets of clinical and administrative data. HL7 supports the exchange of information between computer applications while preserving the meaning of the original message or data. The primary focus of HL7 is clinical and administrative data. For example, HL7 supports transmission of medical orders, nursing documentation, and medication administration records. http://www.hl7.org/
LOINC (Logical Observation Identifiers Names and Codes)	LOINC provides a standard set of universal names and codes for identifying individual laboratory and clinical results and allows users to merge clinical results from many sources into one database for patient care, clinical research, and management. LOINC provides the translation of laboratory data, which are usually transmitted using the internal codes of the specific laboratory system. LOINC codes allow the data to be read and stored in the electronic medical record. LOINC is also designed to code hemodynamic and other clinical and medication data. http://www.regenstrief.org/loinc/

have embedded icons in EMR systems, demonstrating an immediate level of support for practitioners. This type of knowledge representation brings the most recent medical literature to the fingertips of the practitioner, thereby enabling the practitioner to evaluate the information in the literature and appropriately weave it into patient care as the individualized plan of care is developed.

An exciting next-generation dimension of clinical practice guidelines is evolving. Generally, implementation of practice guidelines beyond the local setting has been severely limited. One limitation is the lack of standards to support representing guidelines in a machine-readable format. A second limitation is that guidelines are not documented in a language that is nonambiguous, with clear and nonredundant definitions. Third, clinical practice guidelines must have access to stored data of the patient, and that data repository must contain the necessary clinical data that will support decision making. Clinical practice guidelines to date have been created using the relative simplicity of "if-then" statements. More recent research, devoted to creating software that will enable practitioners to query large databases for best practices, structuring the query to consider information and context specific to the subject patient, offers the promise of a much more dynamic, real-time clinical decision support system (Institute of Medicine, 2004).

Terminologies

Terminology standards are part of health-care data standards. Nursing terminologies have special meaning to nursing practice. A suitable summary for why nursing terminologies are needed is that "if we cannot name it . . . we cannot control it, finance it, research it, teach it or put it into public policy" (Royal College of Nursing [UK], 2004). This quote is an apt distillation of the importance of nursing terminologies and the work that is being conducted in this field. Collectively, nursing does not have standard terminology, and this is readily evidenced within any given hospital or nursing unit that does not have an electronic documentation system. To a significant extent, nursing has followed the medical model, failing to articulate clearly a precise, unique name and definition for much of the work of nursing.

Nursing terminology is another critical standard necessary to the evolving medical record. Nursing terminology is a standard that is generally more functionally apparent to practitioners than other standards because users interact with the terminology throughout the electronic documentation experience. The underlying terminology guides the selection of data elements to be included in the documentation screens, the definition of those elements, and the selection options available to the nurse.

Standardized nursing terminologies, or languages, provide important benefits to nursing practice, which include:

- Consistency in documentation resulting from the ability to trend or evaluate data longitudinally

- Nursing clinical decision support
- Significantly enhanced nursing research ability resulting from easier and more comprehensive data retrieval from EMRs and use of data from multiple geographic sites in research studies
- Evidence-based nursing practice resulting from EMRs that support the process of developing evidence
- Quality assessment and evaluation of practice resulting from the ease of data retrieval and subsequent analysis
- Professional billing for nursing services; unambiguous, consistent, comprehensive documentation is a necessary prerequisite to bill for nursing services, and standardized languages are a cornerstone to realization of that documentation
- Creating visibility for the care provided by nurses; the terms, definitions, and classifications that are inherent in standardized terminologies will ensure that care provided by nurses will be definitively incorporated in the patient medical record
- A bridge between the different terms used by the various care provider professions as well as a bridge between regional terminology differences across the country; as our society becomes increasingly multicultural, the need for a clearly defined and consistently employed terminology system becomes more urgent to help reduce communication ambiguity and increase patient safety.

Given the benefits that standardized terminologies offer the nursing profession, it may be surprising to learn that consensus on nursing terminologies has not been achieved. Nursing is a very complex and diverse profession, and no single terminology has been created to meet the data collection and documentation needs of the profession.

There is some agreement regarding the functional characteristics and structural attributes of terminologies. These features include (Henry & Mead, 1997):

1. The system should be **complete** and have sufficient in-depth coverage and granularity (depth and level of detail) to depict nursing care processes. For example, the full spectrum of nursing diagnoses needs to be incorporated.

2. The system needs to be **comprehensive,** including each facet of the nursing care process. For example, it should include risk factors or the recipient or target of the education that is to be provided.

3. Concepts should be **nonredundant,** without vagueness or ambiguity, and there should be no overlapping meanings.

4. Concepts should be **atomic,** or separable into their constituent components. For example, a category should not be "pain" but instead subdivided into chronic pain or acute pain.

    Atomic elements must be able to be combined (**compositional**) to create concepts. For example, an atomic element could be chronic fatigue, which, combined with acute fatigue, would create the larger concept of fatigue.

5. The system needs to be able to support **hierarchies** of concepts, allowing linking of general and more specific terms, and support multiple "parents" and "children." For example, incontinence may be due to neurogenic causes or bladder prolapse.

6. Each term and concept must have a clear and concise **definition**.

7. The above list is a sample of the considerations and criteria employed in evaluating or creating a terminology system. This brief overview provides some insight into a complex process that is highly collaborative, requiring consensus building and continual review.

In 1995, the ANA established the Nursing Information and Data Set Evaluation Center (NIDSEC) to evaluate standardized nursing and other terminologies that have been developed by professional groups or information system vendors. The purpose was to identify and recognize those terminologies that effectively represent nursing practice and support documentation of nursing practice in computer information systems. NIDSEC evaluation criteria incorporate nomenclature, data repository (how data are stored), clinical content, and general characteristics of the system (NIDSEC - Nursing Information and Data Set Evaluation). As of February 24, 2006, NIDSEC recognized two minimum data sets, eight nursing interface terminologies, and three multidisciplinary terminologies. A brief description of each is included in Table 9-2.

Nursing documentation in the paper medical record has traditionally included one or more flow sheets as well as narrative notes. Documentation of patient care in a paper medical record is relatively unstructured, most specifically within the narrative notes. Clearly, many health-care organizations have documentation standards, such as documentation by exception; however, within the defined standard there is generally significant flexibility. Narrative notes have a number of limitations, including:

- Differences in terminology between care providers, even when the providers are referencing the same topic
- Use of abbreviations and acronyms, resulting in confusion and misinterpretation
- Differences in writing style and content that limit the development of continuity and the ability to trend the clinical condition and responses of the patient
- Illegible handwriting
- Difficult, very costly, and limited data retrieval ability

Consequently, employing the use of terminologies represents a significant change in documentation practice. Documentation in a well designed EMR is completed largely by selecting the appropriate option from prepared selection lists that are coded to ensure consistent data storage.

Information System Goals for the Early 21st Century

The report of the Institute of Medicine (IOM), *Crossing the Quality Chasm,* identified six major aims for improving the health-care system of the 21st century. Targeted to all health-care organizations, professional groups, and private and public purchasers of health-care services, the focuses are: safety, effectiveness, becoming patient-centered, timeliness, efficiency, and equitability (Institute of Medicine, 2001). Although not a panacea, the EMR and the work of nurse informaticists in collaboration with clinical nurses can make significant contributions to the agenda set forth by the IOM. Patient safety can be significantly enhanced through the use of EMR systems. Some examples in which EMR systems support these goals include:

chapter star

Concerned about the variable computer skills and documentation practices demonstrated by unit coworkers, ABC, RN, made an appointment with the nurse manager to discuss his observations. During their meeting, ABC shared his concerns and indicated he would like to work on supporting his peers and resolving the problems he had noted. ABC also shared that his concern was predicated by his understanding that nursing documentation in the EMR would provide for better understanding of the outcomes of patient care delivery on the unit and that he would support quality improvement and nursing research in the months and years to come. But, he said, those goals would not be realized if the staff feared or were uncomfortable with the system and did not use it in the way it was designed to be used. The manager asked ABC if he could be more specific in describing his concerns. ABC shared the following observations made over the past 10-12 weeks, since implementation of the most recent functionality of the hospital EMR system. He indicated that each instance involved a small subset of the staff. Although some staff members had been observed having difficulty in more than one of the situations, the situations represented a cross-section of the unit staff:

- Difficulty navigating the EMR and finding key laboratory data
- Reluctance to use the nursing documentation system, often reverting to paper documentation, indicating no functional computers were available prior to the end of the shift
- Reluctance to document at the bedside, preferring to record assessment and clinical data on paper and subsequently transfer the information to the EMR later in the shift
- No changes in documentation of the clinical assessment of the patient despite knowledge of significant changes in the patient's condition
- Detailed recording of all the clinical tasks ordered for the patient during shift report

The nurse manager shared that she had noted similar behaviors and was concerned about supporting the staff to ensure they effectively integrated the EMR into their workflow. She asked ABC to prepare recommendations regarding how he believed the problems he had noted should be addressed. They agreed to meet again in 10 days to discuss his recommendations.

At their next meeting, ABC presented to the nurse manager his recommendations, addressing each of the concerns noted. ABC's recommendations included:

1. Offer a basic computer skills class to staff. Rather than focus the class on use of the EMR, he suggested they frame the class as a "life skills" computer class, building skill sets through use of simulated on-line banking, personal budget development, computer-based recipe files, etc.
2. Prepare and distribute a survey regarding concerns and personal weaknesses in use of the EMR. The survey would be anonymous, asking only for job title.
3. Collaborate with technology staff responsible for hardware and software support to create routine preventive rounds on the unit, ensuring that all computers would be assessed for performance at least once a month. At the same time, post signs at each computer listing the number of the Help Desk for immediate reporting of computer malfunctions.
4. Host a unit patient safety fair. Include in the fair a poster and other information regarding how real-time documentation supports patient care, other practitioners, and safety.
5. Request information from the EMR staff regarding documentation performance of the unit. Provide feedback to staff, celebrating the areas of high performance. Share the areas where there are opportunities for improvement, and commit time during the staff meeting over the next 6 months to discuss the data and discuss how performance can be improved.

The nurse manager was pleased with the thoughtful recommendations ABC prepared. They discussed accountabilities, priorities, plan details, resources that would be required, and a timeline. At the conclusion of their discussion, the nurse manager committed to ABC that 20% of his working time (8 hours each week) would be scheduled as nonpatient care time. During that time, ABC would prepare resources and execute the plan. The nurse manager and ABC agreed to meet weekly to discuss the progress of the plan, resources, and support that ABC needed. They would evaluate the plan and continuation of the 20% release time from patient care in 6 months.

- Legibility of handwriting and ready identification of the authors of documentation are fully supported in an EMR system. Error reduction is achieved because drug dosages are clearly written and documentation standards, such as the use of leading zeros preceding decimals, are ensured
- Clinical alerts, such as drug-drug and drug-allergy interactions, provided to the physician at the time an order is entered in the EMR save pharmacists and nurses time clarifying orders and enable the appropriate medication intervention to reach the patient more quickly
- Nurses receive allergy interaction information at the time of medication administration
- Positive patient identification systems, such as bedside bar-code scanning of patient wristbands, medications, and the medication administration record, can support consistent and clear verification of the five patient rights and can help to avoid medication errors.

Effective care can be supported by access to evidence-based practice databases and up-to-date protocols, helping to make sure that patients are receiving care based on the most recent scientific information. Presenting the most recent evidence to practitioners can be achieved by clinical decision support systems that offer recommendations or that suggest treatment modalities based upon the clinical condition and clinical data of the patient. Effectiveness can be further supported through data-mining (retrieval of selected clinical data from the EMR), for example, some systems analyze the response of patients with similar clinical presentations and diagnoses to specific clinical interventions.

EMR systems can also offer reminders to clinicians regarding best-practice recommendations for laboratory testing, such as monitoring therapeutic blood levels of an antibiotic or anticoagulant. Preventive care screening recommendations, such as annual mammograms or initial colonoscopy for patients who have reached the age of 50, are another example of assuring that patients receive timely interventions. Patient-centered care is enhanced as documentation by various practice disciplines, such as physicians, nurses, therapists, and pharmacists, is integrated, and practice silos are diminished or eliminated. For example, EMR systems support patient-focused problem lists, interdisciplinary communication through integration of documentation entries, and elimination of redundant documentation through presentation of previously documented data when and where they are needed in data screens.

Computer Hardware

Computer technology is changing rapidly, and the half-life of what is considered to be a sophisticated computer has become very short. Within that context, this section will briefly discuss the components of a computer. Perhaps the place to begin is to clarify that hardware refers to all of the physical

Practice to Strive For 9-1

The data collected, stored, and retrieved from the EMR comprise an important key to the future of nursing and the care delivered to patients. However, data depend on the value and respect individual practitioners have for what the data represent for the patients for whom they care. Nurses need to embrace accurate, complete, and real-time documentation. This documentation will enable them and their peers and colleagues to make effective decisions for their patients. This documentation will also serve as the database for research and quality improvement efforts that will guide the development of new evidence on which to base practice. Nurses need to become involved in the design, development, and feedback of the EMR systems in their hospitals. They need to develop an understanding of the design and underlying care philosophies that are used as guideposts in the design of the EMR. Nurses need to articulate their workflow needs in order to influence the design of documentation and related policies so that they are realistic. Nurses need to advocate for collection of baseline data prior to implementation of major new functionality so that nursing will be able to measure the changes that result from the new documentation processes and workflow. Nurses need to support their peers and reinforce the benefits of electronic documentation systems. Nurses must become involved; through involvement they participate in shaping their future, rather than respond to what others think the future should be. The data nurses choose to collect and the accuracy of those data will significantly influence how nursing is able to articulate the contribution of nursing care to patient outcomes.

components of the computer. This hardware is often classified as processing components, memory, and input and output devices. Familiarity with these terms can diminish some of the mystery of computers for those who are not accustomed to using them or their component parts.

PROCESSING COMPONENTS

The central processing unit (CPU) is the brain of the computer. Think of the CPU as the control center, directing the flow of information while also interpreting, directing, and monitoring the execution of instructions received from memory. The CPU is also responsible for arithmetic logic, the foundation of computer function.

The motherboard is another key element, providing the connective infrastructure of the computer. The CPU, chips, hard drives, and disk drives are mounted on the motherboard, and the motherboard creates the internal organization and is the location for addition of new components.

An important feature of any computer is the speed at which the computer processes information. Speed is usually described as clock speed, or the number of electric pulse cycles that occur in a defined period. Hertz is the term used to measure clock speed, and 1 hertz is 1 cycle per second. Megahertz (MHz) is 1 million cycles per second, and gigahertz (GHz) is 1 billion cycles per second.

INPUT AND OUTPUT DEVICES

In order to work and accomplish tasks using the computer, input devices are necessary. Input devices enable the user to enter data, such as numbers or words, that the computer then uses to perform computations based on commands that are also entered by input devices. Another way of perceiving input devices is that they enable two-way communication between the user and the computer. Commonly used input devices include the keyboard, mouse, and scanner; some computers support the use of light pens or touch-screens and other devices. In most cases, a combination of input devices, such as the keyboard and mouse, is needed for entry of data and commands.

A means of extracting data from the computer is also necessary; output devices are required for this purpose. Output devices include disks, CDs, flash

drives, electronic transmission to another computer, and printers, to name the more commonly used devices.

MEMORY

Computer memory consists of read-only memory (ROM), random access memory (RAM), and storage memory. ROM is memory used only by the computer and is protected from alteration, including erasure, by the user. The information stored in ROM supervises the overall function of the computer and enables certain computer functions, such as starting computer operation, often referred to as booting.

RAM is usually called the working memory of the computer, and it is RAM that supports the various applications used, such as spreadsheet and word processing. Another term associated with RAM is volatile memory, a reference to the temporary nature of RAM storage. Instructions needed to operate an application are retrieved from permanent storage, such as the hard drive, CD, or diskette, and used by RAM while the application is in use. Because RAM loses the information stored in it each time the computer is turned off, any work completed using applications must be saved to permanent storage so that it can be retrieved later.

The files created and saved while working on the computer are placed in storage memory, sometimes called permanent memory. The term permanent memory should not be misleading; the files stored in permanent memory reside there until such time as they are erased or overwritten by new files. Hard disks, CDs, and diskettes are used to store files. Another, more recent, innovation for file storage is the flash drive, also known as a thumb drive or memory stick. These highly portable devices are available in ever increasing memory capacities (Saba & McCormick, 2006; Thede, 2003).

COMPUTER POWER

The way in which the computer works with and stores data is based on the binary system. A bit is the smallest unit of storage in the computer. It has two possible values, zero and one (0 and 1). If you think of the bit as an on-off switch, the "on" position is equal to 1, and the "off" position is equal to 0. Bits are combined in groups or units of eight bits,

TABLE 9-4	Computer Memory in Bytes	
PREFIX	UNITS (# OF BYTES)	NUMBER
Kilobyte	Thousand	1,000
Megabyte	Million	1,000,000
Gigabyte	Billion	1,000,000,000
Terabyte	Trillion	1,000,000,000,000
Petabyte	Quadrillion	1,000,000,000,000,000
Exabyte	Quintillion	1,000,000,000,000,000,000
Zettabyte	Sextillion	1,000,000,000,000,000,000,000
Yottabyte	Septillion	1,000,000,000,000,000,000,000,000

which are known as a byte. A byte represents a single character, such as an M or the number 4 (Saba & McCormick, 2006).

The number of possible combinations of 0 and 1 in a byte is 255, and in the early days of computer technology 255 was the limit of the number of characters a computer could represent. With the advent of newer technology, computers are able to express increasingly more characters and graphics, greatly expanding the flexibility for image and other visual displays. One expression of power today is to indicate the number of bytes the computer can handle: Table 9-4 is a scale of the actual and theoretical storage capacity of computers; for example, at the time this chapter was written, the yottabyte was theoretical storage capacity.

Privacy and the Protection of Health-Care Data

The Health Insurance Portability and Accountability Act (HIPAA) was enacted by Congress in 1996 to protect workers by limiting employer denial of health insurance coverage to employees with preexisting medical conditions. Interestingly, because the act also directed the Department of Health and Human Services to develop privacy rules for health data contained in EMRs, HIPAA indirectly promoted significant impetus for development of a number of standards to support data transmission. The privacy portion of this act, often referred to as the Privacy Rule, affects all health-care providers and health plans and specifically indicates that pro-

tected health information (PHI) may not be disclosed without the permission of the patient (Flores, 2005).

HIPAA, although referred to as an act or government regulation, is more appropriately characterized as a process. As the years have passed since the law was enacted in 1996, HIPAA has gradually become recognized as a significant source of change in the culture of health care . The accountability for protection of PHI has resulted in a changed organizational focus that extends beyond the tenets of the original act. For example, quality assurance data designed to monitor and improve patient safety often include PHI information to enhance and strengthen data analysis. The need to assure that PHI is appropriately protected and that data are effectively de-identified has resulted from the evolving awareness of the need to respectfully protect information that could be traced back to individual patients.

The future challenge for the health-care industry will be to balance the need to protect the PHI with the contrasting advantages that could be gained for streamlined patient care as a result of access to medical record information. For example, in the event of a widespread health emergency, access to personal medical record information would support creation of aggregate data pools or databases that would greatly speed understanding and insight into the problem and accelerate identification of preventive or treatment solutions.

Nurses have historically advocated for and protected patient privacy. HIPAA supports and increases the accountability of the nurse, as a health-care provider, to protect the privacy of the patient. There are personal measures that are deeply embedded in nurses' daily practice to protect patient privacy. For example, nurses can make certain that they protect the privacy of personal security passwords to information systems and refuse to share their passwords. Experts advise against writing down passwords due to the risk of discovery by others. All practitioners are responsible for all documentation made under their password, even if they did not make the entry. This sobering fact offers a compelling rationale for not sharing passwords and assuring that they cannot be discovered by others.

Another example of protecting the privacy of the patient occurs when using the EMR. By ensuring that each session is closed and logged out each time one leaves the computer, the nurse is demonstrating respect for this important patient right. Each of these measures is part of the overall strategy present in health-care organizations to honor and respect the trust relationship with patients.

All Good Things...

Nursing informatics is a new and important part of the nursing care arsenal. Working in partnership with the other members of the team, informaticists help the team define the clinical, administrative, and research outcomes and how those outcomes can be supported with comprehensive clinical data. Informaticists assist in creating an infrastructure that supports clear communication through the design of documentation consisting of nonredundant data elements with nonambiguous definitions. Nurse informaticists guide nursing leadership through the selection of a terminology system that meets the clinical and strategic goals of nursing practice and supports patient care. Nurse informaticists actively participate with clinical and information systems leadership in designing the strategic direction of the EMR system, ensuring the practice needs and imperatives of nursing are incorporated.

Nursing informaticists also communicate and interpret the role of nursing informatics to the nursing community. Effective staff training in effective use of information systems is an ongoing focus of nurse informaticists. An important facet of the role is translation of key accountabilities of practicing nurses as they use information systems and assisting the nursing community to perceive and understand the importance of its ongoing engagement and input to the work of nursing informaticists.

Let's Talk

1. Describe at least three situations or examples in which clinical decision support benefits patient care.

2. Discuss the value that a terminology system provides to nursing practice.

3. What are the drawbacks and limitations of terminology systems?

4. How do EMR systems that are designed using a terminology system differ from paper medical record documentation?

5. Describe the role of a nursing informaticist. Consider the educational preparation for such a role in your response.

6. HIPAA was discussed as a motivating factor for patient privacy concerns. Discuss the ways in which patient privacy could be jeopardized in the health-care environment.

NCLEX Questions

1. The Institute of Medicine (IOM) established six major aims for improving the health-care system in the 21st century. One major goal is improving patient safety. Identify two of the remaining goals.
   A. Increase numbers of nurses and increase efficiency.
   B. Enhance patient-centered focus and protect privacy.
   C. Improve effectiveness and reduce costs.
   D. Increase timeliness and enhance patient-centered focus.

2. Computers have several types of memory to support their function. Which of the following options is not a type of memory?
   A. Flash drive.
   B. ROM: read-only memory.
   C. RIM: read internal memory.
   D. RAM: random access memory.

3. Which of the following features is not an example of knowledge representation?
   A. E-mail.
   B. Clinical practice guidelines.
   C. Systematic reviews of the literature.
   D. Clinical decision support.

4. Nursing terminology systems support nursing documentation in several important ways. Identify the option that is least important in the benefits offered by terminology systems.
   A. Ensure the value and visibility of nursing in the medical record.
   B. Eliminate lengthy narrative notes.
   C. Support nursing research.
   D. Support quality assurance and improvement activities.

5. Which response is the most accurate regarding the purpose of data standards for information systems?
   A. Data collection and storage.
   B. Data retrieval and transmission.
   C. Both of the above.
   D. Neither of the above.

6. Standardized nursing terminology affords nursing a number of benefits. The benefits include:
   A. Increased medical record visibility of nursing contributions to patient care.
   B. A database that supports clinical research.
   C. The ability to implement clinical decision support.
   D. A and B.
   E. A, B, and C.

7. Nursing science serves as the foundation of nursing informatics. The domain of informatics exists as the intersection of what other three sciences?
   A. Communication, cognitive, and computer sciences.
   B. Information, programming, and communication sciences.
   C. Cognitive, computer, and information sciences.
   D. Computer, information, and communication sciences.

8. Protected health information (PHI) is individually identifiable health information. Which of the following data elements is/are considered PHI data?
   A. Name and address.
   B. Birth date.
   C. Telephone number.
   D. Social security number.
   E. A, B, and D.
   F. A, B, and C.
   G. A, B, C, and D.

9. Patient safety can be improved through the features of an EMR system by a number of means. Which of the following are patient safety outcomes of an EMR?
   A. Legibility of the data entered.
   B. Drug-allergy alerts at the time of medication administration.
   C. Costing of medications at the time of ordering.
   D. A and B.
   E. A, B, and C.

10. Which of the following dimensions of computer hardware and function is/are not correct?
    A. Hertz is the term used to represent the speed of the computer.
    B. Data are permanently stored in the hard drive or output device.
    C. A byte is eight bits.
    D. A byte represents eight characters.
    E. A and D.
    F. B and C.

REFERENCES

ACS (The Accredited Standards Committee). (2003). *ACS X12*. Retrieved May 1, 2006, from http://www.x12.org/x12org/subcommittees/sc_home.cfm?sendTo=PurposeAndScope%2Ecfm&doSet=TRUE&CFID=1748141&CFTOKEN=8624906

American Nurses Association. (2001). *Scope and standards of nursing informatics practice*. Washington, D.C.: American Nurses Publishing.

Flores, J.A. (2005). HIPAA: Past, present and future implications for nurses. *Online Journal of Issues in Nursing, 10*(2), 131–147.

Graves, J.R., & Corcoran, S. (1989). The study of nursing informatics. *Image: Journal of Nursing Scholarship, 21*(4), 227–231.

Henry, S.B., & Mead, C.N. (1997). Nursing classification systems: Necessary but not sufficient for representing "what nurses do" for inclusion in computer-based patient record systems. *Journal of the American Medical Information Association, 4*(3), 222–232.

Institute of Medicine. (2001). *Crossing the quality chasm*. Washington, D.C.: National Academy Press.

Institute of Medicine. (2004). *Keeping patients safe: Transforming the work environment of nurses*. Washington, D.C.: National Academies Press.

Mayes, R. (2001). Data standards. In Saba, V.K., & McCormick, K.A. (Eds.). *Essentials of computers for nurses: Informatics for the new millennium*. (3rd ed., pp. 167–176). New York: McGraw-Hill.

NIDSE—Nursing Information and Data Set Evaluation. Retrieved May 3, 2006, from http://www.nursingworld.org/nidsec/

Office of Civil Rights. (May 2003). *Summary of the HIPAA privacy rule*. Retrieved May 12, 2006, from http://www.hhs.gov/ocr/privacysummary.pdf

Royal College of Nursing (UK). (April 15, 2004). *Defining nursing*. Retrieved May 5, 2006, from http://www.rcn.org.uk/news/display.php?ID=448&area=Press

Saba, V.K. (2001). Historical perspectives of nursing and the computer. In Saba, V.K., & McCormick, K.A. (Eds.). *Essentials of computers for nurses: Informatics for the new millennium*. (3rd ed., pp. 9–45). New York: McGraw-Hill.

Saba, V.K., & McCormick, K.A. (Eds.). (2006). *Essentials of nursing informatics*. (4th ed.). New York: McGraw-Hill.

Sensmeier, J. (2006). Healthcare Data Standards. In Saba, V.K., & McCormick, K.A. (Eds.). (2006). *Essentials of nursing informatics*. (4th ed., pp. 217–228). New York: McGraw-Hill.

Thede, L.Q. (2003). *Informatics and nursing: Opportunities & challenges.* (2nd ed.). Philadelphia: Lippincott Williams & Wilkins.

Turley, J.P. (1996). Toward a model for nursing informatics. *Image: Journal of Nursing Scholarship, 28*(4), 309–313.

Washington Publishing Company. (1998). *Overview of healthcare EDI transactions: A business primer.*

Whitten, J.L., Bentley, L.D., & Dittman, K.C. (2000). *Systems analysis and design methods.* (5th ed.). Boston: McGraw-Hill Irwin.

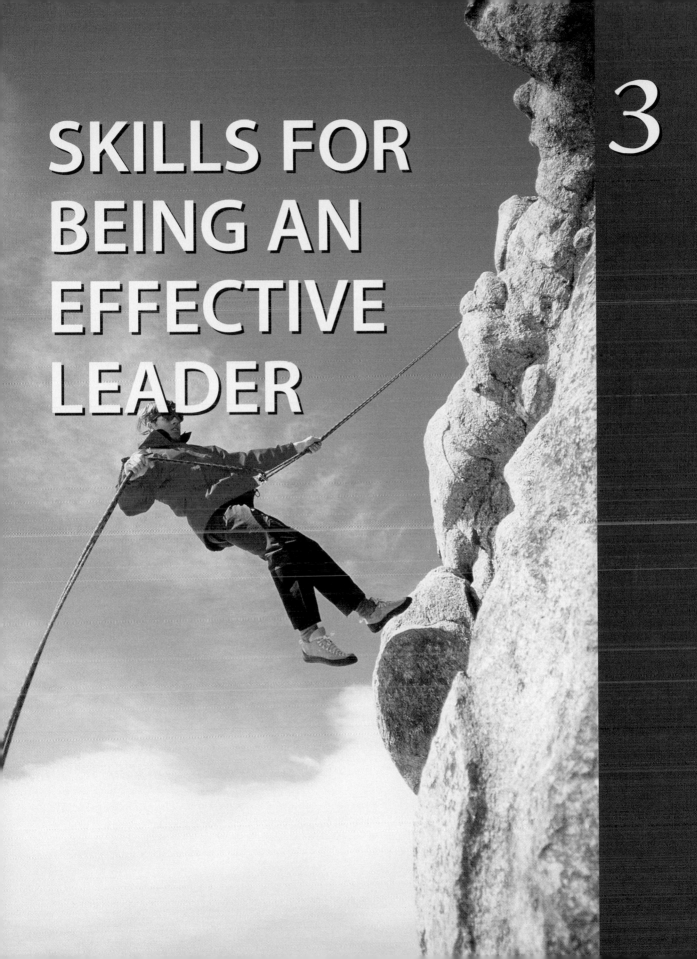

SKILLS FOR BEING AN EFFECTIVE LEADER

3

chapter 10

Enhancing Your Critical Thinking, Decision Making, and Problem Solving

DEBORAH A. JASOVSKY, MSN, PHD, RN, CNAA, BC

MARY KAMIENSKI, PHD, RN, APRN-C, FAEN

CHAPTER MOTIVATION

"Successful problem-solving requires finding the right solution to the right problem. The problems we select for solution and the way we formulate them depends more on our philosophy and our world view than on science and technology."

Russell Ackoff, a social systems scientist

CHAPTER MOTIVES

- Identify the relationships between critical thinking, decision making, and **problem solving**.
- Discuss various decision-making and problem-solving **models**.
- Utilize various **tools** to make good decisions and solve complex problems.
- Utilize group techniques to enhance problem solving.

Decision making is one of the most frequent activities performed by a professional nurse. At the bedside or in the boardroom, nurses must make decisions and solve problems to produce outcomes that enhance patient care. Some decisions, like when to brush your teeth, become habits, so one does not think about them. Other decisions become life-altering events that should be made with structured thought or after utilizing problem-solving techniques. All decisions are not made in response to problems, but all problems were resolved because of decisions made along the way.

Driven by critical thinking and using a multidisciplinary knowledge base, nurses need to make decisions that are appropriate to the context of the situation and considerate of the culture where the services are being provided. These decisions need to be based on knowledge of the individuals, relationships, ethics, politics, and financial considerations of the situation. **Decision making** can be simple or complex. The situation may require a quick response or allow for reflection, collaboration with others, and a carefully considered response. Nurses need to develop and enhance ways to see all sides of an issue, find various approaches to solve problems, and make careful, intelligent decisions. Critical thinking is the foundation for examining all possibilities and arriving at reasonable and justified conclusions. This chapter will explore various ways to make good decisions and solve problems effectively by using creative critical thinking skills.

Critical Thinking

Critical thinking is a complex process that has many definitions. Some authors state that it is a reflective and reasonable way of thinking; others see it as an attitude of inquiry. Still others describe it as a disciplined, self-directed thinking process. Most agree that critical thinking does entail an orderly investigation of ideas, **assumptions**, principles, and conclusions. Critical thinking is the process that guides scientific reasoning, the nursing process, problem solving, and decision making. The cognitive skills attributed to the critical thinking process include divergent thinking, reasoning, reflection, creativity, clarification, and basic support (Green, 2000).

- Divergent thinking is the ability of an individual to analyze a variety of opinions and judgments.
- Reasoning involves the use of logic and the ability to discriminate between observation and inference, fact and guessing.
- Reflection allows one to deliberate about something, whereas creativity enables one to produce ideas and alternatives and consider multiple solutions.
- Clarification includes identifying similarities, differences, and assumptions and defining terms.
- Basic support involves the use of known facts and background knowledge.

CRITICAL THINKING PROCESS

Critical thinking is a process that entails identifying assumptions, considering context and meaning of issues, and gathering data to consider alternatives and outcomes (Box 10-1).

Identifying Assumptions

The critical thinking process begins by exploring the assumptions underlying a situation. These assumptions may be beliefs that influence how an individual will reason or understand a situation and may reflect a person's point of view or perspective. These assumptions may not necessarily be grounded in reality. For example, administering medications is a common activity of nurses, and finding strategies to avoid medication errors has become an important concern and problem-solving initiative in many organizations. If a patient assumes the nurse will always administer the correct medication, it is unlikely that the patient will

---

Box 10-1

Critical Thinking Process

1. Identify assumptions underlying the issue.
2. Consider the context and meanings of the issue to all of the individuals.
3. Gather enough data to allow for consideration of alternatives and prediction of multiple possible outcomes.

question any medications the nurse offers. This assumption will have an impact on any efforts to include the patient in a program to decrease medication administration errors.

Considering the Context

The critical thinking process involves considering the context of the present problem or situation. Analysis and interpretation of the meanings of the present issue or situation are essential to developing a conclusion. Returning to the patient taking medication, a context could be when the patient is not responsive or not physically or mentally capable of being involved in taking the medications and cannot be safely included in the process. Another context is the patient taking medications at home without direct nursing supervision. All these situations might involve different strategies to try to avoid medication errors.

Data Collection

Data collection is the next step in the critical thinking process. All too frequently, snap decisions are made based on first impressions. Leaders who use critical thinking skills do consider first impressions, but they are always careful to continue to gather data and carefully evaluate all the alternatives and possible outcomes. Nurses are often faced with clinical situations that require gathering assessment data and considering various alternative interven-

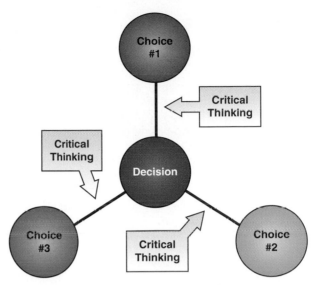

FIGURE 10-1 Decision model.

tions while balancing the needs of the individual patient and predicting potential outcomes. For example, making a patient assignment involves reviewing the acuity of the patients and where the patients are geographically located, reviewing the staff mix based on status of the nurses, the experience of the individual staff members, and the numbers of staff available.

Making Decisions

All nurses make decisions frequently. Making many decisions, however, does not necessarily guarantee that an individual will make good decisions. This section will discuss ways to enhance decision-making skills and strategies. Because decision making is a complex, abstract process, individuals may have many different ways of thinking about it. A discussion of various decision-making models can be helpful in explaining and understanding this phenomenon (Fig. 10-1).

MODELS RELEVANT TO MAKING DECISIONS

Brief snapshots of the following models are intended to guide readers to an understanding of the decision-making process:

To Adapt or Innovate

According to McNichol (2002), individuals either adapt or innovate when faced with new or unknown situations that may require problem solving or decision making. **Adaptors** are naturally convergent thinkers, whereas innovators are divergent thinkers. Adaptors fit the new situation into known structures, systems, and models. These people control activity and follow through on tasks but tend to be stressed when lots of changes and uncertain outcomes occur. On the other hand, **innovators** enjoy experiencing new situations and look for opportunities to do things differently. While valued for generating ideas and identifying possibilities, these workers are viewed as chaotic and unable to complete their tasks.

chapter star

Dawn Wise is the nursing manager of a 40-bed medical/surgical unit. Recently, full-time staff resignations for relocation or retirement reasons have created many openings on the 3 p.m. to 11 p.m. and 11 p.m. to 7 a.m. schedule. Although the positions have been posted on the hospital Website, Dawn decides she needs to have her staff assist in filling the open positions on a temporary basis. The problem of staffing offers several options for the manager to consider: additional part-time coverage, per diem staff, agency staff, overtime, or flex-time with change to 12-hour coverage. Dawn's hospital does not have a central staffing office, nor are there extra nurses from any other department who can work.

Using critical thinking skills, Dawn identifies the underlying assumption that the staffing decision needs to provide cost-effective and safe care for the patients on the unit. She understands that the decision how to provide the necessary coverage will be of great concern to the staff, who want adequate numbers of people to work each shift but will not want coverage decisions mandated by management. Information about how to make this decision will need group input to consider all the possible alternatives.

She decides to discuss the problem and potential solutions with her staff. After the staff meeting, in which brainstorming took place, Dawn talks to each part-time RN and receives a commitment for extra time. As the staff requested, Dawn posts the remaining openings in the next schedule for interested staff to sign up for overtime before seeking per diem or agency staff. The staff agreed with Dawn not to consider 12-hour shifts unless the positions remained open for more than 2 months.

Dawn sums up the decision-making process in this way: "Our philosophy includes shared governance, and our nurses know how important their input is to the work environment. Sharing the decision making increases our shared accountability to the public for providing qualified, competent staff. We rely on administration to support our joint efforts in problem solving and decision making."

- Information processing model: Continuum consisting of short- and long-term memory using a four-stage process, including weighing the pros and cons of each decision alternative
- Wheeler's model: Knowing the context in which choices can be made from options that affect the individual and up through the society at large as represented in concentric circles
- Nursing process: Evaluation process allows for continual assessment of the response to any

decision, with new plans being implemented for alternative responses

Information Processing Model

In this model, decision making is seen on a continuum and not as an either/or process (Thompson, 1999). This model consists of two components: short- and long-term memory. Short-term memory contains the stimuli information necessary to "unlock" factual and experimental knowledge that is stored in the long-term memory. The clinician uses a four-stage process to make decisions in this theory:

1. Gather clinical patient data.
2. Generate hypotheses or predictions about the issue.
3. Interpret the data and confirm or refute the hypotheses.
4. Weigh the pros and cons of each decision alternative.

One of the strengths of this model is that it allows the use of all types of assessment data, including individual "memory" data, which is the information each person carries consisting of previous knowledge and experiences. An experienced clinician can use experience and knowledge to predict that a decision will or will not work. For example, an experienced nurse manager is faced with completing the summer vacation schedule for the unit. The manager is aware of the restrictions placed by administration about the number of individuals who may be on vacation for each shift and other issues regarding seniority. After weighing the pros and cons of the choices (allowing employee choice takes more time; allowing employee choice makes the nurses happier; allowing choice could propel arguments), the manager could decide to:

1. Complete and post the vacation schedule.
2. Ask for requests in advance and post the vacation schedule.
3. Post a tentative schedule and ask for comments and suggestions.
4. Post a blank schedule and ask everyone to complete this schedule within the required administrative restrictions by a certain date.

Based on experience and knowledge of human nature regarding choice, he rejects options 1, 2, and 3 and decides to post a blank schedule. It is a good model to use to process information because it offers the opportunity to consider many alternatives and demonstrates the importance of a thorough assessment in order to develop alternative choices.

Wheeler's Model

Wheeler (2000) suggests that having choices and knowing the context in which choices are made are the most important elements of proactive decision making. Being proactive allows the anticipation of an event and allows one to generate actions before the event. For instance, planning for staff replacement during a maternity leave provides options: temporary replacement with additional part-time use, agency nurses, overtime use, extended shifts, and so on (Fig. 10-2).

Having a choice involves having at least two options. One of the options may be not to act at all, but that does constitute a choice. In that situation, the decision maker allows other people or events to determine the outcome. Wheeler uses concentric circles to conceptualize the relationships between the five primary areas (contexts) for consideration when determining choice and context. Knowing the context helps to put the choices in perspective. The personal arena is the first level. Here, decisions occur that pertain solely to the individual. The second level is the family arena. The third is the social arena, where decisions can affect business associates and close friends. The fourth level is the community arena, which includes cultural, ethnic, religious, and national groups. The fifth level is the global or international arena, involving philosophical, political, and financial issues.

Wheeler's model might have limited usefulness in a nursing environment as it is described; however, changing the labels of the circles (see Fig. 10-2) might allow one to use it to determine context and how far-reaching an anticipated decision might be. For example, levels could be changed to reflect unit personnel, patients/families, budget, the nursing organization, the entire agency, and so on. Circles could be added to indicate a more complex decision. The strength of this model is the fact that it is graphic. In the example presented in Figure 10-2, choice #1 will affect the unit staff and may also influence the budget to some extent. Choice #2 will definitely affect the budget and may affect patient care if staff becomes overextended or fatigued. Choice #3 affects the existing staff to orient the agency and traveling staff; patient care might be affected, and the budget will be affected because of the increased cost in hiring nurses. The nursing department will become involved because these nurses will be processed through other departments, such as Employee Health and Nursing Education. Finally, choice #4, which is actually a choice not to make a choice, will affect the entire agency. After all, failing to provide adequate staffing can result in poor clinical outcomes, dissatisfied patients and nurses, increased complaints, the possibility of risk of liability to the agency, and damage to the agency's reputation. All the individuals involved in the decision can judge what the impact of the decision might be on their part of the entire organization. This model allows one to look at the perspectives of others and what their concerns and issues might be. Finally, it encourages one to consider as many alternatives as possible to satisfy the needs of everyone involved.

Staff Replacement for a Maternity Leave

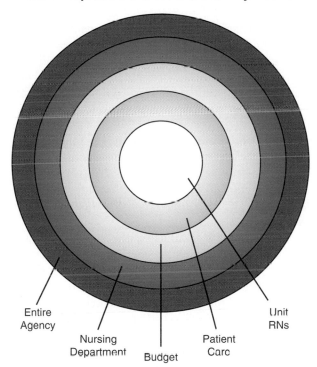

Entire Agency

Nursing Department

Budget

Patient Care

Unit RNs

Choice #1
Use existing part-time staff to take on additional shifts.

Choice #2
Use planned overtime and extended shifts.

Choice #3
Use agency staff and traveler RNs.

Choice #4
Provide no additional coverage.

FIGURE 10-2 Wheeler's model.

Nursing Process

Although there are many decision-making models, the nursing process may be the most familiar and comfortable model for nurses to utilize to make decisions.

The nursing process is ongoing and begins with phase I, assessment, according to Figure 10-3. This phase includes defining the assumptions and context, collecting data, identifying and naming the problem(s), and deciding on actions or interventions. Phase II is implementation or intervention as planned in phase I. Phase III is evaluating the outcomes. Based on the evaluation, the process begins over again with more data collection, if indicated. For example, during a home visit to a patient, the nurse is concerned about the safety of an elderly man who is post–cerebral vascular accident (stroke) with some mobility problems. She observes many throw rugs on the floor, extension cords that are visible in the walking areas, and several cats who roam around the patient when he gets up to walk into the kitchen or bathroom. The nurse identifies all these as safety hazards and labels the problem "Alteration in safety related to environmental hazards." She makes a plan to review the environment with the patient and make necessary changes by eliminating the throw rugs or anchoring them to the floor, removing the extension cords or taping them down, and discussing how the cats can be controlled when the patient is walking through the house. The nurse then discusses the problems and possible solutions with the patient, comes to consensus about the changes, and makes arrangements for the alterations. This is the implementation phase. Short-term evaluation of the changes will occur on her next home visit; long-term evaluation will be measured by the lack of falls by the patient. This nurse used the nursing process to make decisions about the care of this patient. The same process can be used to make all decisions, even those that do not involve patient care.

Using the nursing process as a guide, start the decision-making process by collecting data and assessing the situation. It is important to make decisions with as much information as possible. Leaders make their most successful decisions when they assess the strengths and weaknesses of the people and the environment. Good decision making relies on building relationships, knowing the politics of the players, understanding the time and other envi-

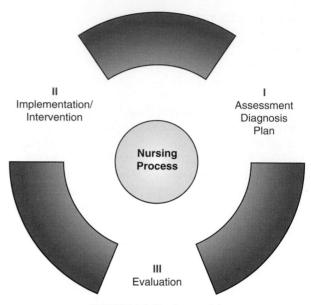

FIGURE 10-3 Nursing model.

ronmental constraints, integrating cultural values, and staying true to personal and organization ethics. Furthermore, the cultural diversity found in any organization needs to be considered in any decision that affects more than one person. Differences in frames of reference, perspectives, norms, values, and communication style are often aggravated by prejudices, stereotypes, and misunderstandings (Broome, et al., 2002). In the home care nursing example, major misunderstandings could occur if the nurse did not include the patient in any environmental alteration. The cats may be very important to the patient, who may be willing to risk falling rather than confining them to a separate room.

Aside from its familiarity, the strength of this model is its feedback mechanism. If evaluation reveals an unanticipated or unacceptable outcome, the assessment begins again. In today's health-care environment, the concept of evidence-based practice supports the need to gather as much evidence as possible to make a decision that can lead to best practices. Sources of data for decision making come from more formal sources such as quality assurance, benchmarking, and risk management data (see Chapter 15). Observation and inquiry can also yield information about a situation. Finally, scientific research data make excellent assessment data and should be the basis for much of decision making in nursing whenever possible.

TYPE OF DECISIONS

Not all decisions are critical or global in their impact. Decisions are made at all levels of the hierarchy in organizations. Some experts believe that a decision should be made as close to the action as possible. At the same time, however, as demonstrated in the Wheeler model, good decision making also means considering the impact the decision will have beyond the immediate environment.

Routine decisions can be used to respond to frequently occurring, common, and reasonably well-defined issues. Policies and procedures and established rules can be used to guide the decision-making process. The level of personnel that makes routine decisions can range from the staff nurse to top administrators. For example, when a patient falls, there is a clearly defined process to follow regarding immediate intervention, reporting, and follow-up. Decisions about who will do what and when can be made easily, based on the incident. Leaders should attempt to determine quickly if there are established guidelines for a particular situation and apply them as soon as possible. Leaders should be careful, however, to avoid generalizing every situation and should make decisions that are appropriate in the context of each event.

Innovative decisions are made when the situation or problem is unusual and the rules and guidelines do not clearly define or dictate a course of action. Nurses, from the bedside to top administration, need to make these kinds of decisions frequently. For innovative decisions, it is helpful if the nurse understands the art of decision making. In any event, there is work to be done before implementing the decision-making process at any level. Innovative decisions generally take longer to make and require more attention to data collection and assessment. Without rules and policies to guide the decision-making process, the leader must be sure to view all possible alternatives.

PRE–DECISION MAKING

Before making a decision, ask several questions based on the assessment data. First, is there really a need to make a decision? Is there a problem that needs to be solved? The perception of a problem is relative. A headache is painful to the individual but is good for the pharmacist. A wise leader needs to determine first how the issue is affecting the current situation and if it truly requires intervention.

Another pre-decision question involves timing: how quickly does the decision need to be made? One of the characteristics of leadership is the ability to think critically and make difficult decisions quickly and effectively. But delaying decision making or not making a decision is actually making a decision not to take any action. Striking a balance between a knee-jerk response and a delayed or non-response is one hallmark of an effective leader. If the decision will affect others and represent a change in procedure, it might be necessary to assess the readiness of others to accept the decision or change (see Chapter 11).

Nurses are very aware of modifiable and nonmodifiable risk factors in relationship to cardiac health. The same concept can be applied to decision making. Some situations are controllable, and some are uncontrollable. Before making a decision, a wise leader will identify uncontrollable factors and avoid spending time trying to alter them. Additionally, leaders need to identify situations where factors can be modified but not by them. It is difficult for some leaders to let go of situations that do not fall under their authority. For example, an emergency department manager may be able to control the process by which laboratory diagnostic test requests are made but cannot control the volume of requests that are made from within the department or throughout the hospital.

TOOLS FOR MAKING DECISIONS

After determining that a decision must be made, the effective leader turns to the decision-making tools. The *traditional problem-solving process* is well known and was the basis for the development of the nursing process. This traditional model is a seven-step process:

1. Identify the problem
2. Gather data

> **Pre–Decision Making Questions**
>
> Does a decision need to be made?
> 1. How soon does the decision need to be made?
> 2. Who has the power to make the decision?
> 3. What are the controllable and uncontrollable factors?

TABLE 10-1	Comparison of the Traditional, Managerial, and Nursing Process Models for Decision Making and Problem Solving

TRADITIONAL	MANAGEMENT	NURSING
1. Identify problem	1. Set objectives	1. Assessment
2. Collect data	2. Search for alternatives	2. Identify problem
3. Explore alternatives	3. Evaluate alternatives	3. Plan
4. Identify alternatives	4. Choose	4. Implement
5. Evaluate alternatives	5. Implement	5. Evaluate
6. Select alternative	6. Follow up	
7. Implement	7. Control	
8. Evaluate results		

3. Explore alternatives
4. Evaluate alternatives
5. Select the appropriate solution
6. Implement the solution
7. Evaluate the results

The *managerial model* is similar to the traditional model and comprises the following steps:

1. Set the objectives
2. Search for alternatives
3. Evaluate alternatives
4. Choose an alternative
5. Implement
6. Follow up
7. Control the outcomes

Decision making occurs at step four when a choice is made.

Table 10-1 compares the traditional managerial, and nursing process for decision making and problem solving. There are strengths and weaknesses in each model. For example, in the managerial model the objective is determined at the beginning. Sometimes it is difficult to know what the objectives need to be to reach an outcome, and this model does not focus on data collection in order to identify the alternatives. The traditional model requires problem identification as a first step, whereas the nursing process collects data to determine if there is a problem. Both methods can be useful in making a decision, yet the nursing process allows for the possibility that there is no problem or no need to make a decision or take any action. Problem identification is the foundation of good decision making. If the correct problem is not identified initially, a very good decision can be made for the wrong problem.

Specific Decision-Making Tools

The use of tools is a systematic way to collect the data necessary for making a good decision. Specifically, pros and cons, SWOT analysis, and 2 × 2 matrix are recommended for beginning nurse managers.

Pros and Cons

A simple strategy is to make a list with one side labeled "Pro (or Advantages)" and the other side "Con (or Disadvantages)." Writing down options helps to clarify the decision that needs to be made. More accurate decisions can be made by assigning weights to each factor, with 5 representing very significant and 1 representing minor significance. Table 10-2 illustrates the use of this strategy to make a decision about which shifts might be appropriate for a particular nursing unit. The use of a

TABLE 10-2	Moving From 8- to 12-Hour Shifts		
PROS	WEIGHT	CONS	WEIGHT
Staff satisfaction	5	Increased fatigue	4
Ease of scheduling	3	Need more full-time employees	3
Patient satisfaction	5	Increased absences	4
		Patient satisfaction	5
Totals	13		16

weighting system allows the decision maker to determine what the most important factors are.

SWOT Analysis

Once the problem has been identified, the **SWOT analysis** can be extremely useful for decision making. SWOT stands for Strengths, Weaknesses, Opportunities, and Threats. For example, a SWOT analysis can be used to assess:

- A nursing unit and its position in the agency
- A nursing care delivery system
- A scheduling process
- A recruitment idea
- A strategic option, such as developing a specialty unit
- A new management hierarchy
- Outsourcing a service
- A new documentation method
- A different communication system
- A job description for unlicensed personnel

For example, if a nursing department needs to determine the most effective and efficient method for providing ongoing professional education and development for staff, it can use a SWOT analysis to identify the risks and benefits in outsourcing this service. Strengths include not paying benefits and having specialists to provide specific services as opposed to generalists, yet there is a risk that the individuals may not have a commitment to the organization and may not be familiar with or comfortable with the culture of the organization. They may be perceived as "outsiders," which can pose a threat to employee satisfaction. Making the final decision may involve determining how important each strength, weakness, opportunity, and threat is to the department. The final decision can be made only in the context of that nursing department, within the financial constraints of the organization, and in consideration of the culture of the organization.

2 × 2 Matrix

Similar to the SWOT approach is the use of a 2 × 2 **matrix**. The 2 × 2 matrix is a relatively simple way to visualize issues or concerns. It conveys the choices available in relationship to a goal. According to Lowy and Hood (2004), the x and y axes are used to clarify issues; a complicated situation can be reframed to allow everyone to understand all aspects of the issue. Instead of looking for a single right answer, conflicting goals are identified and labeled. Rather than discouraging differing perspec-

Sample SWOT Analysis: Outsourcing Nursing Education

STRENGTHS	WEAKNESSES
■ Providing no benefits will decrease overall costs ■ Can use specialists who may be more competent than generalists ■ Eliminates need to perform non-core activities	■ Vendors may be dissociated from the goals of the organization ■ Because vendors are off site, there may be a time or scheduling issue ■ Need to learn culture of units
OPPORTUNITIES	**THREATS**
■ Allows focus on core activities, i.e., patient care ■ May lead to other outsourcing opportunities ■ Allows access to other highly skilled individuals	■ May lose information or intellectual property ■ Employee satisfaction issues ■ Lose management control

tives, this approach encourages these differences in order to work toward a decision. A common issue confronting individuals personally and professionally is that of too much to do and not enough time in which to do it. Table 10-3 is an example of the use of a 2 × 2 matrix to assist with decisions about time management. The axes in this matrix are the importance of the tasks described versus the urgency of completing these tasks. Striking a balance between getting things done on time and doing important work becomes the goal. Individuals can include items in the matrix based on personal choice. For instance, a nurse leader may include resolving a crisis and meeting deadlines as having high importance and high urgency but planning for the future, preventing crises, and preserving relationships as having high importance but low urgency. Another individual may put planning and prevention in high importance and high urgency boxes. This matrix becomes a quick and visual method of deciding what to do next.

Using a simple matrix model consistently can help a novice leader develop these skills quickly and continue to make good decisions in all areas. Even

TABLE 10-3	Sample Matrix: Time Management	

	High		
Importance	Unexpected crisis Deadlines 1	Planning Prevention Relationships 2	
	3 Returning calls Approving schedule change requests	4 Reviewing mail and e-mail Answering telephone	Low
	High	Low	

with the best of models, however, there are some common mistakes made by even the most experienced leaders. The following is a discussion on how to recognize and avoid making some of these mistakes.

AVOIDING COMMON DECISION-MAKING MISTAKES

According to Anderson (2004a), emotions can bias rational judgment because people have a subconscious tendency to decide what they want to do before they know why they want to do it. Another tendency is for people to be more engaged with things they like than with things they dislike. Anderson describes a number of traps into which people may fall when making decisions. One is the confirming evidence trap. She suggests that individuals check for this trap by examining all the evidence with equal rigor. Seek people who can offer independent information and opinions to play devil's advocate.

The framing trap occurs when a decision is made based on how the choices are viewed or framed. For example, in Hospital A, the postanesthesia recovery unit (PACU) nurses who have been employed for more than 10 years are no longer required to be on call. But they are required to work a certain number of holidays each year. Because the unit is closed on holidays except for on-call emergencies, they are required to work on another unit in order to fulfill this obligation. The PACU nurses are not happy

Practice to Strive For 10-1

The nurse executive of a very successful nursing agency is being interviewed. When asked how he makes decisions, he responds that he walks and talks with his people. They know what he is thinking and envisioning for the company. They also know they can tell him what they see as the future for the agency. When they have a problem, they share the problem and the solution. He does not always have the last word, even when making financial decisions. He also gives people the power to make decisions that need to be made quickly and always backs them up even when he would not have made the same decision or carried one out the same way. His guideline for decision making is well known by everyone who works for the agency. It includes:

- *Making an analysis of all the components of the issue*
- *Thinking of all the people who will be affected by the decision*
- *Thinking everything through*
- *Having the self-confidence to make a short- or long-term decision and the strength to stand by it*
- *Communicating the decision to others*
- *Having the ability to overcome the conflict that may arise from the decision*

He cautions never to forget evaluation after the decision is made. The information obtained from evaluation can be used to help make decisions in the future. This mantra is posted throughout the agency. There are times when he has to make a decision that will have far-reaching effects on the agency and even beyond. He uses a graphic presentation of his decision-making process and posts the analysis. He often uses the SWOT analysis and even invents his own graphics to reflect his thinking process and encourages the staff to do the same. He frequently asks individuals to show everyone the process that was used to arrive at different decisions. He believes that when the process is shared, individuals understand the thinking and are more likely to support the solution or decision. Using this method also helps others to develop better decision-making skills by example.

about this arrangement. In Hospital B, the same rules apply. However, operative cases requiring PACU nurses on a holiday are called "unscheduled" rather than "emergencies." PACU staff rotates coverage for unscheduled holiday cases with an option to stay home and wait for a case or come into the hospital and perform other duties in the PACU. Those who choose to stay home are paid a percentage of their regular hourly rate plus a holiday bonus; those who come into the hospital are paid at their regular hourly rate plus a holiday bonus. Simply using different terms to describe the pay rate and the obligation has resolved the on-call problem, and the nurses are happy with the arrangement. Try to reframe the problem or opportunity in several ways to maximize understanding and potential solutions.

The status quo trap occurs when people look for decisions that involve the least amount of change (Anderson, 2004b). Keep in mind, however, that change is necessary for growth. Look at possible future situations when considering a change. Even the status quo will change over time. The status quo should never be the only alternative to consider.

It is difficult to change course or deviate from a decision whenever an investment of time, money, personal reputation, or other resources is at stake. Making similar decisions that justify past actions is comfortable but can become a trap (Anderson, 2004b). It can be risky to step off the path and decide that decisions need to be made to go in a different direction. Cultivate a climate where individuals can admit mistakes without enduring penalties. Do not apply sanctions or punishments when an individual admits making a mistake. Analyze the issues, and move on to different decisions.

The prudence trap intervenes when estimates are made (and then making decisions based on these estimates) using the worst case scenario (Anderson, 2004a). This is sometimes called the knee-jerk response. When a situation has occurred with a negative outcome, it is tempting to make a global change or decisions based on this one bad event. For example, in an agency a patient fell in the shower and was injured. The agency immediately instituted a policy that patients could no longer shower. Careful consideration should be given to making any decisions based on one bad event. Again, analyze the issue, and consider many scenarios. Similarly, individuals may fall into the "recallability" trap, when overwhelming events and experiences influence decision making, even though the events are inapplicable to the current decision.

Other mistakes can include relying too much on "expert" information, overestimating the value of information received from others, highly selective hearing or seeing and, most important, not listening to one's own feelings or "gut reactions." Whenever possible, delay the decision, and the right choice may become obvious. See Box 10-2 for some effective decision-making tips.

Problem Solving

The term "problem solving" is often used synonymously with decision making, but the processes are not the same. Decision making may or may not involve a problem but always involves selecting one action from several alternatives. Problem solving involves diagnosing or identifying a problem and solving it and includes making decisions along the way (Sullivan & Decker, 2001). In other words, problem solving is broader in scope than decision making in that it may include making many decisions in order to resolve the problem (Fig. 10-4). But problem solving is also more narrow in scope than decision making in that decisions are made about many different issues, not just about problems.

Box 10-2

Decision-Making Tips

- Do not make decisions that are not yours to make, and do not waste your time making decisions that do not have to be made.
- Not making a decision is a decision; it is a decision to not take action.
- When making a decision, a choice is made from options. A choice is not being made between right and wrong.
- Avoid snap decisions. Move quickly on the reversible ones and slowly on the nonreversible ones.
- Make decisions on paper. Make notes, and keep ideas visible so all the relevant information can be viewed
- Be sure to choose what is right, not who is right.
- Make decisions as you go along. Do not let them accumulate.
- Consider those affected by a decision. Whenever feasible, get people involved to increase their commitment.
- To be effective, a manager must have the luxury of having the right to be wrong.
- Once the decision has been made, do not look back. Never regret a decision; it was the right thing to do at the time.
- As part of the decision-making process, always consider how it will be implemented.

(Liraz Publishing Co., 2001)

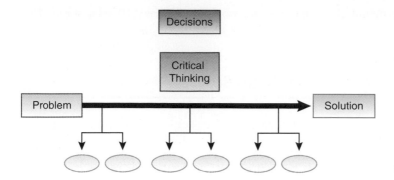

FIGURE 10-4 Decision model.

The problem-solving process can take some time to define the problem and its scope and the goal for problem solving. Problem solving should be a group process, involving all individuals or groups affected by the problem. Problems can also be viewed as opportunities to make change and improve outcomes. Start the investigation with who, what, when, where, why, and how. Either or both of the following techniques present effective ways to explore all aspects of the problem and obtain feedback about the decisions that are made along the way.

BRAINSTORMING TECHNIQUE

Using the basic brainstorming technique to solve problems can be a very powerful strategy. This is a group process using a strong facilitator who can control the discussion while allowing each individual the freedom to meet and express ideas without threat of ridicule or sanction. The purpose of the meeting must be clear to everyone involved, and the facilitator has the task of keeping everyone focused on that purpose. Deciding how much time will be allowed to brainstorm is critical, and the facilitator or leader should be prepared with ideas to get the process started and keep it moving. Frequent clarification and summary will help keep the discussion on track, and the outcomes should be apparent and flow logically from the discussion. The process begins with defining and agreeing on the objective and continuing as follows:

- Brainstorm ideas and suggestions with an agreed upon time limit.
- Categorize/condense/combine/refine.
- Assess/analyze effects or results.
- Prioritize options/rank-list as appropriate.
- Agree on action and period.
- Control and monitor follow-up.

SEVEN HAT TECHNIQUE

A parallel thinking technique introduced by deBono (1985) can enhance problem solving. DeBono identified six thinking hats, with each colored hat representing a different viewpoint. This deliberate method encourages a group to think along similar lines at the same time so that personal egos do not interfere in the creation of facts, information, or solutions. Each individual in the group is expected to take a particular position or "wear a different color hat." Individuals may be asked to change hats and review the issues from a different perspective.

- Blue Hat thinking provides a formal structure to the thinking at all times. One person, usually the group facilitator, wears this hat. The blue hat is responsible for focusing the thinking at all times and keeping the various thinking hats trained on the correct tasks. One suggested sequence, controlled at all times by the blue hat, is to start with the white hat, followed by the red, yellow, green, and black hats.
- White Hat thinking deals with figures and facts in an objective or neutral way. Individual opinion is excluded. It provides an opportunity to move back down the abstraction ladder to the data, or lowest-rung, level. An example of white hat thinking is "There are RNs and UAPs in all nursing departments." It would be unacceptable to say "I think all nursing departments should consist of RNs and UAPs."
- Red Hat thinking involves emotion and is not rational. It is based on feelings and intuitions that can be positive or negative. The key to red hat thinking is that explanations are unnecessary. The red hat puts positive and negative feelings out in the open so they do not lurk in the background and cloud the thinking

process. The red hat acknowledges the fact that feelings can shape perceptions.

- Yellow Hat thinking is visionary. It is about constructive thinking and making things happen. Here, alternatives are discussed and may be speculative in nature. "Long shots" are included because they expand the thinking and provide the opportunity to clarify other ideas. Ideas do not have to be new or unique; yellow hat thinking is concerned about finding effective ways to accomplish the task.
- Green Hat thinking involves the creation of new ideas or thinking about things in different ways. This hat legitimizes the wild and crazy ideas. It involves movement in a forward direction. Here, the fact that that there is more than one right answer to a problem is acknowledged.
- Black Hat thinking is logical and negative, never emotional. This hat does not consider arguments for or against, only negative statements that are based on reason and logic. Facts produced in the white hat thinking can be challenged when wearing the black hat. Statements take the form of "I am concerned about" and "Can you help me with this concern?"

All Good Things...

- Critical thinking is the process that guides scientific reasoning, the nursing process, problem solving, and decision making.
- Critical thinking involves the use of the cognitive process, which includes divergent thinking, reasoning, reflection, creativity, clarification, and basic support.
- Decision making and problem solving are not synonymous.
- Decision making involves identifying and selecting a course of action from several alternatives.
- Problem solving requires identifying a problem and finding a solution.
- There are many decision-making models, which are derived from theories to guide the process.
- There are two types of decisions: routine and innovative.
- The problem-solving process involves identifying the problem, gathering and analyzing

information, developing and implementing the solutions, and evaluating the outcomes.

Let's Talk

The coordinator of a home care team has been informed by administration that the team must begin to care for patients who have external defibrillators in the home. The nursing staff is not familiar with this technology. The team leader must decide who to assign to care for these patients.

1. Use the pre–decision making process to analyze this issue.

2. How soon does a decision need to be made? Determine when the agency will be accepting patients for home care who have external defibrillators.

3. Who has the power to make the decision? Obviously, the administration made the decision about accepting this type of patient. Determine if you will be able to decide when and how many of these patients are accepted for home care.

4. What are the controllable and uncontrollable factors? After gathering this information, you will be able to determine what you can control. You can then move on to decide how best to prepare the nurses to care for these patients.

NCLEX Questions

1. When the nurse manager of a busy rehabilitation unit decided the best way to reward staff was to give a monetary bonus rather than time off, many of the staff became upset and went to administration with complaints. This manager skipped which step of the critical thinking process?
   A. Obtaining a majority consensus of all of the staff.
   B. Considering the context and meaning of the issues to each individual.
   C. Not asking the staff how much money would be considered an adequate reward.
   D. Identifying assumptions underlying the issue.

2. The manager of a unit was concerned about the plans for unit renovations. In an effort to be sure

the renovations would be "nurse-friendly" he asked the staff to make a wish list of everything they would like moved or fixed on the existing unit. This is an example of which part of the decision-making process?

A. Assessment/data collection.
B. Planning.
C. Data interpretation.
D. Generating hypotheses.

3. S. Adams read the notice about the new intravenous pumps that had been purchased for the unit. She reviewed the information and instructions for use and compared them with the pumps they had been using. She listed all the similarities in her mind and decided these new pumps were not really very different and might be easier to use than the old pumps. She is an example of which kind of individual?

A. Chaotic thinker.
B. Innovative thinker.
C. Negative thinker.
D. Adaptive thinker.

4. A good decision maker is one who:

A. Uses various models to guide the process based on the situation.
B. Adopts one model and uses it to guide all decision making.
C. Does not use any models because they are not at all useful.
D. Develops a model each time a decision needs to be made.

5. Using Wheeler's decision-making model with concentric circles is useful only if:

A. One applies the model exactly as it is presented in the textbook.
B. One can absolutely predict the outcomes in any given situation.
C. Everyone understands the model.
D. The labels are changed in the circles to represent the situation.

6. J. Strong, manager of an orthopedic unit, drafted a policy to be used in his department to define the process to have laboratory tests completed on his unit. This policy included the times of regular collection and the process for emergency or STAT laboratory testing. The policy and procedure were never followed because:

A. The policy was too complicated and included too much information.

B. The policy and procedure made decisions for another department.
C. The staff did not believe it was necessary to follow any procedure.
D. None of the above.

7. Amazing fell into what trap when she decided that all staff would be required to pick up all medications from the pharmacy for their patients because the unit secretary brought the medications from a different unit, which caused a half-hour delay in administering medications on the unit?

A. Status quo.
B. Framing.
C. Expert.
D. Prudence.

8. All nurses were advised to register any additional vehicles they might drive to work with security. JJ could not decide which other car to register so he did not register any additional automobiles with security. When his primary car was in the shop, he could not park in the employee area and had to pay visitors' parking fees. This was what kind of decision making?

A. Not making a decision results in a decision being made for you.
B. Making a decision that is not yours to make.
C. Relying on too much expert opinion.
D. Innovative decision making.

9. There were many new nurses working on the unit, and many of them were from other countries. The manager became aware of many difficulties that seemed to be arising from this cultural diversity. She decided to get the staff together to talk about the differences and commonalities and decide on a plan to educate every one working on the unit about the different cultures. This is an example of what kind of problem-solving technique?

A. Seven hats.
B. Pros and cons.
C. Brainstorming.
D. Concentric circles.

10. When confronted with the controversy and apparent poor morale of the 3-11 p.m. staff, the manager decided the staff needed to take vacation days and began to schedule these days for them. Many nurses became very upset with this, and finally one nurse said that the problem

was not the schedule but the difficulties the nurses were having with the charge nurse with the patient assignments. This is an example of what kind of error in problem solving?

A. Not using a problem-solving model.

B. Poor evaluation of outcomes.

C. Not considering several alternatives.

D. Incorrect problem identification.

REFERENCES

Anderson, K. (2004a). More of the most common decision-making mistakes people make. Accessed August 31, 2004, at www.pertinent.com/articles/communications/KareCom

Anderson, K. (2004b). How we sometimes fool ourselves when making decisions: Part I. Accessed August 31, 2004, atwww.pertinent.com/articles/communications/KareCom1.asp

Broome, B.J., DeTurk, S., Kristjansdottir, E.S, et al. (2002). Giving voice to diversity: An interactive approach to conflict management and decision-making in culturally diverse work environments. *Journal of Business and Management, 8*, 239–264.

deBono, E. (1985). *Six Thinking Hats.* Boston: Little, Brown & Co.

Decision Making Tips. (2001). Liraz Publishing Co. http://www.LIRAZ.com/tdecision.htm

Fralic, M.F., & Denby, C.B. (2000). Retooling the nurse executive for the 21st century practice: Decision support systems. *Nursing Administration Quarterly, 24*(2), 19–28.

Lowy, A., & Hood, P. (2004). *The Power of the 2 × 2 Matrix.* San Francisco: Jossey-Bass.

Marketing Teacher, (n.d.). *S.W.O.T. Analysis.* http://www.marketingteacher.com/index.html

McNichol, E. (2002). Thinking outside the box: Encouraging flexible thinking for problems and decisions. *Nursing Management* (London), 9(4), 19–22.

Sullivan, E.J., & Decker, P.J. (2001). Problem solving and decision making. *Effective leadership and management in nursing.* (5th ed.). Upper Saddle River, NJ: Prentice Hall.

Thompson, C. (1999). A conceptual treadmill: The need for "middle ground" in clinical decision making theory in nursing. *Journal of Advance Nursing, 30,* 1222–1229.

Wheeler, R. (2000). Being proactive, not reactive. In Fay L. Bower (Ed.) *Nurses taking the lead: Personal qualities of effective leadership.* Philadelphia: W.B. Saunders.

BIBLIOGRAPHY

Benner, P. (1984). *From novice to expert: Excellence and power in clinical nursing practice.* Reading, MA: Addison Wesley.

Bruhn, J.G. (2004). Leaders who create change and those who manage it: How leaders limit success. *The Health Care Manager, 23,* 132–140.

Carlson, R. (1997). *Don't Sweat the Small Stuff . . . and It's All Small Stuff.* New York: Hyperion Press.

Clancy, R.R. (2003). The art of decision-making. *Journal of Nursing Administration, 33,* 343–349.

Fraser, K.D., & Strang, V. (2004). Decision-making and nurse case management: A philosophical perspective. *Advances in Nursing Science, 27,* 32–43.

Green, C. (2000). *Critical thinking in nursing,* Upper Saddle River, NJ: Prentice Hall Health.

Janis, I.L., & Mann, L. (1977). Decision making: A psychological analysis of conflict, choice, and commitment. New York: Macmillan.

Johnson, L.J. (1990). The influence of assumptions on effective decision-making. *Journal of Nursing Administration, 20*(4), 35–39.

Kay, S. (1998). How employees process information. *Supervision, 59*(12), 6–7.

Kikuchi, J.F., & Simmons, H. (1999). Practical nursing judgment: A moderate realist conception. *Scholarly Inquiry for Nursing Practice, 13,* 43–55.

Lindner, K. (2004). *Crunch Time: 8 steps to Making the Right Life Decisions When It Counts.* New York: Gotham Books. Accessed March 31, 2005, at http://www.msnbc.com/id/6766123/

McGraw, P.C. (2000). *Life strategies.* New York: Hyperion Press.

Peterson, T.O., & Lunsford, D.A. (1998). Parallel thinking: A technique for group interaction and problem solving. *Journal of Management Education, 22,* 537–554.

Rausch, E. (1999). Management/leadership decision guidelines: Critical ingredients for competitiveness. *Competitiveness Review, 9*(2), 19–27.

Smith, G.F. (2003). Beyond critical thinking and decision making: Teaching business students how to think. *Journal of Management Education, 27*(1), 24–51.

Tucker-Ladd, C.E. (2002). Decision-making and problem-solving. *Psychological Self Help.* Online book: Mental Health Net. http://mentalhelp.net/psyhelp/chap13/chap13o.htm

Wheeler, J. (2001). Thinking your way to successful problem-solving. *Nursing Times, 97*(37), 36–37.

Nurses Leading Change

DEBRA A. MORGAN, EDD, RN
JEWETT G. JOHNSON, NSN, RN
DEBORAH R. GARRISON, PHD, RN

CHAPTER MOTIVATION

"Nothing is permanent but change."

Heraclitus (c. 500 BC)

CHAPTER MOTIVES

- Apply change theories to clinical situations.
- Identify strategies to overcome barriers to change.
- Discuss the role of the change agent.
- Identify common characteristics among various change theories.
- Use various change theories as frameworks for initiating change.

*C*hange is nothing new. In fact, it is often said that change is the only constant. Change, particularly in the health-care environment, is complex and is occurring at an unprecedented rate. Change is driven by many factors: the increasing cost of health-care delivery, the nursing shortage, the rapid advancements in technology and information management, and new expectations by the public to have a more active role in health-care decisions. Meeting the health-care needs of the world requires that the nurse be proactive and creative in guiding change. The ability to create and manage meaningful change is an essential skill for nurses in the 21st century.

Change fosters growth and innovation; progress cannot occur without change. If nurses are to be leaders of change, it is imperative that they understand the changes occurring in the health-care arena, use political clout to have a hand in the changes, and master the change process. This chapter will introduce readers to the principles of planned change, barriers commonly encountered when introducing change, strategies for overcoming barriers, and the role of the nurse as the change agent.

Elements of Change

Change is an integral part of any organization, and the process can be uncomfortable and disturbing to those who are affected. An awareness of the elements common to the change process is important.

DEFINING CHANGE

Change means to be different, to cause to be different, or to alter. Change may be personal or organizational and can occur suddenly or incrementally. Change may be planned or unplanned. Unplanned change, or reactive change, usually occurs suddenly and in response to some event or set of circumstances. For example, an unanticipated rise in patient census may precipitate the need for a change in patient assignments. Decisions are made—and change follows—as a reaction to an event. Planned change, however, entails planning and application of strategic actions designed to promote movement toward a desired goal. Planned change is deliberate and proactive. For example, changing staffing patterns from extensive use of unlicensed assistive per-

sonnel to an all-professional staff requires time and planning. Specific strategies need to be developed and implemented before such a sweeping change is adopted. Generally, planned change is more likely to occur incrementally, over time. Planned change responds to anticipated events in the environment or community.

Change may be initiated in response to internal or external forces. Internal forces stem from within the organization. Internal forces include organizational values and beliefs, culture, and past experiences with change. External forces come from outside the organization. These can be social influences, economic factors, or legislation. For example, a 1996 legislative mandate put the federal Health Insurance Portability and Accountability Act (HIPAA) in place (Public Law 104-191). This piece of legislation forced all health-care agencies, schools of nursing, and their governing bodies to plan and implement major system-wide changes in the way personal information is collected, handled, and stored.

Another factor essential to change is the presence of a change agent. A **change agent** is one who generates ideas, introduces the innovation, and works to bring about the desired change. In fact, the one who assumes the leadership role of change agent in today's health-care environment is the nurse. Members of an organization assume different roles in a change, depending on the nature of the change and their role in the organization. A leader often assumes the role of change agent and initiates change; an effective follower actively participates in the change effort and is essential to the successful implementation of change. Registered nurses are frequently in a position of leadership within health-care organizations and, as such, are well positioned to be the leaders of change.

ASSUMPTIONS REGARDING CHANGE

When initiating change, the following assumptions are important to consider.

Assumption 1

Change of any kind represents loss. Even if the change is positive, there is a loss of stability. This loss of the familiar may produce anxiety and even grief in many individuals. The leader of change must be sensitive to the loss experienced by others.

Assumption 2

The more consistent the change goal is with the individual's personal values and beliefs, the more likely the change is to be accepted. Likewise, the more different the goal is from the individual's personal values, the more likely it is to be rejected. The change agent needs to know and respect the values and beliefs of those most affected by the change.

Assumption 3

Those who actively participate in the change feel accountable for the outcome. The more people who are involved in the process, the more the group will feel responsible for the outcome.

Assumption 4

With each successive change in a series of changes, individuals' psychological adjustment to the change occurs more slowly. It is for this reason that the leader of change must avoid initiating too many changes at once. Timing is important.

Assumption 5

Power is important to the change process. Organizations with many layers of hierarchy between the initiator of change and the ultimate decision makers may have difficulty with implementing change. The shorter the distance the change proposal must travel from the initiator to the decision maker, the greater the likelihood that the change will be accepted. Conversely, the greater the distance, the more likely resistance will occur.

ASSESSING READINESS FOR CHANGE

Assessing readiness for change is generally the first step in any change project. Until participants are ready for change, little can be done to bring about change. According to Terry (1993), readiness for change is assessed by answering the following questions:

1. What is the ultimate purpose of the action/change?
2. Why might I lead or be involved in this change?
3. What is at stake if I lead or participate in this change action?

4. What structures are in place either to foster success or hinder the change?
5. Are the necessary resources available to achieve this change action?
6. What is the stakeholders' level of commitment to the change?

Practice to Strive For 11-1

Betty R. is a practicing registered nurse who has worked in the intensive care setting for several years and is highly respected by her peers, supervisors, and hospital administrators. She is also a graduate student in a family nurse practitioner program and has developed strong rapport with the faculty in the program. Being in graduate school has given her new perspective on the value of research-based practice. Her clinical manager has also been attending graduate classes in nursing education and likewise values research as a basis for practice. Betty has implemented a new evidence-based patient care initiative at work. The facility is not new to change as it recently underwent a massive redesign in facility and organizational structure. We will use Betty's questions in the analysis of this new evidenced-based change initiative.

The purpose of the change is to enhance patient care by using evidence based practice in the delivery of care. Betty is in a position to lead this change because she can use the information she gained in her master's program to help other nurses use research findings concerning patient care. School has given her a fresh perspective on the nursing profession and the importance of using research rather than tradition in providing patient care.

One of Betty's concerns was that her peers might view her as a "prima donna" or "stuck up." Her motivation was that patients would receive care based on evidence, which would result in optimal patient outcomes. Betty has a good rapport with individuals who are the informal leaders. Her clinical manager and the vice president for patient services have already indicated their support for this change. The organization has demonstrated an ability to manage other types of change effectively.

Betty's relationships with faculty in the graduate program also provided resources. One of her faculty members works part-time at the hospital as a house supervisor and is respected for her knowledge and expertise. Betty's clinical manager is prepared at the graduate level in another discipline and is currently pursuing a master of science degree in nursing as a nurse educator. Moreover, as a stakeholder, Betty herself is committed to the project as a part of her graduate degree requirements. The administration has a very high level of commitment as it is committed to achieving the best patient outcomes through excellent nursing care.

Strategies for Leading Planned Change

Those wishing to bring about change must develop strategies to foster change. Bennis, Benne, and Chin (1969), in their classic text, *The Planning of Change*, identified three strategies to promote change: rational-empirical, normative-re-educative, and power-coercive. Decisions about which strategies to employ depend, to a great extent, on three factors: the type of change planned, the power of the change agent, and the amount of resistance expected. These strategies may be used independently or together. More often than not, some combination of strategies is indicated: the larger the change and the more resistance expected, the more strategies the change agent must employ.

RATIONAL-EMPIRICAL

This strategy assumes that people are rational beings and will adopt a change if it is justified and in their self-interest. When using this strategy, the change agent's role includes communicating the merit of the change to the group. If the change is understood by the group to be justified and in the best interest of the organization, it is likely to be accepted. This strategy emphasizes reason and knowledge. It presents those affected by the change with the knowledge and rationale they need to accept and implement the change. This strategy is most useful when little resistance to a change is expected. The power of the change agent is typically not a factor in changes amenable to this strategy. This strategy assumes that once given the knowledge and the rationales, people will internalize the need for the change and value the result.

NORMATIVE-RE-EDUCATIVE

A second strategy takes into account social and cultural implications of change and is based on the assumption that group norms are used to socialize individuals. This strategy requires "winning over" those affected by the change. Success is often relationship-based; relationship, not information, is the key to this strategy. The success of this approach often requires a change in attitude, values, and/or relationships. Sufficient time is essential to the successful use of the normative-re-educative strategy. This strategy is most frequently used when the change is based in the culture and relationships within the organization. The power of the change agent, both positional and informal, becomes integral to the change process. For example, one of the most powerful changes in recent history occurred when the norm changed regarding when to wear surgical gloves for preventing the spread of infection. More than knowledge (rational-empirical) and administrative directives were needed to bring about this change: it took a change in cultural values that redefined the practice norms.

POWER-COERCIVE

This strategy is based on power, authority, and control. Political or economic power is often used to bring about desired change. The change agent "orders" change, and those with less power comply. This strategy requires that the change agent have the positional power to mandate the change. Change effected by this strategy is often based either on the followers' desire to please the leader or fear of the consequences for not complying with the change. This strategy is very effective for legislated changes, but other changes accomplished using this strategy are usually short-lived if people have not embraced the need for the change through some other mechanism (Table 11-1).

Barriers to Change and Strategies to Overcome Them

All changes have the potential for both gain and loss. It is important to *identify* all the potential barriers to change, to *examine* them contextually with those affected by the proposed change, and to *develop* strategies collectively to reduce or remove the barriers. Barriers most common to change within the health-care environment are discussed below, along with some strategies to overcome them. Additional barriers appear in Table 11-2.

Change requires movement, which, as physics indicates, is a kinetic activity that requires energy to overcome resistance. Also, as in physics, an object at rest (and that includes an organization) prefers to remain at rest. Movement over barriers requires an

TABLE 11-1	Change Strategies	
SITUATION	**CHANGE STRATEGY**	**DISCUSSION**
HIPAA	Power-coercive	Agencies were mandated to implement policies and practices to bring them into compliance with legislation. There are negative consequences of not following the mandate, including legal actions and financial sanctions. Therefore, personnel have no choice but to accept the change.
Changing visitation hours in ICU	Normative-re-educative	This policy change, driven internally, represents social and cultural adaptation within the organization. As society has become less structured, visitation policies need to adapt to allow interaction between family members and the critically ill patient.
Changing from centralized to decentralized staffing	Normative-re-educative	As nurses gain more autonomy in the profession and in their roles in patient care settings, they also desire more autonomy in scheduling their work hours. The formal and informal leadership collaborate to foster and lead change.
Implementation of evidence-based research in practice	Rational-empirical	As nurses become more immersed in and committed to evidence-based practice, the knowledge gained from research drives change.

TABLE 11-2	Common Barriers to Change and Strategies to Overcome Them	
BARRIER	**DISCUSSION**	**STRATEGY**
Desire to remain in our comfort zone.	Those who become increasingly attached to a familiar way of doing things (comfort zone) often view change as an unwelcome disruption.	Rational-empirical strategies can be used effectively to allow people to become comfortable with exploring new ideas. Give people all the information available. For example, a change in staffing patterns would be sooner accepted if the nursing staff was part of the change process from the beginning. As invested players in the change, staff nurses are more likely to accept a change in staffing pattern if they know and understand what the policies are and the rationales for them.
Inadequate access to information.	Do not rule out a lack of information as a barrier to change. Just because information has been made available does not mean it has been read and understood by all.	This is one of the easiest barriers to overcome. Use the rational-empirical strategy. Provide information to the members of the organization through every possible means: e-mail, phone calls, memos, staff meetings, mail, and informal gatherings to be sure everyone knows about the change that is under way.
Lack of shared vision.	It is critical to have widespread involvement, input, and ownership of the change. The lack of a shared vision will cripple a change effort.	The normative-re-educative strategy work effectively to remove this barrier. Through dialogue and discussion, the affected members can gain new insights and new perspectives on the change proposal. This process is an integral part of building trust and sharing vision and values.

(Continued on following page)

TABLE 11-2	Common Barriers to Change and Strategies to Overcome Them *(continued)*

BARRIER	DISCUSSION	STRATEGY
Lack of adequate planning.	To manage change well, ensure that the people affected see it coming. Involving people in the planning gives them a sense of control and decreases their resistance to the change.	Rational-empirical and normative-re-educative strategies are helpful in overcoming this barrier. The leader's role in envisioning the future is vital. Efforts must be made to keep all members of the organization informed about and involved in organizational changes.
Lack of trust.	Trust is key to bringing about change. People must trust the change agent; they must also trust that the change is in their best interest.	Use both rational-empirical and normative-re-educative strategies to develop trust. Provide all the information people need. Include all individuals who are willing to participate in the planning of change.
Resistance to change.	Achieving lasting and effective change requires the cooperation and involvement of the whole team, not isolated individuals.	The normative-re-educative strategy is needed to help overcome resistance to change. Work to empower people. Offer them opportunities to develop skills and to use those skills to become leaders in the change process.
Poor timing or inadequate time planned.	Even desired change can fail due to poor timing or a lack of planning.	It is important to predict and anticipate system responses to change. For instance, when planning how fast the change will occur, remember that the larger the change, the more people will be affected, and that more time will be required. Timing is everything. It is imperative that careful attention be given when a change plan is made public and when it is implemented. Introducing a change at a time when the staff is already feeling overwhelmed is a certain guarantee for failure. Likewise, do not move too quickly. Change that is made too rapidly removes the opportunity for meaningful dialogue and discussion that is essential for planned change to occur effectively. Conversely, do not lag. When people are ready to move, get moving.
Fear that power, relationships, or control will be lost.	Every change represents the potential for loss to someone.	Normative-re-educative strategies are needed to alleviate these fears. Employ strategies that include all those for whom the change seems to represent loss. Help members of the organization reframe the change so they can see that what will be gained is greater than what will be lost. (Emphasize direct and open communication and addressing of fears here. Maybe individual meetings would prove most effective)
Even when a change is desirable, the amount of personal energy required for the change to occur is deemed too great.	Sometimes change is desired but people are not willing to do what is necessary to effect the change.	This is not the time to give more information or employ peer pressure. The best strategy may simply be to slow the change process. Give people a chance to catch up and reenergize. Remember the power of timing.

even greater expenditure of energy. The very energy requirement to change may be too much of a drain on an already overtaxed organization, and the energy required to be a leader of change in a resistant group can be overwhelming. For this reason, timing is a critical element of the change process. Correctly determining when people are most receptive to the initiation of change can be the determining factor in the success or failure of the change process. When people are dissatisfied with the status quo and yet not too overwhelmed with merely trying to keep up, the time for change is ripe.

People become comfortable with what "is." The functional parameters are clear as are expectations and rewards. Change, by its very nature, moves people away from their comfort zones. By providing realistic planning of and adequate information about how the impending change will affect each of those areas, some—probably not all—of this resistance can be minimized.

Although legendary heroes and heroines led massive societal changes, within an organization change rarely occurs without the assistance of others. Frequently, individuals have great ideas that would truly improve the function of the organization, but because the idea cannot be implemented by one person, it becomes lost to the organization. The support of both formal and informal leaders can be a critical element to successful change. Both types of leaders have their own audiences and their own abilities to sway groups and influence the "buy-in." That buy-in and ownership of the change will become a shared vision for the organization that will draw in other supporters. Because the formal and informal leaders have, in essence, "blessed" the change, a number of trust issues for subordinates will also have been overcome.

Change Theories

A number of theories exist to explain the change process. These theories provide a framework within which to guide change efforts. They are useful for planning both personal change and organizational change. Tiffany et al. (1994) surveyed 176 nurse-authored journal articles dealing with planned change. This study identified the type and frequency of planned change theories found in the nursing literature. Lewin's Change Theory was most com-

monly used as a framework for change. Several other change theories were also frequently referenced. A brief description of Lewin's theory, along with Lippitt's Phases of Change, Havelock's Six Step Change Model, and Rogers' Diffusion of Innovations Theory, follows. These models of change are a mere sampling of change models. They provide a strong basis for understanding change theory. Before exploring the change theories, consider this brief discussion of change agents, an element in any change theory.

CHANGE AGENTS

A **change agent** is the individual or group that seeks to lead change. The change agent may be from inside or outside the organization. Change agents may have formal lines of authority or may be informal leaders. In either case, the change agent is responsible for moving those affected by the change through the process and implementing the change. Effective change agents are masters of change. They do three things correctly: they sense the right moment to initiate the plan, they find supporters for their ideas, and they have vision (Bruning, 1993). The successful change agent earns the respect and trust of the target system (individuals, groups, or organizations) by communicating openly and honestly, offering assistance, and demonstrating ability. A change agent's success depends on communication and consultation style, interpersonal skills, and expert power. Ongoing communication is integral to the role of the change agent (Box 11-1).

Becoming a Change Agent: A Practical Guide

Change is an inevitable part of life; learning to lead change effectively is a skill that can be cultivated

Box 11-1		
Roles of the Change Agent		
VISIONER	**FACILITATOR**	**IDEA PERSON**
Communicator	Challenger	Problem solver
Advisor	Advocate	Objective observer
Coach	Educator	Resource linker
Provider of feedback	Empowerer	Problem finder

and mastered with practice. If you have been given the responsibility of leading an organizational change, there are several practical steps you can take to increase your chance for success.

1. Begin by articulating the change vision clearly and concisely.
2. Select the change project team carefully.
3. Identify the formal and informal leaders who can help you implement the change successfully.
4. Stay alert to political forces, both for and against the change.
5. Develop communication skills. Keep communication lines open.
6. Practice problem-solving skills.
7. Develop conflict resolution skills.
8. Learn to trust yourself and your project team.

Functioning effectively as a change agent requires the nurse to have an understanding of the theoretical frameworks of change. A discussion of several classic, as well as emerging, theories of change follows.

KURT LEWIN'S FORCE FIELD ANALYSIS

Lewin's **Force Field Analysis** is probably one of the best known and frequently used change theories (Tiffany et al., 1994). This theory conceptualizes change as movement across time. Lewin views behavior as a dynamic balance of forces working in opposite direction within a field (individual or organization). According to Lewin, change occurs in response to disequilibrium within a system (Lewin, 1951). Therefore, in order to effect change, there must be an imbalance between the forces that push for change (driving forces) and those forces that oppose change (restraining forces) staving to maintain the status quo. Basically, strategies for change are aimed at increasing driving forces and decreasing restraining forces. Lewin identified three phases of change: unfreezing, moving, and refreezing.

Unfreezing

Unfreezing the existing equilibrium involves motivating others for change. The change agent must loosen, or "unfreeze," the forces that are maintaining the status quo. This involves increasing the perceived need for change and creating discontent with the system as it exists. If individuals do not see a need for change, they are not likely to be motivated or ready for change and may even hinder change. Assessment of readiness for change is critical in this phase.

Moving

During the **moving** phase, the change agent identifies, plans, and implements strategies to bring about the change. The change agent must do all that is possible to reduce restraining forces and strengthen driving forces. It is critical that the change agent continue to work to build trust and enlist as many others as possible. The more ownership there is in the change, the more likely the change will be adopted. Timing is also important during this phase. People need time to assimilate change; therefore, the change agent must allow enough time for people to redefine how they view this change cognitively.

Refreezing

During the **refreezing** phase, the change agent reinforces new patterns of behavior brought about by the change. Institutionalizing the change by creating new policies and procedures helps to refreeze the system at a new level of equilibrium. Refreezing has occurred when the new way of doing things becomes the new status quo.

LIPPITT'S PHASES OF CHANGE

Lippitt's Phases of Change Theory (1958) is built on the Lewin model. He extended the model to include seven steps in the change process. Lippitt's model focuses more on the role of the change agent than on the evolution of the change process. Communication skills, team building, and problem solving are central to this theory. The participation of key personnel, those most affected by the change, and those most critical in promoting the change is essential to the success of the change effort (Noone, 1987). The seven steps of Lippitt's phases of change are:

Step 1: Diagnosis of the Problem

The person or organization must believe there is a problem that requires change. The change agent helps others see the need for change and involves key people in data collecting and problem solving. The ideal situation exists when both the organization and the change agent recognize and accept the need for change.

Step 2: Assessment of the Motivation and Capacity for Change

Determine if people are ready for change. Assess the financial and human resources. Are they sufficient for change? Analyze the structure and function of the organization. Will it support the change, or does there need to be organizational redesign? This process is essentially defining the restraining and driving forces for change within the organization.

Step 3: Assessment of the Change Agent's Motivation and Resources

This step is crucial to achieving change. The change agent (either an individual or a team) must count the personal cost of change. The change agent must be willing to make the commitment necessary to bring about the planned change. He or she must have the energy, time, and necessary power base to be successful. The change agent may take on the role of leader, expert consultant, facilitator, or cheerleader, but whatever role is assumed, the change agent must be willing to see the change through.

Step 4: Selection of Progressive Change Objectives

The change is clearly defined in this step. Establish the change objectives. Develop a plan of action; include specific strategies for meeting the objectives. Decide how to evaluate the change plan and final result.

Step 5: Implement the Plan

It is critical to remain flexible during implementation. If resistance is higher than anticipated, slow down. Give others a chance to catch up. On the other hand, if all is going well and the momentum is good, keep the plan moving ahead.

Step 6: Maintenance of the Change

During this phase the change is integrated into the organization. It is becoming the new norm. In this phase, the role of the change agent is to provide support, positive feedback and, if necessary, make modifications to the change.

Step 7: Termination of the Helping Relationship

The change agent gradually withdraws from the role and resumes the role of member of the organization (Lippitt, Watson, & Wesley, 1958).

HAVELOCK'S MODEL

Havelock's Six Step Change Model (1973) is another variation of Lewin's change theory. The emphasis of this model is on the planning stage of change. Havelock's model asserts that with sufficient, careful, and thorough planning, change agents can overcome resistance to change. Using this model, essential to the success of change is inclusion. It is imperative that the change agent encourage participation at all levels. This follows the assumption that the more people are part of the plan, the more they feel responsible for the outcome, and the more likely they will work to make the plan succeed.

The planning stage of Havelock's model includes: (1) building a relationship; (2) diagnosing the problem; and (3) acquiring resources. This planning stage is followed by the moving stage, which includes choosing the solution and gaining acceptance. The last stage is stabilization and renewal (Havelock, 1973).

ROGERS' DIFFUSION OF INNOVATION

Everett Rogers (1983) developed a diffusion theory, as opposed to a planned change theory. It is included with change theories because it describes how an individual or organization passes from "first knowledge of an innovation" to confirmation of the decision to adopt or reject an innovation or change. Rogers defined diffusion as "the process by which innovation is communicated through certain channels over time among the members of a social system" (as cited in Hagerman and Tiffany, 1994, p. 58). Rogers' framework emphasizes the reversible nature of change. Initial rejection of change does not mean the change will never occur. Likewise, the adoption of change does not ensure its continuation. Rogers' five-step innovation/decision-making process is:

Step 1: Knowledge

The decision-making unit (individual, team, or organization) is introduced to the innovation (change) and begins to understand it.

Step 2: Persuasion

The change agent works to develop a favorable attitude toward the innovation (change).

Step 3: Decision

A decision is made to adopt or reject the innovation.

Step 4: Implementation/Trial

The innovation is put in place. Reinvention or alterations may occur.

Step 5: Confirmation

The individual or decision-making unit seeks reinforcement that the decision made was correct. It is at this point that a decision previously made may be reversed.

EMERGING MODELS OF CHANGE

The classic models of change are linear. While they have been used successfully in many situations, they may not be as useful as they once were in the complex, ever-changing health-care arena. Because health care is changing so rapidly, health-care organizations must be able to organize and implement change quickly. The linear models of the past may not be sufficient to meet this challenge. Two models

> **Characteristics Common to Change Theories**
>
> Problem identification
> Plan for innovation
> Strategies to reduce resistance
> Evaluation plan

> "Life uses messes to get to well ordered solutions. Life doesn't seem to share our desires for efficiency or neatness. It uses redundancy, fuzziness, dense webs of relationships, and unending trials and errors to find what works. Life is intent on finding what works, not what's "right." It is the ability to keep finding solutions that is important; any one solution is temporary. There are no permanently right answers. The capacity to keep changing, to find what works now, is what keeps any organism alive" (Wheatley & Kellner-Rogers, 1996).

of change that are quickly becoming recognized in leadership circles are the Learning Organizations and Chaos theories.

Learning Organizations Theory

The Learning Organizations Theory is based on systems theory. It is a framework for seeing the interrelatedness of relationships; the whole is not just the sum of its parts, because each separate part affects the whole. Indeed, each part is essential in defining the whole. Peter Senge (1990) described learning organizations as organizations where people at all levels are collectively and continuously working together to improve what they do. Learning organizations celebrate differences and recognize that every member of the organization has something to contribute to organizational growth. Over time, a learning organization embraces change as a means of creating the organizational environment it desires. A learning organization develops the capacity to recreate itself in response to change. Senge describes five disciplines that must be mastered if an organization is to achieve the status of a learning organization. Learning organizations model the change process (Table 11-3).

Discipline 1: Personal Mastery

First, the members of a learning organization must develop personal mastery. Personal mastery involves clarifying and deepening a personal vision. There must be personal vision before there can be shared vision. People with a high level of personal mastery are continually expanding their ability to create the results they want in life. Two important characteristics of personal mastery are a clear vision of what one wants and the ability to see cur-

TABLE 11-3	Senge's Five Disciplines of Learning Organizations
Discipline 1: Personal mastery	Developing and clarifying a personal vision
Discipline 2: Mental models	Building an internal picture of the world; the lens through which the world is viewed
Discipline 3: Building shared vision	Translating personal vision into a collective vision and developing a culture of common caring
Discipline 4: Team learning	Fostering shared, participative decision making
Discipline 5: Systems thinking	Shifting from fragmentation to holism

rent reality accurately. Creative tension exists when there is a gap between the vision and the current reality. In order to shorten the gap, change must occur.

Discipline 2: Mental Models

A mental model is an internal picture of how one views the world. Mental models are deeply held thoughts or beliefs about how the world works. They are the filters for everything one sees or hears. Often, mental models are so deeply engrained that individuals are not consciously aware of them. Mental models shape action. Learning to recognize and question mental models is crucial to becoming part of a learning organization. Change will require the development of new mental models.

Discipline 3: Building Shared Vision

Shared vision is translating a personal vision into a collective vision, created together. Shared vision derives its power from a common caring about something the organization truly wants. Individuals do not have to give up their personal beliefs or passions, but instead continue to learn and grow together. Shared vision is essential if members of an organization are going to work well together. Shared vision takes time and ongoing conversation to create. When building shared vision, the goal is to create the most inclusive environment possible. It is a process that requires commitment, not just compliance. Shared vision does not require knowing how

to get where you want to go; it does require knowing where you want to go.

Discipline 4: Team Learning

Team learning is the process of aligning and developing the capacity of organizational members to achieve the vision. This requires much communication. It involves examining all ideas. It requires listening to others' ideas and suspending judgment for a time. When people suspend judgment and think together, new ideas arise. The objective is to go beyond personal understanding and gain new insight into the issue. When this process is used, people become observers of their own thinking, and that leads to greater insight. Learning teams, as the name implies, are highly participatory in decision making. One person is not the teacher or leader; rather, all members have something to teach and a responsibility to lead. Team learning accepts both individualism and collectivism.

Discipline 5: Systems Thinking

Systems thinking is the cornerstone for learning organizations. This fifth discipline weaves the other four disciplines together into a cohesive body of theory and practice. It is a shift from seeing "parts" to seeing "wholes." When problems are identified in the organization, they are examined through the lens of a system. The question asked is, "What is wrong with the system?" Systems thinking is about finding solutions to problems, not placing blame.

Learning organizations are distinctive because of their ability to learn and not simply be content with what they are doing (Senge, 1990). The capacity to reflect and to see patterns of interdependency is critical. Senge states "Systems thinking is the discipline for seeing wholes. It is a framework for seeing interrelationships rather than things, for seeing patterns of change rather than static snapshots" (p. 68). The art of systems thinking lies in being able to recognize increasingly complex and subtle structures amid the wealth of details, pressures, and cross-currents that exist in real management settings. The essence of mastering systems thinking as a management discipline lies in seeing the patterns where others see only singular events. Senge lists some of the laws of the fifth discipline:

1. Today's problems come from yesterday's "solutions."
2. The harder you push, the harder the system pushes back.

3. Behavior grows better before it grows worse.
4. The easy way out usually leads back in.
5. The cure can be worse than the disease.
6. Faster is slower.
7. Cause and effect are not closely related in time and space.
8. Small changes can produce big results—but the areas of highest leverage are often the least obvious.
9. You can have your cake and eat it too, but not at once.
10. Dividing an elephant in half does not produce two small elephants.
11. There is no blame.

Chaos Theory (1995)

Chaos Theory has its genesis in quantum physics. The universe does not run rigidly in accordance with the laws of classic physics. Hawking (1987) noted that this uncertainty was likely the result of tiny fluctuations that interacted within systems and resulted in large-scale effects. The result stems from multiple interrelated changes within the universe.

Chaos Theory hypothesizes that chaos actually has an order. Changes that seem to occur at random are, in reality, the result of a complex order. Complex systems give rise to complex and interrelated behaviors. The paradox that disorder can be a source of order is particularly encouraging to nursing and to health care in general. Health care is in chaos. Instability is caused by many interrelated variables, including managed care, shifting demographics, age, gender, and ethnicity. According to Valadez and Sportsman (1999), three principles can be drawn from quantum/chaos theory to help leaders in nursing manage the environment: "a) the world is unpredictable, b) the world is not independent of the observer; rather, the intent of the observer influences what is seen; and c) the relationships among things are what counts, not the things themselves" (p. 210). While strategic planning remains important to the life of an organization, the plan cannot remain static; it must change, take into account new data, examine the relationships inherent in the system, and allow for the exploration of differences of multiple perspectives of stakeholders in the organization. Pascale (2002) states that innovation increases near the edge of chaos. In the face of threat or opportunity, organizations move into mutation and experimentation.

The challenge is to disturb the system in a manner that will push the system in the direction of a desired outcome. Just as the path of the universe cannot be changed with complete accuracy, neither can the path of health care be directed. But it can be nudged in the right direction.

Example of Chaos Theory in Action

Consider this example of Chaos Theory in action at Medical Surgical Services of Utopia Medical Center:

Mission Statement

It is the mission of our collaborative, interdisciplinary health-care team to provide holistic care for the patients on our units and their families. We will support each other in the accomplishment of our responsibilities through open communication and by striving for flexibility through which to manage the multiple priorities of our service.

Members of the Medical Surgical Services Team

Nurses
Physical therapists
Respiratory therapists
Radiology technicians
Physicians
Unlicensed assistive personnel
Registered dietitians

Situation

The nurses have approached their manager about the problems associated with nursing care that are caused by professionals from other disciplines who appear on the unit and commandeer the patients. These situations have been long-standing, are interrupting patient care, are causing delays in administration of medication, and have resulted in the inability of the nurses to conduct patient education sessions on much needed topics, such as diabetes care.

Problem Solving

The Director of Medical Surgical Services has called a team meeting to discuss potential solutions to these problems. Each discipline voices understanding of the problem, but there seems to be no solution to which everyone can agree immediately. This is an example that the world is not independent of the observer and that the intent of the observer influences what is seen. Each discipline agrees there is a problem but views it primarily from its own frame of reference. The director asks one of the charge nurses for ideas about how to solve the dilemma. The charge nurse suggests that the group focus on the mission statement for the area. As the team discusses the implications of the mission statement, it is reminded that holistic patient care is the ultimate goal, and the members recognize that fragmented care is not holistic care. They also recognize that their environment is complex and rapidly changing. Their worldview recognizes unpredictability. They recall their commitment to supporting each other through open communication and a flexible approach. They decide that, together, they can make a general schedule for when certain activities will occur and that through communication about exceptions or crisis situations they can arrange to provide patient care in a more organized, synchronized fashion. The relationships among things is what counts, not the things themselves. In this situation, the mission statement served as the "strange attractor" that brought the team together to meet a common goal.

Eight Basic Lessons of the Paradigm of Change

Michael Fullan, in his classic book *Change Forces*, outlined eight lessons of change. Although Fullan's work is not technically a theory for change, it does offer wisdom for understanding change. Taken together, these lessons help define the new paradigm of change (Fullan, 1993).

Lesson One: You can't mandate what matters.

"When complex change is involved, people do not and cannot change by being told to do so. Effective change agents neither embrace nor ignore mandates. They use them as catalysts to examine what they are doing" (Fullan, 1993, p. 24).

Lesson Two: Change is a journey, not a blueprint.

"Change is nonlinear and is loaded with uncertainty and excitement. Even well-developed innovations represent journeys for those who are encountering them for the first time" (p. 25).

Lesson Three: Problems are our friends.

Problems are inevitable, and learning cannot happen without them. In fact, avoiding problems is the enemy of productive change. Openness and a spirit of inquiry are essential to learning and therefore to change.

Lesson Four: Vision and strategic planning come later.

"A shared vision is vision that many people are truly committed to, because it reflects their own personal vision" (Senge, 1990, p. 206). Vision requires reflection. Reflection requires time. Spending too much time preplanning early in the change process is a mistake. Ownership seldom occurs in advance. Flexibility is needed early, vision will follow. Then planning can occur.

Lesson Five: Individualism and collectivism must have equal power.

The creative tension between individualism and collectivism can be a great asset to change. Typically, collectivism (collaboration, participation) is touted as good, and it is. One must be careful, however, not to allow collectivism become group-think. Likewise, the ability to think and act independently is good. The danger here is isolation. The best strategy is to recognize that one does not have to be exclusive of the other. Embrace them both.

Lesson Six: Neither centralization nor decentralization works alone.

Both top-down and bottom-up strategies are necessary. There needs to be a balance of pressure, control, and support.

Lesson Seven: Connection with the wider environment is critical for success.

The best organizations learn externally as well as internally. "To prosper, organizations must be actively plugged into their environments, responding to and contributing to the issues of the day" (Fullan, 1993, p. 39).

Lesson Eight: Every person is a change agent.

Change is too important to leave to the experts. "Since no one person can possibly understand the complexities of change in dynamically complex systems, it follows that we cannot leave the responsibility to others" (Fullan, 1993, p. 39).

All Good Things...

It is important to remember that change is a journey, not a destination; it is a process, not an outcome. It is less important to know how many steps are in the change process than it is to understand the process of change. With this in mind, recognize that change theories, regardless of the number of steps involved, have several common elements. All change theories begin with diagnosing a problem, identifying what requires change. They provide a thoughtful plan for an innovation—the change idea. Change theories develop strategies to bring about the change. These strategies include a plan for implementation, and contingency plans for overcoming obstacles to change. Finally, they should provide a means for evaluation of the change.

Pascale (2002) wrote that "ships can't steer if they are not moving, and living systems—such as organizations—can't survive without change, challenge, variety, and surprise" (p. 17). Learn to lead change, rather than let change lead you.

Let's Talk

1. *You are the nurse manager responsible for implementing a change from total patient care to a case management model of patient care on your unit. Using Lewin's Force Field Analysis as a framework for implementing change, respond to the following.*
   A. *Describe the process you will undertake.*
   B. *Identify the stage represented by each step you plan.*
   C. *What do you see as driving forces for this change?*
   D. *What are potential restraining forces inhibiting this change?*

2. *Assume you are leading a task force to explore the possibility of changing ICU visiting hours from set times (such as 10 a.m. to 2 p.m.) to open visitation.*
   A. *Who are the stakeholders in this situation?*
   B. *What would be the barriers to overcome?*
   C. *What strategies would best be used to overcome these barriers?*

3. *You are the charge nurse on a medical-surgical unit. You wish to implement a new method of "flagging" charts that contain new doctors' orders. Your staff members complain that they like things the way they are and are openly resistant to implementing this change. What can you do to decrease resistance and win your staff over?*

4. *What role does Chaos Theory play in innovation in nursing?*

NCLEX Questions

1. Which activity would be considered expected behavior during the refreezing phase of planned change?
   A. Developing policies and procedures
   B. Working to develop trust
   C. Identifying restraining forces
   D. Allowing time for people to assimilate the change

2. The change agent can increase the likelihood of the success of planned change by:
   A. Implementing the change rapidly to prevent development of the objections
   B. Including only formal leaders in planning the change to ensure management support
   C. Instituting the change process during a period of low staffing so fewer people will be affected
   D. Being sensitive to the internal and external environment of the organization to ensure the change will be culturally acceptable

3. Which change strategy is represented by changing the location of unit patient information boards so the information cannot be seen except by those who need the information in order to provide patient care?
   A. Rational-empirical
   B. Normative-re-educative
   C. Notional-intuitive
   D. Power-coercive

4. Gaining trust is a fundamental element in planned change. Which process or behavior would hinder the development of trust?
   A. Providing all necessary information
   B. Providing only information deemed necessary by formal leaders
   C. Achieving buy-in from formal and informal leaders
   D. Including all interested parties in the planning of the change

5. An organization that celebrates differences and embraces change is known as:
   A. An externally sensitive organization
   B. An internally sensitive organization

C. A learning organization

D. A collective vision organization

6. Chaos Theory embraces which of the following principles?

A. It is important that the observer not influence what is being observed

B. Certain parts of the world interact predictably with certain other parts

C. Relationships between objects are more important than objects themselves

D. Change occurs following certain sequential steps

7. Achieving a shared vision requires which of the following?

A. That individuals sublimate their individual goals and desires

B. That one individual champion a personal vision

C. The exclusion of some individuals from the collective

D. Commitment rather than compliance

8. Which of the following is best described as change that applies strategic actions to promote movement toward a specific goal?

A. Reactive change

B. Planned change

C. Internal force change

D. External force change

9. Which of the following is an important assumption to make about change?

A. A positive change represents a gain for everyone affected by the change

B. The fewer the people involved in the process, the more likely the change will be accepted

C. The shorter the gap between change initiator and decision maker, the more likely the change will be implemented

D. When a series of changes is desired, it is more efficient to implement them all at once

10. The change agent must do which of the following?

A. Have a formal line of authority

B. Have a disregard for organizational politics

C. Be a member of the organization

D. Possess conflict resolution skills

REFERENCES

Baulcomb, J. (2003). Management of change through force field analysis. *Journal of Nursing Management, 11*, 275–280.

Bennett, M. (2003). The manager as agent of change. *Nursing Management, 10*(7).

Bennis, W., Benne, K., & Chin, R. (1969). *The Planning of Change,* (2nd ed.). New York: Holt, Rinehart and Winston.

Bruning, L. (1993). Managing change in a changing environment. *Today's OR Nurse,* 9-11.

Fullan, M. (1993). *Change forces.* London: Falmer Press.

Hagerman, L., & Tiffany, C. (1994). Evaluating plan change theories. *Nursing Management, 25*(3), 54–57.

Havelock, R. (1973). *The change agent's guide to innovation in education.* New Jersey: Educational Technology Publication.

Hawking, S. (1988). *A brief history of the universe: From the big bang to black holes.* NY: Bantam Books.

HIPAA Legislation Retrieved February 29, 2005, from aspe.hhs.gov/adminsimp/p1104191.htm

Lewin, K. (1951). *Field theory in social service: Selected theoretical papers.* New York: Harper Brothers.

Lippitt, R., Watson, J., & Westley, B. (1958). *The dynamics of planned change.* New York: Harcourt, Brace.

Noone, J. (1987). Planned change: Putting theory into practice. *Clinical Nurse Specialist, 1*(1), 25–29.

Pascale, R., Milleman, M., & Gioja, L. (2002). *Surfing on the edge of chaos: The laws of nature and the new laws of business.* NY: Three Rivers Press.

Rogers, F. (1983). *Diffusion of innovations.* New York: Free Press.

Senge, P. (1990). *The fifth discipline: The art and practice of learning organizations.* New York: Doubleday.

Terry, R.W. (1993). *Authentic leadership.* San Francisco: Jossey-Bass.

Tiffany, C., et al. (1994). Planned change theory: Survey of nursing periodical literature. *Nursing Management, 25*(7), 54–59.

Valadez, A.M., & Sportsman, S. (1999). Environmental management: Principles from quantum theory. *Journal of Professional Nursing, 15*(4), 209–213.

Wheatley, M., & Kellner-Rogers, M. (1996). *A simpler way.* San Francisco: Berrett-Koehler.

chapter 12

Building Teams for Productivity and Efficiency

CAROL SEAVOR, EDD, RN

"People make fewer errors when they work in teams. When processes are planned and standardized, each member knows his or her responsibilities as well as those of teammates, and members 'look out' for one another, noticing errors before they cause an accident. In an effective interdisciplinary team, members come to trust one another's judgments and attend to one another's safety concerns."

Institute of Medicine, 2000

CHAPTER MOTIVES

- Describe the contributions of teams and teamwork to quality patient care.
- Discuss the relationship between good communication, healthy group dynamics, and effective teamwork.
- Understand the competencies needed for successful team building and effective team leadership.

Delivery of health care is quite complex. Even though nurses may deliver care as individuals, they are usually part of a caregiving team working in concert. Even care delivered to patients by an individual nurse or other caregiver has probably been influenced by others, through diagnosing, planning, referral, or other types of collaboration. The admitting physician provides the initial medical diagnosis, the admitting nurse establishes the initial nursing care plan, and other health-care disciplines, such as social work, physical therapy, diet therapy, and occupational therapy, may influence the plan of care. Treatments, equipment, and medications have been developed over time and studied and tested by unknown numbers of professionals (many working in teams) to develop the best models of care. Many nursing interventions are also the result of nurse researchers working in teams to broaden the repertoire of evidence-based practice. The complexity of both the health-care arena and the nursing profession challenges nurses to become proficient in the skills of collaboration and team building. Most health-care delivery agencies employ nurses with varying credentials and levels of education. The existence of multiple levels of nursing personnel requires that all nurses understand the various roles performed at each level. Doctoral, master, bachelor, and associate degree nurses work along with licensed practical nurses (LPN) and certified nursing assistants (CNA) in large medical centers. In order for patients to receive effective, coordinated optimal care, smooth teamwork must exist. Table 12-1 summarizes the levels of educational opportunities in nursing and the roles associated with each.

As multiple roles have evolved within nursing, so too have the roles within other health-care disciplines. For example, respiratory therapists, physician assistants, occupational therapists and occupational therapy assistants, surgical technologists, radiological technicians, and a myriad of other supportive technicians are likely to be part of the health-care team. Never has mutual understanding, mutual respect, group work, and teamwork been more important and more crucial to the well-being of patients receiving care within the health-care system. Table 12-2 provides examples of the roles played by some of the health-care disciplines likely to be included in the care of hospitalized patients.

This chapter will review the importance of teamwork in nursing and health-care delivery. Learning to be an effective team member and/or team leader will serve you, your patients, and their loved ones well. Understanding the dynamics that occur within teams, the roles that members play, and the patterns of communication that develop will help you be an effective team member. Learning about these dynamics will prepare you to ease some of the friction, avoid some of the conflict, and learn from both. You will see that partnerships and collaboration are essential for safe, efficient, and effective health care. Teamwork with other nurses, teamwork with other disciplines, and multidisciplinary teams will help you provide the best possible care for your patients. Good teamwork is essential for good nursing, and good teamwork begins with good group work.

Group Work

Nurses usually work in diverse caregiving groups and are expected to collaborate with others to produce positive patient care outcomes. The popular adage "A camel is a horse designed by a committee" is a reminder how ineffective group work may have unintended and unwanted outcomes. Groups consist of people in relationships. As the size of the group grows, group dynamics become more complex, and the opportunities for misunderstanding, friction, and conflict grow. Those who share a household with their children may recall the simplicity of life prior to parenthood. Similarly, those who are oldest children in the birth order of their family may harbor fond memories of a time when sharing was not necessary or when negotiating was not a daily event. Students expected to work within a study group or required to complete group projects have experienced how group work can be fraught with pitfalls and frustration. Although groups may differ in their **purposes**, **structure**, and **processes**, most groups do have one characteristic in common: the possibility of conflict. Understanding the phenomena associated with good group functioning facilitates good group work and eases frustration and conflict. When group members are aligned about their purpose, work within a well-understood structure, and have a strong and healthy group process, their group is poised to function as an effective health-care team.

TABLE 12-1	Levels of Nursing Education

CAREGIVER	ROLE
Nurse's aide (NA)	Assistants who work under the direction of an LPN, registered nurse (RN), or physician provide basic care for patients. Most states require a minimum number of hours of clinical practice and classroom instruction in a formal program, usually at a community college, in adult education, or in a hospital or nursing home. The program usually lasts for several weeks. In most states, an examination must be passed for certification, and the aide is designated as a CNA.
Licensed practical nurse (LPN) or licensed vocational nurse (LVN)	The LPN or LVN is an entry-level nurse who is responsible for providing basic nursing care, working under the direction of a physician or RN. Educational programs usually last about 1 year and are given in community colleges or hospital settings. LPN educational content is similar to that for RNs but the amount of time, the number of hours required, the prerequisite courses, and the responsibilities and decision-making expectations are reduced. A national examination (NCLEX-PN) must be passed for licensure.
RN	Requires completion of a formal education program in nursing at a community college, state university, or private college. A national licensing examination (NCLEX-RN) must be passed for licensure as an RN. Graduates of the following nursing programs are allowed to sit for the NCLEX-RN examination: associate degree, baccalaureate degree, or entry level master's degree. Associate degree nurse (ADN) programs typically require 2 years of course work. Bachelor of science nurse (BSN) programs require 4 years for completion. In some states, hospital-based programs (diploma programs) offer training required for licensure without an academic degree, usually lasting 3 years. An entry-level master's degree is a graduate program that admits students with bachelor or higher degrees in other fields and prepares graduates with an initial degree at the master's level in nursing.
Master of Science in Nursing (MSN)	Usually requires students to have a BSN degree and includes 1 or more years of course and clinical work, offered by private and state universities. MSNs are prepared in several specialties, including nursing education, nursing administration, medical/surgical, family, psychiatric, community, and pediatrics obstetrics health nursing. They are also prepared for various practice roles such as clinical nurse specialist (CNS), nurse practitioner (NP), family nurse practitioner (FNP), certified nurse midwife (CNM), and certified registered nurse anesthetist (CRNA).
Doctoral prepared nurse (for example, PhD, DNS)	Usually requires 3 or more years of education at a doctorate granting institution. These nurses have strong research, theory, and practice skill and serve in nursing faculty positions, research positions, direct research-based clinical specialty practice, or administrative positions.

GROUP PURPOSE

In caregiving agencies, groups (often in the form of committees) exist or are created to fulfill an ongoing function, responsibility, or task within the organization. Managers also create short-term groups (often called ad hoc groups or task forces) to accomplish a specific task or outcome. Long- and short-term groups created and supported by the organization are called **formal groups**. **Informal groups** may also form within caregiving agencies. These groups are not officially designated or supported by the organization but exist because the participants chose to be in a relationship to share a common interest. Effective informal groups that demonstrate

a contribution to an organization may become a formal group. Groups containing members who are clear about their purpose and are committed to working toward achieving their purpose have the best potential for success. Some illustrations of formal and informal groups include:

Formal:

- A group of nurses assigned to the recovery room or a surgical floor
- A group of nurses employed by a visiting nurse agency
- The institutional research board of a community hospital
- The curriculum committee of a nursing education program

TABLE 12-2   Examples of Team Member Roles

TEAM MEMBER	EXAMPLES OF PRACTICE ROLES
Patient/consumer/client	Participates to extent possible in plan of care and goal setting; identifies cultural needs and practices; reports own experience of progress
NURSING	
RN, doctorate	Conducts clinical research; provides consultation to clinical staff and administrative leadership within agency; serves as nursing faculty
RN, master's	Within a specialty, provides comprehensive nursing care, health promotion, histories, and physicals in outpatient and acute/home/long-term care settings; teaches and counsels; if certified as an advanced practice nurse may order, conduct, and interpret laboratory and diagnostic tests as allowed by state nurse practice act; provides consultation support for nursing staff; serves as nursing faculty; provides administrative leadership within agency
RN, bachelor's	Develops and implements comprehensive nursing care in all settings; provides leadership for health-care teams
RN, associate	Develops and implements nursing care usually in settings where patients have stable and predictable health needs
LPN	Delivers basic nursing skills as defined by the facility under the supervision of an RN or physician
CNA or NA	Assists with basic nursing skills as defined by the facility under the supervision of an RN; see Chapter 22 for additional examples of unlicensed assistive personnel (UAP)
MEDICINE	
Physician	Diagnoses and treats diseases and injuries, provides preventive care, prescribes drugs, and performs medical or surgical specialty care according to preparation
Psychiatrist	Medical doctors who diagnose and treat mental, emotional, and behavioral disease and conditions
ALLIED HEALTH	
Dietitian	Evaluates the nutritional status of patients; works with family members and medical team to determine appropriate nutrition goals for patient
Occupational therapist	Utilizes therapeutic goal-directed activities to evaluate, prevent, or correct physical, mental, or emotional dysfunction or to maximize functions for optimal independence
Pharmacist	Devises and revises patient's medication therapy to meet medical and therapeutic needs; information resource for the patient and medical team
Physical therapist	Evaluates, plans, utilizes exercises, rehabilitative procedures, massage, manipulations, and physical agents such as mechanical devices, heat, cold, air, light, water, electricity, and sound in the aid of diagnosis or treatment
Physician assistant (PA)	Practices medicine under the supervision of licensed physicians; provides a broad range of diagnostic and therapeutic services
Speech language pathologist	Assesses and treats speech, language, and swallowing disorders; provides individual or group therapy to maximize functional communication and swallowing ability
OTHER PROFESSIONS	
Chaplain	Provides spiritual support and ministry to patients and families
Psychologist	Assesses, treats, and manages mental disorders; provides psychotherapy with individuals, groups, and families
Social worker	Assesses individual and family psychosocial functioning and provides care to help enhance or restore capacities, including locating services or providing counseling

- The annual dinner ad hoc committee
- A committee assigned to research the factors related to an increased incidence of patient falls on a nursing home unit

Informal:

- A lunch group with an interest in starting a local chapter of a nursing specialty group
- A mutual support group of new employees
- A group interested in research on empathy in nursing

GROUP STRUCTURE

Formal and informal groups may be highly structured or have very little structure or few rules that guide their collaboration. Formal groups with longevity are apt to have more rules and provide more guidelines for the expectations of behavior of group members. The amount of structure in a group is reflected by its written guidelines, record keeping, style of leadership, process of decision making, and membership. A highly structured group maintains by-laws or other documents that define expectations of the group's functions. These documents may address, for example: purpose; goals; roles and responsibilities of members; time, place, and order of meetings; and how minutes will be recorded and filed. The leadership structure and process will be defined clearly as will lines of authority and responsibility. The process of decision making will be clear and consistent. Members of structured groups are usually chosen because of their competence or ability to meet the goals and purposes of the group and are apt to have the same or similar backgrounds and educational levels.

Groups with little structure take a more laissez-faire approach; roles and responsibilities are not spelled out clearly, and group members decide among themselves, often through trial and error, how to proceed. The role of leader may rotate among members, or a leader may evolve. Decision making may be by consensus or fiat by a leader or member. Perhaps little decision making will occur or be needed. Members may not always be the same, and backgrounds and educational levels may vary.

The extent of structure within a group has a significant impact on the group's productivity and effectiveness. For example, groups with clearly communicated guidelines for membership, roles, respon-

sibilities, meeting schedules, tasks, goals, purpose, minutes, and agendas help members understand the expectations of membership. These expectations suggest appropriate and productive group and homework activities. Groups with a purpose but little or no structure are likely to have confused and frustrated members. Productivity and achieving goals become more difficult.

GROUP PROCESS

A group usually exists to get a job done a job that is often referred to as the **group task**. **Group process** comprises the dynamics that occur between and among group members as they work to complete the group task. Group process encompasses patterns of behavior and issues that occur as a group forms and develops over time. Just as an individual develops from infancy to adulthood and moves with some predictability through patterns of behavior and stages of development, so do groups. Having an understanding of what to expect of an individual's development helps parents to guide children through each stage and successfully negotiate growth and development. Understanding the dynamics of group process and what to expect as groups grow and develop will help group members function more effectively and more comfortably.

Group Stages of Development

Decades ago, Homans (1950, 1961) proposed a concise and easily understood process that described the predictable progress and process of groups. His thesis has stood the test of time and has been reviewed and expanded by others (Tuckman, 1965; Tuckman & Jensen, 1977; Lacoursier, 1980; Drinka & Clark, 2000). Homans' theory suggests that groups move through four stages: forming, storming, norming, and performing.

STAGE 1: FORMING

In this initial stage, group members look to the leader for guidance. If there is no designated leader, one may emerge, or several members may take a leadership role at various times. Conversation is polite; the goal is to create a safe environment and find common interests and areas of acceptance.

Group Members' Thoughts in the Forming Stage

I wonder what they are thinking about me?

Will I be accepted or rejected?

Will they think my ideas are stupid?

Will they pressure me to talk?

Will I fit in?

Will I say too much?

What if they find out what I am really like?

What if I say the wrong thing?

What if they ask me to do something I don't want to do?

Members are alert to similarities and differences that they will note for future reference when forming subgroups later. The group avoids controversial or serious subjects. Discussion centers around how to define the scope of the task, how to approach it. See Box 12-1 for some of the thoughts and private concerns that members are likely to be having at this stage.

Characteristics of this stage can include impatience, confusion about group purpose, anxiety, silence and awkwardness, and off-topic chatter. General issues of trust are being considered as the group struggles to find a level of ease. To grow from this stage to the next, each member must relinquish the comfort of nonthreatening topics and risk the possibility of conflict. As members take small steps risking sharing their substantive ideas and begin to experience positive reactions, group comfort will grow, and the group will move to the next stage of development. Consider the following example:

During the first week of fall semester, eight members of a new junior-level class of nursing students have agreed to join their college chapter of the Nursing Student Association (NSA). They have been told by the seniors who are the leaders of the NSA that they should meet regularly and work toward enrolling all of their junior-year classmates into the NSA. They are expected to be the "front runners," who will convince their classmates of the benefits of joining this organization, and they need to learn as much as they can about the organization as quickly as possible so they can be effective mentors for others. The president of the NSA, Kerry, has asked Kathryn to call the first meeting as soon

as possible and to take responsibility for leading future meetings. The goal is to enroll at least 75 of the 100 juniors by November 1.

Kathryn has assembled the group of eight for the first meeting. Most are chatting quietly about the courses they are taking, the faculty they have, and their concerns about the seniors telling them how difficult the next 2 years will be. Kathryn tells everyone what Kerry expects them to do during the next 6 weeks. All are quiet; sidelong glances are passing through the group as each waits to see who will be the first to speak.

Amy thinks, "There's no way anyone is going to come up with $20 to join NSA because I ask them to. I am a total failure at selling anything." She says edgily, "Why do we have to get members? Why don't the seniors do their own work? They are the NSA officers." More time passes quietly, and Greg thinks "I know I won't fit in here because I'm a guy, and they probably don't even care if guys join or not." Lindsey thinks, "I never should have come to this school; too many spoiled children will see me as the 'old lady' with children of my own and think I have nothing important to say." Shanna says, "Can anyone tell me where the bookstore is? I haven't bought my books yet." Trent says, "Sure, I'll show you where it is. Where are you from?" Kathryn asks tentatively, "Well, I know we have a big job to do. Is anyone willing to help work on a plan for how to begin?" Jane thinks, "I knew I shouldn't have come here. I'm already sure I'm going to fall behind in my schoolwork and part-time job, and here I am being asked to do more work. What's wrong with me?"

Superficial remarks go on for the course of the meeting as members learn about each other's towns, mutual friends, dorms, and so on. Eventually, Greg and Shanna agree to meet with Kathryn the next day and work on a plan of activities to move them toward their goal. All agree to meet at least once a week until November 1, when their list of new members and the money must be turned in. Over the next 2 weeks, there are three meetings of the core group and two more where all eight attend. By then, when all are gathered, there is more comfortable conversation. Some have met for dinner and arrived together; two others have joined an aerobics class together and have arrived energized. Others are trading notes from their leadership class. Some are still shy, but most are ready to talk about the next steps of their plan for approaching new NSA members.

STAGE 2: STORMING

As work begins on the job at hand (group task) and the group tries to get organized, competition and conflict develop among personal relations (group process). This conflict occurs because many individuals attempt to contribute, blend, and mold their ideas, feelings, attitudes, and beliefs as they try to find a way to approach the task at hand. As each individual contributes to the group, there may be fear of rejection, fear of failure, tentativeness, frustration, and a growing desire for structure, clarification, and sense of direction. Questions will arise about the rules, who is responsible for what, what the goals are, and how goals will be evaluated. These questions and comments reflect emerging conflicts over leadership, purpose, structure, authority, and influence. As these areas of difference emerge, there will be varying levels of comfort within the group as well as wide differences in behaviors. Some members may become very silent and withdraw; others will attempt to dominate. Cliques and subgroups will develop as agreement and disagreement over issues become apparent. Trivial matters may become the focus of attention but may be masking frustration and an inability to deal openly with larger issues.

In order to progress to the next stage, group members must move from a "testing and proving" to a problem-solving mentality. Leadership and the ability of group members to listen to each other are critical for groups to move on to the next stage of development. An effective group leader will utilize skills of negotiation and consensus building, to help group members develop greater tolerance for diverse views, and the varying roles and contributions of all the members. Think about the NSA group as they continue developing into the storming stage.

The group has been experiencing some rocky times. The meetings are often fraught with sullen silences and sarcastic remarks. Frustration and anger seem to be frequent visitors, and members are sometimes missing with no explanation. Some of the remarks heard during the last few meetings include:

"It would be nice if someone would give us the right information once in awhile. Are we supposed to be collecting money from our classmates or not?"

"Looks like someone wants to take all the credit for herself" (glancing sidelong at Kathryn, who had just reported on the number of members joined).

"Just because someone happens to be dating a senior, he thinks he knows what is going on better than the rest of us."

"I have lots of people who want to join. Why do we have to collect the money and be so strict about keeping a record? Why can't we just take their word for it and put their names on the new member list?"

"I think the four of us who live in Windsor Hall should be a team and not have to keep meeting with everyone every week."

"If we can't figure out a better way to work together, we aren't going to come anymore."

After a couple of such discouraging meetings, Kathryn talks with Greg and Shanna about what to do next. They approach Dr. X, one of the NSA faculty advisors they trust, and explain the situation and ask for help. The advisor explains she thinks the group behaviors may reflect positive group growth and signify that the group is moving out of the "I"-centered forming stage and beginning to test the tolerance of others. Some are showing their frustration with the group's lack of productivity by angry silences or by angry remarks. Dr. X agrees to try and help. At the next meeting, Kathryn explains they talked with Dr. X and asked her to help the group get better organized. She asks if the group is willing to have Dr. X work with them. The response is lukewarm but, hearing no strong objections, Dr. X thanks the group, hands out an agenda, and explains some ground rules for the meeting. The ground rules ask that all stay focused on the agenda items, agree to speak only when recognized by the leader, promise to make an effort to listen carefully with an open mind to the person who is speaking, to make notes for reference if they have something to add when it is not their turn to speak, and to contribute with serious, thoughtful, suggestions focused on the problem being discussed. All agree to follow the ground rules. Dr. X then shares her impressions of the situation. She acknowledges the group's frustration. She also notes the commitment of everyone, as reflected by consistent attendance. She tells them that their willingness to voice their frustration is very likely related to their being people who do not like to waste time and who are conscientious and goal-oriented and want to get the job done well. There are nods of agreement.

She passes out a feedback form, asking everyone to take a few minutes to write about what they value about this group, what they wish was different, what they would like to accomplish, and what suggestions they have to accomplish the goals. They spend the rest of the evening discussing the collective feedback of the group and brainstorm a list of goals, a list of short-term objectives, a detailed plan of tasks, and a list of volunteers to work on each task. Finally, they develop a time line for the completion of each task. The next few meetings are less chaotic, becoming more focused on the group purpose.

STAGE 3: NORMING

The next stage is called norming because, as the group becomes more cohesive and tolerant of differences, the group process becomes calmer. Members have had time to become more familiar with each other and are better able to predict each other's reactions and behaviors. This normalcy lessens anxiety and builds trust as group norms begin to develop. Over time and with good group leadership, roles and responsibilities become clearer, and members begin to feel less tension. More productive patterns of behavior develop. Cliques dissolve, and members listen to and value facts, ideas, and opinions brought to the group. Problem solving improves. The **group job** during this stage entails actively engaging in problem solving, sharing ideas, doing research, and producing facts and information. The group members share feelings and ideas, solicit and offer feedback to one another, and explore actions related to the task. Creativity is high. At this stage, interactions (**group process**) are characterized by more acceptance, openness, and sharing on both a personal and task level. Consider the NSA group as it embarks on group norming.

Over the next couple of weeks, group members have additional interaction as they compare notes and communicate between classes and in the evenings about how well tasks are being completed. Greg is feeling more comfortable that his classmates appreciate his record-keeping skills, even though he does not share their interest in the shopping trip they are planning. Jamie has experience selling books door-to-door and is teaching the group the art of how to convince others of the value of what you are selling and how to follow through with collecting the money. Amy keeps everyone informed by e-mail of the progress being made. Trent takes responsibility for safeguarding the money collected and issuing receipts. Lindsey plays the role of being the sounding board for the latest gripes, ideas, and suggestions. She strives to keep everyone motivated and encourages those who may be having less than stellar results. Dr. X attends meetings for a few minutes each week to offer her help but observes that the group has shifted its focus from individual needs to the group job. Many good ideas for ways to encourage their classmates to join NSA are generated, and members are often heard complimenting each other for their successes.

STAGE 4: PERFORMING

Not all groups reach the performing stage. If they do, the capacity of the group members and the depth of their relationships become truly interdependent; the group has established a highly functioning team. Group members can work independently, in subgroups, or as a total unit with equal facility. Roles, authority, and responsibilities easily adjust to the changing needs of the group and of individual members. Members feel secure, and the need for group approval is no longer an issue. Members have become highly task-oriented and people-oriented. Morale and group identity are strong; group loyalty is intense. The group is productive, engages in genuine problem solving, and creates effective solutions. The transformation from being a group of individuals to being a highly functioning team is complete.

November 1 was celebration day for the group. Through the weeks, members produced steady results and rallied around each other to overcome obstacles. As midterm approached, all were challenged by increased demands on time. Greg admitted that he was behind in his research paper for adult nursing; Shanna volunteered to keep records for a week so he could catch up. Lindsey's father suffered a serious illness that required all her attention. The rest of the group took turns baby sitting each evening for her and involved her two children in stuffing membership envelopes. Trent took on Lindsey's role of encourager by making a large chart showing progress toward the goals for the week. Jamie invited a different senior to come each week to talk about the fun and professional activities that membership in the NSA offers. At one point, it became clear to the group that several juniors wanted to join NSA but could not afford membership. Kathryn, Jane, and Shanna had an idea that was quickly embraced by the entire group. Kathryn approached the manager of the local music store where she worked, and he agreed to donate a $50 gift certificate to the group. The group organized a raffle. Each member committed to sell at least 12 tickets for $2 each, and they raised $200 from students, friends, family, and faculty. With the help of Dr. X, the money was discreetly distributed to 10 qualified students to help them pay membership dues. During this process, it was clear that the group members were willing to work together toward group goals, and each knew he or she could count on teammates for help with tasks and personal support.

Not all groups develop to the performing stage, but those that do become highly functioning, highly effective teams. Many groups form and accomplish a task without investing the time and energy necessary to become a team. But when work groups do become teams, they return the highest level of productivity to their employers and the highest level of service to their clients. The difference in effectiveness of teams versus lower-functioning groups that have not negotiated through the group development stages can mean the difference between optimal nursing care and care fraught with inefficiency and

error. Consider the level of nursing care that might be delivered by a group at an early stage of development, perhaps at the storming stage, compared with a team at the performing stage. See Table 12-3 (adapted from the Web page of Nondestructive Testing, Teamwork in the Classroom [2004]).

Interdisciplinary Teams

As society has experienced a knowledge and technology explosion, the number of health-care disciplines has increased, and coordination of care has become more complex. A patient entering the health-care delivery system, even for an overnight stay, is likely to be observed, interviewed, examined, tested, treated, discharged, and monitored by a dozen different caregivers representing several medical, nursing, and allied health disciplines. This process offers the patient a breadth and depth of

TABLE 12-3   Group Versus Team Characteristics

STORMING STAGE GROUPS	PERFORMING STAGE TEAMS
Members work independently and may not be working toward the same goal.	Members work interdependently and work toward both personal and shared team goals and understand these goals are accomplished best by mutual support.
Members focus mostly on themselves and are not involved in the planning of their group's objectives and goals.	Members feel a sense of ownership toward their role in the group because they committed themselves to achieving goals they helped create.
Members are assigned tasks or told what their job is, and suggestions are rarely welcomed.	Members collaborate and use their multiple talents and experiences to meet the team's objectives.
Members are cautious about what they say and are afraid to ask questions. They may not fully understand what is taking place in their group.	Members base their success on trust and encourage all members to express their opinions, varying views, and questions.
Members do not trust each other's motives, and roles are not clearly understood.	Members make a conscious effort to be honest and respectful and listen to every person's point of view.
Members may have a lot to contribute but hold back because of superficial relationships with other members.	Members are encouraged to offer their skills and knowledge, and in turn each member is able to contribute to the group's success.
Members are bothered by differing opinions or disagreements because they consider them a threat. There is no group support to help resolve problems.	Members consider conflict as a part of human nature, and they react to it by treating it as an opportunity to hear about new ideas and opinions. Everybody wants to resolve problems constructively.
Members may or may not participate in group decision making, and conformity is valued more than positive results.	Members participate equally in decision making, and each member understands that the leader might need to make the final decision if the team cannot come to a consensus.

comprehensive knowledge and expertise and requires a high level of communication, collaboration, mutual understanding, and respect among the caregivers. Caregivers may include a physician (perhaps multiple specialists); physician assistant; nurses; respiratory, occupational, or physical therapist; social worker; nutritionist; and a myriad of administrators, aides, and technicians. Clerical employees and other support persons may be assisting each discipline. This plethora of personnel presents a serious challenge to effective communication and efficient teamwork.

Health-care agencies expect their caregivers to be competent practitioners and effective team members. To be effective, each team member must understand the various roles played by each discipline. Physicians are trained and educated to be the central hub of the health-care team. They are likely to be the first point of contact, and they focus on the disease process or condition that has caused the patient to seek health-care services. Nurses are educated and trained to focus on the holistic needs of the patients as they respond to the stresses associated with their disease or condition.

The critical importance of teamwork and communication in health care has been underscored by several published reports in the last decade. These studies document the association between quality patient care and effective teamwork (Firth-Cozens, 2001; Institute of Medicine Study, 1999; Kaissi, Johnson, & Kirschbaum, 2003; Majzun, 1998; Sexton, Thomas, & Helmreich, 2000). The findings suggest that teamwork enhances efficiency, contributes to improved morale and job satisfaction, lowers stress, and improves patient satisfaction. Risser et al. (1999) points out that effective teamwork provides a safety net against patient care errors because it allows for coordinated and integrated clinical activities and gives caregivers more control over their work environment. An earlier study by Williamson et al. (1993) and cited by Kaissi reported that 70%–80% of medical errors are related to interpersonal interaction issues. Communication and teamwork issues have been often cited as shortcomings in the health-care system. Caregiver errors contribute to compromised patient safety and diminish job satisfaction among health-care professionals. A recent report, entitled "Silence Kills," (2005) published by VitalSmarts in collaboration with the American Association of Critical Care Nurses (AACN), addresses the need for health team members to communicate better.

The study points out the need for professionals to confront each other about detrimental caregiving behaviors that contribute to hundreds of thousands of patients being harmed each year. In addition, it notes that 1 in 20 hospitalized patients will be given a wrong medication; 3.5 million will get an infection due to lack of handwashing or good precautions (Wenzel & Edmond, 2001); and 195,000 will die because of other mistakes made by caregivers (HealthGrades Quality Study, 2004).

Practice Proof 12-1

Article: Silence Kills, The Seven Crucial Conversations for Healthcare

Author: Maxfield D., et al. Source: VitalSmarts in Partnership with the American Association of Critical Nurses, www.silencekills.com

This study addressed communication patterns among caregivers in hospitals. Researchers collected data from a sample of 1700 nurses, physicians, and other health-care personnel in 13 U.S. hospitals during 2004. Data collection methods included interviews, surveys, and observations. They examined how caregivers communicate their concerns to their coworkers when they observe them providing care in ways that contribute to errors, reduced productivity, poor morale, and high turnover. Results suggest that the majority of health-care workers practice safely and competently. More than half the caregivers surveyed, however, reported observing some number of workers who exhibit problem behaviors continuing over long periods who were not held accountable. They reported witnessing policy infractions, incompetence, and mistakes. Yet fewer than one in ten discussed their concerns with the coworker, and most indicated they did not think it was possible to change and felt no responsibility to raise their concerns. Twenty percent of the physicians said they saw harm come to patients as a result of these concerns, and 23% of nurses reported considering seeking new positions as a result of these concerns. About 10% of the respondents reported willingness to raise their concerns with their coworkers and as a result observed better patient outcomes, more satisfaction, and commitment to staying in their positions. The study results suggest that if more health-care workers would communicate their concerns when they see inappropriate practice behaviors, there would be significantly fewer errors, higher productivity, and lower turnover.

Most health-care workers want patients to get good care yet they are reluctant to confront their coworkers when they see risky behaviors. Why does that happen and can you describe some examples of similar situations?

Another significant published work that calls attention to the need for teamwork in the context of patient safety is "To Err is Human: Building a Safer Health Care System" prepared by the Institute of Medicine (1999). This report cites many factors related to health-care errors and makes many recommendations for improvement, including the need for excellent communication among health team members and effective teamwork training. The report calls for health-care organizations to implement patient safety programs that promote team functioning and to train in teams those who are expected to work in teams. Drinka and Clark (2000) support the "training in teams" concept. They recommend that students participate in interdisciplinary courses during college. In their courses, the goal is to develop an appreciation for and an understanding of the differences and similarities among their professions. Students could engage in learning about the theoretical and value orientations of other professions and develop a foundation for continued understanding and collaboration that will transfer to practice. McPherson, Headrick, and Moss (2001) also support educational strategies that prepare learners to collaborate and provide a comprehensive review of recent literature that identifies the issues, examples, methods, and conclusions about "interprofessional education."

Kaissi, Johnson, and Kirschbaum (2003) conducted a survey that explored the attitudes of nurses related to patient safety and teamwork. The nurse respondents were members of teams practicing in high-risk areas, such as operating room, emergency room, and intensive care units. These nurses believed that effective teamwork was as important as clinical competency with respect to patient safety. They also reported the need for clearer team leadership roles, more team input into patient care decisions, and better teamwork relations between nurses in high-risk areas and with anesthesiologists and nurse anesthetists. These reports strongly support the need for health caregivers to be proficient and effective team members and continually to build skills needed to be successful team leaders. Effective teams need the structure of clear **ground rules** that all members know, understand, and support. Teams with good structure, good communication, and good leadership will far exceed the accomplishments of an individual. Teams that invest the time and energy to learn and execute team skills will provide uncommon results.

Practice to Strive For 12-1

The team must have clear goals. Team goals should call for a specific performance objective that is expressed so concisely that everyone knows when the objective has been met.

The team must have a results-driven structure. Teams need latitude to organize themselves in a way that will let them produce results. Teams needs space, resources, members with expertise, self-defined roles, and time.

The team must have competent team members. The problems given to the team should be those the members can solve given their level of knowledge and experience.

The team must have unified commitment. This does not mean that team members must always agree. It means that all individuals must be directing their efforts toward the goal. If a member's efforts are going toward personal goals, the team should address this and communicate the need for commitment to goals from all.

The team must be collaborative. Trust produced by honest, open, consistent, and respectful behavior and communication is required. With trust, teams perform well; without it, they fail.

The team must have high standards that are understood by all. Team members must know what is expected of them individually and collectively. All are responsible for clarifying confusion and giving and asking for guidance when needed.

The team must receive external support and encouragement. Encouragement and praise work just as well to motivate teams as they do individuals.

The team must have principled leadership. Teams usually need someone to lead the effort. Team members must know the team leader is competent and is working for the good of the team. Team members will not support the leader motivated primarily by the need to achieve personal recognition or other benefits not related to achieving team goals.

Note some best practices based on the work of Larson and LaFasto (1989).

Effective Communication Within Teams

Many of the problems that occur within teams are the direct result of people failing to communicate effectively. **Effective communication** takes place only if the **receiver** understands the exact information or idea that the **sender** intended to transmit. Most literature about effective communication agrees that the communication process begins with the sender having information in his or her mind. It may be a thought, a conceptual idea, technical information, or a feeling. The sender "sends" this communication, using observable behaviors, to the receiver, and the receiver "gets it" using senses, and translates the words or message into information in the receiver's mind. This could be described as a "mind to mind" transmission. During the process, the receiver will receive a message about both the content and the context of the message. **Content** is the actual spoken or written language that can be understood by those who speak the same language. Misunderstandings or confusion may occur when senders and receivers apply different interpretations or usage to the same words. **Context**, sometimes referred to as paralanguage, includes the additional messages that may be sensed or perceived through nonlanguage behaviors. Context may include tone of voice, the look in the sender's eyes, body language, hand gestures, or real or perceived state of emotion (anger, fear, uncertainty, confidence, etc.). These multiple variables of paralanguage can easily cause misinterpretation of or confusion about what may appear to be clear content. Individuals believe what they see over what they hear and tend to trust the accuracy of nonverbal behaviors more than verbal behaviors (Schuster, 2000, p.13). Several nonverbal contextual behaviors that have a significant influence on the way messages are received are described in Box 12-2 (Arnold & Boggs, 1995; Burgoon et al, 1996; Riley, 2000; Schuster, 2000).

In the process of communication, there are many opportunities for a message to become distorted or altered between the sending and receiving. For example, many team leaders think they have communicated once they have told someone to do something ("I don't know why it did not get done, I told Jim to do it.") Perhaps Jim did not hear or understand the message. The message has not been communicated unless the receiver has received and understood it exactly as the sender intended it to be understood. Communicators can validate if a message has been properly received by engaging in two-way communication (**feedback**). Communication is an exchange, not just a one-way give, and both parties must participate in the feedback process to be sure nothing was "lost in translation." One excellent way to ensure effective two-way communication is with **active listening** and feedback.

Box 12-2
Common Nonverbal Behaviors

Vocal: Tone, pitch, rhythm, timbre, volume, and inflection are nonverbal gauges of enthusiasm and interest. A monotone sends a signal of boredom, dullness, and disinterest.

Facial expressions: Smiling signals happiness, friendliness, warmth, and liking to Smiling is likely to create comfort and willingness to listen.

Eye contact: Signals interest in others. Initiates flow of the message and conveys interest, concern, warmth, credibility, and presence.

Personal space: Dictated by cultural norms to signify a comfortable physical distance for interaction with others. Signals of discomfort caused by invading one's space include moving away, turning away, rocking, leg swinging, finger tapping, averting eyes.

Speaking style: A lively speaking style captures the listener's attention, makes the conversation more interesting, and facilitates understanding. Lack of animation while speaking may be perceived as boredom, ill ease, and disinterest.

Posture and body orientation: Standing erect and leaning forward communicate approachability, receptivity, and friendliness. Interpersonal closeness is created when sender and receiver face each other. Turned to side or back, looking at the floor or ceiling communicate disinterest and discomfort.

Active listening is listening with full attention with the intention of understanding. It requires a conscious focus of energy and concentration and full engagement of the listener. It requires listeners to listen as if they will be asked to repeat every word they have heard. Not only will this level of attention promote effective communication of the message, it will also nonverbally communicate full attention and interest back to the sender. Some signs of active listening appear in Box 12-3 (Arnold & Boggs, 1995; Burgoon et al, 1996; Riley, 2000).

Feedback is another powerful communication tool because it helps to verify that the message received was the one sent. Providing feedback may entail the receiver paraphrasing or restating what was perceived, such as "This is what I understood you to say" or "This is what I understand you are feeling. Am I correct?" The feedback process can identify the need for further discussion to prevent misunderstanding. Communication "in a hurry" and without feedback can lead to errors, hurt feel-

Box 12-3

Signs of Active Listening

Spends more time listening than talking.

Notices own biases. (We all have them. We need to recognize them, acknowledge them, and ask ourselves how they affect what we are hearing.)

Does not daydream or become preoccupied with own thoughts when others talk.

Allows time for other speaker to talk. Does not dominate the conversation.

Creates responses after the other person has finished speaking, <u>not</u> while the person is speaking.

Provides feedback but does not interrupt incessantly.

Analyzes by looking at all the relevant factors and asking open-ended questions. Reflects, summarizes, asks for more information.

Stays attentive to what the speaker says; does not shift to what interests the listener.

May take brief notes, which requires concentration on what is being said.

---

ings, wasted time, and an inefficient and ineffective work environment. When providing feedback, it is important to stay positive and **nonjudgmental**. Being nonjudgmental requires conscious effort on the part of the listener. The listener must attempt to resist being distracted by inner thoughts and judgments that arise in reaction to the message being heard. Attending to these inner thoughts and judgments, instead of giving full attention to the message, distracts the listener and may create misunderstanding. For example, if the listener experiences anger at what is being said during the first part of the message, it is likely that the feeling of anger will become the focus of the listener, and the rest of the message may be distorted or lost. If the listener can make a conscious effort to wait until the entire message is heard before attending to any emotions that may be associated with the message, it will improve the effectiveness of the communication.

Dr. Carl Rogers, a noted psychologist during the first half of the 20th century, was an advocate for nonjudgmental communication. He advocated using several deliberate techniques to provide feedback. He recommended paraphrasing, interpreting, providing supportive statements, probing for more information, reflecting back the same words and/or feelings, and sharing feelings. He advised that the

techniques be practiced and utilized with genuineness by the communicators. He cautioned that utilizing feedback techniques in a mechanical way or as manipulations would likely be recognized as such by the communicators and interfere with clear communication and trust building. Effective communication is a cornerstone of effective teamwork, and it works best when those involved are committed to utilizing excellent communication skills, attempt to suspend personal judgments, and extend respect and positive regard for their teammates.

Good communication is a rare and precious talent and requires practice. Nurses working together must apply best practices of good communication to minimize opportunities for errors or omissions in care based on misunderstandings. Communication skill is foundational to professionals being able to share, collaborate, delegate, and integrate their knowledge, expertise, and experiential wisdom. Professional expertise that is shared and blended among colleagues optimizes benefits to patients. Each discipline must understand its own roles as well as the roles of other team members so that appropriate referrals can be made and specialized expertise applied.

Team Leading

Effective team leaders must understand the concepts and theories that explain how teams function so they can meet the challenges inherent in this complex leadership role. Adjusting to the complexities of caregiving settings, negotiating development through group stages, facilitating effective communication, and maintaining patient safety is work to be guided by the team leader. In fact, one of the most important factors in overcoming these challenges and rising to the opportunities is having a competent team leader.

LaFasto & Larson (2001) note "Your purpose as a leader is to add value to your team's effort" (p. 99). The team leader's primary job is to stay focused on the results that the team has been charged to produce. As tasks are shared, different points of view are expressed during planning, or conflicting feelings are shared about group events, and the leader must react appropriately. The challenge will be to interpret and react while keeping the ultimate goal of the team in mind. The best leaders will consistently monitor the progress toward the goal and plan actions accordingly. The leader must "keep an eye on the prize" and rally team members to do the same.

Some skills to assist the leader to stay focused on the goal include:

- Define the goal often to the team and ask the team to do the same.
- Provide visual reminders of the goal.
- Explain how tasks or assignments will contribute to accomplishment of the goal, and ask members to do the same.
- Keep the goal alive by discussing it frequently and in different ways.
- Use frequent examples of how all contributions are moving toward the goal.
- Share examples of reports/stories/literature of how others reached similar goals.
- Help all to understand how/why difficult tasks may be the key to creating the change.
- Value team members, and trust them.

Team leaders must also invite active participation of all team members and make it clear that all members' input is valued. Team leaders should be honest when providing feedback to members. Ground rules must call for the expectation of honest communication delivered in a respectful manner. The leader must set the tone and example for communicating honestly and respectfully and must calmly and respectfully confront others not observing this rule. In most circumstances, the leader should expect, acknowledge, and reward **collaboration** over competition (see Chapter 21). Providing guidance in using a methodical and clear problem-solving method is essential. A balance between tending to the need for technical knowledge and expertise and tending to interpersonal group process needs must be met. There will be times that team effectiveness is blocked because a deeper level of knowledge is needed or times when progress is impeded because team members are not working well together. The good team leader will constantly monitor the team's progress toward its goals and provide the skill and support that are needed to help the team progress. This may take the form of exposing the team to new information, or it may require mediating a disagreement between team members who are not working well together. Providing effective leadership will require diligent monitoring and holding high expectations of team members. Encouraging task assignments that have high expectations but are doable will stretch the team's ability. Success with stretch-

ing will build confidence and create the opportunity to experience a "win." A leader who is fair and impartial, shows no favoritism, and facilitates inclusiveness will create a team that is willing to take greater and greater risks. **Building confidence** will create more motivation for positive action. A good leader says "thank you" in as many verbal and nonverbal ways as can be imagined.

Effective leaders are mindful of the need for good **technical expertise**. Teams need to have the necessary knowledge, experience, and background necessary to reach the goal. Hard work goes a long way toward success, but without the right knowledge in the right areas effective problem solving is unlikely. A team leader who recognizes that a team has knowledge deficits will search for assistance. Possible solutions include adding more knowledgeable team members or providing the team with strong consultation to assist members with building the competence needed.

While keeping the team's ultimate goal in mind, a wise leader will also develop interim steps designed to move toward goal achievement and will assist members with prioritizing each step. To focus energy and ensure efficiency, leader and members must be clear about what work is essential and what is not. Effective leaders set priorities by asking, "What are the three most important steps for us to achieve today (or by our next meeting)?" Teams cannot reach goals, work collaboratively, build confidence, or apply their expertise if they are not clear about the priorities or if they have too many priorities. The team leader must consistently **communicate the priorities** to be met and help envision how the step-by-step priorities fit within the big picture of goal attainment.

Finally, the team leader must apply management skills to facilitate effectiveness and productivity. **Nonperformers** must be managed in a positive way. The leader must communicate concern to nonperformers and provide clear descriptions of expected performance. Nonperformers must be made aware of expected time lines and the rewards and consequences that will be applied for improved or continued lack of performance. Lack of response by nonperformers will create deterioration of team morale and will soon affect team productivity. Nonperformers will likely appreciate guidance toward better performance or will welcome the opportunity to acknowledge they would prefer not to be part of the team. Team leaders who guide their team to stay focused on the goal, stay in a collaborative rather than competitive mode, maintain confidence, provide or build the necessary technical knowledge for goal attainment, set priorities, and manage performance will find themselves in constant demand for service. They will also be appreciated by their team members and will make a lasting contribution to the safe and effective care of health-care consumers.

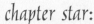

chapter star:

Two nurses and a physician have led formal performance improvement teams, created with the approval and support of hospital administration, to improve patient care outcomes. Issues of care addressed by the teams included length of stay and care of patients at risk for or experiencing deep vein thrombosis, cardiac care, pneumonia, and infections. Team membership varied with the condition being addressed and involved a wide variety of levels and disciplines, including physicians of multiple specialties, nurses of multiple units and specialties, case managers, pharmacists, compliance officers, education consultants, telephone operators, unit secretaries, health information managers, and technology support. Team leaders unanimously agreed that their experience with leading interdisciplinary teams left them with the beliefs that good teams create safer and better patient care, improve resource utilization, improve collaboration, and contribute to more satisfied caregivers. Informal conversations with these team leaders also revealed eight recurring themes that exemplified the challenges, opportunities, rewards, and value of effective team leadership in caregiving settings. These themes are:

1. **The need for clear goals.** Leaders emphasized that a condition for success was the identification of clear goals and the need for leaders to facilitate the "buy-in" of goals by all team members. Asking each team member to commit to the success of the team one by one was noted as a successful strategy within one team. The importance of leaders having public support of the team goals from highly regarded influential hospital leaders was also noted as crucial. Adopting national quality indicators for patient care issues was also noted as an important element in goal setting. Leaders also noted the need to revisit goals and articulate the vision loudly and often.

2. **The need for ground rules.** Leaders agreed that members need to know expectations for structure and behavior and that leaders must make these clear. Ground rules that were considered most important included: clear expectations for time and place of meetings, attendance, communication, collaboration, and mutual respect among members. Examples of interventions that were applied by leaders to address the need to follow ground rules included the next five themes.

3. **Need for attendance.** A leader discussed pattern of poor attendance privately and respectfully with a member and requested better performance in future. After little improvement, member was confronted again and given the opportunity to withdraw from the team with the promise of joining at a future time when she would have more time to devote to teamwork. This proved to be an acceptable solution to all and preserved integrity of team and member.

4. **Need for mutual trust.** Members expressed concern that data-gathering protocols were not followed by some group members. Leader acknowledged the concern and evaluated data-gathering process. Leader used the incident as an opportunity to facilitate open discussion among team members about the need to respect, trust, and value the competence and contributions of all caregiving disciplines while acknowledging the responsibility of the team to identify concerns about inadequate performance.

5. **Need for effective communication.** Leaders believed the need for good communication was imperative. They noted that willingness to communicate created opportunity to solve problems effectively within the team. They also noted that when team members became more familiar with each other's roles, communication improved as did respect and collaboration.

6. **Need for recognizing progression from norming to storming.** One member consistently monopolized team time to criticize progress. Reactions from other team members reflected frustration, sarcasm, defensiveness, and clique formation. Leader led discussion with reminders for respect and focus on issues. Resolved by giving the criticizer the responsibility for a new task that would improve productivity and take advantage of his talent for attention to detail and doing it his way.

7. **Need to facilitate scholarship oriented collaboration:** Improved relationship and respect for others led to sharing of professional literature and ideas. Assessment tools and protocols were developed reflecting interdisciplinary interests. Team members reported more collaborative care and more satisfaction with their work environment.

8. **Need to communicate across generations:** New team approach seemed to threaten autonomy and "old way of doing things" for some practitioners. Team agreed to enlist key peers of older generation (who were accepting of changes) to communicate rationale for changes.

All Good Things...

This chapter has explored the value of team building and teamwork in health care. The innumerable numbers and types of health-caregivers create potential for chaos and require coordination of care for patient safety. Coordination of care occurs best with teamwork, and the elements of good teamwork include good communication and good group work. Effective communication is based on intentional application of good sending and receiving techniques. Effective group work occurs when group members understand group structure and process and are committed to achieving group goals. Groups grow through stages of development; those that are highly developed become productive teams. The best teams have effective leaders, excellent communication, group loyalty, clear goals, flexibility, competence, and members who care about each other. Teams are the cornerstone of high-quality patient care and satisfying work environments.

Let's Talk

1. Think about the various health-care workers you have met. How well informed do you feel about the roles they fill? How does the nursing role differ from the respiratory therapist role? How are they the same? How could you find out more about their role and the roles of other health-care disciplines?

NCLEX Questions

1. The situation that best exemplifies why nurses must be skilled in functioning as an interdisciplinary team member is:
   A. Nurses are frequently expected to serve as a team leader on their nursing unit, which may include several levels of nurse caregivers.
   B. Most practicing nurses are expected to be a member of or provide leadership for formal nursing committees.
   C. Nurses must be prepared to participate in nursing research groups to improve nursing care.
   D. Most nurses function in hospitals that employ specialists from many different caregiver groups who must work together to provide coordinated care.

2. Pick the situation below that would provide the greatest opportunities for misunderstanding, friction, and conflict based on the concepts described in this chapter.
   A. Ms. Hassad, AS, RN; Mr. Krank, CAN; and Dr. Arrington, ER physician, are applying a cast to Steven, a 4-year-old accident victim. Steven's mother, father, and grandparents are present. The family is very anxious and watching to be sure that Steven receives the best care.
   B. The staff members of the NICU (six BSN, RNs; two CNAs, one medical director, one surgical director, two respiratory therapists, two unit administrative assistants, one pharmacist, and one MSN nurse manager) are working as a team to lower the nosocomial infection rate on their unit.
   C. Ms. Carmen, BSN, RN, is a home health nurse caring for Mr. Wolinski who lives alone and is very depressed, argumentative, and hard of hearing.
   D. Six BSN nursing students enrolled in Nursing 301, Healthy Communities, have been assigned to work as a group to develop a teaching plan for smoking cessation.

3. Which of the statements below best describes the relationship between nursing care, groups, and teams?
   A. Good teamwork is dependent on understanding how groups work
   B. Good nursing care is dependent on good teamwork, and good teamwork is dependent on good group dynamics.
   C. All three are equally important, and it is not necessary to understand their relatedness.
   D. Good group work has nothing to do with good teamwork

4. All of the following groups are considered "formal" groups except:
   A. The nursing research committee of the NICU
   B. Nurses who are friends and have a walkers' group at lunchtime
   C. Memorial Hospital Nursing Safety Committee
   D. The IRB of University Medical Center

5. Consider the following description of the NICU staffing group in Question 2 above: All staff members have been employed on this unit and have been working together for at least 6 months. All the staff caregivers deliver conscientious quality care each day. Part of their caregiving plan follows a special protocol that the group developed (based on research about nosocomial infections in the NICU). It includes careful hand-washing, careful adherence to sterile technique and universal precautions, careful adherence to proper equipment use, and careful observation of all caregiver behaviors to be sure they are aligned with agreed upon standards of care. Disagreements occur and are discussed and resolved at team meetings. When illness requires a change in staff workdays, someone volunteers to cover; members celebrate holidays and birthdays; they do their homework and they work together to screen new applicants for open positions to protect the collaborative culture and effective caregiving model they have developed. This group best exemplifies what stage of group development?
   A. Norming
   B. Forming
   C. Storming
   D. Performing

6. The critical importance of teamwork and communication in health care has been documented in many published reports. These reports support the positive association between effective teamwork and:
   A. Quality patient care
   B. Higher medication errors
   C. Compromised patient safety
   D. Lower staff morale

7. The best way to check to see if what you have communicated has been understood the way you meant it to be is to use:
   A. Content and context clues
   B. Nonverbal communication
   C. Reliance on paralanguage
   D. Active listening and feedback

8. Effective communication is a cornerstone of effective teamwork and it works best when those involved are **committed** to all of the following except:

A. Utilizing mechanical techniques
B. Attempting to suspend personal judgments
C. Extending respect and positive regard for their teammates.
D. Utilizing excellent communication skills

9. Skills of good team leaders include all of the following except:
   A. Clearly defining the goal and providing frequent visual reminders of the goal
   B. Ignoring nonperformers and expecting others to do so
   C. Explaining how tasks or assignments will contribute to accomplishment of the goal and asking members to do the same
   D. Using frequent examples of how all contributions are moving toward the goal

10. When a team leader recognizes a need for improved technical expertise in the team, the leader may address this problem by:
    A. Demanding that the team members work harder to gain more knowledge and experience in the necessary technical areas
    B. Sharing disappointment with the team and requesting that members solicit assistance from a colleague to help them become more competent
    C. Adding a new team member who is knowledgeable and can provide the team with strong consultation to assist other members
    D. Explaining to the employer that the team does not have the necessary knowledge and skills to meet the team goals

REFERENCES

Arnold, E., & Boggs, K. (1995). *Interpersonal Relationships* (2nd ed.). Philadelphia: W.B. Saunders.

California Strategic Planning Committee for Nursing. Retrieved September 9, 2004, from http://www.csuchico.edu/nurs/levelsofnursed.htm

Burgoon, J.K., et al. (1996). Deceptive realities: Sender, reviewer, and observer perspectives in deceptive conversations. *Communication Research, 23,* 724–748.

Drinka, P., & Clark, P. (2000). *Health care teamwork: Interdisciplinary practice and teaching.* Westport, CT: Auburn House.

Firth-Cozens, J. (2001). Cultures for improving patient safety through learning: The role of teamwork. *Quality in Health Care, 10*(Suppl II), 1126–1131.

Geriatric Interdisciplinary Team Training: A Curriculum from the Huffinton Center on Aging at Baylor College of Medicine. (2001). Long, D.M., & and Wilson, N.L. (eds.) New York: John Hartford Foundation, Inc. Retrieved

November 5, 2004, from http://www.hospice.va.gov/Bronx/module_3.htm

HealthGrades Quality Study (2004). *Patient safety in American hospitals.* HealthGrades, Inc.

Homans, G. (1950). *The human group.* New York: Harcourt Brace Jovanovich.

Homans, G. (1961). *Social behavior: Its elementary forms.* New York: Harcourt Brace.

Institute of Medicine (1999). *To err is human: Building a safer health system.* Washington, DC.: National Academy Press.

Kaissi, A., Johnson, T., & Kirschbaum, M. (2003). Measuring teamwork and patient safety attitudes of high risk areas. *Nursing Economics, 21*(5), 211–218.

Lacoursiere, R.B. (1980). The life cycle of groups: Group development theory. New York: Human Sciences Press.

LaFasto, R., & Larson, C. (2001). *When teams work best.* Thousand Oaks, CA: Sage.

Larson, C.E., & LaFasto, F.M.J. (1989). *Team work: What must go right/what can go wrong.* Newbury Park, CA: Sage.

Majzun, R. (1998). The role of teamwork in improving patient satisfaction. *Group Practice Journal, 47.*

McPherson, K., Headrick, L., & Moss, F. (2001). Working and learning together: Good quality care depends on it, but how can we achieve it? *Quality in Health Care, 2110*(10): 47–53.

Nondestructive Testing (2004). Teamwork in the Classroom. Retrieved October 29, 2004, from http://www.ndted.org/TeachingResources/ClassroomTips/Teamwork.htm

Riley, J.B. (2000). *Communication in nursing* (4th ed.). St. Louis: Mosby.

Risser, T.R., et al. (1999). The potential for improved teamwork to reduce medical errors in the emergency department. *Annals of Emergency Medicine, 34*(3): 373–383.

Rogers, C.R. (1961). *On becoming a person.* Boston: Houghton Mifflin.

Schuster, P.A. (2000). *Communication: The key to the therapeutic relationship.* Philadelphia: F.A. Davis.

Sexton, J., Thomas, F., & Helmreich, R. (2000). Error, stress, and teamwork in medicine and aviation: Cross sectional surveys. *British Medical Journal, 320,* 745–749.

Silence kills: The seven crucial conversations for healthcare (2005). Retrieved July 2, 2005, at http://www.silencekills.com

Stout, R., Salas, E., & Fowlkes, J. (1997). Enhancing teamwork to complex environments through team training. *Group Dynamics: Theory, Research & Practice 1*(2): 169–182.

Tuckman, B. (1965). Developmental sequence in small groups. *Psychological Bulletin, 63,* 384–399.

Tuckman, B., & Jensen, M. (1977). Stages of small group development. *Group and Organizational Studies, 2,* 419–427.

Wenzel, R., & Edmond, M. (2001). The impact of hospital acquired bloodstream infections. *Emerging Infectious Disease, 7*(2).

Williamson, J., et al. (1993). Human failure: Analysis of 2000 incident reports. *Anesthesia Intensive Care, 21*(5): 678–683.

chapter 13

Power, Politics, and Policy

CAROLINE CAMUÑAS, EDD, RN

CHAPTER MOTIVATION

"Never doubt that a small group of thoughtful, committed citizens can change the world; indeed it is the only thing that ever has."

Margaret Mead

"The ultimate measure of a person is not where one stands in moments of comfort and convenience but where one stands in times of challenge and controversy."

Martin Luther King, Jr.

CHAPTER MOTIVES

- To define power, politics, and policy.
- To investigate and discuss power, politics, and policy in relation to nursing and health care.
- To examine outcomes of the workings of power, politics, and policy.
- To develop an understanding of how effective use of power, politics, and policy can enhance nursing and health care.

Power, politics, and policy should be familiar concepts for all nurses and are especially important for nursing leaders. Power, politics, and policy influence nursing practice, education, and research, which in turn influence health care. Power and politics are intricately entwined concepts and are sometimes difficult to differentiate. Both are used to achieve ends or goals, and both do so through manipulation of others. Power and politics also interact. People who are powerful are able to exert more political pressure; political success brings power that allows people to accomplish goals through policy development and implementation.

Power is the ability to do or act; it is a state in which one can manipulate others. Politics is negotiation for (scarce) resources; it is a process through which one tries successfully or unsuccessfully to reach a goal. Policy is the "consciously chosen course of action (or inaction) directed toward some end" (Kalish & Kalish, 1982, p. 61). Obtaining and allocating resources are two examples of possession and use of power. They also exemplify the use of politics in that influence is needed to get what you want and need. Policies are guidelines that tell us how we obtain and allocate those resources. Understanding power, politics, and policy is crucial to effective patient care because these concepts have a significant impact on access to care, allocation of funds, and standards of care.

Power

There are multiple definitions of power. Some assert that power is an overall concept that includes authority and influence. Others see authority and influence as separate ideas or concepts; as such, they require individual consideration. Power is the ability to influence other people despite their resistance and may be actual or potential, intended or unintended. It may be used for good or evil, for serious purposes or for frivolous and selfish ones. Power is the ability to control, dominate, or manipulate the actions of others or, as Rollo May stated, "power is the ability to cause or prevent change" (1972, p. 99). It is a term used freely by politicians, policy analysts, and many others. Power is important to nursing because having it is necessary to achieve goals as individuals, professionals, and lead-

ers. There are no definitive models of power, which often makes aspects of power complex and contradictory. Power can shift; it is dynamic.

There are a variety of sources (types or bases) of power that have been identified, as derived from the work of French and Raven (1959), Hersey, Blanchard, and Natemeyer (1979), Ferguson (1993), and Joel and Kelly (2002). Understanding sources of power facilitates analysis of individual and organizational behavior and enables prediction in specific situations. Power sources or types are presented below.

TYPES OR SOURCES

Power can be either positional and personal. Positional power is awarded or granted to a person, but it is derived from a person's position, office, or rank in a formal organization system. Personal power, on the other hand, is derived from followers. Leaders who act in ways that are important to followers are given power. An example is the nurse managers who have power because they are seen as highly competent, are good role models, or have some personal attribute that makes them effective in their roles. Expertise (which is discussed below) is a way to gain personal power. Common types of power include (a) authority, (b) expertise, (c) reward, (d) coercive, and (e) referent.

Authority and Administrative

Administrative (sometimes called legitimate) or positional power requires that one serve in a line position and have responsibility for management and actions of other employees. This kind of authority is given to a position rather than to a particular person, for it is part of a role regardless of who fills that role. For example, although the chief executive officer (CEO) in a health-care organization has the most power, the CEO is still answerable to the board of trustees or directors. The chief nurse executive (CNE) has the most power relative to the nurses who are situated further down the chart of the organization, such as supervisory staff, nurse managers, and staff nurses. It is power accorded to a person by virtue of the position held by that person. Nurse managers and team leaders have more power than do staff nurses. CNEs, deans, senators, mayors, governors, presidents, and other elected officials have administrative power.

Administrative authority is the power or right to give orders or commands, to enforce compliance, to take action, and to make final decisions. For example, the dean of a nursing school has authoritative power from her position. As dean, she has the power to make decisions that have both short- and long-term consequences and that directly affect education and student life. Similarly, the primary nurse has more authority in regard to her primary patients than do other nurses or nursing assistants.

Authority can also be personal and as such is defined as power or influence that results from knowledge or expertise. Professional authority is granted by choice, not position, and applies to competent professionals, whereas administrative authority depends upon job descriptions and place in the organization.

Authority has been a problem for nursing since at least the Victorian Era, when nurses were first seen in the aggregate. For most of nursing's modern history, nurses were kept under the authority of physicians. Reverby (1987a, b) states that nurses had to limit revelation of the scope of their knowledge and the effectiveness of their care. They had the responsibility for patient care without needed authority. Reverby asserts that nurses are ordered to care by a society that does not value care. Nurses gained authority through knowledge, feminist influences on society, and slow increases in the scope of practice. Nurse leaders worked hard to gain the power of authority. Judicious, skilled use of power and politics in an environment set for change helped them to change policy with legislation and regulations to achieve their goals. Nursing leaders fought hard for standardization of nursing education, development of knowledge, and professionalization.

Feminism from the late 19th century to the present helped achieve increasing professionalization and improved status. As education and professionalization grew, so did nursing's scope of practice. In 1972, New York State passed the first nurse practice act. For the first time, the essential role of nursing in dealing with human response to illness or treatment was stated, debated, and legislated (Diers & Molde, 1983). The nurse practice act conferred authority on nurses and nursing. Authority was, and is, necessary to nursing as it gives status and power within institutions and communities to mobilize resources to achieve health-care goals.

Expert

Expert power is influence that results from knowledge or expertise that is needed by others. It is similar to personal authority, but it is gained and affirmed through respect for expertise. Expertise can be an indispensable source of power within health-care organizations. Such power is granted by choice to a person, not to a position, and applies to competent professionals.

Nurses work in dynamic environments where change is rapid and where power and influence often take new forms. Expertise brings knowledge and skills to the assessment of problems and issues, which brings about solutions and change. Those who are lifelong learners have an important effect on deliberations and decision making because they understand those changes and can participate fully and find and implement important and creative solutions to situations or problems. Those who do not keep their knowledge current fail to earn or retain expert power. Continued acquisition of new knowledge and skills is essential to maintain this form of power. Expert nurses, nurse practitioners, clinical specialists, and other nurses have power based on their knowledge and expertise. Benner (1984) asserts that nurses can use this power source as they become expert practitioners. This is a source of power that nurses can and must use, because they have expertise that policy makers generally lack. Such professionals have power to exert successful change. Expert power follows the person as long as the person maintains his skills.

Reward

Reward power is the ability to offer rewards, which is a potent type of power. It is the promise or perception of money, goods, services, recognition, and other recompense in exchange for some action that benefits the powerful person. Behavior is affected in that a person will often honor wishes or demands for the potential (or actual) rewards from the powerful person. Managers, supervisors, and administrators have access and ability to use this power through their authority to reward people with bonuses, salary increases, promotions, and recognition. Appropriate use of reward power is the promotion of a nurse who has earned and is qualified for a new position. Inappropriate use of rewards is the assignment of a rotating nurse (bypassing others) to the day shift in return for favors or friendship.

Power to punish is included in the concept of reward. Those who have the capacity to reward also have the ability to punish. In organizations the person with reward power can usually also discipline and fire employees.

Lobbyists often use reward power. They educate legislators and other government officials. Lobbyists bring a high degree of access to and accountability from elected officials. They form coalitions to influence needed legislation and policy change and development. The American Nurses Association (ANA) lobbies for legislation that is important to patient care and nursing. Lobbyists or advocates can have relationships with legislators where one rewards the other. For example, lobbyists promise monetary support for reelection campaigns in exchange for favorable votes on beneficial legislation. Legislators who are found to participate in this kind of power brokering are prosecuted.

Coercion

Coercion is the real or perceived threat of pain or harm of one person by another. Coercive power may be physical, psychological, social, or economic and involves the use of force in the form of penalties and rewards to effect change. It shows a lack of respect for the autonomy of others and is seen in sexual harassment and threats to livelihood. Those who use coercion are interested in their own goals and are rarely interested in the wants and needs of subordinates. An example is the threat by a supervisor to fire whistle-blowers (people who speak out about a wrong). The threat of a state health commissioner to implement onerous regulations for nurse practitioners or visiting nurses if some action is not done is coercion. A volunteer religious group that demands religious conversion by threatening to withhold or withdraw education, expertise, materials, or care coerces the people it is there to help.

Referent

A leader who is followed based on admiration and belief has referent power. The chair of a committee, for example, has referent power for those who work closely with her. Referent power is gained through association with a powerful person or organization. Selection of a powerful person as a mentor and working on powerful committees are ways to develop and hold referent power.

THE NEED FOR POWER

Nurses are predominantly women and provide the most direct patient care in male-dominated organizations. Nurses have rarely had significant power in health-care organizations. Over the past 15 years, nurse administrators have made progress in gaining recognition at the top levels; some have even made inroads to governance. These leaders are all too often terminated, however, which is an all too graphic indication that role acceptance has not been accomplished (Camuñas, 1994a, b, 1998; Carroll, DiVincenti, & Show, 1995; Donnelly, 2006; Kopala, 2001; Sabiston & Laschinger, 1995; Vestal, 1990; Vestal, 1995).

Power commensurate with knowledge and expertise is needed to enable nurses to provide competent, humanistic, and affordable care to people; to participate in health-care policy development; to gain leverage proportionate with their numbers; and to ensure that nursing is an attractive career choice for all who want to provide care, influence, and improve nursing, health care, and health policy.

WAYS TO ACHIEVE POWER

There are multiple ways to accumulate, or gain, power. Some may be more appropriate at higher positions in an organization. Skills to achieve and maintain power take time and patience to learn, develop, and refine. Methods to acquire power include the following:

- Broad human networks: the more networks and the more extensive they are, the more power potential.
- Broad information networks: the more diverse types of information controlled, the more power.
- Multiple formal and informal leadership roles: high engagement and visibility bring increased power.
- Ability to assess situations accurately (especially unstructured ones) and to solve problems.
- Authority over others and resources via legitimate work organizational roles.
- Vision for the future and creativity.
- Ability to grant services to others, which builds debts.
- Expertise that is sought by others.

Ways to Increase Expert Power

There are many ways to enhance your power, for example. Professionals, to maintain their competence and develop their careers, use these tactics:

- Participate in interdisciplinary conferences to broaden knowledge, develop skills, and build networks
- Keep knowledge and skills current to maintain and extend power. Continuing education offerings, books, and journals are effective means.
- Earn higher degrees; education brings expertise and enhances credibility.
- Participate actively in professional associations such as the ANA, state nurses associations, and specialty groups to broaden networks, hone expertise, and develop legitimate and referent power.
- Participate in nursing research to develop knowledge and increase expertise.
- Problem-solve with colleagues in nursing and other disciplines to develop expertise and networks and to polish skills.
- Participate in nursing and interdisciplinary committees to develop and enhance expert, referent, and legitimate power.
- Publish to develop expert power.
- Learn from mentors; be a mentor (Flynn, 1997; Vance & Olson, 1998) to develop expertise and connections or referent power.

EMPOWERMENT

Empowerment is a sense of having both the ability and the opportunity to act effectively. Empowerment is a process or strategy the goal of which is to change the nature and distribution of power in a specific context. It is a group activity that increases political and social consciousness, is based on the need for autonomy, and is accomplished with continuing cycles of assessment and action. Nursing organizations seek to empower nurses; nurses endeavor to empower patients to seek and adopt healthy lifestyles. Likewise, nursing managers and administrators take actions to empower nurses to achieve effective, rewarding, competent practice.

Empowered nurses have three required characteristics that enable them to participate in policy development. The first is a raised consciousness of the social, political, and economic realities of their situation or environment and society. They are aware of culture and diversity and of gender, race, and class biases, prejudices, discrimination, and stereotyping that produce the need for policy development or change. Such nurses can evaluate and understand the dynamics of a situation or issue in which they find themselves and can more readily find or help to find remedies..

The second quality empowered nurses have is a positive sense of self and self-efficacy regarding their ability to effect, or facilitate, change. They value themselves and have voice to articulate and effect change. Within an institution, for example, they can identify situations that constrict professional practice, lower quality of care, waste resources, and cause myriad other problems. They can also contribute to the resolution of problems that affect health at the community, state, and national levels.

Development of skills that allow active participation in change processes is the third important characteristic. Empowered nurses know how to use traditional methods of power and politics in policy making. Concrete knowledge and information are necessary, as is understanding interpersonal communication skills, politics, and power and how to use them (Kuokkanen & Katajisto, 2003; Manojlovich & Laschinger, 2002).

Abuse of Power

Abuse of power is the control of people by some kind of force. It is the use of power for one's own benefit (individual or group) and can be present in families, organizations, and all levels of domestic and international government. It is always unethical. Poor, developing nations around the world are obvious examples. Dictators abuse their people often to the point of genocide. Industrialized nations engage in unfair trade and often exploit workers.

Abuse of women, children, the elderly, the sick, and innumerable others who cannot assert themselves is not uncommon. To combat these types of abuse of power, we use political negotiations to develop policies to assuage or eliminate the problem. We have child protection laws, laws to protect people with disabilities, and laws that prevent emergency patients from being transferred to other health-care organizations when doing so puts the patient at risk. Around the world, abuse of power causes violence, human suffering, and tragedy on unimaginable scale (Farmer, 2005). Violence can be physical, psychological, or structural (the absence of health care, education, and just law enforcement for the poor, for example). Leaders who enforce structural and societal inequalities abuse power.

Power and politics are often discussed together in the nursing literature. The linkage may be due to the difficulty that arises in attempts to distinguish them. Those with power find it easy to participate in politics, and those who participate in politics gain power. Both power and politics serve to achieve goals, and both do so through the ability to use skills to convince others to serve the power holder's purposes. Power and politics are the means to achieve health-care goals in a compassionate and humane way. Application of power and politics through collaboration, creativity, and empowerment are effective ways to influence policy.

Politics

Politics is the negotiation for, or influencing of, allocation of scarce resources. Influence is the act or power to produce an effect without apparent use of force or direct command. Politics is a neutral term and a process. Flexibility is perhaps the most important trait of a good politician.

POLITICAL ACTION SPHERES

The process of influencing others, or politics, in order to achieve ends can be seen in relation to four arenas, spheres, or domains. These spheres are (a) the workplace, (b) professional organizations, (c) community, and (d) local, state, and federal governments. Although the ranges of these domains differ, and the target publics to be influenced differ, the political tactics and strategies are similar. These spheres overlap; what happens in one affects the other. Ignoring one can jeopardize outcomes in the others. The fact that nurses have not consistently paid attention to this has contributed to the fact that the level of influence nurses possess is not com-

chapter star:
Florence Nightingale (1820–1910)

Florence Nightingale had a major impact on health-care policy in the British army, in India, as well as on the development of nursing. Indeed, her effect on nursing and health care is still felt today; her book, *Notes on Nursing,* is still in print. That she was Victorian has special significance. She gained power and affected policy in ways that were unheard of for a woman to accomplish. Her leadership skills were formidable.

Nightingale was born into a wealthy, educated, extended family. The women especially were social activists whose thinking was ahead of their time in significant ways. Women had no public role and received education only insofar as it would increase marriage possibilities. Florence was a talented, gifted child who was educated by her father. She learned Latin, Greek, mathematics, and religion; read English classics; and learned controversial topics such as poetry, philosophy, science, economics, and political theory. Her Greek, which is more difficult than Latin, was at the level where scholars consulted with her (Gill, 2005, p. 128). From her father she learned to excel and to compete with the men who ruled the British Empire. And she nursed people in her family and on family estates and towns, which taught her a great deal about caring for the sick.

Nightingale understood when she was in her early 20s that the women she knew had no desire or want of power; but she did want power. "In pursuit of knowledge Florence was remorseless. She was brilliant, she was focused, she was competitive, and she identified learning, correctly, as an avenue to power" (Gill, 2005 p. 129). Nightingale also understood that knowledge would not be enough "considered how she, a woman of high social status, could use her personal friendships and family alliances to effect larger social goals such as improvement in national health care" (p. 177). Her intellectual skills, family connections, and understanding of power and politics enabled her to go to Turkey to improve and reform care for the wounded of the Crimean War. She was successful, had tested her abilities, and had gained powerful authority in the highest reaches of government, including Queen Victoria and Prince Albert.

Upon her return to England, she was appointed to two commissions to reform public health. Nightingale was the "chief strategist, chief correspondent, chief worker; in other words, the one essential person upon whom the whole male team of experts relied." The work Nightingale accomplished had significant effect on the army's support services, public health in England and India, and the development of professional nursing. Even without consideration that she was a Victorian woman, her work was enormous. Understanding and use of power and politics in development of effective health policy, which is rare even in the early 21st century, made her a hero for the ages.

mensurate with the numbers of nurses, their abilities, and their responsibilities and contributions.

Workplace

Nurses work in organizations with varied characteristics—private or public; profit, nonprofit, or charitable; large, small, or medium; and in large or small cities, towns, small towns, or rural areas. In the workplace, there are many issues with which nurses are involved. Power and politics may be necessary to resolve issues. Some issues that may be found in some, or all, workplaces include the following:

■ Mandatory overtime work requirements.
■ A nursing clinical ladder program that rewards excellence with promotions and pay incentives.
■ Work scheduling length of shift, evening and night rotation, vacation priority.
■ A smoking ban in the entire facility; designation of smoking areas.
■ Visiting hours in special care units.
■ Identification and security procedures.
■ Authority to delay discharge from or admission to special care units based on professional nurse assessment.
■ Authority to refer patients to a home health-care agency.
■ Decisions regarding substitution of unlicensed personnel for RNs to provide care.

Politics are part of *every* organization; nurse executives have to use politics to administer their areas of control. They have to negotiate with CEOs and other administrators (their peers) for budgets to meet organizational goals.

Professional Organizations

Professional organizations have been essential to the "professionalization" of nursing. The modern nursing movement began in 1873 in response to the changing role of women. Pioneers of this movement worked for a new profession for women and for better health for the public (Reverby, 1987a). These women used political power to open nurse training schools, organize professional associations, and participate in social issues such as women's suffrage, public health, and integration (Rogge, 1987). These leaders sharpened their political expertise in nursing organizations they created beginning in 1893.

Professional organizations have made significant contributions in developing nursing practice. They have set standards of practice, advocated for change in the scope of practice and passage of nurse practice acts, and advocated for nurses in collective action in the workplace. Such organizations have an ever-increasing role in health policy development.

Fewer than 10 % of nurses belong to the ANA, even though it represents the interests of all nurses in the United States (Foley, 2001). Membership in specialty nursing organizations rarely exceeds 30 % of those eligible to join (Foley, 2001). These organizations are essential for advocating for nurses and for humanistic health promotion. A strong professional organization needs to be a visible force: a national organization should have national visibility; a local organization should be known locally. For example, the ANA works on national issues in Washington, DC; the state nurse associations work on state-wide issues; and the local districts work on issues in the local community. These three levels of the ANA work in concert. Organizations can identify issues that concern nursing and health care, bring them to the public, and take a leadership role in advocating for development of policies that improve health and ensure high-quality nursing care. To achieve this, organizations need support of nurses through their membership and through their political acumen.

The New York State Nurses Association (NYSNA), for instance, developed and championed the legal definition of professional nursing in New York State. The New York State Nurse Practice Act was passed in 1972 and was the first law to define nursing as an independent profession. This definition of nursing still stands and has served as the model for nurse practice acts in the other states. The ANA is working to influence legislation to deal with overcrowded emergency departments (Trossman, 2006).

Community

Community is most often defined as a geographic area with boundaries, but during the 1960s the idea of community empowerment grew to define a group with a common good that required coordinated action. Power, politics, and policy became attached; community, in this context, is defined as a population, a neighborhood, a state, a nation, and the world. It can be a nursing organization or an online group. An individual is usually a member of more than one community. The other three political action spheres exist in the sphere of community. For example, an individual can be a member of the education, religious, and nursing communities. The countries of Western Europe have joined together to become the European Economic Community; they are also joined with the United States in the North Atlantic Treaty Organization.

Nurses are members of a community with the responsibility to promote the wellbeing of the community and its members. In exchange, the community provides important resources for nurses' work in health promotion and health-care delivery. Many of the people who live in a community, such as health-care administrators, corporate managers, industrial leaders, elected and career government officials, and patients, have power. These people can, and do, participate in community activities; they have status, expertise, and connections. By building relationships with community members, nurses can gain supporters to achieve goals. The connections they make can transform into networks, and the people in the networks can be asked to support agendas.

In exchange, nurses should support community agendas to work to improve community life. There are innumerable ways to participate actively in the community. Groups such as parent-teacher associations, community boards, councils, conservancies, civic groups, and soup kitchens are but some groups that need and welcome participation and help. Nurses can help mobilize communities on issues such as recycling, environmental clean-up, safety, energy conservation, health screening, and the like. Although activism may grow out of private interests, it can affect professional life with increased skills, knowledge, experience, and power development. In addition, nurses who are active and form connections in their communities become role models and represent the whole profession.

Government

Government affects most aspects of our lives. We must document births, marriages, and deaths; the buying and selling of real estate; and mandatory childhood immunizations. Government establishes the age at which people may drink alcohol, drive a car, cast a vote, and join the military. Laws determine the health services and social security available to people in old age. Our collective society is organized in ways that make us interdependent; the health and welfare of each of us are dependent on the health and welfare of all. Government is needed to ensure that what we need to get done is accomplished.

Government plays an essential role in nursing and in health care. State government defines what nursing is, and it defines what nurses do. It influences how our health-care system is organized. Government influences reimbursement systems, such as Medicare and Medicaid. Government influences and supports the current managed care arrangement, which provides for reimbursement for health and nursing care. To a large extent, government determines who has access to care and to what type of care. Federal, state, and local governments make decisions about major health issues in our society. Recent decisions include:

- The kinds of foods and snacks available to children at schools
- Prohibition of smoking in some public places
- The initiation and continuation of Head Start
- Provision of meals for the poorest children
- The health services available at schools and whether schools may provide sexual and reproductive information; whether schools may provide condoms to sexually active students to prevent the spread of human immunodeficiency virus (HIV) and acquired immunodeficiency syndrome (AIDS)
- Whether public funds can be used to distribute clean needles to intravenous drug users to reduce the spread of HIV and AIDS
- Whether women can receive full information about reproductive rights and who can provide that information
- Whether violence is treated only as a crime or also as a public health issue and whether to regulate the use of hand guns
- Allocation of funds for housing development and maintenance

POLITICAL ANALYSIS

Effective use of power and politics to facilitate strategy development for the policy process requires systematic analysis of the issues. The following is a framework for systematic analysis. Adroit use will increase nurses' political leverage. Although this is directed at broad political action in government and the community, it is also applicable to workplace and organizational policy processes (see Box 13-1).

Box 13-1

The Problem

What is the scope, duration, and history, and whom does it affect?

What data are available to describe the issue and its implications?

Are there gaps in existing data? What else do we need to know?

What types of additional research might be useful?

Components of Political Analysis

Identify and Analyze the Problem

Identification and analysis of the problem or issue is the first step. The problem must be understood in order to frame it in ways that will move elected officials to action. It must be carefully crafted in terms that make sense; calls for public action must be clearly justified. Use of public relations theory will help with the expression of, or framing, the issue.

To frame the problem adequately, state the scope, duration, and history of the problem. An important point is to be explicit about whom this problem affects. Then collect all data that are available to describe the issue and its implications. Identify any gaps in the data. Identify whether more research might be useful and, if so, what types would help.

Outline and Analyze Proposed Solutions

Present possible solutions to public officials along with the identified problem. It is best to develop more than one solution because costs, effectiveness, and durability differ from approach to approach. For example, an enduring problem is the nursing shortage; multiple proposals have been developed to correct it and its effects. If increased access to nursing education is a proposed solution, then the proposal must include how this is to be accomplished. The federal budget is limited; there are many demands for funding for worthy goals, and they must be considered. Competition for federal funds is stiff; nursing education and health care are only two goods among many. Each funding solution—grants, tax incentives, and other sources—has different implications, and each must be understood before making a proposal for federal aid.

A proposal for addressing safe patient handling and prevention of musculoskeletal disorders (MSDs) among nurses was promoted by NYSNA and proposed for legislation. Research showed that promoting proper body mechanics alone is an ineffective way to reduce MSDs in health-care workers. The governor signed a measure for funding a demonstration project. A change in policy will protect patients and health-care workers. Added benefits include increased employee retention and reduced worker replacement and compensation costs (ANA, 2005, p. 4). The ANA and NYSNA performed an effective problem analysis based on solid data. They now have state funding to gather more data and ultimately work for a change in policy.

Understand the Background, Including Its History and Attempts to Solve the Problem

It is important to understand what attempts have been made to address an issue. The history, including why and how previous attempts failed, will provide an estimation of the potential success of the current proposal. For example, the reform of our health-care system, especially implementation of a national health service, would require a review of the background of the Medicare/Medicaid system and also a review of President Clinton's Health Security Act. Assessment of the public's perceptions of public funding and American emphasis on individualism is needed so that political action can be planned thoroughly. Knowledge of positions of key public officials will also assist in planning.

Even in a workplace context, understanding the background of an issue is important. If you believe that the staffing on a unit needs to be changed to improve patient care, efficiency, and nurse satisfaction, you must assess how the staffing was structured, why it was done in that particular way, and why and how that format is outdated before you present your proposal to the nurse manager or appropriate committee.

Locate the Political Situation and Its Structure

After the problem and solutions have been delineated, assess and choose the appropriate political venues. The choice is between the private sector and government. If the decision made is to approach government, decide on the level and branch. There are times when both the public and private sectors are involved, but in that case, only one has the decision-making responsibility. When all sectors have equal power, no one sector has the responsibility to make a decision nor the vested interest to prevent a decision. Be sure to identify the political setting accurately, because making an error can cause you a loss of credibility and a loss of power. For example, if nurses are concerned about an aspect of patient care, the employer must be approached through the organization structure. It is unfair and impolitic to go to public officials before internal mechanisms have been exhausted. It is also imprudent to exclude the nurse manager and go directly to the chief nurse executive or a supervisor. Again, so doing will cause loss of face, credibility, and power.

Evaluate the Stakeholders

The next step is to identify the stakeholders. Stakeholders are those who are affected by or have influence over an issue or who could be recruited to care about it. Stakeholders include policy makers who have proposals related to the issue, special interest groups, and those with a position on the issue. For example, after her husband was fatally shot and her son seriously wounded, Congresswoman Carolyn McCarthy, an LPN, became a respected and powerful proponent for gun control. She was able to recruit other stakeholders, such as victims of gun violence, during her campaign. One of the most important stakeholders she identified was the American Academy of Pediatrics, which has significant power and resources. The congresswoman recently established the Carolyn McCarthy Center on Gun Violence and Harm Reduction to mobilize public support at the grassroots level for new gun safety legislation.

Conduct a Values Assessment

All political issues have value or moral aspects. Human rights, international health law, the right to health, genetic engineering, embryonic stem cell research, genetic technologies, terrorism, abortion, and the death penalty are among the most visible moral issues today (Annas, 2005). Issues necessitate that stakeholders assess their own values and those of their opponents.

Ascertain Financial and Personnel Needs to Attain Goals

Any effective political strategy must include assessment of resources needed to reach goals. In addition to money, other needed resources include time, connections or network, volunteers, contributors, and intangibles, such as people who are strategists and those with creative ideas. Short- and long-term tactics and goals must be considered in resource analysis.

The budget structure within an organization or government agency must be considered. It is important to understand the budget process, including how money is allocated to a cost center or line budget, who makes decisions regarding expenditures, how use of funds is evaluated, and how an individual or group can influence budget development and implementation.

Analyze Power Bases

In any setting, assessment of power bases of both proponents and opponents is essential. Review the section on power for further discussion.

After the political analysis is accomplished, it is time to plan political strategies and identify tactics and guidelines.

POLITICAL STRATEGIES

After the political analysis is completed, a plan of action with strategies is developed. Strategies are the plans to achieve political and policy goals. One strategy does not work in all situations. To achieve goals, it is useful to follow these tactics:

- Persistence. Change takes time; conflict is almost always part of policy change. Usually there is much discussion, negotiation, and col-

---

Practice to Strive For 13-1

Many nurses and nursing associations voice the importance of political participation and activism to improve health care for all people. This is not an easy task as our culture urges that health care should be organized as a commodity. Professional nurses must be politically active to change the ethos of health care as commodity to the ethos of health care as a right. Although the right to health care is not in the constitution, society can make it so if it chooses. To achieve this, nurses must become activists and move beyond the passive activities of letter writing and slogans. Nurses must assume broader roles to improve access to and standards of care for all. Nurses must prepare themselves to be capable in the world of power, politics, and policy. As novices, nurses must learn subjects such as women's studies, ethics, communication, economics and politics of health care, history of social movements and reforms, and strategies and tactics of politics. There are so many with vested interests in health care that the system, health care, and nursing are in danger and require reform. Nurses must be visionary and politically skilled.

laboration with attendant delays, retrenchment, and realignments. Policy change or new policy development and implementation is a long-term commitment and requires commitment and endurance.

- Look at big picture. Always prepare for the political process of policy development by clarifying aspects of the issue. This includes knowing your position and possible solutions supported by data, assessing your power base and that of others involved, planning strategies, and knowing the opposition and their plans and rationales. Understand the context of the issue.
- Frame issue adequately. Understand the stakeholders and target audience to present the issue in ways that are congruent with their values.
- Develop and use networks. Use power that accrues through personal connections, which requires keeping track of what you have done for others and asking them to reciprocate.
- Assess timing. Consider carefully when is the most opportune time to act. Knowing when the time is right requires accurate assessment of the values, concerns, goals, and resources of those you have to convince that your way is best.
- Collaborate. Work with others to achieve policy goals. Collaboration usually achieves goals more effectively than does individual action.
- Prepare to take risks. Do a risk-and-benefit analysis of an action. This analysis entails consideration of the benefits gained or goals achieved in relation to the expenditure of all resources, including personnel, money, time spent that could have been used on another endeavor, and coherence with values.
- Understand the opposition. Put aside emotional positions, focus on the issues, and try to understand the fears and concerns of the opposition. Educate the opposition to appreciate the nursing position.

Political Tactics

The effective functioning of an organization depends on the relationships between individuals and groups. Effective use of politics in the workplace can facilitate achievement of goals. A characteristic of political action is that it creates obligation; that is, to get something, something may be expected in return. Such an approach may achieve only part of a goal, but that partial achievement is a step toward the goal.

- Employ opportunism; act when the time is right.
- Use trade-offs; support a cause or person in exchange for the goal at hand.
- Sell votes on one issue for votes on another.
- Negotiate; each side gives up lesser values to achieve greater values.
- Form coalitions; two or more smaller groups band together to defeat a larger power.
- Compromise; each side settles for a partial win or part of what it hopes to achieve.
- Lobby; attempt to build collectible debts with persons who may influence (or vote) in your favor.

Skills and Tactics in the Workplace

The effective functioning of an organization depends on relationships between individuals and groups. Often, problematic conflicts arise that are threatening to groups. Resolution of these conflicts requires significant managerial skill. Effective use of politics can facilitate conflict resolution and achieve goals. Not all the following skills and tactics may be acceptable, useful, or necessary in a particular situation, but they are useful and have a high probability of success:

- Build your own team. Executives, administrators, and managers are often defeated in their roles because persons from the previous team are unhappy, jealous, and disgruntled and do not support, or actively sabotage, the work of the new boss.
- Choose your second-in-command carefully. "An aggressive, ambitious, upwardly mobile number two man (or woman) is dangerous and often difficult to control" (McMurray, 1973, p. 70).
- Establish alliances with superiors and peers. Determine expectations and motivations of others before you form true friendships. Alliances with superiors and peers are needed to achieve goals.
- Use all possible channels of communication. Develop and maintain open, effective channels of communication to avoid isolation,

pre-emption, and loss in power struggles. Be fair, but learn to recognize aggressive, manipulative people.

- Do not be naïve about how decisions are made. Learn and understand the preferences and the way powerful people act in the organization in order to predict how they will make a decision; then plan accordingly.
- Know what takes priority. Know what the goals are and how the organization generally works to achieve those goals. In other words, know the *modus operandi.*
- Be courteous. Treat others with respect. Respect can prevent feelings that can lead to sabotage and retaliation.
- Maintain a flexible position and maneuverability. Identify what is ethically important and nonnegotiable. Then you can maneuver confidently to change and power.
- Disclose information judiciously. In order to work effectively, it may be necessary not to disclose how power strategies are used.
- Use passive resistance when appropriate to gain time. Delay can be useful when time is needed for gathering information.
- Project an image of confidence, status, power, and material success. The image of weakness conveys a lack of power and decreases ability to act and achieve goals.
- Learn to negotiate and collaborate. Do not be ingratiating or conciliatory.

COALITIONS

Coalitions have great power to achieve a specific, common goal. They bring diverse people together, with different worldviews, and encourage collaboration, creativity, and empowerment. There is strength in numbers, so coalitions increase the probability for success in political and policy processes.

Coalitions take many forms and usually arise out of a challenge or opportunity. They are often disbanded when the goal is achieved, but sometimes they can be long-term and function for years. When they stay together, it is generally because after they achieve their goal, another goal becomes apparent and they choose to continue to work together.

Effective coalitions have three important characteristics that are necessary to use power and politics

skillfully and to influence policy processes. These characteristics are (a) leadership, (b) membership, and (c) creativity. Without these attributes, a coalition cannot identify, assess, plan, and implement or seize opportunities to further its goals.

A coalition needs two types of leaders. One has to have spirit and passion for the cause. This leader has to motivate the membership to get the job done. The second leader must be an organizational leader who is adept at administration that supports the coalition. This leader may be paid if the coalition has funds; other leaders and members are volunteers.

The more members, the more effective the coalition becomes. Without members, the coalition would not exist. Members do the work of the coalition and increase its visibility. Members benefit the coalition, but the coalition also benefits them because they learn and hone skills (Berkowitz & Wolff, 2000).

The ability to recognize and seize an unexpected opportunity and make the most of it is essential. This requires creativity, innovation, and the willingness to take risks. It also requires that leaders and members continually assess their environment, use and enlarge their networks, and keep track of politics associated with their goals in their community.

It is hard work to keep a coalition on target to achieve goals. Effective leadership, management, and active, interested, and participating membership are essential to success. Coalitions bring diverse people together for a common cause. They meet regularly and implement or act on their plans. Members must be active and receptive to fresh ideas and innovations. Nurses and nursing must participate in coalitions to improve health care through policy change. An example of an effective coalition is that formed by nurse practitioners and nurse midwives in Maine. Although they had won a change in the nurse practice act, they did not have third-party reimbursement. A coalition was formed and after much work, they finally won payment (Leavitt, 2002).

CONFLICT RESOLUTION

We have defined power as the ability to act and politics as the allocation of resources that are used for an identified end, goal, or policy. Often during this process, conflicts develop and must be resolved. The resolution process includes negotiation, which can result in one side winning or both sides getting something (often referred to respectively as win-lose and win-win resolutions, discussed in Chapter 20). A summary of win-lose methods was identified and characterized by Roe (1995): (1) denial or withdrawal, (2) suppression or smoothing over, (3) power or dominance, and (4) compromise.

Win-Win Solutions

Win-win solutions, on the other hand, manage conflict in a way that neither party loses and the outcome is creative and productive. Collaboration and principled negotiation are two approaches to win-win resolution to conflict. See Chapter 20 for further discussion.

Collaboration

The goal of collaboration is for parties to work cooperatively with one another in a way that everyone wins and no one has to give up anything. Marquis and Hurston (1994) explain that in collaboration "both parties set aside their original goals and work together to establish a supraordinate goal or common goal. Because both parties have identified the joint goal, each believes they have achieved their goal and an acceptable solution. The focus throughout collaboration remains on problem solving, and not on defeating the other party" (p. 290).

Collaboration requires time and full commitment to the resolution process. Mutual respect, communication skills, and an environment where all are heard and considered are necessary for successful collaboration. Collaboration is the ideal solution where all parties are satisfied and all win. Senators from opposite sides of the aisle collaborate when they jointly propose a bill in the U.S. Senate.

Principled Negotiation

Principled negotiation is a form of conflict resolution developed at the Harvard Negotiation Project and has four basic steps as identified by Fisher, Ury, and Patton (1992). These steps are as follows.

- Separate the people from the problem. This step strives to depersonalize the argument. All parties in the negotiation are persons with feelings, needs, values, experiences, and percep-

tions and come from different backgrounds. Each person has a personal worldview that must be respected. Because negotiation is easily influenced by the relationships and the problem, it is essential to keep to the issues and not let personalities and feelings intervene in the conflict in such a way as to cut off communication and productive search for a solution. Again, U.S. Senators may fight on the floor but it is done in a way that keeps the person out of the argument. Mutual respect is a must.
- Focus on interests, not positions. Interests define the problem and are the motivators. Positions are generally conflict needs, wants, discomforts, and fears. For example, nursing staff suffers because patients are difficult, abusive, and manipulative, and they are increasingly unhappy. Staff members believe that they do not matter as people, that they cannot continue to act in professional ways. The interests are adequate staff, material resources, and support to care for these patients. The positions of the staff are anger at administration for allowing the situation to persist, anger at patients who do not appreciate their hard work, fears that they are inadequate, and so forth. The administration fears for their jobs if they do not allocate resources to in a responsible way. Positions are the objectives that arise out of interests. Identification of interests leaves room for alternative positions that serve mutual interests. It is important to identify the facts and feelings behind each party's wants and fears. Doing so will identify shared and compatible interests. To focus on positions limits ability to consider other options as parties will be too engaged in defending their positions to negotiate in a meaningful way.
- Invent options for mutual gain. Develop a large number of possible solutions to avoid stymied, narrow negotiations. The more options identified, the greater the possibility of creative, productive solutions.
- Brainstorming is a frequently used successful method to create options free of judgment. Participants in the negotiation identify as many ideas as possible without critique. The expectation is that ideas should be congruent with shared interests. These interests are goals and need to be made explicit.

Box 13-2

Steps to Conflict Resolution

Identify who is involved in or the source of the conflict.

Identify interests and clarify issues.

Build mutual trust.

Separate the persons from the conflict (depersonalize the conflict).

Stay in the present or look to the future; do not dwell in the past.

Avoid placing blame.

Remain focused on the identified issues or problems.

Discover options; brainstorm.

Develop objective evaluation criteria.

Come to a consensus.

■ Insist on using objective criteria. Use of objective criteria such as research findings will ensure a better agreement. The criteria must be based on a fair standard and should be identified before agreement. Discuss criteria rather than positions to be gained or lost. Focus on objectives will preserve ego and keep relationships intact.

Nurses will continue to need expertise in conflict resolution as change continues to challenge health care. After all, so much is at stake. Negotiation often occurs with participants of unequal power, which puts the less powerful at a disadvantage that is not often acknowledged. Justice, equity, and fairness are uncertain or unlikely in such situations. Successful negotiation requires broad and deep knowledge, the ability to synthesize diverse components of a situation in order to bring trust and respect needed for conflict resolution. Adversity can be a good teacher and impetus for change. Conflict provides an opportunity for personal growth and development, creativity, and innovation that nurses would do well to use to improve health care. The steps outlined in Box 13-2 are useful in conflict resolution.

Power and politics are used to achieve goals. In nursing and health care, the goals are policies that help nurses to deliver appropriate care to persons in local, state, national, and international communities.

Policy

Policies are written directives or actions to follow to meet identified ends or goals. Policies reflect values; stakeholders work for policies that are morally congruent with their values. A policy is a guideline that has been formalized by administrative authority and guides or directs action to an identified purpose or specific goals. Policies are developed within organizations, associations, and governments at local, state, federal, and international levels. Values and goals are reflected in the choices an organization, community, and society make. In nursing and in health care, major choices relate to policies governing access to care, allocation of resources, and standards of care. Policies help organizations run smoothly and protect both health-care providers and patients.

A policy system is the total group of events and rules to that policy. The three major parts of a policy system are (1) a purpose or goal, (2), a policy rule, or how to achieve the goal, and (3) a written directive (procedure) on actions to follow in implementing the rule. For instance, an institution may have a policy that all nurses must participate in continuing education each year. This policy rule requires a written directive on the actions to be taken because the policy is still open to many interpretations. What is the content to be required? Can it be done in-house or outside? When must it be done? How many hours are needed?

In the United States, health-care policy is particularly rife with disagreement because of four goals that are in conflict. These conflicting goals are (1) provision of the best possible care for all, (2) provision of equal care for all, (3) freedom of choice on the part of health-care providers and consumers, and (4) containment of costs. These conflicting goals and values demonstrate the reasons we have not been able to develop satisfactory health-care system reform. Accessible, cost-effective, equitable, and high-quality care has been elusive. The power, politics, and interests of the special lobbies of big business, such as the insurance, pharmaceutical, and supply industries, champion the free market for health-care system reform. These industries have great wealth and therefore great power to gain and keep control of reform. Weakest in this equation are the poor, the underinsured and the uninsured, and increasingly the working and middle classes who have little or no voice and power. Research has consistently demonstrated prevalent race and gender discrimination in health-care allocation (Bach et al., 2004; Bloche, 2004; Jha et al., 2005; Shischehbor et al., 2006; Smedley, Stith, & Nelson, 2003; Steinbrook, 2004.)

The free market reforms that were implemented have failed to achieve important goals of the system. The amount of money spent on health care now exceeds 15% of the gross domestic product (Centers for Medicare & Medicaid Services, 2003). The Kaiser Family Foundation found that health care grew to over 16% in 2006. Administration costs of third-party payers have risen sharply. Both providers and consumers have little, if any, choice regarding care. Disparities in standards of care are growing. Fewer people have access to care; the number of people in 2004 without access was 45.8 million (*American Journal of Nursing*, 2006), which is up from 37 million in 1990 (Kaiser Commission, 2004). These statistics reveal that the free-market reforms have failed to improve access to care, control costs, and maintain standards of care. With increased free-market policies, the number of people without access to care has increased, costs have increased, and quality of care has decreased.

The health-care system is extremely complex and is not wholly amenable to free-market forces. The marketplace has failed to reform the health-care system because of six characteristics or factors (Alward & Camuñas, 1991). These factors are (1) imperfect information, (2) third-party payers, (3) gatekeepers, (4) forced purchase, (5) lack of competition, and (6) distorted profit motives. These factors are discussed below.

In the free market, consumers have the ability to gather all of the information they need to make informed choices. This is not the case in health care. It is difficult to obtain and understand all of the relevant information. In many cases, data simply do not exist.

Third-party payers remove the issue of cost for users (patients) and the direct providers of the service (physicians, nurses, hospitals). It is possible for consumers of goods, such as televisions, compact discs, clothing, or services such as lawn and hair care, to shop for what they can afford and for that which meets their wants and needs. When shopping for health care, it is the third-party payer who pays, which decreases the importance of price as a criterion regarding choice. Third-party payers also allow providers, such as physicians and hospitals, to charge what the market will bear. The patient is not the consumer who pays, so there is little incentive on the part of providers and consumers alike to contain costs. And yet, if individuals were left to pay all the costs, only the very rich could afford health care, as is the case in many developing nations. The system would be tattered indeed; modern health care and innovations would not be available and health-care science would falter. Gatekeepers have a profound effect on the efficacy of the free market in health care. When consumers decide to eat in a restaurant, buy a new car, or see a movie, they decide when, where, and how to make the purchase. In regard to health care, it is the physician, nurse, or hospital insurance company who decides.

Very often, the purchase of health care is forced. The woman who has a heart attack, the man who has prostate cancer, the child who breaks a leg cannot plan, delay, or reasonably refuse or postpone the purchase of care. Persons need health care when they are hurt or sick. It is hard and often deadly to put off health care in the face of illness and injury.

The lack of competition in health care further distorts the marketplace. Insurance is most often bought by employers who want to minimize costs, bypassing patient choice. Patients do not know with certainty if they will need health care, when, and what type. When patients are given a wide choice, it is confusing and difficult to make sense of all the options. The plethora of drug prescription plans available to Medicare recipients clearly demonstrates this.

A case in point is the diabetes epidemic. In New York City, diabetes centers that delivered comprehensive care to diabetics had to close because they could not financially keep afloat. Good care means bad business (Urbina, 2006). Care that keeps people well is not affordable; insurance does not adequately reimburse preventive care, such as hypertension, diabetic, and cardiac chronic care. They do reimburse for care that deals with the complications of diabetes (and other chronic illnesses) such as renal dialysis and amputation.

POLICY DEVELOPMENT

The specific steps taken from identification of a policy problem to a functioning program to solve the problem are referred to as the policy process.

Several models have been developed to implement the policy process. These models include Kingdon's policy stream model (1995), Cohen, March, and Olsen's "garbage can" model (1972), and the stage-sequential models of Ripley (1996) and Anderson (1996). Stage-sequential models are systems-based approaches and may be more accessible and useful to the novice. A discussion of the stage-sequential approach to the policy process follows.

A series of stages constitutes stage-sequential models. These stages are analogous to the nursing process (see Table 13-1).

A policy problem is identified and added to the policy agenda. Then the policy is developed, accepted, implemented, and evaluated. As with the nursing process, the policy process is dynamic and cyclical. Both are cyclical in that evaluation often leads back to assessment, and so the process continues. Areas that are not well delineated by the stage-sequential model are (a) who gets what and why, and (b) the effect of stakeholder wants and the implications of their ideas, values, and agendas during policy development. The growing problem of childhood obesity and its solution can be examined from a stage-sequential model. Childhood obesity and its attendant risks are identified and are added to the policy agenda. Assessment revealed that easy access to junk food, high-calorie soft and sports drinks, and poor school cafeteria menu choices are major contributors to obesity. Additionally, lack of knowledge of good healthy food choices and lack of exercise worsen the problem. Policies that change foods available at schools, educate students and families about good nutrition, change gym and sports requirements, and educate regarding exercise are developed and implemented. Outcomes of new policies are evaluated for effectiveness, which brings the process back to assessment.

Aspects of Policy Development

Health-care agencies, organizations, institutions, and associations make private policy. Such policies include directives that govern employment conditions and service guidelines or provisions. For example, there are policies that stipulate licensure, education, and experience requirements for specific nursing positions. Other policies provide guidelines for patient care: the use of side rails and methods for dispensing medications are examples of service provisions.

Local, state, and federal governments make public policy. Included are legislation, regulation, and court rulings that are made at respective levels and jurisdictions. In New York City, for example, a local policy regarding health care is the no-smoking law in public and workplaces. States control licensure for professional practice, and the federal govern-

TABLE 13-1	Comparison of Nursing Process and Policy-Setting Process

	NURSING PROCESS	POLICY-SETTING PROCESS
Assess	Physical, emotional, psychological needs	Situation needs or dissatisfaction; identify context: social, economic, ethical, legal, political stakeholders
Plan	Develop care plan	Identify options, goals, and objectives, a policy rule, policy formulation
Intervention	Link patient to services; implement plan	Implement program, policy
Evaluate	Ensure needs are met	Ensure program efficacy
Reassess	What, if any, changes needed	Should program continue; sections of policy to remain, discard, revise
Plan	Develop care plans, critical pathways	Revise policy as needed
Intervention	Implement changes; advocate	Continue, revise, terminate
Evaluation	Monitor and document progress; include cost-effectiveness, quality	Monitor program; assess outcomes

ment controls Medicare. Private and public policy have a linked relationship because public policy directly affects private policy, and the need for new or changed public policy arises from private institutions. Included in health policy are the private and public policies that control service delivery and reimbursement,

Government also develops and implements policies at the local, state, and federal levels. Health-care organizations must develop and implement internal policies as well. All policies have unanticipated outcomes that have both detrimental and positive effects. Within an organization, positive outcomes of a policy include rules that protect departmental autonomy, provide support when making unpleasant decisions, and help decide between choices when one does not have a clear advantage.

Unanticipated effects of policies are seen when the original purpose is covert, unknown, or forgotten. Organizations sometimes have policies that are blindly followed long after their usefulness has been outgrown. An example is taking temperatures at 5 a.m. even when not warranted by patient condition because it is policy and procedure. Change in circumstances without concomitant change in policy can have detrimental consequences. Detrimental effects also occur when policies are implemented in ways not intended.

Despite the difficulties, risks, and hazards of policy change, change is often necessary. Change is a better alternative than continuing with outdated policies or working without a policy when one is clearly needed. Given the difficulties of change, it is essential to adhere to two rules before implementing the change: (1) test any new policy on a small group or unit; this is similar to conducting a pilot or feasibility study before initiating a research project or study; and (2) identify the purpose of the policy in the procedure or action directive. These steps will identify problems with the new procedure early so that changes may be made and will help with the implementation of the new policy as intended. This information will also be used in measuring the effectiveness of the policy.

All Good Things...

From the beginning, nurses have used power, politics, and policy to further and achieve their goals. It is important for nurses to develop group process, problem-solving, conflict management, crisis intervention, and communication skills to effectively help move toward goals to improve health and health care. These human relation activities are essential to exert such influence to make a positive impact on policy. Collectivity and collegiality help to empower nurse leaders who must position themselves to act to make policy rather than to react to policy proposals of others.

Calls for health-care delivery reform are coming from all segments of society. Big and small businesses want reform because the current system is costly and in many ways ineffective, resulting in reduced competitiveness. The high cost of health care is passed on to the consumer and makes products more expensive. Providers of health care have greatly reduced resources with which to provide care. Fewer resources jeopardize access and quality of care, resulting in less healthy populations, which decreases productivity and increases costs throughout the economy.

Patients, families, and communities are increasingly dissatisfied with the quality and kinds of health care and services available and received. Frustration, fear, and helplessness are growing in the face of a system unresponsive to needs. The health-care system is in dire need of major policy change. Health-care professionals must be proactive and participate in health-care reform.

Nurses can and should be major participants in reform. They know well the problematic areas, the gaps, the weaknesses, the dysfunctionalities, and the strengths of the current system. Nurses have insight and knowledge of what works and what does not in setting standards of care, access to care, and allocation of resources. With adroit use of power and political theory, nurses can participate in shaping health policy to improve efficacy and distribution in an equitable way.

Health-care reform is a major challenge. With increased scope of knowledge and skills, coupled with conscious and conscientious development and use of political action, nurses can participate in and support policy development. Nurses are needed to change and improve health care at the institutional, community, state, and national levels. Nursing provides abundant resources to do so; nurses must develop and use political know-how to influence important needed changes and reforms.

Let's Talk

1. List and describe types of power.

2. List several ways that a staff nurse might achieve power and discuss.

3. List and describe ways to increase expert power.

4. List and discuss the components of a political analysis.

5. What are the steps involved in conflict resolution?

6. Describe coalitions as a skill or tactic for use in the workplace.

7. List and compare the steps in the nursing process with the steps in the policy-setting process.

NCLEX Questions

1. Empowerment is an important concept in nursing. Nurses often talk about empowering patients. Empowerment is also important in leadership as it influences:
   A. Social and political reform
   B. Productivity and effectiveness
   C. Individual attributes
   D. A and B
   E. All of the above

2. Three characteristics of empowered nurses are:
   A. Raised consciousness of social, political, and economic realities
   B. Confidence in self as a change agent
   C. Motivation to develop skills
   D. All of the above
   E. B and C

3. Power can be defined as:
   A. Authority or influence
   B. Ability to cause or maintain the status quo
   C. A negative attribute related to authoritative leadership and hierarchical organization
   D. All of the above
   E. A and B

4. Politics are used in the following arena(s):
   A. Federal and state government
   B. Workplace
   C. Organizations and associations
   D. All of the above
   E. A and C

5. Among decisions that politics influences are:
   A. Allocation of resources such as staffing in hospitals
   B. Vacations
   C. Scope of professional practice
   D. All of the above
   E. None of the above

6. In solving a problem, it is important to:
   A. Identify your position and stick with it
   B. Present your solution as best
   C. Identify flaws in other positions
   D. Seek a compromise
   E. Collaborate

7. When evaluating courses of action, it is important to:
   A. Identify your values and those of stakeholders
   B. Recognize that values are not important
   C. Recognize that values confuse the issue and increase difficulties
   D. Always insist on your values
   E. B and D

8. Policies in the workplace are:
   A. Not needed; no one ever looks at the policy and procedure book
   B. Common sense
   C. Not important to patient care
   D. All of the above
   E. None of the above

9. Policies:
   A. Eliminate disparities in care
   B. Do not need to be reviewed and revised
   C. Are inflexible
   D. All of the above
   E. None of the above

10. All of the following are true about power except:
    A. Used to enable nurses to provide optimal care
    B. Used to influence national health policy
    C. Is increased with an authoritarian approach to leadership
    D. Is not always commensurate with position
    E. Is enhanced with education and continuing education

REFERENCES

Alward, R.R., & Camuñas, C. (1991). *The Nurse's Guide to Marketing*. Albany, NY: Delmar.

American Journal of Nursing (2006). The US health care system in crisis. *American Journal of Nursing, 106*(1), 20.

American Nurses Association. (Nov/Dec. 2005). In brief: New York & safe patient handling. *American Nurse, 37*(6), 4.

Anderson, J.E. (1990). *Public policymaking*. Boston: Houghton-Mifflin.

Annas, G.J. (2005). *American bioethics: Crossing human rights and health law boundaries*. New York: Oxford University Press.

Bach, P.B., et al. (2004). Primary care physicians who treat blacks and whites. *New England Journal of Medicine, 351*, 575–584.

Benner, P. (1984). *From novice to expert: Excellence and power in clinical nursing practice*. Menlo Park, CA.

Berkowitz, B., & Wolff, T. (2000). *The spirit of coalition*. Washington, DC: American Public Health Association.

Bloche, M. (2004). Health care disparities: Science, politics, and race. *New England Journal of Medicine, 350*, 1568–1570.

Camuñas, C. (1994a). Ethical dilemmas of nurse executives Part 1. *Journal of Nursing Administration, 24*(7/8), 45–51.

Camuñas, C. (1994b). Ethical dilemmas of nurse executives Part 2. *Journal of Nursing Administration, 24*(9), 19–23.

Camuñas, C. (1998). Guest Editorial: Managed care, professional integrity, and ethics. *Journal of Nursing Administration, 28*(3), 7–9.

Carroll, T.L., DiVincenti, M., & Show, E.V. (1995). Nurse executive job loss: Trauma or transition. *Nursing Administration Quarterly, 19*(4), 11–17.

Centers for Medicare & Medicaid Services (2003). *National health expenditures and projections, 1990–2013*. Baltimore, MD: Author. Retrieved April 16, 2005, from http://www.cms.hhs.gov/statistics/nhe/projections-2003/tl.asp

Cohen, M.D., March, J.G., & Olsen J.P. (1972). A garbage can model of organizational choice. *Administrative Science Quarterly, 17*, 1–25.

Diers, D., & Molde, S. (1983). Nurses in primary care: The new gatekeepers? *American Journal of Nursing, 83*, 742–745.

Donnelly, G.F. (2006). *A futurescan of nursing: A journey to tomorrow*. Paper presented at the 43rd Annual Isabel Maitland Stewart Conference on Research in Nursing, New York, NY.

Farmer, P. (2005). *Pathologies of power*. Berkeley, CA: University of California Press.

Ferguson, V.D. (1993). Perspectives on power. In Mason, D.J., Talbott, S.W., & Leavitt, J.K. (Eds.). *Policy and politics for nurses: Action and change in the workplace, government, organizations, and community* (2nd ed.). Philadelphia: Lippincott.

Fisher, R., Ury, W., & Patton, B. (1992). *Getting to yes: Negotiating agreement without giving in* (2nd ed.). New York: Penguin.

Flynn, J.P. (Ed.). (1997). *The role of the preceptor: A guide for nurse educators and clinicians*. New York: Springer.

Foley, M. (2001). ANA: Preserving the core while preparing for the future. *American Nurse, 33*(2), 5.

French, J.R.P., & Raven, B. (1959). The basis of social power. In Cartwright, D. (Ed.). *Studies in social power*. Ann Arbor, MI: University of Michigan.

Gill, G. (2005). *Nightingales: The extraordinary upbringing and curious life of Miss Florence Nightingale*. New York: Ballantine Books.

Hersey, P., Blanchard, K., & Natemeyer, W. (1976). Situational leadership: Perception and impact of power. *Group Organizational Studies, 4*, 418–428.

Jha, A.K., et al. (2005). Racial trends in the use of major procedures among the elderly. *New England Journal of Medicine, 353*(7), 683–691.

Joel, L., & Kelly, L. (2002). *The nursing experience: Trends, challenges, and transitions* (4th ed). New York: McGraw-Hill.

Kaiser Commission (2004). *The Kaiser Commission on Medicare and the uninsured*. (Fact sheet #1420-06) Washington, DC: Kaiser Family Foundation. Retrieved April 21, 2005, from http://www.kff.org

Kaiser Family Foundation. (2006). Snapshots: Health care costs. Washington, DC: Author. Retrieved May 10, 2006, from www.kff.org

Kalish, B.J., & Kalish, P.A. (1982). *Politics of nursing*. Philadelphia: Lippincott.

Kingdon, J.W. (1995). *Agendas, alternatives, and public policies*. Boston: Little, Brown.

Kopala, B. (2001). Professional nursing: Issues and ethics. In Chaska, N.L. (Ed.). *The nursing profession: Tomorrow and beyond*. Thousand Oaks, CA: Sage.

Kuokkanen, L., & Katajisto, J. (2003). Promoting or impeding empowerment? Nurses' assessment of their work environment. *Journal of Nursing Administration, 33*(4), 209–215.

Leavitt, P. (2002). Managed care mandated coverage in Maine: A grassroots success story. In Mason, D.J., Leavitt, J.K., & Chaffee, M.W. (Eds.). *Policy & politics in nursing and health care* (4th ed.). St Louis: W.B. Saunders.

Manojlovich, M., & Laschinger, H.K.S. (2002). The relationship of empowerment and selected personality characteristics to nursing job satisfaction. *Journal of Nursing Administration, 32*(11), 586–595.

Marquis, B., & Hurston, C. (1994). *Management decision-making for nurses* (2nd ed). New York: J.B. Lippincott.

May, R. (1972). *Power and innocence*. New York: Dell.

McMurray, R.N. (1973). Power and the ambitious executive. *Harvard Business Review, 52*(6), 69–74.

Reverby, S. (1987a). *Ordered to care: The dilemma of American nursing, 1850–1945*. New York: Cambridge University Press.

Reverby, S. (1987b). A caring dilemma: Womanhood and nursing in perspective. *Nursing Research, 36*(1), 5–11.

Ripley, R.B. (1996). Stages of the policy process. In McCool, D.C. (Ed.). *Public policy theories, models, and concepts: An anthology*. Englewood Cliffs, NJ: Prentice-Hall.

Roe, S. (1995). Managing your work setting: Positive work relationships, conflict management, and negotiations. In Vestal, K.W. (Ed.). *Nursing management: Concepts and issues* (2nd ed.). Philadelphia: Lippincott.

Rogge, M.M. (1987). Nursing and politics: A forgotten legacy. *Nursing Research, 36*(1), 26–30.

Sabiston, J.A., & Laschinger, H.K. (1995). Staff nurse work empowerment and perceived autonomy. Testing Kanter's theory of structural power in organizations. *Journal of Nursing Administration, 25*(9), 42–50.

Shishehbor, M.H., et al. (2006). Association of socioeconomic status with functional capacity, heart rate recovery, and all-cause mortality. *Journal of the American Medical Association, 295,* 784–792.

Smedley, B.D., Stith, A.Y., & Nelson, A.R. (2003). *Unequal treatment: Confronting racial and ethnic disparities in health care.* Washington, DC: National Academies Press.

Steinbrook, R. (2004). Disparities in health care: From politics to policy. *New England Journal of Medicine, 350,* 1486–1488.

Trossman, S. (2006). A state of emergency: Nurses continue to contend with crowded EDs. *American Nurse, 38*(1), 1, 7–8.

Urbina, I. (2006). In the treatment of diabetes, success often does not pay. *The New York Times,* pp. A1, A22–23.

Vance, C., & Olson, R.K. (Eds.). (1998). *The mentor connection.* New York: Springer.

Vestal, K. (1990). Fired! Managing the process. *Journal of Nursing Administration, 20*(6), 14–16.

Vestal, K.W. (1995). Nurse executives: Career derailment, success, and dilemmas. *Nursing Administration Quarterly, 19*(4), 83–88.

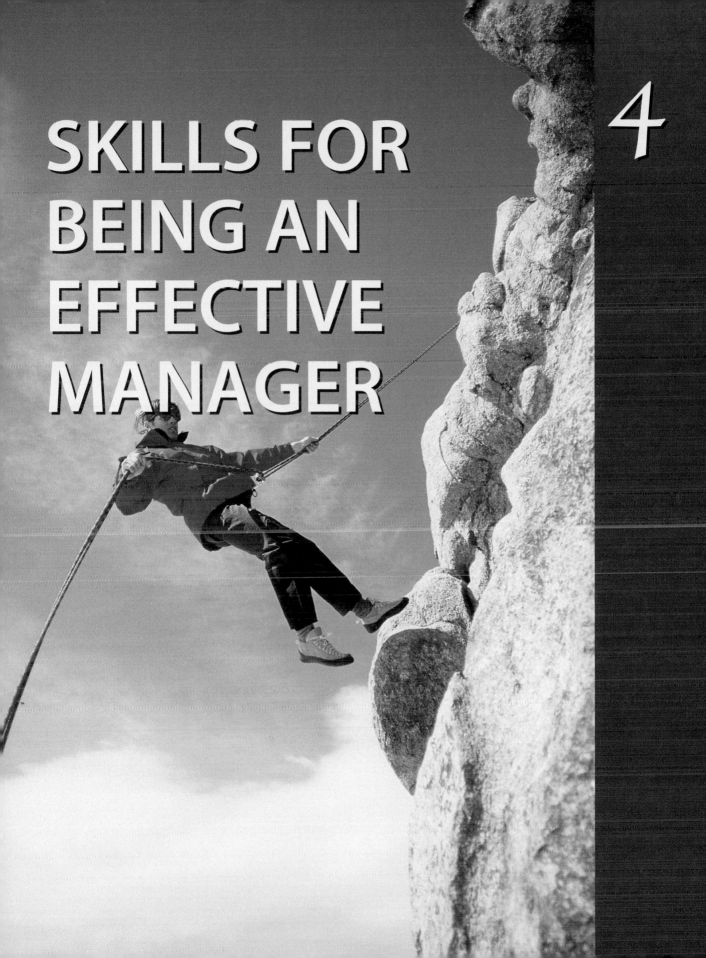

SKILLS FOR BEING AN EFFECTIVE MANAGER

chapter 14

Planning and Marketing for a Healthy Organization

ESPERANZA VILLANUEVA JOYCE, EDD, RN
PATRICIA MARTINEZ, MD

CHAPTER MOTIVATION

"A man who does not think and plan long ahead will find trouble right at his door."

Confucius

CHAPTER MOTIVES

- Define planning, project planning, operational planning, and strategic planning.
- Describe the elements of the strategic planning process.
- Recognize your organization's mission statement.
- Identify your unit's/organization's strengths and weaknesses.
- Discuss the differences between threats and opportunities.
- Discuss the relationship between goals and objectives.
- Identify effective approaches in writing objectives.
- Define marketing within the health-care setting.
- Identify the components of marketing.
- Identify specific marketing principles that transfer to the health-care environment.

The environmental challenges of providing health care in the 21st century require more sophisticated problem-solving solutions. With shrinking fiscal resources and increasing demands in the work place, it is imperative that planning become a major element in any manager's job description. It is easy to lose sight of the big picture when we are so busy focusing on the small one. In our daily nursing routines, we sometimes fail to understand overriding nursing administration goals and objectives. We become so consumed with our shift's activities that we cannot see beyond them. As a result, we are not always prepared to deal with situations that arise, and we fail to anticipate situations that may have benefited from advance thought and planning.

Nurses are familiar with the process of planning. Planning is an integral step in the nursing process. We understand that without planning, our patients would not fare well. We plan for patient care on a short-term basis, and we anticipate needs on a long-term basis.

Planning differs with the job. A nurse at a unit level may be concerned with daily operations so the period for planning may be a few days, a week, or a month. Middle managers generally plan for 1 to 3 years, whereas top executives plan for 3 to 7 years. Middle managers, because they are involved at the unit level, plan for unit activities such as length of hospital stay, seasonal changes, staff assignments, and so on. On the other hand, top executives plan for activities that involve the entire hospital (both physical and fiscal) operations, that involve larger sums of money, and that require longer time to complete. At the unit level, a 1-day retreat devoted to planning may be sufficient. In larger organizations, it may take weeks to accomplish all of the planning in various departments. This chapter discusses various types of planning in an organization. It explores elements of the strategic planning process and defines the components of marketing.

Types of Planning

There are various types of planning such as:

- Business planning, to plan a business organization, plan to test a product, plan a budget

- Program planning, which involves a major internal or external function such as planning for the hospital's 25th anniversary
- Career planning, which involves educational milestones for individuals or groups
- Performance planning, which involves development, implementation, and evaluation of job descriptions
- Disaster planning, which involves guidelines, protocols
- This chapter covers project planning, operational planning, and strategic planning.

PROJECT PLANNING

Project planning entails planning for a project. Project planning involves a one-time effort, for example, to gather a team of nurses to conduct a community fundraising event. Most unit managers will involve their staff in project planning. This type of planning requires that one:

- Identify the problem that the project will ultimately address.
- Name the project. Selecting a name for the project is important. For example, if your department wants to recruit foreign nurses, you may want to name it the Foreign Nurse Exchange Project. Choose a name that will help members quickly identify your project. Once a project has been created, the name cannot be changed.
- Determine the project goals. Setting goals and measurable objectives will guide you through the completion of the project. For example, if a goal is to decrease the vacancy rate of nursing staff, your objective may read: within 6 months, staff will increase by 15%.
- Specify tasks for each member. Determine the size of the project team, and then distribute the necessary tasks. For example, if you plan to recruit foreign nurses, you may want to designate a person to review the literature to specify which countries export the largest number of nurses. Another project member may meet with the marketing department to start an advertising campaign.
- Identify resources needed. It is essential to list the resources needed, such as travel monies if the project manager is involved in interview-

ing staff nurses in another country or release time for all team members to be able to plan and monitor the project.

- Indicate timelines for completion. To keep all members aware of the progress of the project, it is advantageous to display a chart or timeline that provides the status of each activity and its completion.
- Implement the project. Once you have gathered all the data and know which group of nurses to target, your team will determine by whom and where the project will be implemented.
- Evaluate the project. It is important to assess the progress of the project so that evaluation becomes a natural step in the process. Evaluation of the project should always go back to the objectives. Were the objectives accomplished? For example, if you were successful with your recruitment, at the end of the 6-month period, your evaluation should read: 35 (15%) nurses from the Philippines were recruited.

One of the most common problems surrounding plans for projects is the potential for procrastination. Some individuals tend to leave an assignment for the last minute. Thus, it is extremely important to identify a leader when planning a project. The responsibilities of the project leader include clarifying the purpose of the project to all project members, identifying the roles and responsibilities of each of the members, and keeping members on track. The project leader needs to facilitate and help the project members overcome barriers to the project's success. The leader is responsible for providing necessary financial and human resources to accomplish the project. The leader should recognize members for a job well done.

OPERATIONAL PLANNING

An operational plan is a detailed work plan for a coming year. It is the blueprint by which the objectives of a unit, for example, are put into measurable actions. It also describes the short-term (a fiscal year) organizational objectives (Table 14-1). Operational planning involves the day-to-day execution of objectives that assist in accomplishing the organization's mission. This plan is used to identify the responsibilities and resources needed to accomplish the department/unit priorities in the current fiscal year. Operational planning focuses on sustaining the course of action and ensuring the employees' ability to perform the designated tasks. Middle managers generally get involved in operational planning. Managers examine measures that can reduce the obstacles employees may encounter; this type of planning should not be considered a rigid process. The manager must ensure that all aspects of the operational plan are implemented; the strategies to accomplish the plan may need to change over time. Like project planning or strategic planning (discussed below), operational planning addresses questions such as:

TABLE 14-1	Operational Plan in a Medical-Surgical Unit		

Mission: To provide high-quality care to patients
Vision: To become the leader in health care in the Southwest.

GOAL	OBJECTIVES	STRATEGIES	OUTCOMES
Improve patient satisfaction on 3 West.	Within 6 weeks, 85% of patients will report satisfaction with care provided.	Orient patients on admission to the unit. Inform patients of the unit's policies and procedures. Answer patients' call light within 2 minutes.	87% of patients in the unit reported satisfaction with care provided.
Improve unit staff's cross training.	Within 4 months, 50% of staff members will cross train to at least one other unit.	Provide a minimum of 30 clock hours of training in mental health, obstetrics, and pediatrics. After training is completed, rotate two staff to identified unit for 2 weeks.	62% of staff cross trained to one unit.

TABLE 14-2	**Gantt Chart**								
WEEK									
1	2	3	4	5	6	7	8	9	10
Recruit staff Market center	Hire staff	Assess staff's strengths	Train staff Order furniture and equipment	Train staff	Install furniture and equipment	Install information system	Prepare patient medical records	Hold open house	Admit patients

- Where is the unit/organization now? (assessment of the environment)
- Where do we want to be? (goals and objectives)
- How do we get there? (strategies)
- How do we measure progress? (outcomes)

To answer such questions, the middle manager must gather data (such as budget, patient, and quality improvement data) from both previous and current fiscal years. The operational plan must link goals and objectives to the organization's strategic plan and link the strategies to the performance indicators or outcomes.

Managers must ensure that employees at the unit/department level are involved in the operational plan. This means that all employees determine together what objectives need to be accomplished in that particular unit and understand the strategies that need to be implemented in order to meet the unit's goals. A variety of tools, such as flowcharts, diagrams, and matrices, can assist managers as they create detailed operational plans. These tools use arrows, lines, boxes, circles, and other symbols to communicate processes. Some of the common tools that managers use to create operational plans include the Gantt chart (Finkler & Kovner, 2000), critical path method (Baker 2006), and program evaluation and review technique (McGuffin,1999), which is a variation of the critical path method.

Gantt Chart

The Gantt chart is useful for planning and scheduling projects. It allows the manager to assess how long a project should take, determine the resources needed, and lay out the order in which tasks need to be carried out. Gantt charts help the manager monitor the project's progress and stay on track. Gantt charts help the manager plan out the tasks

that need to be completed by scheduling times that the tasks will be carried out and allocating resources. When establishing a surgical center, for example, the manager's ideal plan may include the timeframe in Table 14-2.

The chart is also useful when working with multiple projects. See Table 14-3. An advantage of the chart is the ability to review projects that are progressing in a timely fashion.

Critical Path Method

The critical path method (CPM) is another tool that helps managers prepare a schedule and plan resources. During the management of a project, the CPM allows a manager to monitor achievement of project goals and take remedial action if the project is not going well. The CPM consists of diagrams that depict the activities and the time line required (Fig. 14-1).

The diagram shows the start event (step 1) and the completion of the task of recruiting staff and

TABLE 14-3	**Gantt Control Chart**							
Cumulative weeks	1	2	3	4	5	6	7	8
Project 1 orientation SNII	X				X			
Project 2 orientation SNII		X				X		
Project 3 SWOT seminars	X		X		X		X	
Project 4 establish surgical center								X

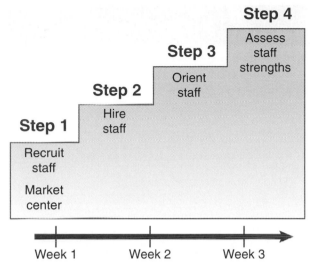

Step 4
Assess staff strengths

Step 3
Orient staff

Step 2
Hire staff

Step 1
Recruit staff

Market center

Week 1   Week 2   Week 3

FIGURE 14-1 Critical path method.

marketing the center (step 2). This activity should take 1 week. One activity cannot start until another is completed. Assessing the staff strengths (step 4) cannot be done until completion of step 2 (hiring staff) and step 3 (orientation). In the event that the task is completed in less time, such as hiring staff, the time of completion can be adjusted in the diagram. If you are not graphically oriented, this diagram can be difficult to draw without using commercial software.

Program Evaluation and Review Technique

The program evaluation and review technique (PERT) calculates a realistic timeframe by using the shortest possible time each activity will take, the most likely length of time, and the longest time it might take. Managers can input these figures into PERT to calculate the time to use for each project stage. The formula follows:

$$\frac{\text{Shortest time} + 4 \times \text{likely time} + \text{longest time}}{6}$$

Example:

$$\frac{6 \text{ weeks} + 4 \times 12 \text{ weeks} + 24 \text{ weeks}}{6} = 24 \text{ weeks}$$

Using the formula helps to bias time estimates away from the unrealistically short time scales often assumed. Using a realistic timeframe is helpful when developing the strategic plan for your unit or department.

STRATEGIC PLANNING

Strategic planning is a systematic process that emphasizes assessment of the environment (economic, political, social, and technological) both internally and externally. It focuses on performance improvement and utilizes strategies to accomplish the organization's desired outcomes. Business organizations embraced the idea of strategic planning in the 1950s. And in the last 20 years, even institutions of higher education have attempted to implement strategic planning out of a need to respond to challenges with finances, student attrition, and educational demands.

Strategic planning is a management tool that helps organizations set long-term goals. It assures that the individuals working for the organization work together to accomplish set goals and objectives. Executives in the organization are generally responsible for initiating the strategic planning process. The current trend in business is to plan for 2 to 3 years. Because of employee mobility and the changing economy, industry usually is not able to plan for more than 3 years. Strategic plans in certain organizations may be drafted for 10 or more years.

The strategic plan, just like the project or operational plan, should be simple and easily understood by the participants. The way a strategic plan is developed depends on the nature of the organization's leadership, culture of the organization, complexity of the organization's environment, size, and the expertise of the planners. Strategic planning models can be issue-based, goal-based, and scenario-based.

Issue-based strategic planning utilizes a very focused approach as is used in manufacturing businesses (Hiam, 1990) to improve productivity over a specified period. Scenario-based strategic planning is used frequently in human resources or marketing operations (Hiam, 1990) to improve decision making and sales forecasting. The goal-based model is the most widely used in organizations. Its key elements include: the organization's assessment of the environment, mission statement, vision, development of goals and objectives, strategies to accomplish the goals and objectives, and outcomes (Table 14-4).

Unlike project planning or operational planning, strategic planning requires a multidisciplinary approach. Every single department or unit in an organization must be involved in the plan to ensure that staff members comply with goals and objectives and that strategies are implemented. Managers may initiate the strategic planning process by communicating the initiative in their monthly meetings. They may invite an expert to provide a seminar to inform all the employees about the process. Once the employees are oriented to the strategic plan, they volunteer to work with specific sections. Without this involvement, employees may not buy into the organization's goals and objectives and may hinder the plan's success.

One benefit of strategic planning is that it helps managers make current decisions in light of future consequences. For example, if your unit plans for expansion from 16 to 32 beds within 6 months, you need to start planning for staffing now. Planning helps managers develop a comprehensive basis for decision making and exercise maximum direction in organizational control. In addition, strategic planning assists managers to:

- Resolve organizational problems goals; they are shared with the entire organization

TABLE 14-4	Strategic Planning Process

External assessment
      Opportunities and threats
Internal assessment
      Strengths and weaknesses
Mission
Vision
Goals
Strategic
      Organization
Operational
      Department
      Unit
Objectives
Strategies
Implementation
Outcomes
Evaluation

- Improve performance strategies; they are accepted by all staff
- Build teamwork expertise; staff must work together to identify goals and objectives and determine strategies.

Strategic Planning Process

Strategic planning is a step-by-step process that delineates ongoing group activity. Table 14-4 demonstrates the steps of the process.

ASSESSMENT OF THE ENVIRONMENT

The first step of any planning process is assessing the environment. At any level, the assessment conducted is both external and internal (Table 14-5). At the unit level, an environmental assessment includes assessment of employees, for example. The manager needs to examine how the staff is likely to feel and react to the contents of the project, operational, or strategic plan. Even at an organizational level, a nursing executive needs to know the staff in the departments he/she oversees. Because staff plays a crucial role in strategic planning, some key questions that a manager should ask before any type of planning occurs include:

- Who are the best, most interested staff members in your unit/department?
- What is the emotional or financial interest they have invested in the organization?
- What motivates them?
- Are there staff members who are not ambitious, who do minimal work?
- What do staff members think about administration?
- Who are the informal leaders who influence the unit/department?
- How can everyone be engaged in the planning process?

Once they have answered these questions, managers need to inform all staff members about the necessity of planning, answer the "what's in it for me" questions, and guide the staff toward the realization of the plan. Managers must talk to staff directly if they perceive a lack of interest or a lack of understanding of the process. Most people are willing to share their views, and asking their opinions will make them feel like they are contributing to the organization's plans.

When creating a project or operational plan, it is important to assess the department's/unit's immediate physical environment as well. When developing a staffing plan at the unit level, for example, you must determine future patient census on the unit based on past data. When does the patient census peak? When does it drop? In which months of the year does a particular disease become prevalent? What kind of financial resources will be required? Based on these data, you can make projections and continue in the planning process

When preparing a strategic plan, the assessment becomes a bit more expansive. The manager must assess the internal and external environment of the organization thoroughly.

The external assessment should include the competition for services in the community. For example, determine which hospitals are around the area and what kind of specialized care they offer and compare it with yours. Take a look at the markets, and identify your customers. Health-care trends also influence planning. If the elderly population in your community indicates an upward trend, your organization may choose to accommodate the elder's needs by planning a skill care unit or expanding the cardiac care unit.

In order to assess the internal environment, strategic planners must identify a variety of systems within the organization. Important to assess are patient care standards, not only to comply with accrediting organizations but also to improve the care offered. Other assessments include financial resources, information systems, research capabilities, staff development, and educational systems. In any health-care organization, nursing is the largest human resource group. Thus, it is imperative that this segment of employees be taken into consideration as the organization conducts strategic planning. The quantity and quality of staff development and educational systems need to be assessed, especially when considering expansion of services.

Environmental Assessment Techniques

One technique used to assess the environment is the PEST, which stands for political, educational, social, and technology factors that affect an environment. In the political realm, managers analyze factors such as legislative activities, antitrust regulations, and environmental protection laws that may affect the organization. In the economic environment, analysis includes trends, events, and economic indicators specific to the marketplace in

TABLE 14-5	Environmental Assessment	
ASSESSMENT OF EXTERNAL ENVIRONMENT	**ASSESSMENT OF INTERNAL ENVIRONMENT**
Competition	Patient care
Markets	Financial resources
Health-care trends	Human resources
Economic factors	Information systems
PEST: Political, Educational, Social, Technology factors	Research capabilities
	Staff development
	Educational systems

which the organization operates. The PEST also assesses areas and services of potential growth and monitors trends in industry, global economy, interest rates, and energy availability. In the societal environment, it analyzes population growth, age distribution, regional changes, health status of the population (death rates, communicable diseases, Medicare/Medicaid resources), and safety issues. In the technological environment, it helps managers focus on what the organization has or lacks in terms of current technology as well as on what is available.

The SWOT technique is another tool to help managers conduct a thorough environmental assessment. The acronym stands for the strengths, weaknesses, opportunities, and threats in an organization. SWOT requires analysis of multiple factors related to the health-care industry: human resources, the physical facility, the population, and the economic stability of the organization, for example. Table 14-6 presents a brief example of a SWOT analysis.

The risk analysis, another environmental assessment technique, helps the manager spot project risks, weaknesses in the organization, and external risks. For example, suppose an organization discovers that a group of physicians plans to build a neurology center and recruit nursing staff from your

units. This has the potential for affecting not only the finances of the hospital but also the patient care offered. Conducting a risk analysis helps the manager to make additional plans to neutralize some risks.

MISSION AND VISION STATEMENTS

Mission statements identify why the organization exists (see Chapter 4). They encapsulate the overriding purpose of the organization. Vision statements identify the future of the organization. They provide the ultimate level the organization aims for. Mission and vision statements can be one sentence, a number of phrases, or multiple sentences. When creating a mission statement, it is imperative that all individuals in the organization understand the purpose of the content. For example, the mission statement at a hospital in Ashland, Kentucky, reads: "To Care. To Serve. To Heal." These phrases summarize why the hospital exists. Such statements are generally simple so that employees can identify with and remember them. A children's hospital's mission statement in Virginia reads: "To provide the highest level and quality of pediatric care available in our community." This statement is concise and easy to interpret. St. George's Hospital Medical School University of London has a mission statement that reads: "To promote by excellence in teaching, clinical practice, and research the prevention and understanding of disease." This statement lets you know that this is a teaching hospital with a medical school where research is a priority. The vision statement accompanies the mission statement but is more future-oriented. It states where the organization is going, the ultimate position that the organization plans to achieve: "To achieve a local, regional and national reputation as leader in health care." This could be a vision statement of an organization that has been operating only at the local level. A hospital could have a vision statement that reads: "To provide world-class care in our communities." This is a very clear, self-explanatory statement.

GOAL SETTING

Goals, in general, are global statements that help an individual or an organization plan for the future in a constructive way. Goals should delineate clearly

TABLE 14-6	SWOT Technique

STRENGTHS	WEAKNESSES
10-year- old facility	Nursing staff turnover at 36%
Experienced senior staff	Lack of staff development
Strong information system	High nurse/patient ratio
Quality of clinical resources	

OPPORTUNITIES	THREATS
Increase in the aging population	Construction of three specialty hospitals
Partnerships with diverse groups	Urban population declining
Develop mentor programs	High unemployment rate
Develop student preceptorship programs	Salary competition between hospitals

the desired end product. Goals may be short-term, to be accomplished within a week, a month, or a year. Or they may be long-term, indicating what the organization aspires to become 5 to 10 years from now. For planning purposes in organizations, goals are written for the operational plan and the strategic plan.

Operational goals at the unit or department level are statements that indicate future directions. Goals are more specific statements of the organization's vision, enumerating the accomplishments to be achieved if the vision is to become real. Strategic plan goals are institutional goals often written by executives or upper-level administration members who oversee the organization's activities and are able to conduct environmental assessments. A current trend encourages all individuals in the organization to participate in the goal-setting process, but involvement depends on the size of the organization. For large companies, involving all employees may be next to impossible. Operational plan goals are congruent with strategic plan goals (Table 14-7).

OBJECTIVES

Objectives are descriptions of performances or activities. They are statements that make goals more specific and measurable and give managers the ability to evaluate goal achievement. For this reason, over the last two decades organizations have included objectives in their operational and strate-

TABLE 14-8	Objectives	
OBJECTIVES	**STRATEGIES**
By 2007, provide well-qualified College of Medicine faculty in all departments.	Recruit board-certified physicians. **a.** Partner with university to offer curriculum on site.
By 2009, all nursing staff at the Medical Center will be pursuing or have a baccalaureate degree.	**b.** Negotiate tuition reimbursement.

gic plans. When incorporating objectives into plans, keep asking yourself, "Are you sure we can do this?" Objectives are the specific, measurable results produced while implementing strategies (Table 14-8).

As you work with objectives, state them separately, and show related information that is linked to strategies. This means that if you listed a number 1 under objectives, make sure you have a number 1 in the strategies. Objectives are written in a logical sequence, preferably in numeric order. For example, all objectives related to human resources (individuals), staff development, or clinical practice should be grouped under those sections. Be sure that the period for the objective is clear and realistic. The time line ensures achievement of the outcome by the target date. If there is no time line stated in an objective, that objective is assumed to be bound by the fiscal year covered by the plan.

STRATEGIES

Strategies are a series of actions or behaviors that assist planners in achieving the objectives. Strategies link to a particular objective and intended outcomes. Well-planned strategies provide specific directions to achieve objectives (see Table 14-8; 14-9). Strategies are not static. They can change and be modified during the implementation of the plan. Strategies may be clustered under a common objective. For example, if the Human Resources department has an objective to increase the diversity of the staff, the strategy may be to (a) travel to the South to recruit minority physicians, and (b) advertise nursing positions in minority nursing journals. Strate-

TABLE 14-7	Strategic and Operational Goals	
STRATEGIC GOALS	**OPERATIONAL GOALS MEDICINE UNIT**
1. Optimize the resources of the medical center.	**a.** Increase nursing visibility within the medical center and the community.
2. Emphasize clinical excellence.	**b.** Assure cost containment at the unit level. Evaluate the performance of all employees in a manner that produces growth in the employee and upgrades service standards.

TABLE 14-9	Outcomes	

DEPARTMENT GOAL: OPTIMIZE TECHNOLOGY RESOURCES

OBJECTIVE	STRATEGY	OUTCOME
1. Within 2 years, provide state-of-the-art computer enhancement in the department	1 a. Solicit input from vendors. b. Assess staff's knowledge of computers. c. Purchase wireless computers.	1 a. Within 6 months, at least six vendors will visit the hospital and demonstrate their products. b. Within a year, at least 50% of the staff will receive computer training. c. Purchase seven computers by the end of the fiscal year
2. Nursing staff vacancy rate will decrease below the national standard of 12%.	2 a. Plan recruitment and retention activities. b. Address workplace issues such as mandatory overtime, staffing, and quality care. c. Address compensation and benefit packages.	2 a. Within 6 months, recruitment activities will be conducted in 19 adjacent counties. b. Within a year, RN staff:patient ratio will be 1:6. c. Annual RN salary will increase to $52,000.

gies must be resource driven and sequential. Being resource driven means that the constraints of people, equipment, operating systems, money, and other resources are considered when developing a strategy. Strategies must be designed after the desired outcomes are written. Managers must assess whether the strategies produced the desired outcomes.

IMPLEMENTATION

In the implementation phase of the strategic plan, all the strategies planned are carried out. The success in the implementation of the strategies depends on the involvement of managers who must monitor all the activities to ensure accomplishment of the objectives.

OUTCOMES

Outcomes are the results that you plan to accomplish. Outcomes must be realistic and achievable. If the vision is an expansive one, such as "to offer the best service in the world," managers need to determine how to write goals and objectives to assure outcomes are achieved. Otherwise, outcomes may fall short of expectations. Outcomes are indicators against which you measure the success in meeting your objectives (see Table 14-9). Outcomes reflect

the effectiveness in meeting the expectations of the planners. It is important to select benchmarks, measures that compare the organization with others. For example, if your objective reads that the nursing turnover rate in your facility will decrease below the national standard, then your outcome would be measured by comparing your rate with the national average as a benchmark.

EVALUATION

The evaluation determines the organization's progress toward attaining the identified outcomes. How did the organization respond to the implementation of the plan? How was productivity achieved? To what level? Was the budget sufficient? The evaluation compares outcomes or results with objectives.

Dashboards and scorecards (Table 14-10) are tools that help organizations to achieve strategic outcomes. These software application tools have been used extensively in the last few years because of their ability to amass large volumes of information, making it easy to monitor trends and to respond to time-sensitive events. Dashboards and scorecards can promote performance visibility and effectiveness.

The purpose of the dashboards is to foster better communication between managers and staff. The

Table 14-10	Dashboards and Scorecards	
CHARACTERISTIC	DASHBOARD	SCORECARD
Purpose	Measures individual or group performance	Charts the progress of a planned strategy or objective
Users	Supervisors	Executive leadership, middle managers, staff
Data	Specific events	Summarizes the progress or the accomplishment of goals
Display	Graphs, data	Graphs, tables

dashboard enables the user to communicate via threaded discussions, and employees can monitor metrics that are relevant to their roles. Supervisors generally used scoreboards to measure individual or group performances. These performances measure productivity related to specific events. The dashboard evaluates performance against metrics (measurements) using predefined goals. For example, in a hospital setting, a supervisor will use the dashboard to determine patient care hours during the months of December through February, when most cardiac patients increase the census on a medical floor. These dashboards will give the nursing staff an idea of how the unit should be staffed to maintain quality of care.

Scorecards are used by executives and middle managers to monitor the progress of planned goals and objectives. The executive or the manager presents summaries monthly or quarterly of unit goals accomplished. The length of stay, for example, can be measured by using the scorecards. If a unit's goal is to keep inpatients diagnosed with cellulitis for only 2 days, the manager can compare the current length of stay with that of the previous month or quarter. In addition, the scorecards can be used to compare the unit's data with national benchmarks. Other benefits of the scorecards include increase in employee participation, elimination of initiatives that do not contribute to the unit or the organization's goals, and development of consistent key performance indicators.

Marketing

A marketing plan is important for an organization to succeed. It should form part of the overall strategic plan because marketing can make a large contribution to the profitability and success of an organization. Whereas strategic planning is an overall organizational plan, marketing can be organizational or departmental. It is the process of exchanging resources for goods and services to meet the needs and wants of the individual as well as of society. In this sense, marketing fits in with the strategic plan because an organization such as a hospital has to be able to function by meeting the needs of individuals. At a departmental level, marketing is a tool used to advertise services or to recruit staff.

The health-care industry embraced marketing concepts in the 1970s. Marketing concepts are methods that create awareness about a particular organization. Their purpose is to attract customers, to sell their products, or to offer services. These methods include public relations, such as news releases, feature stories, press conferences, or open houses; advertising and mass media, such as newspapers, magazines, and journals; broadcasting, such as radio and television; or electronic, like banners, links, and directories.

In a hospital setting, marketing means that the hospital must produce services that the consumer needs. To this end, many hospitals maintain a marketing department. The marketing manager must understand financial analysis because it is important to know the financial impact of proposed marketing strategies. In addition, the marketing manager must possess skill in market research, product development and management, pricing, negotiating, communicating, salesmanship, and recognizing new opportunities.

The basic components of a formal marketing plan include a situational analysis, goals and objectives, marketing strategies, and evaluation.

MARKETING'S SITUATIONAL ANALYSIS

The SWOT analysis (see Table 14-6) is a very simple but effective means of carrying out an analysis of the hospital or a product for marketing purposes. Very specific questions that managers need to answer include:

hot topic:
Marketing Your Hospital

The Magnet Hospital Recognition Program is a prestigious honor, that recognizes hospitals that are successful in recruiting and retaining nurses. The award is the highest level of recognition awarded by the American Nurses Credentialing Center (ANCC). Hospitals that achieve magnet status have a working environment that supports nursing excellence. This award can be used as an effective marketing tool by hospitals. Hospitals that have received this honor display the ANCC logo on their Web sites as well as in the hospital units. This advertisement attracts nurses who are looking for environments that provide independence, respect, and satisfaction in delivering patient care. It also attracts physicians and other health-care workers because of the team approaches that magnet hospitals expect. From a patient's perspective, going to a magnet hospital eases anxiety about the care provided. Research has verified that hospitals that are magnets have higher patient satisfaction, lower rates of infection, fewer complications, and improved morbidity and mortality rates. In addition, this status can also be used as a marketing tool by hospitals when applying for funding, because ANCC certifications are highly regarded across the nation by federal, state, and local agencies.

- Who are the hospital's main competitors?
- How do they position themselves?
- What is their pricing structure?
- What are the standard terms of business for the health-care industry?
- How does the hospital compare with its competitors?

The strengths of the hospital should be communicated in marketing promotional materials and all advertising. The weaknesses that managers may discover need to be corrected.

Hospitals operate in dynamic environments. External influences (opportunities and threats) over which managers have little or no control can make or break the hospital. Marketing managers must identify opportunities in order to exploit them and anticipate threats in order to plan to handle them. Some examples of opportunities or threats include:

- Economic: unemployment rates, poverty, price rise of equipment
- Patients: know the current patient base: age, gender, income, ethnic background, neighborhood, increase in the chronic nature of diseases, preventive care patterns or habits
- Politics: changes in the legislature, decrease in funding for Medicare/Medicaid
- Technology: rapidly changing technology that is costly; know how it affects your services; know when it will become obsolete; know if the hospital is equipped to adapt quickly to changes
- Competitors: establishment of new hospitals or specialty centers, know exactly which services they offer, number of beds, number of employees, know their location and the potential population from which they will draw

The challenge of the marketing plan is to monitor the external environment continuously to anticipate threats and opportunities and set interventions in place that will protect the hospital from the worst and enable the organization to profit from the best.

MARKETING GOALS AND OBJECTIVES

Major overall goals of health-care marketing include: (1) maximizing the marketplace's consumption of an organization's products; (2) maximizing consumer satisfaction; and (3) contributing to the quality of life. Thus, marketing plays an important role in the entire health-care industry. Hospitals offer a myriad of services in order to satisfy patients' needs and increase their quality of life. An example of a hospital marketing goal could be to enhance its cardiovascular program. A marketing objective could be: "within a year, increase by 20% the number of open heart surgeries."

Nursing departments can assist the organization to accomplish marketing goals. Increasing the awareness of patients for the services that the units provide (Table 14-11), tracking costs at the unit level, and assuring that length of stay is congruent with diagnosis are examples of important nursing activities that will affect patient outcomes. Providing nursing care with respect, courtesy, and safety will improve customer satisfaction. Increasing the

TABLE 14-11	Unit-Specific Goals and Objectives

| Goal: Increase patient awareness of department services. | Objectives: 1. Within 8 weeks, develop and print brochure. 2. Provide brochure to patients on admission. 3. Explain to patients which services are offered within the department and the hospital. |

educational level of the nursing staff will directly and indirectly affect patient quality of life as well.

MARKETING STRATEGIES

Marketing strategies are actions intended to accomplish the marketing plan objectives. Marketing has been identified mostly with promotions and advertisement. But according to Philip Kotler (2002), one winning marketing strategy is to "define the target market." In hospitals, the target market is patients. At the department level or in a specialty hospital or community-based program, the market may be more specific, such as adolescents with eating disorders, people with heart problems, and children. A hospital should strive to offer quality and unique services to patients if the goal is to remain ahead of the competition. In order to remain viable, an organization must remain knowledgeable of the changes in the population. For example, if the elderly become the majority of the population, the organization must develop services to target that population.

Marketing strategies that a hospital can employ to remain visible and competitive include:

- The design of a Web page that expresses the hospital's mission, vision, services, and other attributes. The Web page should be attractive and easily accessible, with links to questions and answers related to hospital services or with links to common disease information.
- Offering free, on-site, classes for various age groups. Through this effort, more potential customers will be attracted.

- Conducting other activities in the community at large to publicize the hospital, including health fairs, fundraising events, speaker's bureaus, and recruitment activities.
- Promoting hospital services is another marketing strategy. Promotional methods include newspaper articles, public service announcements, printed materials, newsletters, billboards, paid advertisement, and introductory offers of special services, such as massage therapy in conjunction with physical therapy, and free demonstrations, consultations, and seminars.

MARKETING EVALUATION

The nurse manager communicates with the marketing manager to receive periodic feedback evaluation throughout the planning and implementation period. As with other plans, evaluation includes a comparison of objectives with outcomes to assess success. In marketing evaluation, actual figures are compared with the figures determined in the environmental assessment to highlight any significant changes, trends, or results. The nurse manager notes the trends and communicates these to staff to incorporate in future plans.

Marketing Plan Sample

Marketing Plan Regional Medical System Surgical Center

Market Summary: Include information about potential patients

Population characteristics (age, ethnicity, sex, income, education)

Market needs: Accessibility, services, competitive prices for procedures

Market trends: Patient census, need for services

Market growth: Determine factors such as various seasonal services

SWOT Analysis:

Competition: Describe who your competitors are, especially during seasonal variations; which organizations offer what services and their capacity to decrease the numbers of patients that your organization can attract.

(Continued on following page)

Marketing Plan Sample *(continued)*

Services: Describe the services provided and the environment in which the services are delivered.

Marketing: Determine your advertisement needs and the venues to advertise, such as the Web, radio, billboards, television. Describe the Center's relationship to the regional medical system.

Mission: The Center's mission must align with the regional medical system's mission.

Marketing objectives: Need to be specific and outcome-oriented.

Financial objectives: Need to be specific to the Center.

Budget: Determine your potential expenses and revenues.

Controls: Monitor monthly expenses.

All Good Things...

In this chapter we addressed the importance of planning at any level in an organization. Planning is a systematic process in which all employees must be involved to be able to accomplish the mission and the vision of the organization. Identification of strengths, weaknesses, threats, and opportunities will help employees understand the organization and help them to establish realistic goals and objectives. A variety of tools for planning and scheduling projects are available for managers to use in developing and implementing their operational or strategic plans. In addition, knowledge of marketing concepts will prove essential for managers who wish to capture a share of the target population and stay ahead of their competitors in the demand for health-care services.

Let's Talk

1. *Think about the marketing methods that your employer uses. Have you seen a billboard on your way to work? What kind of ad does it use in the phone directory? How do you greet patients when they are admitted to your unit? What do you provide for the patients?*

2. *When was the last time that your organization reviewed the strategic plan? Does it have a strategic plan? How are you involved in the planning?*

3. *Identify some issues that you have questioned in your workplace. What type of planning can resolve your issues?*

NCLEX Questions

1. One of the most critical criteria in the establishment of a hospital's strategic plan should be:
   A. Based on the nature and number of employees
   B. The involvement of every department or unit
   C. The involvement of executives only
   D. Based on the number of patients per department

2. A major challenge of strategic planning is to:
   A. Assure commitment from top administrators
   B. Delegate tasks to staff
   C. Monitor all meetings and write reports
   D. Involve all physicians

3. The most common strategic plan model employed by hospitals is:
   A. Issue-based
   B. Goal-based
   C. Scenario-based
   D. Conflict-based

4. Marcus and his staff have been asked to participate in the plan to merge two outpatient units and determine which services should be offered. The priority task in this planning process is:
   A. Evaluation
   B. Implementation
   C. Assessment
   D. Categorizing services

5. Which of the following is an accurate statement of an objective used in planning?
   A. The hospital will achieve magnet status
   B. Within 7 years all the staff in Unit D will be baccalaureate-prepared
   C. Most of the physicians will attend the planning meetings
   D. Salaries for nursing staff will increase tremendously

6. Hospital B has reduced the patient's stay in the emergency department from 5 hours to 3.5 hours. Hospital A states in the strategic plan that an outcome in the emergency department will be patient stay of 3.0 hours. How is hospital A using hospital B's outcomes?
   A. To benchmark
   B. To collaborate
   C. To differ
   D. To antagonize

7. The Gantt chart, the performance evaluation and review technique, and the critical path method are used most commonly in:
   A. Strategic planning
   B. Operational planning
   C. Conventional planning
   D. Best practice planning

8. Placing an ad in the newspaper, sending a card to recruit new graduates, or advertising new hospital services are methods related to
   A. Planning
   B. Buying
   C. Surveying
   D. Marketing

9. Which of the following is useful for planning and scheduling projects? It allows the manager to assess how long a project should take, determine the resources needed, and lay out the order in which tasks need to be carried out.
   A. Critical chart
   B. Diagnosis chart
   C. Gantt chart
   D. mplementation chart

10. The program evaluation and review technique calculates a realistic time frame by using the shortest possible time each activity will take, the most likely length of time, and the longest time it might take.
    A. True
    B. False

REFERENCES

Ackermann, F. (2005). *The Practice of making strategy: A step by step guide.* Thousand Oaks, CA: Sage.

Anderson, L., & Krathwohl, D. (2001) *A taxonomy for learning, teaching and assessing: A revision of Bloom's taxonomy of educational objectives.* New York: Longman.

Baker, S. (2006). www.hadm.sph.sc.edu/COURSES/J716/CPM/CPM.html; accessed October 20, 2006.

Children's Hospital of the King's Daughters. www.chkd.org/aboutus/overview.asp; accessed March 29, 2005.

Crossan, F. (2003). Strategic management and nurses: building foundations. *Journal of Nursing Management, 11*(5): 331–335.

Dienemann, J.A. (1998). *Nursing administration: Managing patient care.* (2nd ed.). Stamford, CT: Appleton & Lange.

Eckerson, W. (2005). *Performance dashboards: Measuring, monitoring, and managing your business.* Indianapolis: John Wiley & Sons.

Ellis, J.R., & Hartley, C.L. (2000). *Managing and coordinating nursing care.* (3rd ed.). Philadelphia: Lippincott.

Finkler, S.A., & Kovner, C.T. (2000). *Financial management for nurse managers and executives.* (2nd ed.). Philadelphia: W.B. Saunders.

Grant, R.M. (2005). *Contemporary strategy analysis.* (5th ed.). Malden, MA: Blackwell Publishers.

Grossman, S.C., & Valiga, T.M. (2005). *The new leadership challenge: Creating the future of nursing.* (2nd ed.). Philadelphia: F.A. Davis.

Harrison, J.S., & St. John, C.H. (2004). *Foundations in strategic management.* (2nd ed.). Cincinnati: South Western.

Hayes, R. (2005). *Operations, strategy, and technology: Pursuing the competitive edge.* Hoboken, NJ: Wiley.

Hiam, A. (1990). *The vest pocket CEO.* Englewood Cliffs, NJ: Prentice Hall.

Kotler, P. (2002). *Marketing management.* (11th ed.). Upper Saddle River, NJ: Prentice Hall.

Liedtka, J.M., & Majluf, N.S. (1996). *The strategy concept and process, a pragmatic approach.* Upper Saddle River, NJ: Prentice Hall.

Lighter, D.E., and Fair, D.C. (2000). *Principles and methods of quality management in health care.* Gaithersburg, MD: Aspen Publication.

McGuffin, J. (1999). *The nurse's guide to successful management.* St. Louis: Mosby.

Mintzberg, H. (1994). *The rise and the fall of strategic planning.* New York: Free Press.

Roney, C.W. (2004). *Strategic management methodology: Generally accepted principles for practitioners.* Westport, CT: Praeger.

Roussel, L. (2006). *Management and leadership for nurse administrators.* (4th ed.). Boston: Jones & Bartlett.

Smith, C. (2004). New technology continues to invade healthcare: What are the strategic implications/outcomes? *Nursing Administration Quarterly, 28*:92–98.

St. George's Hospital Medical School University of London. www.sghms.ac.uk; accessed March 29, 2005.

Tappen, R.M. (2004). *Essentials of nursing leadership and management.* (3rd ed.). Philadelphia: F.A. Davis.

VA Healthcare Network Upstate New York. www1.va.gov/visn02/network/strategic/missionplans.html; accessed November 14, 2005.

Managing Quality and Patient Safety

BARBARA B. BREWER, MBA, PHD, RN

CHAPTER MOTIVATION

"Quality: a way of thinking, not a recipe."

Dobyns & Crawford-Mason, 1991

CHAPTER MOTIVES

- Define health-care quality and risk management.
- Define patient safety and its relationship to quality.
- Define standards and benchmarks.
- Synthesize classic quality theories.
- Describe the need for quality in nursing and health care.
- Describe select quality tools and strategies.
- Identify key elements of a successful quality program for nursing and health care.

Providing evidence of the quality of our service has become an important responsibility for all nursing leaders. Traditionally, quality in health care was judged by reputation, program features, and compliance with policies and procedures. These traditional methods fall short of providing the level of assurance that society currently demands. In today's environment, nurses and other health-care leaders are expected to identify evidence-based process and outcome indicators of importance to their patient populations, to measure current performance relative to those indicators, and to continuously improve the care provided to their patients (Mitchell, Ferketich, & Jennings, 1998).

Galvanizing these already existing efforts is the patient safety initiative. The Institute of Medicine report *To Err is Human* reframed the quality dialogue around its startling finding that 48,000 to 98,000 lives are lost each year due to medical errors (Kohn, Corrigan, & Donaldson, 2000).

And 5 years later, despite an engaged public and industry-wide attention, there is still much work to be done. Dr. Robert Wachter (2004) of the University of California, San Francisco, challenges us with the following question: "What is the right mix of financial, educational, research, regulatory, organi-zational, and cultural activities and force to catalyze the far greater investment (in money, time, and attention) that will be needed to make health care significantly safer?" Although major national and international players, such as the Institute of Medicine, the Institute for Health Care Improvement, and the Joint Commission on the Accreditation of Healthcare Organizations, address the issues this question raises, nursing needs to be diligent in advocating for quality patient care and must continue to educate the greater community on how to achieve quality and thus a safer environment for our patients. This chapter will provide background information about theorists who pioneered performance improvement, theoretical frameworks for use in practice, and basic tools and techniques for improving quality and patient safety in everyday health-care practice. See Box 15-1 on the words frequently used when discussing quality.

Drivers of Quality

An important indicator of quality is meeting customer expectations. Some organizational leaders take that a step further; they are not satisfied until they have exceeded customer expectations. Meeting customer expectations can be a bit more difficult in health care because, unlike in other industries, the purchaser of health-care services is rarely the consumer of those same services. Nurse leaders play a pivotal role in these efforts and therefore must understand consumer quality expectations.

PATIENTS

As patients are exposed to more media attention to health care, advertisements from hospitals and pharmaceuticals, and access to information on health care, they are becoming more discriminating in what they expect and demand from providers. Patients have a choice about health-care providers. Customer satisfaction surveys are beginning to capture better what patients want and how they are making their choices. Most recently, patients as consumers have indicated that compassion, caring, and excellence are what make a hospital the hospital of choice (Lee, 2004). Nursing is a vital component of all three. Laschinger et al. (2005) found patient satisfaction with nursing care to be a strong

---

Box 15-1

Quality Terms

To make certain we have an understanding of terms commonly used in quality, we provide some definitions:

1. Quality health care: The degree to which health services for individuals and populations are safe, timely, efficient, equitable, effective, and patient-centered (Institute of Medicine Committee on Quality of Health Care in America, 2001).
2. Error: "The failure of a planned action to be completed as intended (i.e., error of execution) or the use of a wrong plan to achieve an aim (i.e., error of planning)" (Kohn, Corrigan, & Donaldson, 2000, p. 23).
3. Adverse event: "An injury caused by medical management rather than the underlying condition of the patient" (Kohn, Corrigan, & Donaldson, 2000, p. 23).
4. Benchmarking: A process used in performance improvement to compare oneself with best practice.
5. Standards: Minimum levels of performance set by the community, regulatory bodies, or professional organizations.

predictor of satisfaction with overall hospital care and with patient intention to recommend the hospital to family and friends. A recommendation from a trusted family member or friend can be an important influence on selection of a care provider, particularly for someone new to a community or who has little or no experience maneuvering through complex health-care systems.

Laschinger's findings provide evidence of the link between nursing and patient recommendations. With nursing playing a key role in achieving patient satisfaction with the overall organization, it becomes most important for nurses to understand patient preferences. In their book *Through the Patient's Eyes*, Gerteis and colleagues (1993) suggest that patient-centered care consists of the following seven patient preferences:

1. Respect for patient values, preferences, and expressed needs
2. Care coordination and integration
3. Education, communication, and information
4. Physical comfort
5. Emotional support
6. Involvement of family and friends
7. Transition and continuity

These preferences are applicable across all settings and patient populations. As you read about the other drivers of quality, you will see that they all tie themselves in some way to the patient. The patient remains the center of all quality efforts.

THE REGULATORS

Regulators have been involved in setting minimum standards for quality measurement for many years. In more recent years they have joined forces with other professional organizations and payers to drive public reporting of quality measures.

Joint Commission on Accreditation of Healthcare Organizations

The Joint Commission on Accreditation of Healthcare Organizations (JCAHO) is the primary accreditation organization for health-care institutions. Through its published standards of care, periodic onsite inspections, and collection of quality data, it helps drive providers to a higher level of care. Achievement of accreditation provides evidence that a health-care organization is meeting minimum standards of care. Accreditation by either JCAHO or a state health department is required for eligibility to receive Medicare reimbursement. Accreditation is therefore critically important to the financial health of most health-care providers, whether they are inpatient or outpatient.

In 1997, the Joint Commission launched its ORYX initiative, which integrates outcomes and other performance measurement data into the accreditation process. A component of the ORYX initiative is the identification and use of standardized—or core—performance measures (core measures). In 2002, hospitals began collecting core measure data on two of four initial core measurement areas: acute myocardial infarction, heart failure, community-acquired pneumonia, and pregnancy and related conditions. In 2003, hospitals began quarterly transmission of their measurement results to JCAHO. In 2004, another core measurement area was added—surgical infection prevention—and hospitals were required to submit to JCAHO another core measure, for a total of three measures. Using data submitted to JCAHO by 223 hospitals, Fonarow, Yancy, and Heywood (2005) evaluated compliance with the heart failure core measures and found improvement in compliance with three of the four measures. The researchers, whose study covered the period from July 2002 through December 2003, found that compliance with discharge instructions improved from 28% to 56%, measurement of left ventricular function improved from 83% to 86%, and smoking cessation instructions improved from 38% to 66%.

More recently, JCAHO introduced the Tracer method of evaluation, where a reviewer follows one patient and one provider, such as a nurse. By using the Tracer method, JCAHO expects to gain a more comprehensive understanding of staff and organizational processes used to ensure quality patient care. More and more, JCAHO is moving inspections from the boardroom to the patient's room, aligning itself closer to the consumer movement. JCAHO has also introduced failure mode and effects analysis (FMEA). FMEA, which is explained further in the section on quality tools, is a technique by which process flowcharting and risk categorization are used to prioritize and redesign weak points within care processes in order to reduce vulnerability to committing serious medical errors. This comprehensive approach to understanding error is required only once a year but can serve as a model for understanding multiple patient care services.

JCAHO (2005) has also incorporated National Patient Safety goals into its accreditation criteria. Goals are specific to the different care settings that fall under its surveillance process. The settings include ambulatory care and office-based surgery, assisted living facilities, behavioral health, hospitals, disease-specific care, home care, laboratories, long-term care, and networks. For 2006, the hospital goals encompass six areas: patient identification, communication between caregivers, infection control, patient falls, medication reconciliation, and standardization of drugs. It is important for nurse leaders to remain current on JCAHO standards in order to ensure that their patients are receiving care that is safe as well as evidence-based. By incorporating evidence-based care indicators, such as the core measures, and improvement tools, such as FMEA, into their accreditation standards, JCAHO has brought focus to care processes supported by research and the expectation of continuous improvement.

Centers for Medicare and Medicaid Services

The Centers for Medicare and Medicaid Services (CMS) is the government institution that oversees both Medicare and Medicaid programs, large consumers of health care. CMS can be considered a driver of quality both from the perspective of a regulator and the perspective of a payer. Often, the two perspectives meet to form one very powerful constituent and a heavy influence on health-care organizations. As a regulator, CMS not only looks at JCAHO accreditation but requires quality indicator reporting of its own, such as its Hospital Compare initiative. Hospital leaders, who voluntarily submit data on such indicators as the proportion of acute myocardial infarction patients who receive aspirin on admission to the hospital, receive a small percentage increase in their reimbursement. CMS then publicizes these finding so consumers can compare hospitals on a number of quality indicators. CMS also has Nursing Home Compare and Home Health Compare. CMS is also preparing to launch the first national survey of patients' perception of hospital care (Centers for Medicare and Medicaid Services & Agency for Health are Research and Quality, 2005).

CMS has played a major role in influencing quality throughout its history. It contracts with state-level organizations that oversee quality for Medicare beneficiaries within their state. These groups provide oversight of nursing home quality, home health services, physician office practices, and hospitals. The state level organizations are called quality improvement organizations (QIOs). The QIOs are the link between CMS officials in Washington, DC, and local patients, providers, their communities, and the press. Before, they were known as peer review organizations. QIOs also have educational programs to assist providers with compliance and to help Medicare beneficiaries understand their benefits.

As the largest payer for individuals with limited financial resources, Medicaid has provided access to services to many individuals who would not otherwise have been able to afford them. Since the mid-1990s, states have become much more active about monitoring the quality of services provided to Medicaid beneficiaries. Quality indicators monitored by Medicaid programs include patient satisfaction, early prenatal care, childhood immunizations, waiting times, diabetes control, cancer screenings, and the availability of translators. Beneficiaries in the majority of states are enrolled in managed care plans administered by multiple health plans within each state. Although states require managed care plans to provide them with quality data, use of the data by the states is variable (Landon et al., 2004).

State Regulators

In addition to meeting quality standards set by accreditation and federal agencies, health-care providers are required to meet standards set by state regulators. Typically, state oversight falls under the state's department of health, which administers licenses to hospitals, day-care facilities, long-term care, home care, laboratories, behavioral health facilities, and freestanding surgery centers.

State departments of health oversee quality in several ways. They investigate patient or family complaints regarding substandard care. They inspect facilities to evaluate compliance with state regulations. The state inspections are generally unannounced and may or may not be in association with annual licensure. As with JCAHO, state surveyors look for evidence of self-monitoring of quality, a continuous improvement program, and policies and procedures directed at providing safe care by competent caregivers.

PAYERS

Employers constitute a large proportion of the payers of health-care services. Competition in global markets, combined with escalating health-care costs, is driving Fortune 500 companies to join consumers on the quality bandwagon. In fact, 170 of these companies have formed the Leapfrog Group, the largest purchasing group of health care. The Leapfrog Group wants a system that keeps employees healthy, gets them back to work earlier, and keeps costs down. Some Leapfrog initiatives include support of computerized order entry systems, evidence-based hospital referral, and the use of intensivists in critical care units.

Employers who are not part of the Leapfrog Group are interested in the same issues. Through managed care plans and other forms of health insurance arrangements, employers help to bring focus to inefficiencies of the health-care system. For example, after learning about the long-term effects on health of tight blood glucose management, a large employer in Connecticut challenged the three local hospitals that provided the majority of care to their employees and their families to work together to develop an integrated program of diabetes management. Moreover, an employers' group in Indianapolis formed a coalition to put pressure on hospitals and physicians to provide it with outcome data that will be publicly displayed at benefits enrollment fairs. They are also discussing ways of structuring their benefits programs to have different co-payments, depending on the provider's outcomes. In this type of a program, employees who choose providers with better outcomes would be responsible for lower co-payments than employees who choose providers with poor outcomes. These types of efforts on the part of employers are putting tremendous pressure on providers to improve outcomes.

PROFESSIONAL GROUPS

The Institute of Medicine and National Quality Forum consist of representatives across professional disciplines that have had tremendous influence on shaping the national quality agenda.

Institute of Medicine

The Institute of Medicine (IOM) was chartered in 1970 as an arm of the National Academy of Sciences. Members of the IOM serve as advisors in health, medicine, and biomedical science. Members are volunteers who are recognized experts in their areas (Institute of Medicine, 2005). The IOM has taken a leadership position in raising national awareness of patient safety issues in hospitals and has therefore spurred the quality movement. The IOM has published several seminal reports: *To Err is Human,* in which it reported that annual deaths of hospitalized patients as a result of errors number between 48,000 and 98,000; *Crossing the Quality Chasm* (Institute of Medicine Committee on Quality of Health Care in America, 2001), in which it recommended health-care reform to improve patient outcomes and reduce error; and the most recent report, *Keeping Patients Safe: Transforming the Work Environment of Nurses* (Page, 2004), in which it reported patient safety issues and recommendations for change to reduce the negative consequences nurses' work environments have on their ability to provide safe care. In *Crossing the Quality Chasm*, the Committee on Quality of Health Care in America recommended six aims for improvement: systems should be redesigned to provide care that is safe, timely, efficient, effective, equitable, and patient-centered.

The IOM has been influential in shaping the national agenda for improving quality and safety outcomes for patients. The shocking nature of its report attributing death of hospitalized patients to medical error captured the attention of the media, which provided wide public exposure beyond the health-care community. The combination of loud public outcry, personal influence of IOM members, and the movement toward pay for performance has contributed to current demands for greater accountability of providers, hospitals, and other health-care agencies.

National Quality Forum

The National Quality Forum (NQF), a nonprofit public-private partnership that works to improve the health-care system through development and dissemination of voluntary consensus standards, recently recommended nursing performance standards (National Quality Forum, 2004). Member organizations represent health-care providers, educational institutions, consumers, employers, state and federal agencies, and research. Four nursing organizations (American Nurses Association,

American Academy of Nursing, American Association of Colleges of Nursing, and American Association of Nurse Anesthetists) are represented among NQF member organizations. The NQF consists of councils, which provide the opportunity for member organizations to discuss issues with each other, and sets consensus standards on issues of current relevance. Examples of these types of consensus standards are Cancer Care, Hospital Standards, Patient Safety Standards, and Nurse-Sensitive Quality Indicators (National Quality Forum, 2000-2004). The nursing standards are the first nationally standardized set of performance measures to assess the effect acute care nurses have on patient health and safety outcomes. Measures evaluate eight patient outcomes (failure to rescue; pressure ulcer prevalence; falls prevalence; restraint prevalence; falls with injury; and three infections: urinary tract, central line, and ventilator-associated pneumonia [VAP]), three process indicators (nurse counseling of smoking cessation for patients with an acute myocardial infarction, congestive heart failure, or pneumonia), and four structural measures (skill mix, nursing hours per patient day, nursing work environment, and voluntary turnover). The 15 indicators are intended to be an initial set.

The notion behind the consensus standards is that all of the NQF member organizations would incorporate the consensus measures into the quality measures they require. By doing so, measurement would become standardized and consistent across organizations and settings, which would allow comparison. Additionally, inclusion of the measures in the Medicare and Medicaid programs gives them the power of regulation for those organizations and individual practitioners participating in these programs. For example, JCAHO has incorporated the NQF nursing-sensitive indicators into its staffing effectiveness measures. Organizations accredited by JCAHO must evaluate nurse staffing effectiveness on at least two of its units by collecting and analyzing two human resource indicators and two clinical service indicators. The indicators must be trended and are to be used internally to evaluate performance. The 15 NQF indicators are included in the set approved by JCAHO for meeting this standard. As a result, use of these indicators has spread quickly across multiple settings and organizations; however, because the standard requires internal monitoring, data are not sent to JCAHO, and no comparison data are available for organizations wishing to use external databases for quality improvement.

American Nurses Association

In the mid-1990s, the American Nurses Association (ANA) published a report containing process, outcome, and structural measures that have been shown through research to be related to acute care nursing (American Nurses Association, 1995). These indicators are a subset of the larger set subsequently published by the National Quality Forum. Some of the outcome indicators contained in the report include patient mortality, length of stay, adverse incidents such as medication errors and patient falls, and complications such as nosocomial infections and decubitus ulcers. Examples of process measures are pain management, use of restraints, and discharge planning. Process measures are phenomena associated with nursing interventions. Structural measures involve, for example, nurse staffing, such as skill mix, experience, and hours per patient day. The report contains operational definitions for all quality indicators as well as references for all evidence linking the indicator with nursing. Quarterly submission of these data to the National Dataset Nursing Quality Indicators is a requirement of Magnet certification. In return for data submittal, nurse leaders receive a quarterly report that shows their data broken down by type of unit, with comparisons with the average performance for all like units in the database. Having such data allows nurses to understand how the results of their care compares with that of other nurses, helps focus attention on care processes that might be substandard, and highlights areas where performance is stellar. By using these types of data to determine where the greatest gaps exist between their performance and that of other like units, leaders can prioritize improvement projects and direct resources to those outcomes where the gaps are greatest.

In addition to the acute care report card, the ANA has published numerous standards of nursing practice. Scope and standards documents have been published for nurse administrators, clinical specialty areas, and nursing informatics. The standards do not replace state law or regulations of individual nurse practice acts; they serve as consensus standards of nurse experts in the areas of the published standards (American Nurses Association, 2004). The criteria for measurement of excellence in nursing care used by the Magnet Recognition Program are based upon the ANA scope and standards for nurse administrators (American Nurses Credentialing Center, 2004). The standards also serve as the basis for specialty certification examinations (Box 15-2).

Models of Quality

Quality models serve as frameworks for diagnosing and finding solutions to performance problems. Often, organizational leadership sets the choice of a model. This section describes models frequently used in health-care settings.

PLAN, DO, STUDY, ACT CYCLE

The Plan, Do, Study, Act (PDSA) cycle is an improvement model that is still practiced widely. Dr. Deming advocated for this method of continual improvement. Each step of the model contains a distinct improvement phase. The model is meant to be repeated over multiple improvement cycles.

Use of the PDSA cycle assumes that a problem has been identified and analyzed for its most likely

---

Box 15-2

Baldrige National Quality Award

Accrediting bodies and state and federal regulations set minimum standards of quality. Organization leaders who wish to be recognized for providing services of the highest quality measure themselves against more rigorous standards, such as those developed for the Baldrige National Quality Award.

The Baldrige National Quality Award program, named for Malcolm Baldrige, a former Secretary of Commerce, is administered through the National Institute of Standards and Technology. The award is based on meeting rigorous quality standards that show an organization has achieved an integrated approach to performance management. The award criteria differ for different sectors of the economy. There are specific health-care criteria, which use a systems perspective to identify relationships among seven criteria for performance excellence. The seven categories encompass:

1. Leadership
2. Strategic planning
3. Focus on patients, other customers, and markets
4. Measurement, analysis, and knowledge management
5. Focus on staff
6. Process management
7. Results of organizational performance (National Institute of Standards and Technology, 2004).

Only one health-care system and four hospitals have achieved this distinction (National Institute of Standards and Technology, 2005).

Historical Perspectives Box

The ideas of Deming, Juran, and Crosby underlie much of the theory, tools, and techniques we use in quality today. Understanding their work provides a historical context of the quality movement and the beginning foundation on which the rest of the information in this chapter will build.

Dr. W. Edwards Deming

Dr. Deming (1950) was one of the pioneers of the quality movement. Deming took a systems view of the world. As a systems thinker, Deming understood that manufacturing a product or delivering a service like health care consists of multiple processes and decisions that are related to one another. When we view our work from a systems perspective, we begin to understand how our actions influence others who follow us in providing care to

patients. Deming suggested that the style of management being practiced in his day, which consisted of use of fear to control workers, inspection of work to reduce defects in manufacturing, and use of targets and quotas to drive productivity, should undergo a transformation. He suggested that his System of Profound Knowledge would provide managers with a theoretical map, a tool that would provide better understanding of their organization.

Deming's System of Profound Knowledge contains four interrelated parts:

1. Appreciation for a system: all work consists of multiple interdependent processes.
2. Understanding of variation: differences in work outcomes are a result of the system of work, not individual worker performance.

(Continued on following page)

Historical Perspectives Box *(continued)*

3. Theory of knowledge: when making improvements we test new designs that we predict will produce better outcomes. Our predictions are based on our understanding of how work processes relate to one another.
4. Psychology: understanding what motivates people (Deming, 2000).

Dr. Deming proposed that variation among workers was caused by their work system. Managers need to manage the system of work to reduce variation among workers and improve the consistency of their product. His model for improvement was the Plan, Do, Study, Act (PDSA) cycle. An explanation of how the PDSA cycle is used in practice is in the section of this chapter on quality models. Deming was also known for his 14 Points for Management. The 14 points were developed in response to frequent requests he received about his transformation of Japanese manufacturing (Stoecklein, 2005). Deming believed it was management's responsibility to create an environment where employees could produce high-quality products. This philosophy can be seen in his 14 points, which cover such elements as constancy of purpose for management, working with vendors so that incoming materials are defect-free, driving out fear among workers, continuous attention to improvement of quality and elimination of waste, and use of statistical quality control rather than mass inspection. His theory was instrumental in improving reliability of Japanese products by guiding leaders to foster an environment where front-line workers had the ability to reduce defects in manufacturing by cooperating with each other.

JOSEPH JURAN

Joseph Juran (1950), who was trained as an engineer, was another of the early pioneers in quality. Juran also spent time in the early 1950s consulting with Japanese industrialists. He is best known for his quality trilogy: quality planning, quality improvement, and quality control (Juran & Godfrey, 1999). Juran defined two different but interrelated concepts, those aspects of a product that meet customer needs and those aspects of a product that are free from defects (Stoecklein, 2005).

Similar to Dr. Deming, Juran used statistical thinking to understand process variation. He introduced the Pareto principle as a method for understanding the "vital few" contributors to the cause of a problem. According to Juran,

20% of the causes contributes to 80% of the problem. Pareto diagrams are used to identify the "vital few"; a full explanation of their use is in the section on quality tools.

PHILIP CROSBY

Philip Crosby (1960) was another of the early pioneers in quality. Crosby defined quality as the extent to which processes are in conformance with requirements, i.e., providing what the customer needs and expects. Consistent with the other quality theorists, Crosby believed that leaders were responsible for creating an environment that promoted continuous improvement. He is most famous for two phrases, which are often found throughout the quality literature: "do it right the first time" and "zero defects" (Nielsen et al., 2004). In other words, managers must not tolerate flaws or errors.

Deming, Juran, and Crosby all had a process focus. All three theorists believed that improvement must be continuous and that knowledge of customer needs and requirements is essential. Whereas Deming, Juran, and Crosby pioneered quality improvement in manufacturing, Donabedian was an early quality advocate in health care.

AVEDIS DONABEDIAN

Dr. Donabedian (1960) is best known for the structure, process, and outcome quality paradigm, which underpins much of the health outcomes research performed by nurse researchers and is the framework that underlies the Quality Health Outcomes Model developed by the American Academy of Nursing Expert Panel on Quality Health Care (Mitchell, Ferketich, & Jennings, 1998). A description of the Quality Health Outcomes Model is in the section on quality models. Structure consists of organizational characteristics such as staffing, models of care, patient types, and volumes. Process consists of tools and techniques involved in providing care. Nursing process and interventions are types of process measures. Outcomes involve the results achieved. They reflect the effectiveness of the structural and process components (Donabedian, 1992; Lee et al., 2005). Outcomes are a product of the structure we have put in place and our care processes. Both components need to be in place to achieve optimal outcomes. For example, a medical-surgical nursing unit that wants to improve its fall rate may need to make improvements in staffing as well as develop a sound process for identifying and protecting patients at high risk for a fall.

causes and that changes have been recommended for eliminating the likely causes. Once the initial problem analysis is completed, a plan is developed to test one of the improvement changes. During the

Do phase, the change is made, and data are collected to evaluate results. Study involves analysis of the data collected in the previous step. Data are evaluated for evidence that an improvement has been

Practice Proof 15-1

Article: Comparison of methods for detecting medication errors in 36 hospitals and skilled-nursing facilities.

Authors: Flynn, E.A., et al. *American Journal of Health System Pharmacy 59*(5): 436–446.

Note: This abstract is available online through PubMed. The full-text may be accessed through libraries that have subscriptions to Academic Search Premier.

ABSTRACT

The validity and cost-effectiveness of three methods for detecting medication errors were examined. A stratified random sample of 36 hospitals and skilled-nursing facilities in Colorado and Georgia was selected. Medication administration errors were detected by registered nurses (R.N.s), licensed practical nurses (L.P.N.s), and pharmacy technicians from these facilities using three methods: incident report review, chart review, and direct observation. Each dose evaluated was compared with the prescriber's order. Deviations were considered errors. Efficiency was measured by the time spent evaluating each dose. A pharmacist performed an independent determination of errors to assess the accuracy of each data collector. Clinical significance was judged by a panel of physicians. Observers detected 300 of 457 pharmacist-confirmed errors made on 2556 doses (11.7% error rate) compared with 17 errors detected by chart reviewers (0.7% error rate), and 1 error detected by incident report review (0.04% error rate). All errors detected involved the same 2556 doses. All chart reviewers and 7 of 10 observers achieved at least good comparability with the pharmacist's results. The mean cost of error detection per dose was $4.82 for direct observation and $0.63 for chart review. The technician was the least expensive observer at $2.87 per dose evaluated. R.N.s were the least expensive chart reviewers at $0.50 per dose. Of 457 errors, 35 (8%) were deemed potentially clinically significant; 71% of these were detected by direct observation. Direct observation was more efficient and accurate than reviewing charts and incident reports in detecting medication errors. Pharmacy technicians were more efficient and accurate than R.N.s and L.P.N.s in collecting data about medication errors.

QUESTIONS

1. Why do you think there was such a discrepancy among the three methods of error detection?
2. What were the most two most frequent types of error detected by direct observation?
3. If you were to replicate the three methods of data collection used in this study, would there be a more cost effective way to do data collection?

made. The Act step involves taking actions that will "hardwire" the change so that the gains made by the improvement are sustained over time.

The PDSA cycle has found widespread use in the health-care setting. It is not unusual in such complex environments for multiple extraneous factors to influence results. Through repetition of the PDSA cycle, multiple corrective actions may be taken and evaluated (Kondo & Kano, 1999).

The following example illustrates how the PDSA cycle may be used in health care. A nurse manager notices that the number of patient falls with injury has been climbing steadily over the last few months. She calls her staff together to brainstorm reasons for the higher number of falls. After considering several reasons, the staff develops a process for earlier identification for patients who may be at risk for a fall (the Plan phase of the PDSA cycle). The staff implements its new risk appraisal process and continues to collect data regarding the number of patients who are injured as the result of a fall (the Do phase). After a few weeks of data collection, the staff reviews the injury data to determine if the new risk appraisal process has resulted in fewer injured patients (the Study phase). Finally, the staff members decide that the new risk appraisal process has resulted in fewer falls, but they believe that they could do better if they also added bed alarms to alert them to high-risk patients who are attempting to get out of bed without appropriate assistance. This is the Act phase (making the risk appraisal process a routine for all patients) and the beginning of another PDSA cycle (implementation of bed alarms). Once the bed alarms are put in place, the staff will again collect patient fall data, examine the data for improvement, and then decide whether the bed alarms resulted in enough improvement to warrant permanent implementation. This example illustrates how the PDSA cycle may be repeated over multiple corrective actions to result in better patient outcomes.

THE MODEL FOR IMPROVEMENT

Another model commonly found in health care is the Model for Improvement (Langley et al., 1996). The model uses a systems framework, which adds three questions to the PDSA cycle. The questions are meant to bring clarity to the improvement process. The three questions are:

1. What are we trying to accomplish?
2. How will we know that a change is an improvement?
3. What changes can we make that will result in improvement? (Langley et al., 1996, p. xiv).

Once the three questions have been answered, the improvement cycle proceeds using the PDSA methodology. The three questions are designed to help bring clarity to the PDSA cycle through goal development, to remind people to collect data relevant to the goal and process they are attempting to improve, and to clarify cause and effect. The Model for Improvement is recommended by the Institute for Healthcare Improvement as a way to accelerate improvement (Institute for Healthcare Improvement, 2005). The model may be used for repetitive tests of small changes.

QUALITY HEALTH OUTCOMES MODEL

The Quality Health Outcomes Model developed by the Expert Panel on Quality Healthcare of the American Academy of Nursing was proposed to serve as a framework for quality activities as well as nursing systems research (Mitchell, Ferketich, & Jennings, 1998). The model's four components (Fig. 15-1)—intervention, system, client, and outcomes—were built on Donabedian's structure, process, outcomes paradigm (Mitchell & Lang, 2004). Additionally, the model, which specifies interdependent relationships among the model variables, was designed to allow measurement of the four components at multiple levels. For example, through the relationships specified by the model, it is possible to examine the effect a hospital safety culture (a hospital-level system component) and a "ventilator bundle" intervention (a patient-level intervention variable) have on the rate of ventilator-associated pneumonia (a unit outcome variable) in critical care patients.

SIX SIGMA

Sigma is a letter from the Greek alphabet that is used in statistics to indicate variability. Six Sigma refers to six standard deviations from the mean and is generally used in quality improvement to define

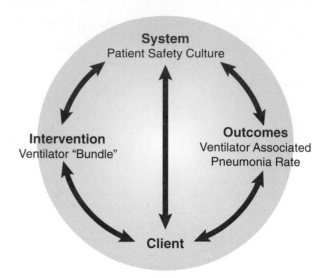

FIGURE 15-1 Quality Health Outcomes Model. (Adapted from Mitchell, Ferketich, and Jennings [1998].)

the number of acceptable defects or errors produced by a process. In the Six Sigma model, the number of acceptable errors is always 3.4 per million occurrences. As a result, it comes closest to Crosby's zero tolerance philosophy. Because this method focuses on outcomes (the number of acceptable errors), it may be used in conjunction with one of the process-focused methods, such as PDSA (Barry, Murcko, & Brubaker, 2002).

Specifically, Six Sigma is a rigorous improvement method tied to key business processes and customer requirements. The method contains five steps: define, measure, analyze, improve, and control (DMAIC). In the define step, questions are asked about key customer requirements and key processes to support those requirements. In the measure step, key processes are identified, and data are collected. In the analyze step, data are converted to information. Causes of process variation are identified. The improve stage generates solutions and makes and measures process changes. In the control stage, processes that are performing in a predictable way at a desirable level are in control. Monitoring to evaluate ongoing performance is done as part of this stage (Lee et al., 2005). For example, if we go back to our earlier example of patient falls with injury, in a hospital where the improvement model was Six Sigma, improvement of the number of patient falls with injury would not be achieved until there were fewer than 3.4 injury falls per one million patient days. Injury falls are typically measured per 1000 patient days. As you can see, the Six Sigma approach is 100 times more stringent. If we were to use the DMAIC model for falls, we might come up with the following:

- **Define:** Patients want to be safe and free from falling.
- **Measure:** Use information from incident reports and clinical experience to identify key processes associated with patient falls. We might consider toileting, medications, frequency of fall risk assessment, etc. We would then collect data about the processes identified in this step.
- **Analyze:** Use the gathered data to evaluate the most frequent reasons patients are falling. Determine which of the causes, if removed, would result in the greatest improvement.
- **Improve:** Design an intervention to remove causes identified in the previous step. Implement intervention, and continue to measure the number of patient falls. Evaluate whether or not the intervention resulted in improvement.
- **Control:** Monitor patient falls to ensure improvements gained following the implementation of the improvement process continue.

LEAN

The final improvement model we will discuss in this section is the Lean methodology. The underlying assumption of the Lean methodology is that all processes contain waste. In their book, *Lean Thinking: Banish Waste and Create Wealth in Your Organization,* Womack and Jones (2003, p. 15) define lean thinking as *"lean* because it provides a way to do more and more with less and less—less human effort, less equipment, less time, and less space—while coming closer and closer to providing customers with exactly what they want." Lean thinking was originated at Toyota and is also known as the Toyota Production System (TPS).

TPS is built on four basic principles:

1. All work processes are highly specified.
2. Every customer and supplier relationship is clear.

3. Pathways between people and process steps are specific and consistent.
4. Improvements are made at the lowest possible organizational level and based on scientific method (Spear & Bowen, 1999).

Toyota's success is based on the idea that each employee identifies problems and is taught how to improve. Front-line workers make the improvements to their own jobs, and their supervisors provide direction and assistance as teachers. The TPS method goes beyond those described previously in this section because it incorporates ergonomics involving the individual workers in its view of work processes. For example, ergonomic process redesign would include such elements as evaluating ways of decreasing the distance of supply carts to point of care or adding computer terminals to patient rooms to decrease the number of steps nurses must make to find a place to chart patient information. Both of these examples involve "waste" in the form of unnecessary steps staff must take to complete their care tasks.

It is difficult to find examples of TPS in health care because processes in health care are far more complex than those found in manufacturing. In addition, it is very difficult for a single individual to redesign a process and test and refine it within the clinical setting without influencing other departments or individuals.

Many organizations have attempted to achieve the exceptional performance Toyota has realized through its TPS, but few have been capable of doing so (Spear, 2004). Health-care organizations within the Pittsburgh Regional Health Initiative have adopted TPS as the improvement methodology. One of the care processes they have redesigned using TPS is medication administration (Thompson, Wolf, & Spear, 2003). The authors described an improvement project that resulted from patient complaints of discomfort following intravenous administration of antibiotics. The major cause of discomfort was the drug concentration, which was irritating patients' veins. Following careful diagramming of all of the pathways required for a nurse to drip a more dilute form of the antibiotic rather than push the form sent by the pharmacy, it was discovered that a small change by the pharmacy (sending the drug vial attached to a minibag of intravenous solution) would result in consistent delivery of the more dilute form of the drug, less patient discomfort, and a savings of 4 minutes of nursing time per dose.

Nursing Quality

Nurse leaders are pivotal to hospital-wide quality initiatives. They must also lead initiatives that improve nursing quality. Using the same tools and techniques but with nurse-sensitive indicators, nursing can improve processes directly related to the practice of nursing. Nurse-sensitive indicators are those that through research have been associated with nursing care. Examples of some of these indicators are patient falls, mortality, failure to rescue, pressure ulcers, deep vein thrombosis, and VAP. A more comprehensive explanation follows below. Nursing quality improvement programs are designed to enhance patient care through systematic assessment and improvement of the quality and appropriateness of care rendered. Opportunities to improve patient care through evaluation of clinical and operational performance measures are integrated into ongoing management processes. For example, some nurse leaders use unit-based report cards to share trended data regularly with their staff. Many of these report cards are produced monthly and contain such data as patient falls, medication errors, turnover and vacancy rates, staff satisfaction, patient satisfaction, and financial indicators such as length of stay or cost per adjusted discharge.

MEDICATION ERRORS AND NURSING QUALITY

Nearly every quality initiative in this country includes attention to medication errors. Nursing leaders must work closely with pharmacists and physicians to reduce medication errors. Leading the nation in this arena is the Veterans Health Administration, well known for its system-wide computerized patient record system and bar code medication administration. Bar code medication administration reduces medication errors by combining positive patient identification (bar code on patient's wristband) with positive drug identification (bar code on medication package). When a bar-coding system is integrated with computerized physician order entry, errors associated with incorrect interpretation of physician medication orders and nonintravenous-related medication errors are eliminated. These types of systems do not address errors associated with intravenous medication rates resulting from incorrect programming of intravenous administration devices, however.

Adverse drug events or injuries caused by drug therapy are frequent in hospitalized patients. In a study performed in 36 accredited and nonaccredited hospitals and nursing homes, researchers found that 19% of medication doses given were in error (Barker et al., 2002, Flynn et al., 2002). Of those errors, 7% were judged by a group of physician reviewers to be potentially harmful. Hatcher and colleagues (2004, p. 438) suggest that more than half of adverse medication errors are associated with drugs administered intravenously. They suggest that a computerized point-of-care intravenous delivery system that "integrates infusion, patient monitoring, and clinical best practice guidelines" is a necessary ingredient to reducing these serious errors. Such systems, sometimes called "smart pumps," provide safety alerts when a nurse attempts to program a dose outside of those established to be appropriate. In addition, they record in an "events" log the number and type of errors averted through use of the device. Data from the events log may be used by nurse leaders to understand the types of medications, time of day, types of patients, and nursing units associated with alarms. Such data may be used to monitor change as a result of quality improvement activities.

Nursing plays a major role in processes such as medication administration. Medication errors must be trended and studied for patterns within the errors. For example, Barker and colleagues (2002) observed nurses administer medications in 36 hospitals and nursing homes in Georgia and Colorado. Researchers observed at least one nurse per institution during an entire pass of medications. This approach allowed them to observe the entire medication distribution process of the observed nurse. Of the 3216 doses observed, 19% resulted in a medication error. Errors by category were wrong time (43%), omission (30%), wrong dose (17%), and incorrect drug (4%).

Nurse leaders may learn about the types of errors within their units by evaluating data from occurrence reports. Error data should be categorized in order to identify the most frequent types of errors. The most frequent types of errors should then be examined for their root causes. In order to uncover the root cause of a problem, it is necessary to ask five "whys" (see root cause analysis below). Accepting explanations before reaching the fifth why may lead to incorrect conclusions regarding cause. Systems for medication distribution are very complex, often involving multiple people and process steps. Unraveling problem causes takes patience and discipline. For example, Thompson, Wolf, and Spear (2003) point out how wrong conclusions about root cause may be reached when explanations short of the fifth why are accepted. They reviewed a root cause analysis of a missing 8 a.m. medication dose to try to understand why the dose was not in the patient's medication drawer so that it could be given by the nurse. The analysis revealed a far different explanation at the end of the fifth why (the first, midnight, dose of medication was in the wrong drawer, causing the 8 a.m. dose to be given at midnight) from what would have been accepted as the explanation (the pharmacy technician returned the midnight dose, which should have been the 8 a.m. dose, for credit) had staff not been disciplined enough to keep pushing for the root cause.

PATIENT SATISFACTION AND NURSING QUALITY

Patient satisfaction with nursing care is an important measure of the quality of nursing care. Because nursing is at the core of the patient care experience, patient satisfaction measures have always been of interest to both hospital and nursing administration. Measures of satisfaction may include patient perceptions of being well cared for, satisfaction with nurse friendliness and timeliness of response to call bells and pain medication as well as explanations given to family and friends. Some organizations have chosen to design and distribute their own measures, and others have decided to use a third-party vendor, such as Press Ganey or NRC Picker, which allows them to compare scores with other like organizations. Whatever measure an organization chooses to evaluate patient satisfaction, it is important to trend results over time so that changes in satisfaction, both positive and negative, may be

spotted early. Moreover, staff satisfaction has been found to be strongly correlated with two patient satisfaction indicators, intent to return and intent to recommend the hospital to others (Atkins, Marshall, & Javalgi, 1996).

One of the most influential books on measuring patient care is *Through the Patients' Eyes* (Gerteis et al., 1993). The book draws on research from the Picker/Commonwealth Program for Patient-Centered Care. The authors suggest that patient-centered care includes the eight dimensions: access; respect for patient's values, preferences, and expressed needs; coordination and integration of care; information, communication, and education; physical comfort; emotional support and alleviation of fear and anxiety; involvement of family and friends; and transition and continuity. See Box 15-3 for a brief description of each dimension.

Box 15-3

Picker Patient-Centered Care Dimensions

1. **Access** (including time spent waiting for admission or time between admission and allocation to a bed in a ward)
2. **Respect for patient's values, preferences, and expressed needs** (including impact of illness and treatment on quality of life, involvement in decision making, dignity, needs, and autonomy)
3. **Coordination and integration of care** (including clinical care, ancillary and support services, and "front-line" care)
4. **Information, communication, and education** (including clinical status, progress and prognosis, processes of care, facilitation of autonomy, self-care, and health promotion)
5. **Physical comfort** (including pain management, help with activities of daily living, surroundings, and hospital environment)
6. **Emotional support and alleviation of fear and anxiety** (including clinical status, treatment and prognosis, impact of illness on self and family, financial impact of illness)
7. **Involvement of family and friends** (including social and emotional support, involvement in decision making, support for caregiving, impact on family dynamics and functioning)
8. **Transition and continuity** (including information about medication and danger signs to monitor after leaving the hospital; coordination and discharge planning; clinical, social, physical, and financial support).

As consumers become more engaged in choosing health care, more patient satisfaction surveys continue to evolve with a focus on the patient experience. Leading this effort is a joint initiative of CMS and the Agency for Healthcare Research. Together, with input from multiple groups, they have developed the Hospital CAHPS, a standardized survey instrument and data collection methodology for measuring patients' perspectives on hospital care. Table 15-1 contains draft questions contained in the survey. The questions in this instrument encompass seven key topics related to patient experience:

1. Communication with doctors
2. Communication with nurses
3. Responsiveness of hospital staff
4. Cleanliness and noise level of the physical environment
5. Pain control
6. Communication about medicines
7. Discharge information

TABLE 15-1   Hospital Consumer Assessment of Health Plans (HCAHPS)*

1. During this hospital stay, how often did nurses treat you with *courtesy and respect?*
2. During this hospital stay, how often did nurses listen carefully to you?
3. During this hospital stay, how often did nurses explain things in a way you could understand?
4. During this hospital stay, after you pressed the call button, how often did you get help as soon as you wanted it?
5. During this hospital stay, how often did doctors treat you with *courtesy and respect?*
6. During this hospital stay, how often did doctors listen carefully to you?
7. During this hospital stay, how often did doctors explain things in a way you could understand?

The Hospital Environment

8. During this hospital stay, how often were your room and bathroom kept clean?
9. During this hospital stay, how often was the area around your room quiet at night?

Your Experiences in this Hospital

10. During this hospital stay, did you need help from nurses or other hospital staff in getting to the bathroom or in using a bedpan?
11. How often did you get help in getting to the bathroom or in using a bedpan as soon as you wanted?
12. During this hospital stay, did you need medicine for pain?
13. During this hospital stay, how often was your pain well controlled?
14. During this hospital stay, how often did the hospital staff do everything they could to help you with your pain?

15. Before giving you any new medicine, how often did hospital staff tell you what the medicine was for?
16. Before giving you any new medicine, how often did hospital staff describe possible side effects in a way you could understand?

When You Left the Hospital

17. After you left the hospital, did you go directly to your own home, to someone else's home, or to another health facility?
18. During this hospital stay, did doctors, nurses, or other hospital staff talk with you about whether you would have the help you needed when you left the hospital?
19. During this hospital stay, did you get information in writing about what symptoms or health problems to look out for after you left the hospital?

Overall Rating of Hospital

20. Using any number from 0 to 10, where 0 is the worst hospital possible and 10 is the best hospital possible, what number would you use to rate this hospital?
21. Would you recommend this hospital to your friends and family?

About You

22. In general, how would you rate your overall health?
23. What is the highest grade or level of school that you have completed?
24. Are you of Hispanic or Latino origin or descent?
25. What is your race? Please choose one or more.

Draft items as of 12/16/04.

Whichever tool a hospital or institution uses, the role of the nurse leader is critical in this area. The nurse leader will have measured information directly linked to the patient experience upon which she can improve patient care on the unit. For example, if the nursing leaders on a unit decide they want to improve pain management for their patients, they may want to measure the level of improvement by evaluating differences in patient pain scores as well as changes in patients' scores on patient satisfaction questions asking them about pain management. The quality of nursing care is of strategic importance to most health-care organizations. A nursing quality program must ensure that standards are in place (quality assurance), but more importantly, it must include a focus on performance improvement. Performance improvement should be geared toward nursing-sensitive indicators as well as patient satisfaction and medication safety.

Margaret Gerteis and colleagues (1993, p. 299) set forth a challenge and an imperative: "Unless we understand and meet patients' subjective needs, we cannot hope to build confidence and trust in any provider, institution, or health care system."

The next section provides information regarding quality tools and strategies nurse leaders may incorporate into their performance improvement programs.

hot topic:
How Do We Stack Up?

We are constantly asked to compare our performance against that of outside bodies, whether as a requirement for Magnet designation or JCAHO accreditation or because we want to understand how our level of performance stacks up against the best. Before we can proceed, we must clarify terms that are sometimes used inappropriately:

Benchmarks reflect outcomes achieved by the best performers. These values must be from the top 5% of all organizations submitting data and, preferably, the highest value of all who submitted. Performance at or better than the benchmark indicates excellence. Comparisons or comparative data may be the benchmark, but not necessarily so. Often, comparative indicators are the mean or median value of all data submitted. When the mean or median is used for comparison, performance better than the comparison reflects performance better than the bottom half of all organizations submitting data; it does not reflect excellence.

Standards are the minimum level of acceptable performance. Meeting standards is not reflective of excellence or best performance.

So now that we have clarity on commonly used terms, how do we decide which to use? The choice depends upon your goal. If the goal is to settle for nothing less than best practice, then a benchmark must be used. If the goal is to provide acceptable care, then a comparison reflecting a mean or median might be an appropriate choice. Your goal must drive your choice.

Finding benchmark or comparative indicators may be challenging. In order to make valid comparisons, the indicators must come from organizations of similar type and size as well as having similar acuity of patients. It would not be valid to compare pressure ulcer data from a nursing facility with data from critical care units. There must be a logical reason for choosing comparisons. Data, whether benchmark or comparative, may be found on Web sites of regulatory agencies, such as JCAHO and CMS. They may also be obtained from population-based registries, such as the National Registry of Myocardial Infarction or from the literature.

Practice to Strive For 15-1

Many acute care and long-term care facilities are evaluating whether they should apply for recognition as a Magnet facility. The Magnet certification program, overseen by the American Nurses Credentialing Center (ANCC), is a rigorous appraisal process to evaluate the quality of nursing programs. Organizations that wish to achieve recognition as a Magnet facility must provide nursing care based on current evidence and must evaluate quality indicators sensitive to nursing. All Magnet facilities and those applying for Magnet recognition submit data regarding patient falls, pressure ulcer prevalence, and hours of staffing. Data are compared with those of similar units in hospitals of similar bed size. In addition, organizations must evaluate performance on two other nursing-sensitive outcome indicators. Among the additional indicators are length of stay, urinary tract infections, pneumonia, deep vein thrombosis, and cardiac arrest. Less than excellent outcomes in chosen quality indicators must be addressed through performance improvement. The ANCC Magnet recognition program provides external recognition of nursing excellence through high-quality nursing outcomes.

Quality Tools and Strategies

Nurse managers have many quality tools and strategies from which to choose. They should be looking at their unit's core processes and making improvements. Tools may be grouped into two categories: (1) process analysis and data display and (2) statistical thinking and control charts. Process analysis and data display involve diagramming processes to understand the current situation and to decide what might be causing wasted efforts, errors, or patient dissatisfaction. Process analysis and data display tools commonly used for improvement include failure modes and effects analysis, root cause or cause and effect diagrams, flowcharts, Pareto diagrams, and histograms. Statistical thinking involves understanding process variation and methods for displaying process capability. Tools in this category are run charts and control charts. The following section will describe each of the major tools and some basic information about variation and control charts.

CHART AUDITS

Until electronic medical records replace paper records, chart audits will remain the most common method of collecting quality data. As anyone who has ever performed chart audits can attest, this is a time-consuming and expensive method of data collection. It is important before beginning an audit to spend time considering the types of data required. Once required data have been established, designing an audit tool to assist in data collection will standardize recording of information and facilitate data entry for analysis.

If multiple staff will do the chart reviews, it is important to define the data elements being audited so all staff collect data in the same way. For example, if the interest is to evaluate improvement in pain scores following administration of pain medication, it is critical that scores immediately before administration are recorded as well as scores following administration of the medication. It might also be useful to include the name and route of medication administered, type and site of pain, and patient age. Collecting all relevant data at the outset will avoid having to repeat the audit for missing pieces of information. Sometimes a concurrent

> **Box 15-4**
> ### Retrospective Versus Concurrent Audits
> Consider doing concurrent audits when evaluating compliance with a change in patient care practices. Concurrent audits allow identification of missing care elements while the patient is still within your care and correction of deficits before discharge. Retrospective audits are valuable tools for data collection, but do not allow for staff reinforcement and correction of omitted care elements.

audit may be more useful than a retrospective chart audit. Box 15-4 provides features of each type of audit.

FAILURE MODE AND EFFECTS ANALYSIS: PROSPECTIVE REVIEW

JCAHO requires leaders to perform a proactive annual failure mode and effects analysis (FMEA) to reduce risk of sentinel events. All systems have design weaknesses. FMEA is tool that takes leaders through evaluation of design weaknesses within their processes, enables them to prioritize weaknesses that might be more likely to result in failure (errors) and, based on priorities, decide where to focus on process redesign aimed at improving patient safety. Known causes for each failure are identified, and a numerical score from 1 to 10 is applied based on the probability of occurrence of the cause (1 being unlikely, and 10 being inevitable). The effects of each failure are listed and ranked from 1 to 10 according to likelihood of detection and severity, 1 reflecting no effect and 10 reflecting very severe effect. Once all causes, effects, and likelihood of detection have been ranked, the product of the three scores results in a risk priority number for each cause and effect. The risk priority number is used to prioritize performance improvement projects aimed at eliminating high-risk failure modes. Leaders should consider high-risk activities within their own organization and those known to have caused problems in other similar health-care settings (DeRosier et al., 2002). For example, we know from the literature that heparin and insulin infusions are associated with high frequency and very severe medication errors in the acute care setting. FMEA should be used by quality leaders in all hospitals to evaluate medication systems associated with these drugs in order to eliminate system weaknesses that increase vulnerability of their patients to injury resulting from an insulin or heparin infusion.

ROOT CAUSE ANALYSIS: RETROSPECTIVE REVIEW

A root cause analysis, or cause and effect diagram, sometimes called a fishbone diagram, is used retrospectively to evaluate potential causes of a problem or sources of variation of a process. Possible causes are generally grouped in four categories: people, materials, policies and procedures, and equipment. Causes are then listed by drawing branches to show their relationship to one of the four categories. More specific causes are shown as bones on its respective branch. Causes are generated by asking a series of "why" questions (Executive Learning, 2002). For example, if a nurse made a medication error, the first "why" question would be: Why did the nurse make the medication error? Assume the answer to that question is because the 9 a.m. dose was not in the medication drawer. The next "why" would be: Why wasn't the 9 a.m. dose in the medication drawer? The answer might be because the 9 a.m. dose was given at midnight. The next question then would be: Why was the 9 a.m. dose given at midnight? The process of asking "why" questions would continue until the root cause for omission of the 9 a.m. dose was identified. As mentioned earlier in the chapter, it is a rule of thumb that the root cause is not reached until the fifth "why" question is answered. Once the causes have become specific enough to be measured, they should be evaluated for cost of correction and potential for improvement.

FLOWCHARTS

Flowcharts are diagrams that represent the steps in a process. They are used to evaluate inefficiencies, describe the current process, and train new staff. It is very important to include "process experts" in the development of flowcharts describing the current process. Process experts are the individuals who are actually performing the work being depicted by the flowchart. They are in the best position to describe what is really happening, which contributes to understanding of rework, non–value-added steps, and complexity.

PARETO DIAGRAM

A Pareto diagram is used to illustrate the 80/20 rule, which states that 80% of all process variation is produced by 20% of items. For example, if a nurse manager had a high prevalence of pressure ulcers, she might review prevalence data from the previous year to evaluate what types of pressure ulcers were occurring on her unit. She would then group the data into categories based on the site of the pressure ulcer. Next, she would place the categories in descending order of frequency and use a bar graph to display these data. She would add a second vertical axis to depict the cumulative percent represented by each successive category (Fig. 15-2). By using this tool, she would see that two pressure ulcer sites, coccyx and heels, represented 80% of the different ulcers occurring on her unit. She would have a place to focus improvement efforts by studying the causes of coccyx and heel pressure ulcers. Pareto diagrams provide a quick way to see where to focus attention.

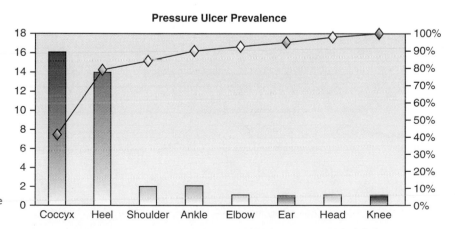

Pressure Ulcer Prevalence

FIGURE 15-2 Pareto diagram of pressure ulcer prevalence.

HISTOGRAMS

Histograms provide another way to view distribution of data. A histogram may be used when a run or control chart is not possible because the time sequence of data has not been preserved (Executive Learning, 2002). A histogram may be useful to understand patterns in data that are not apparent by examining lists or tabled values (Institute for Healthcare Improvement, 2004). For example, if a manager were trying to understand the types of medication errors that occurred on her unit during the previous year, she might use a histogram to display the frequency of different categories of errors. Using a graph rather than a table of numbers to illustrate the frequency of error categories makes it easier to see quickly where most errors are occurring.

RUN CHARTS

Run charts are graphical displays of data over time. The vertical axis depicts the key quality characteristic, or process variable. The horizontal axis represents time. Run charts should also contain a center line representing either a mean or a median. A median should be used if the data contain outliers, which are less sensitive to extreme values. Figure 15-3 illustrates this point. Data regarding the number of patients who left an emergency department without being seen by a physician were collected for 2 weeks preceding and 2 weeks following a process change. The run chart contains two center lines, a mean and a median. In both cases (before and after adding another physician), the mean is greater than

the median because of the 8 days when much higher numbers of patients left. These 8 days represent extreme values and, as illustrated, have a greater effect on the mean score than the median. The run chart also shows a pattern in the data: two extreme days occur in pairs and always following 5 days of lower values. After checking days of the week associated with the extreme days, the manager noted that they were weekends.

Rules may be used with run charts to pinpoint special cause variation. The previous example of the extreme values on weekends represents a special cause. Eight or more consecutive points, either below or above the central line, represent a shift. Six points all going up or all going down represent a trend (Executive Learning, 2002).

STATISTICAL THINKING AND CONTROL CHARTS

The topic of statistical thinking involves three central concepts: thinking about all work as processes; knowing that all processes exhibit variation; and recognizing, appropriately responding to, and taking steps to reduce unnecessary variation (Executive Learning, 2002). When managers do not understand these three fundamental concepts, they tend to react to the "ups and downs" of performance data that they routinely scrutinize in managing their departments. Statistical thinking helps us to understand when and how to react to changes in performance. When we do not use statistical thinking, we can waste a great deal of our valuable time making changes or celebrating "improvements" that are not sustainable. For example, we commonly exam-

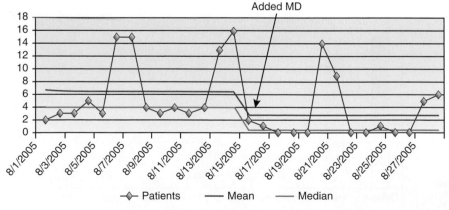

FIGURE 15-3 Run chart reflecting process change.

ine infection data on a monthly basis. We often compare the current month with the previous month or quarter. Some months will have a greater number of infections than others. Some months may have zero infections. A person who understands statistical thinking will know that these monthly fluctuations reflect normal variation inherent in the care processes performed by the individuals caring for the patients on the unit. If studied over time, the monthly values generally will fall within boundaries and fluctuate above and below the mean point of the monthly values. Figure 15-4 illustrates this point. The figure contains a run chart of a critical care unit's VAP rate over an 18-month period. The data reflect a rate varying between zero and five cases. The central line was calculated from the rates during the 12 monthly rates in 2005. On close inspection, one will observe that the rate was zero on two consecutive months, March and April, 2006. Without an understanding of normal process variation, the first month without cases may have caused some excitement, with even greater excitement on the second month of no cases, only to be dashed in May when the rate bounces back to four cases. Once viewed over time in the run chart, it becomes clear that the months where the rate drops to zero are a result of the same process that achieved rates of four and five cases in previous months: no cause for celebration after all.

Run and control charts are two tools that we have at our disposal to help us incorporate statistical thinking in our daily work. They enable us to discern special-cause from common-cause variation. Common-cause variation is "due to the process itself and is produced by interactions of variables of that process" (Executive Learning, 2002). The VAP example above illustrates this point. Special-cause variation is "assignable to a specific cause or causes. It arises because of special circumstances" (Executive Learning, 2002). The higher number of patients on weekend days who left without being seen in the emergency department is an example of special-cause variation. Control charts help us to predict the range of possible values we might expect from a process. Upper- and lower-control limits, based upon statistically calculated values, allow us to predict process capability. Without systematically changing a process, performance may fall anywhere within the upper- or lower-control limits. Choice of appropriate control charts and calculation of control limits will not be covered in this section. The reference list contains resources for those who wish to learn more about their use in health care.

Managers have many quality tools available to them. Choosing the right tool is important and should be based on the type of data or project goal. If the goal is to demonstrate and prioritize problem causes or categories of causes, then a Pareto diagram is the correct choice. If the goal is to examine process variation over time, then a run chart is the appropriate choice. If the goal is to understand where process design weaknesses put you at greatest risk for errors, an FMEA is the most appropriate choice. The next section discusses the role of risk management in identifying sets of conditions that put our patients and staff at risk of experiencing and making medical errors.

Risk Management

Risk management is a process used to minimize the loss of an organization's financial assets subsequent

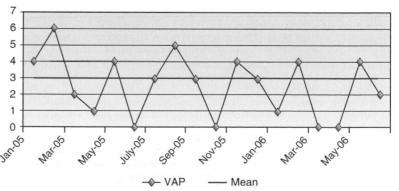

FIGURE 15-4 Run chart reflecting normal process variation.

Ventilator Associated Pneumonia Rate

◆ VAP   —— Mean

to injury to a patient, visitor, employee, or medical staff member. Financial loss also may result from destruction, theft, or loss of property (American Society for Healthcare Risk Management, 2003). Risk managers generally are nurses who have an interest in this area. Some have an advanced degree in law.

Historically, risk managers reviewed the facts after any event thought to put the organization at risk for a lawsuit. They would discuss the case with the caregivers, review the charts for documentation and, if necessary, get counsel from the organization's attorney. A goal of the review was to assess the level of the organization's liability should a suit be filed. If the review resulted in a judgment that the organization was at fault, the risk manager might recommend that any lawsuit be settled out of court. Should the review result in a judgment that the staff had followed policies and procedures and that the poor outcome was not a result of actions taken by the staff involved, the risk manager might recommend that the case go to trial should a suit be filed.

Today, many risk managers take a much more proactive approach by raising awareness of systems issues that might put staff at risk of making an error. This more proactive approach involves performing root cause analyses of near misses of events that might have caused harm had they occurred. A near miss is an event that had it fully evolved would have resulted in a medical error. Organizational leaders who promote patient safety believe that the majority of medical errors made by staff are the result of the design of the systems in place to deliver care, not individual staff negligence. Such leaders devote staff and resources to studying conditions that might result in errors so that processes might be redesigned to reduce the chances of repeating the error. In addition, communication processes are in place to share details of the near miss with staff who work in other areas within the organization in order to raise awareness of the event and the conditions that led up to it. The goal is always to reduce risk of reoccurrence of the error and to improve the level of safety for all patients.

In the event a patient does experience a bad outcome, risk managers evaluate whether care provided was consistent with the standard. A standard of care is the minimum level of service a patient should receive. Standards may be based on scientific evidence, professional society guidelines, regulators such as JCAHO, or traditional patterns of care.

Caregivers and organizations providing care that falls below the standard are putting their patients at risk of poorer outcomes and themselves at risk of legal action.

Using current and best evidence to make patient care decisions minimizes risk of providing care that is substandard. The following section provides information about evidence-based practice in nursing.

EVIDENCE-BASED PRACTICE

According to Melnyk and Fineout-Overholt (2005, p. 6), evidence-based practice "is a problem-solving approach to clinical practice that integrates:

- A systematic search for and critical appraisal of the most relevant evidence to answer a burning clinical question
- One's own clinical expertise
- Patient preferences and values"

What nurse would not want to use the most relevant evidence, clinical expertise, and patient preferences in daily patient care? Yet, as a rule, we do not. Many nurses say that the major barrier to incorporating the latest evidence into their practice is time (Pravikoff, Tanner, & Pierce, 2005). They do not have the time during their busy shifts to review literature or other resources. Pravikoff and colleagues (2005) studied the readiness of nurses practicing in the United States for evidence-based practice. The results of their study indicated that the majority (61%) of nurses require information at least weekly. Of those needing information, two-thirds preferred to seek information from colleagues rather than research. Among the reasons provided for not accessing research were lack of value for research, lack of knowledge regarding electronic databases, lack of access to a computer tied to the Internet, lack of a medical library, and lack of skills regarding reading and critiquing research articles.

Many studies have shown that patients do not receive care consistent with the latest evidence (Kerr et al., 2004). Williams and colleagues (2005) studied improvement in quality indicators submitted to JCAHO for three patient populations: acute myocardial infarction, congestive heart failure, and pneumonia. Eight quarters (third quarter 2002 through second quarter 2004) were analyzed for absolute values and improvement in compliance over time with these evidence-based indicators. One indicator, smoking cessation instruction, is included in each of the patient populations. The mean value at baseline for smoking cessation counseling in each of the patient populations was as follows: myocardial infarction, 65 %; congestive heart failure, 39 %; pneumonia, 34 %. At the end of the 2-year study period, improvements were evident, but still many patients were not receiving benefit of counseling.

Kerr and colleagues (2004) evaluated the percentage of recommended care received by patients residing in twelve communities in the United States. Recommended care fell into one of three categories: preventive, acute, and chronic. The results of their study indicated that, on average, 50 % to 60 % of recommended care was provided to individuals residing in these communities. Communities included major cities from all regions in the country. There are many reasons why patients are not receiving recommended care, but it is the leader's responsibility to create an environment that values and facilitates the use of current evidence.

BUILDING THE ENVIRONMENT

Creating an environment where evidence and best practice are valued requires careful thought and persistence on the leader's part. Creating such an environment involves more than improving access to professional journals and other scholarly materials. Ready access for busy clinicians is critical, but access alone will not result in the behavioral change necessary to incorporate use of evidence in daily practice. Providers must first believe that the effort will improve their practice and allow them to provide better care. Staff and nurse managers will have varying amounts of understanding regarding translation of research into practice. Some staff members will have completed a research course in their basic nursing program, but others may not have done so. Newhouse and colleagues (2005) identified four barriers to implementing evidence-based practice: inconsistency of the clinical question under study and clinical priorities of the nursing unit, staff knowledge deficit concerning critiquing and using research findings, staff feelings of being overwhelmed by the number of studies and different types of evidence associated with each question, and lack of time to focus on this activity so staff could do it correctly.

One idea to combat these barriers and build an environment for best practice is to work with the institution's librarian, if your institution employs one, to subscribe to online databases and electronic journals, arrange for education regarding online searches for research-based articles, and provide education and a framework for making decisions about the usefulness of particular studies to your patient population. Other ideas involve inviting a group of nurses to begin a journal club on a general topic such as critical care or a more specific topic such as care of patients with a tracheotomy or care of patients post myocardial infarction, and then expand to other topics or patient populations. Leaders may also want to develop a relationship with faculty from their schools of nursing who could act as a resource in helping staff develop skills in translation of clinical and administrative research into daily practice.

Outcomes Measurement

Outcomes measurement involves using scientific rigor to evaluate the effectiveness and efficiency of our work. Scientific rigor involves selection of reliable and valid tools to evaluate process and outcomes of care. Measurement is generally performed on a population of patients, such as patients with congestive heart failure or patients who are post hip replacement surgery. Outcomes may also be measured on heterogeneous patient populations, such as all medical-surgical or critical care patients. Outcomes typically measured in acute care are length of stay, mortality, complications, health-related quality of life, functional assessment, and costs.

As discussed earlier in the chapter, quality indicators may include outcome, process, and structure indicators. Unlike measurement of the other two types of indicators, outcome measurement generally requires statistical adjustment for patients' pre-existing conditions and socioeconomic status. Without appropriate adjustment, comparisons among different care providers, patient care units, nursing facilities, outpatient clinics, or hospitals are meaningless. For example, patients who are chronically ill with conditions such as diabetes or congestive heart failure have a much greater chance of developing a complication, such as a myocardial infarction or renal failure, than patients who are newly diagnosed. Socioeconomic factors such as age, income, and insurance status may also affect patient outcomes, independent of the care they received. For this reason, it is necessary to perform a mathematical technique called risk adjustment to "equalize" differences related to the patient's severity of illness.

According to Wojner (2001, p. 126), "Severity is a term used to describe a relative loss of function." Severity adjustment involves accounting for significant physiological changes associated with a disease state. Risk adjustment models, on the other hand, are used to predict the probability that a patient or group of patients will develop a poor outcome. Variables that place a patient at higher risk for an untoward event are identified from statistical analysis of similar cases predictive of the event, such as mortality (Wojner, 2001). For example, conditions that are predictive of death vary by patient population. Factors that might be associated with death of an inpatient may be specific to their illness, such as the presence of metastatic cancer.

There are many commercially available tools for severity and risk adjustment. Such tools are case mix index, all-patient-refined–diagnosis-related-groups (APR-DRGs), Acute Physiology and Chronic Health Evaluation (APACHE) scores, and Medical Illness Severity Grouping System (MedisGroups). For example, APR-DRGs use clinical logic, patient demographic information, comorbidities, and principal diagnosis to assign patients to one of four severity and mortality levels: minor, moderate, major, or extreme. Patients categorized as extreme would use far more resources and be significantly more decompensated than those categorized as minor. The same would hold true for the mortality categories. Patients who are categorized as minor risk for mortality (within their DRG) would be less likely to die than those in the extreme category. Because this type of categorizing system allows sorting of patients by severity class, it "equalizes" pre-existing differences among patients and allows for measurement of legitimate differences in outcomes.

All Good Things...

Quality is not a religion, but it does require a belief and passion, discipline, and the application of learned principles. The most common thread throughout all of the quality literature is leadership. And nurse leaders must answer that call. First, we need to become technically proficient in how to ensure quality in our units. Second, nurse leaders need to begin to see themselves as drivers of quality. That requires additional competencies in risk taking, courage, and political governance. The most important competency might be that of listening. Nurse leaders create the environment that allows the people closest to the work, the ones who "think outside the box," the innovators, to step forward and drive and create change. Finally, nurse leaders need to be acutely aware of, if not personally involved in, the dynamic dialogue in this country on how we are going to manage a health-care system that needs a complete redesign.

This chapter has presented a number of models, tools, techniques, and suggestions for creating an environment of improvement. Understanding quality and making improvements require use of data and a disciplined approach to improvement. A number of tools and models have been provided for that purpose. The chapter has also provided contextual information so that nurse leaders may understand how the current movement toward public reporting of quality data and pay for performance fits within the bigger health-care picture. Nurses must ensure practice is based on the best available evidence that is delivered in a reliable, safe manner.

Let's Talk

1. *Think of a time when you knew your staff members were delivering patient care inconsistently. Perhaps physicians were complaining about differences among the skill level of your staff, or patient complaints began to increase. You want to share your concerns with your staff and, at the same time, encourage members to use current evidence of best practice to redesign care processes. How might the tools and models suggested in this chapter help you "make the case" for improvement to your staff?*

2. *After presenting a Pareto diagram of the most frequent patient complaints received from comments on patient satisfaction surveys and calls to risk management, your staff members decide to set a goal of zero patient complaints by*

end of the year. Together you decide to tackle the issue of untimely response to call lights. Where would you begin?

3. *You might consider using a cause-and-effect diagram to get to the root cause of why response time is long. Once you have narrowed the issue to the root cause, you might want to do a literature review to determine best practice. You might also want to contact the patient satisfaction survey vendor to check if the vendor will give you the names of hospitals that have the best scores for satisfaction with response to call bells. What measures would you use to understand if you were improving timely response to call lights?*

4. *You might want to check if it is possible to get a patient call system report that provides average call bell response time by time of day. If available, you might want to use a run or control chart to examine patterns of either short response times or long response times by time of day and day of week. If patterns exist, you could study them so that you could build on the processes where response times are short and eliminate processes where response times are long. If a report is unavailable, consider collecting data by recording call bell response times for an hour during randomly selected hours of the day and days of the week. You might also use a run or control chart to track patient responses to the call bell question on your patient satisfaction survey. How would you determine if improvements to responsiveness to call bells were sustained?*

5. *Continue to monitor response times and patient satisfaction indicators to determine if the response times are stable (consistent over time) and patient satisfaction scores remain within the goal range. Post the response time and patient satisfaction run charts in a place where they are visible for staff.*

NCLEX Questions

1. Drivers of quality are:
   A. Nurses and physicians
   B. Regulators
   C. Payers
   D. B and C

2. According to Gerteis and colleagues, patient-centered care consists of the following patient preferences:
   A. Respect for patient values, preferences, and expressed needs
   B. Following the physician's orders
   C. Excluding family and friends from any discussions about the patient
   D. Putting the patients' physical comfort above any safety measures

3. Dr. Deming viewed quality:
   A. From a systems perspective
   B. Involving unrelated processes and decisions
   C. Involving management by fear
   D. Based on the biological sciences

4. Joseph Duran is best known for:
   A. The Pareto principle used to identify the "vital few" contributors to a problem
   B. The quality trilogy consisting of plan do, act
   C. Two aspects of the product, quality and cost
   D. Use of statistical thinking

5. Phillip Crosby was another quality theorist who:
   A. Provided the customer with a nondefective product
   B. Involved leaders who practice contingency leadership
   C. Defined quality as the extent to which processes are in conformance with requirements
   D. All of the above

6. Dr. Avedis Donabedian is best known for which perspective on quality?
   A. Structures consist of how organizations develop reporting structures
   B. The structure, process, and outcome paradigm
   C. Processes used to make nursing decisions
   D. Outcomes related solely to the finances of a hospital

7. The model for improvement involves the use of which of the following questions?
   A. How will we know that a change is an improvement?
   B. What are the defects in a process?
   C. Nurse-patient staffing ratios?
   D. All of the above

8. Process analysis and data display as quality tools:
   A. Involve diagramming processes to understand what causes waste, errors, or patient dissatisfaction

B. Involve use of run charts

C. Involve use of control charts

D. All of the above

9. Risk management is a process:

A. In which a risk manager assesses risk due to financial decisions

B. That involves managing problem employees

C. Used to minimize the loss of an organization's financial assessment subsequent to a patient, visitor, employee, or medical staff injury

D. A and C

10. Quality health may be defined as:

A. The patient assuming little risk

B. A zero number of errors made in the provision of patient care by health-care providers

C. Occurring when the patient is cured of any disease or ailment

D. The extent to which health services for individuals and populations are safe, timely, efficient, equitable, effective, and patient-centered

REFERENCES

American Nurses Association. (1995). *Nursing Care Report Card for Acute Care*. Washington DC: American Nurses Publishing.

American Nurses Association. (2004). *Scope and standards for nurse administrators* (2nd ed.). Washington, DC: nursesbooks.org, American Nurses Association.

American Nurses Credentialing Center. (2004). *Magnet recognition program: 2005 application manual*. Silver Spring, MD: American Nurses Credentialing Center.

American Society for Healthcare Risk Management. (2003). Barton certificate in health care risk management program glossary. Retrieved August 28, 2005, from http://www.ashrm.org/ashrm/resources/files/glossary.pdf

Atkins, P.M., Marshall, B.S., & Javalgi, R.G. (1996). Happy employees lead to loyal patients. *Journal of Health Care Marketing, 16*(4), 14–23.

Barker, K.N., et al. (2002). Medication errors observed in 36 health care facilities. *Archives of Internal Medicine, 162*(16), 1897–1903.

Barry, R., Murcko, A., & Brubaker, C. (2002). *The six sigma book for health care: Improving outcomes by reducing errors*. Chicago: Health Administration Press.

Centers for Medicare and Medicaid Services, & Agency for Healthcare Research and Quality. (2005). *Hospital CAHPS® (HCAHPS®): Fact Sheet*. Retrieved June 11, 2005, from http://www.cms.hhs.gov/quality/hospital/HCAHPS FactSheet.pdf

Deming, W.E. (2000). *The new economics: For industry, government, education* (2nd ed.). Cambridge, MA: MIT Press.

DeRosier, J., et al. (2002). Using health care failure mode and effect analysis: The VA National Center for Patient Safety's prospective risk analysis system. *Joint Commission Journal on Quality Improvement, 28*(5), 248–267.

Dobyns, L., & Crawford-Mason, C. (1991). *Quality or else: The revolution in world business*. Boston: Houghton Mifflin.

Donabedian, A. (1992). The role of outcomes in quality assessment and assurance. *Quality Review Bulletin, 18*, 356–360.

Executive Learning, I. (2002). *Handbook for improvement: A reference guide for tools and concepts: Health care* (3rd ed.). Nashville: Healthcare Management Directions.

Fonarow, G.C., Yancy, C.W., & Heywood, J.T. (2005). Adherence to heart failure quality-of-care indicators in US hospitals: Analysis of the adhere registry. *Archives of Internal Medicine, 165*(13), 1469–1477.

Flynn, E.A., et al. (2002). Comparison of methods for detecting medication errors in 36 hospitals and skilled-nursing facilities. *American Journal of Health-System Pharmacy, 59*, 436–446.

Gerteis, M., et al. (1993). *Through the patient's eyes: Understanding and promoting patient-centered care*. San Francisco: Jossey-Bass.

Hatcher, I., et al. (2004). An intravenous medication safety system: Preventing high-risk medication errors at the point of care. *Journal of Nursing Administration, 34*(10), 437–439.

Institute for Healthcare Improvement. (2004). *Histogram*. Retrieved June 5, 2005, from http://www.ihi.org/NR/rdonlyres/82F71CA3-5863-4FB8-9456-B0CB3F289777/1055/Histogram1.pdf

Institute for Healthcare Improvement. (2005). *How to improve: Improvement methods*. Retrieved April 30, 2005, from http://www.ihi.org/IHI/Topics/Improvement/ImprovementMethods/HowToImprove/

Institute of Medicine. (2005). *Institute of Medicine of the National Academies: About*. Retrieved June 11, 2005, from http://www.iom.edu/about.asp

Institute of Medicine Committee on Quality of Health Care in America. (2001). *Crossing the quality chasm: A new health system for the 21st century*. Washington, D.C.: National Academy Press.

Joint Commission on the Accreditation of Healthcare Organizations. (2005). *2006 Critical Access Hospital and Hospital National Patient Safety Goals*. Retrieved June 5, 2005, from http://www.jcaho.org/accredited+organizations/patient+safety/06_npsg/06_npsg_cah_hap.htm

Juran, J.M., & Godfrey, A.B. (1999). *Juran's quality handbook* (5th ed.). New York: McGraw Hill.

Kerr, E.A., et al. (2004). Profiling the quality of care in twelve communities: Results from the CQI study. *Health Affairs, 23*(3), 247–256.

Kohn, L.T., Corrigan, J.M., & Donaldson, M.S. (2000). *To Err is Human: Building a Safer Health System*. Washington, D.C.: National Academy Press.

Kondo, Y., & Kano, N. (1999). Quality in Japan. In Juran, J.M., & Godfrey, A.B. (eds.). *Juran's quality handbook* (5th ed., pp. 4141–4133). New York: McGraw Hill.

Landon, B.E., et al. (2004). The evolution of quality management in Medicaid-managed care. *Health Affairs, 23*(4), 245–254.

Langley, G.J., et al. (1996). *The improvement guide: A practical approach to enhancing organizational performance*. San Francisco: Jossey-Bass.

Laschinger, H.S., et al. (2005). A psychometric analysis of the patient satisfaction with nursing care quality questionnaire: An actionable approach to measuring patient satisfaction. *Journal of Nursing Care Quality, 20*(3), 220–230.

Lee, F. (2004). *If Disney ran your hospital: 9 1/2 things you would do differently.* Bozeman, MT: Second River Health care Press.

Lee, K.W., et al. (2005). Statistical tools for quality improvement. In Ransom, S.B., Joshi, M., & Nash D.B. (eds.). *The health care quality book: Vision, strategy, and tools* (pp. 145–166). Chicago: Health Administration Press.

Melnyk, B.M., & Fineout-Overholt, E. (2005). Making the case for evidence-based practice. In Melnyk, B.M., & Fineout-Overholt, E. (eds.). *Evidence-based practice in nursing & health care: A guide to best practice* (pp. 3–24). Philadelphia: Lippincott Williams & Wilkins.

Mitchell, P.H., Ferketich, S., & Jennings, B.M. (1998). Quality health outcomes model. American Academy of Nursing Expert Panel on Quality Health Care. *Image Journal of Nursing Scholarship, 30*(1), 43–46.

Mitchell, P.H., & Lang, N.M. (2004). Framing the problem of measuring and improving health care quality: Has the quality health outcomes model been useful? *Medical Care, 42*(2 Suppl), II4-11.

National Institute of Standards and Technology. (2004). Baldrige National Quality Program. 2005 Health Care Criteria for Performance Excellence. In Dept of Commerce (ed.): Technology Administration.

National Institute of Standards and Technology. (2005). *Baldrige National Quality Program. Award Recipients.* Retrieved December 6, 2005, from http://www.quality.nist.gov/Award_Recipients.htm

National Quality Forum. (2000–2004). *National Quality Forum Current Activities Archive.* Retrieved December 6, 2005, from http://www.qualityforum.org/activities/ca_archive.htm

National Quality Forum. (2004). *National voluntary consensus standards for nursing-sensitive care: An initial performance measure set.* Washington DC: National Quality Forum.

Newhouse, R., et al. (2005). Evidence-based practice: A practical approach to implementation. *Journal of Nursing Administration, 35*(1), 35–40.

Nielsen, D.M., et al. (2004). Can the gurus' concepts cure health care? *Quality Progress,* 25–34.

Page, A. (2004). *Keeping patients safe: Transforming the work environment of nurses.* Washington, DC: National Academies Press.

Pravikoff, D.S, Tanner, A.B., & Pierce, S.T. (2005). Readiness of U.S. nurses for evidence-based practice. *American Journal of Nursing, 105*(9), 40–51.

Spear, S., & Bowen, H.K. (1999). Decoding the DNA of the Toyota production system. *Harvard Business Review, 77*(5), 96–106

Spear, S.J. (2004). Learning to lead at Toyota. *Harvard Business Review, 82*(5), 78–86.

Stoecklein, M. (2005). Quality improvement systems, theories, and tools. In Ransom, S.B. Joshi, M., & Nash D.B. (eds.). *The health care quality book: Vision, strategy, and tools* (pp. 63–86). Chicago: Health Administration Press.

Thompson, D.N., Wolf, G.A., & Spear, S. J. (2003). Driving improvement in patient care: Lessons from Toyota. *Journal of Nursing Administration, 33*(11), 585–595.

Wachter, R.M. (2004). The end of the beginning: Patient safety five years after 'to err is human'. *Health Affairs, 23,* 4534–4545.

Williams, S.C., et al. (2005). Quality of care in U.S. Hospitals as reflected by standardized measures, 2002-2004. *New England Journal of Medicine, 353,* 255–264

Wojner, A. (2001). *Outcomes management: Applications to clinical practice.* St. Louis: Mosby.

Womack, J.P., & Jones, D.T. (2003). *Lean thinking: Banish waste and create wealth in your corporation.* New York: Free Press.

BIBLIOGRAPHY

Carey, R.G. (2003). *Improving health care with control charts: Basic and advanced methods and case studies.* Milwaukee: ASQ Quality Press.

Ciliska, D., et al. (2005). Using models and strategies for evidence based practice. In Melnyk, B.M., & Fineout-Overholt, E. (eds.) *Evidence-based practice in nursing & health care; A guide to best practice* (pp. 185–219). Philadelphia: Lippincott Williams & Wilkins.

Graham, K., & Logan, J. (2004). Using the Ottawa model of research use to implement a skin care program. *Journal of Nursing Care Quality, 19*(1), 18–26.

Lloyd, R.C. (2004). *Quality health care: A guide to developing and using indicators.* Sudbury, MA: Jones & Bartlett Publishers.

Ransom, S.B., Joshi, M., & Nash, D.B. (2005). *The health care quality book: Vision, strategy, and tools.* Chicago: Health Administration Press.

Stetler, C.B. (2001). Updating the Stetler model of research utilization to facilitate evidence-based practice. *Nursing Outlook, 49*(6), 272–279.

Wheeler, D.J. (1993). *Understanding variation: The key to managing chaos.* Knoxville, TN: SPC Press.

Wheeler, D.J. (2003). *Making sense of data.* Knoxville, TN: SPC Press.

chapter 16

Budgeting

PATRICIA M. HAYNOR, DNSC, RN
STACY GRANT HOHENLEITNER, MSN, RN, CNA, NHA

CHAPTER MOTIVATION

"Dorothy in the Wizard of Oz followed the yellow brick road. Budgets are maps that improve on the yellow brick approach!"

Patricia Haynor

CHAPTER MOTIVES

- Introduce the concepts of budgeting.
- Identify the steps in the budget process.
- Describe the types of budgets.
- Discuss budgeting as a management control process.

Health care is undergoing a transformation that embraces business values while trying to hold onto the professional concept of caring. Health care is a business with limited financial resources. Nurses are finding themselves providing care in an environment where the economics of health care are highly competitive and the costs of health care are closely monitored and frequently contemplated. "Nurses are entering into a new reality of practice that is controlled by costs" (Turkel, 2001, p. 69). Nurses need to keep in mind that money spent in any area must be budgeted. If unbudgeted money is spent, if the category is over budget or over the projected budget, then that money must be subtracted from another area. There is not an infinite supply of money that can be spent, no matter what the reason.

Take for example a personal budget. If you overspend, you try to accommodate this by spending less in another area. Or you go into debt. In contrast, if you spend less than the budgeted amount and are under your budget, you may have money saved for another area or to compensate for overspending. We do, however, have more control over our personal spending than the spending of our organizations. Our organizations are subject to many variables that influence both revenue and expenses. Just think for a minute about the many events that increase labor costs. Sick calls, leave of absence, and an increase in census or acuity are just a few of the incidents that increase the dollars budgeted for staff.

Fiscal Planning and Budgeting

"All planning involves choice a necessity to choose from among alternatives. This implies that planning is a proactive and deliberate process" (Marquis & Houston, 2006, p. 146). Planning skills are an essential function of nursing management so that personal as well as organizational needs and goals can be met. Planning has specific purposes and is one approach to strategy making. Planning also represents specific activities that lead to achievement of objectives.

Fiscal planning is an important, but often neglected, element of the planning process. Fiscal planning must reflect the philosophy, goals, and objectives of the health-care organization. As with all elements of planning, fiscal planning must be proactive, flexible, and clearly stated in measurable terms. The intended goal of fiscal planning is to create a budget that will meet the needs of the nurse manager and unit. When creating the budget, a function within fiscal planning, the nurse manager should take into consideration what may occur in the future that could potentially affect the unit's budget. The nurse manager must be proactive: look to the future and estimate or try to predict the "what ifs" or what could happen during the projected budget period. When predicting the budget for the fiscal year, start with what is currently known and what has happened. Review the previous year's budget to determine where the spending has been within the amount projected as well as areas where the spending has resulted in a surplus or deficit situation. It is important for the nurse manager to realize that there are uncontrollable factors that can affect the bottom line of the budget. The nurse manager must clearly state, in a way that can be quantified or measured, what is to be included within the budget and be flexible to adjust for any unanticipated factors that can influence the budget. Fiscal planning should incorporate short-term and long-term planning. When preparing to create the fiscal budget, nurse managers should involve as many staff in the input process as possible.

Keep in mind that practice makes perfect. Fiscal planning and working with a budget are learned skills. The more times managers plan and work with fiscal budgets, the more they are able to improve their skills and ability to complete the budget process.

"An essential feature of fiscal planning is responsibility accounting, which means that each of an organization's revenues, expenses, assets, and liabilities is someone's responsibility" (Marquis & Houston, 2006, p. 215). This typically means that the individual with the most direct control on any of these financial elements should be held accountable for them. In the department of nursing, this accountability generally is integrated into the responsibilities of the nurse manager. This results in the manager needing to be an active participant in unit budgeting, having a great deal of input into what is to be included in the unit budget, receiving regular budget data reports that compare actual expenses with budgeted expenses, and being held accountable for the financial outcomes that result from the operational budget.

The purpose of budgeting is to define a road map for revenue and expense while identifying cash needs. "A budget is a plan that uses numerical data to predict the activities of an organization over a period of time, and it provides a mechanism for planning and control, as well as for promoting each unit's needs and contributions" (Carruth, Carruth, & Noto, 2000, p. 16).

A budget's value is directly correlated to its accuracy. The level of accuracy is directly connected with the fiscal planning process. The more comprehensive the fiscal planning, the more people who provide input, the greater the amount of information gathered prior to finalizing the budget, the more accurately will the budget reflect the manager, department, and organization. Marquis and Houston tell us "because a budget is at best a prediction, a plan, and not a rule, fiscal planning requires flexibility, ongoing evaluation, and revision" (2006, p. 217). All budgeting is initiated through planning and forecasting. Budgets serve a dual purpose: they are numerical expressions of plans, and they become control standards against which results are compared or benchmarked. Types of budgets and the time frames of the budgets may vary.

Budgets are management tools. Preparing and working with a budget enable managers to reflect upon previous expenses and to be aware of current and future costs as well as the amount of resources that have been and will be utilized. As part of working with and comparing budgets, a manager will review periodic budget reports generally on a monthly basis. As part of this monthly budget review, the manager will compare actual expenditures for the month with the approved budgeted amount and the year-to-date budget status (see Box 16-1).

Box 16-1

Objectives of the Budget Process

- To provide a written expression, in quantitative terms, of the plans of the organization.
- To provide a basis to evaluate financial performance in relation to the plans of the organization.
- To provide a tool to measure fiscal and outcome compliance with the stated plan.
- To create a sensitivity and heightened awareness of costs relative to resources used.

CREATING A BUDGET

Nurses have been expertly educated to use the nursing process. The same type of process is the most widely used approach to preparing a budget:

Assessment → Planning → Implementation → Evaluation

Assessment

The first step within the context of the organization's strategic plan and financial plans is to assess the department and determine what needs to be covered in the budget to meet the organization's goals. The nurse manager assesses the needs of the area for which the budget is being created. It is important to involve as many staff members as possible in the budgeting process so that they have an appreciation for the resources needed to deliver their particular services or product. When nurse managers and their staff are involved in fiscal planning, staff members become more cognizant of what things cost and gain fiscal awareness that will lead to cost-consciousness and potential savings.

In the assessment phase, a significant amount of effort is spent validating the standard of care hours for patients in different cost centers. (i.e., intensive care unit, nursery, etc.). The standard of care hours is most frequently expressed as nursing hours per patient day (NHPPD). In other words, how many hours of care in 24 hours will be available to each patient? This number is used in the budget preparation process as a target. Another term used more recently to discuss the standard of care hours is nurse/patient ratio. This is expressed as one nurse to six patients (1:6), for example, and means that there will be one nurse provided for every six patients. California has legislation that mandates this ratio for medical-surgical patients. Other states are researching the outcomes of this legislative move on patient care and resource use (Garretson, 2004). NHPPD or nurse/patient ratios are calculated into full-time equivalents (FTEs) to plan budgets. An FTE is an accumulation of 2080 paid hours. It is not a person or position. It may be four people being paid for 502 hours each, or two people being paid for 1040 hours each (Fig. 16-1). Rohloff states that the majority of organizations define FTE by using 8 hours/day, 40 hours/week (8/40), and 2080 hours/year. Also common practice is to hire many full-time nurses at 12 hours/day, 36 hours/week (12/36), and

---

Calculation

Average Daily Census (ADC) x NHPPD x 365 = Required Productive Hours

30 x 8 x 365 = **87,600 productive hours**

Productive Hours to FTEs
87600 / 1800 = **48.7 FTEs***

Productive FTE = 2080 paid hours − nonproductive hours
2080 − 280 = **1800 productive hours**

*see Budget Definitions for further explanation of FTE

FIGURE 16-1 Nursing Hours per Patient Day (NHPPD).

1872 hours/year. Finance generally reflects these nurses as 0.9 FTE (Rohloff, 2006).

The FTE calculates the paid hours until the FTE hours of 2080 (or less if a 36-hour week) are reached. These hours are paid but not necessarily worked. Each accumulation of 2080 includes productive (actually worked) and nonproductive (holiday, vacation, sick) hours. The nonproductive hours are also called paid time off. Nonproductive hours become a significant budget calculation because it is time that must have staff coverage, an additional cost. Nonproductive calculations are dependent on benefit time off and vary from employer to employer and personnel category. For example, nonproductive time for a registered nurse may include three weeks of vacation, four holidays, and three education days. This is 28 nonproductive days or 224 hours. Nonproductive time for budget purposes is projected yearly during the planning phase of budget preparation. It is based on the total number of FTEs in each personnel category and their respective nonproductive time based on benefit polices. The salary costs are then calculated and added to the budget.

The assessment phase also entails forecasting and calculating the projected patient days for the new budget period. Projected patient days are based on historical trends, new programs approved for implementation, changes in care delivery, and reimbursement levels. For example, last year's actual days in post partum were 5250. The new budget is using these days and new patient days that reflect the addition of two nurse midwives who have been given privileges to care for and deliver patients. For the new budget year, it is projected that 600 new patient days will result from these new practition-

Budget Definitions

- **Accrual:** An accounting method that records expenses as they happen and revenue as it is earned. In nursing, vacation time is accrued as the employee earns it. This is usually recorded directly on an employee's pay stub in the pay period or month earned.
- **Bottom line:** An expression that discusses the income of an organization that is the result of revenue (money earned) minus expenses: revenue - expenses = income (bottom line)
- **Direct cost:** Items that can be directly attributed to a cost center and related to the service delivered. For example, salaries of personnel and clerical supplies for a particular patient care unit are direct costs.
- **Expense:** This is the amount of money an organization spends to produce its services or products. For example, wages are an expense to produce patient care.
- **Fiscal year:** A business accounting period. It is usually 12 months and is used to report fiscal activity of an organization. This accounting period can start at any month of the year and end 12 months later. For example, it may begin November 1 and end the following October 31, 20XX (the next year).
- **For-profit:** An organization established with the intention of making a profit to share with owners or stockholders.
- **Full-time equivalent (FTE):** An FTE is the equivalent of the cost of one full-time employee working for 1 year. In general practice, this is calculated as 40 hours per week for 52 weeks per year, or a total of 2080 paid hours per year. The 2080 hours include productive (actually worked) and nonproductive time (vacation, sick, holiday, education). More than one employee may work to reach 2080 hours to make up the FTE.
- **Indirect costs:** These costs may not be directly related to the cost center but are for the good of the organization as a whole. For example, costs for an advertisement for nursing positions and for housekeeping of public areas are indirect costs.
- **Nonproductive:** Time not worked but for which the employee receives remuneration, e.g., pay for vacation and sick days.
- **Not-for-profit:** An organization that does not have shareholders and reinvests its profits into the business.
- **Position control:** A monitoring tool to compare actual numbers of FTE employees with the number of FTEs budgeted for the cost center.
- **Productive:** Time actually worked by an employee.
- **Revenue:** The amount of money the organization receives for its services or product.

ers. The projected patient days for the new budget year will be 5850 (5250 + 600).

Planning

The second step in the budgeting process is to develop a plan. The length of time that the budget is to cover must be determined, and this time frame is the budget cycle. Budgets are usually developed to cover a 12-month period, known as a fiscal year. The fiscal year may or may not coincide with the calendar year. A fiscal budget year is broken down into quarters and typically further subdivided into months.

Most budgets are created for a 1-year period; when the budget period is over, the budget planning process starts anew. Although a yearly budget is the most common budget, a perpetual budget may be utilized. A perpetual budget is a continual process by which a budget is created each month so that a continuous 12 months of future budget are always available.

In the planning phase, the required personnel and supply costs are calculated for the projected patient days. This work is completed using a computerized spreadsheet application. The nurse manager begins the planning process by reviewing past budget history to determine average supply costs and the number of patient days or the average daily census for the unit. The nurse manager needs to determine if there will be any significant changes within the unit's supplies, either quantity utilized or if there will be any new supplies or an increase in current supplies related to patient volume, acuity, or diagnosis/procedure specific care. For example, a surgeon has joined the staff and will be performing a highly specialized robotic procedure. The surgeon is projected to perform 1500 procedures per year. The addition of this patient population will thereby: (1) significantly increase the patient days and the average daily census that should be budgeted for the unit, (2) increase the acuity of the patients cared for by the nursing staff, and (3) result in the nurse manager ordering high-cost specialty supplies to care for this patient population. Table 16-1 presents the remaining activities in the planning phase. These activities take the budget plan through its review and approval process. The budget process begins with the organization setting a direction and ends with implementation. This time frame is usu-

ally about 3 months. The activities from budget spreadsheet to final budget listed in Table 16-1 are the mechanics and review process of a budget. Usually the budget parameters are given to the manager as a spreadsheet application, which is the working document for the manager's cost center. The budget is presented to the reviewers; when it meets the operating standards set in the planning phase by revenue and expenses, it goes forward to the board of trustees for the last review. After action is taken by the board, the budget is returned to the manager for implementation.

Implementation

The third step is to implement the budget. Prior to implementing the budget, the nurse manager should thoroughly review the final budget and be certain that the budget is fully understood. The nurse manager will typically meet with her direct supervisor and a member of the finance department to generate the budget for the fiscal year. Being actively involved in the process allows the nurse manager to communicate information about their unit while learning the facility budget creation, approval, and implementation process. A nurse manager who is inexperienced in the area of budgeting should carefully review the budget for her area and ensure that a thorough review of the facility budget process is provided in order to establish a solid understanding of budgeting. The nurse manager should take the initiative to inquire about areas of the budget about which she or her staff members have questions.

During the implementation step of the budget process, the nurse manager must be actively involved in monitoring and analyzing budget activity to remain within the budgeted parameters and to avoid inadequate or excess funds at the end of the budget period. The nurse manager should review the approved budget for the fiscal year with the unit staff. It is especially important for the nurse manager to explain any changes from the previous year's budget. The staff needs to understand projected changes in staffing, patient population, and supply usage. The more the staff understands the budgetary goals and the plans to carry out those goals, the more likely the goal will be attained.

The manager generally is accountable for deviations in the department's budget. Some deviation

TABLE 16-1	Budget Preparation Process	
	ACTIVITY	**RESPONSIBILITY**
A		
Organization	Organizational Plans	Senior Management
Direction	Objectives for Fiscal Year	Senior Management
B		
Planning & Assessment	Preparation	Unit/Dept. Manager
	Care Standard/NHPPD	Policy/Historical
	Nurse/Patient Ratio	Legislation
	Patient Days by Unit	Finance/Budget Manager
	Current Position Control	Human Resources
	Projected Patient Days	Finance/Budget Manager
	New Programs	Senior Management
	Supply Projections	Finance/Budget Manager
	Budget Spreadsheet	Finance/Budget Manager
	Current Data to Spreadsheet	Unit/Dept. Manager
	Presentation of Budget Draft	Director/CNO
	Refine Budget Document	Manager
	Budget Presentation to Finance	Manager &/or CNO
	Budget Review	Finance/Budget Manager
	Organization Budget to Board	CFO/CNO
	Final Budget to Manager	CFO/CNO
C		
Implementation	Implementation of budget for new fiscal year	Unit/Dept. Manager
D		
Evaluation	Ongoing review of budget for new fiscal year	Manager, CNO, finance

CFO = Chief Financial Officer

CNO = Chief Nursing Officer

from the proposed budget can be anticipated, but large deviations must be examined for possible causes, and corrective action must be taken. Box 16-2 lists the rules of budgeting that managers live by. These rules or guidelines are the basic underpinnings that most organizations believe to be essential for sound fiscal responsibility. Budgets should be prepared, explained, and monitored by the same person who will be accountable for compliance with the budget. This person understands the workings of this budget best. This also means that expenses are charged to the cost center (e.g., patient unit) that incurred them (spent the money) and are under the control of the manager. Within

operating budgets for a cost center there are salary, supply, and equipment dollars. These dollars can be used only in these designated areas and cannot be carried over to the next budget year if not spent. Changes from the budget as planned are called variance and must be explained to the department head and have steps taken to correct them.

Evaluation

The fourth step is evaluation. The budget should be reviewed regularly to determine the level of adherence to the budgeted figures. The fiscal budget should be reviewed as often as daily when the newly approved budget is implemented. If variances from the approved projected budget are present, the nurse manager must react quickly by examining the budget closely. The nurse manager should determine what areas within the budget are either above or below the projected budgeted amount. This is accomplished by comparing the projected budgeted amount with the actual amount spent. Modifications in spending should be made throughout the budget period to accommodate for any deviation, and corrective measures should be put in place to bring the year-to-date total into the projected targeted amount. The budget process is continual and cyclical in nature. As the evaluation step is being completed, the nurse manager has begun to assess any deviations from the budget, thereby beginning the cycle once again (Fig. 16-2).

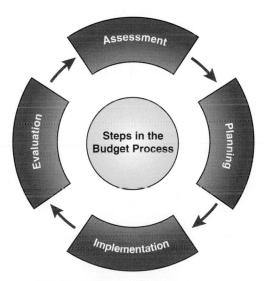

FIGURE 16-2 Steps in the budget process.

TYPES OF BUDGETS

The operating budget is a combination of the revenue and expense budget. It is a forecast of the revenue that is expected to be earned during the defined budget period and the expenses incurred to earn the revenue during the same period. The personnel costs are a significant part of this budget. This budget is a plan for the unit's or organization's daily operating revenue and expenses. It includes the workload budget (FTEs); units of service, such as patients days or visits; and expense budgets with personnel costs, supplies, equipment, and overhead.

A program budget contains all the items that are a cost in a particular care delivery program. This type of budgeting is frequently completed for new programs and expansions of existing programs of care or services. This is usually completed in the early phases of fiscal planning and budget preparation. If the new program is approved for implementation during the budget review process, then its budget becomes part of the operating budget.

Capital budgets summarize the anticipated purchases for the fiscal year and usually have a dollar minimum cost to be included (e.g. > $300). The life span of equipment projected during this phase of budget planning is usually longer than 3 or more years. The capital budget is separate from the everyday operating budget, and the funds for these purchases are usually released by the finance department when available for approved purchases.

The cash budget predicts expected revenue and payments for resource or cash outflow. An example of cash outflow is the payment of salaries for work performed. This budget, is monitored carefully to ensure adequate cash to pay bills in a timely manner and reduce the necessity to borrow funds to pay bills.

Supply Budget

Supply budget predicts the use of medical-surgical supply costs based on predicted case mix of patients for the upcoming fiscal year. The supply budget includes the expense of all supplies that are utilized on the nursing unit to provide patient care. Supplies are the area of the budget in which managers must be actively involved and can make adjustments to remain within the budget. The supply budget reflects expenses that change in response to the volume of service, above or below the budgeted census, and changes in acuity, requiring more, fewer, or completely different supplies. Controlling the number of supplies used in excess or in a wasteful manner is the responsibility of the nurse manager. This is not an easy task; it requires involvement of all staff members at all levels.

Nurse managers must be thoroughly knowledgeable of the supplies that are stocked on their unit, the amount that each supply costs, and the volume of each supply that is used. Each health-care organization will have a different system to ensure that supplies are available for use as well as for tracking the amount used. The nurse manager needs to control the amount of supplies that are available in her department as well as how these supplies are used.

Supplies should be researched to determine their usefulness. Ask the question: is this supply being utilized in the intended manner? Examine supplies that are frequently used and that result in high-volume usage, therefore high cost. Is there a way to decrease the amount of a supply that is used without affecting the quality of care? For example, if the manufacturer recommends applying one incontinence pad to a bed, and an employee applies four incontinence pads, it results in an unnecessary expense that can be prevented or controlled. Perhaps buying one pad of a larger size is cheaper than using two to four pads of a smaller, cheaper vendor. Look at prepackaged supplies. As with many convenience items, these can come with a higher price tag. If prepackaged supplies are being utilized, is every supply item that is included in the package being used? If not, compare cost with convenience; does the expense of the prepackaged supply outweigh the convenience?

Monitoring the supply process within the department must be an ongoing effort. This is not a single-person effort. The nurse manager must educate employees on the importance of utilizing supplies efficiently and encourage them to become actively involved in this cost-saving effort.

THE NURSE MANAGER'S ROLE IN BUDGETING

Historically, nursing management played a limited role in fiscal planning within health-care organizations. The department of nursing was considered to be non—income-producing; therefore, input was not sought or valued. Today, health-care organizations have recognized the importance of nursing involvement in the budget process. Nursing budgets generally encompass the most personnel expenses and are responsible for the largest share of the total overall expenses in health-care organizations. It is imperative that nurse managers gain expertise in fiscal planning and the budget process.

Budgeting is a challenging managerial task because it involves both planning and control functions. A nurse manager must perfect the ability to balance planning skills with control skills. Planning requires an innovative approach to the situation, whereas control can be perceived as restrictive or essentially negative and conservative in nature. In order for a nurse manager to utilize these skills successfully, he must be able to bring balance innovative and conservative view points. A nurse manager could be tempted to request the latest and greatest supplies, furniture, equipment, or increased staffing levels as part of the fiscal planning process for the next fiscal budget. The nurse manager must prioritize what is essential for his unit's functioning in order to deliver high-quality patient care. The nurse manager must ask for what is really necessary or utilize his planning skills while balancing this with control functions or not asking for what would be above what is necessary. This balance entails the ability to look forward or forecast future activities and anticipate what may be needed as well as the ability to look to the past to reflect upon what has already occurred. The manager needs to model scenarios that can change the forecasted numbers. *What if* scenarios offer a snapshot of what may happen if change occurs in the projected patient days, the case mix index, the availability of staff, or reduction in services offered. Forecasting is the selection of the scenario that fits the environment best. Success in budgeting requires thoughtful and deliberate forecasting along with the balancing act of planning and controlling. The staff needs to understand how the budget was planned and its role in using the resources wisely to reach successful outcomes for the patients and the organization.

VARIANCE ANALYSIS

After comparing the budget report, the approved budgeted figure with the actual amount spent, the manager determines if expenses are within, over, or

Budget Approaches

Fixed budget assumes that although there are variations in revenue and expenses through the budget period, they will balance out over time. This is a difficult budget to manage if forecasting of revenue and expenses is not on target. In spite of good planning, the fiscal environment changes many times during the budget year, and balancing over time may not occur without deliberate changes to the revenue and expenses.

Flexible budget is one that is adjusted for changes in the volume of services delivered. This is a reasonable approach that matches revenue and expenses as volume changes, allows for changes in the budget for volume increases, and demands reduction in expenses when volume decreases.

Zero-based budget starts with a blank sheet of paper, and every expense must be justified by the predicted objectives of the program. This type of budget is most often used for new services. This is the most labor-intensive approach to budgeting, but it encourages cost-avoidance activities.

As part of working with and comparing budgets, a manager will review periodic budget reports, generally on a monthly basis. As part of this monthly budget review, the manager will compare actual expenditures for the month with the approved budgeted amount; the year-to-date budget status is also reviewed at this time. Reviewing the outcome of the month's budget allows the nurse manager to identify areas that occur outside of the budget's parameters, either above or below the budget amount, and put corrective measures into place in a timely fashion. A monthly review encourages the nurse manager to utilize the budget as a daily management tool, thereby increasing knowledge and comfort level while working within the budget.

Nurse managers may encounter some difficulty with fiscal planning and the budget process. This may occur because the nurse manager has had little formal education or training in this area. As with any learned skill, practice is essential. Skills will improve with ongoing experience. In an effort to prepare nurses to be involved in the budget process, fiscal planning is included in nursing curricula and in management preparation courses.

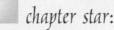 *chapter star:*

"As a new nurse manager, my biggest challenge was the planning and implementation of my first budget. I had excellent support from my new peers, director and budget manager in the assessment and planning phase of the budget. However, the implementation and responsibility to explain any variances from the budget frightened me. I was a firm believer in staff participation and I decided to involve them in the planning phase of the budget. This did require a few education sessions to explain budget terms like full time equivalents (FTEs), NHPPD and others.

"In each of these sessions, we also discussed appropriate use of supplies and I provided examples of products most commonly used. As the planning process proceeded, the staff and I reviewed opportunities to practice with the budget and steps that could be taken if we exceeded the hours of care planned or supply overages. I expected from this process that staff members would understand how a budget was created and implemented and would share responsibility to be accountable for the resources we used. Imagine my surprise when early in the budget year staff members approached me with ideas about how to stay within budget parameters when the average patient census decreased on a day to day basis."

Quoted from a new nurse manager working at an acute care hospital

under the budgeted amount. A deviation from the actual budgeted amount is defined as a variance. Some common reasons for variances are higher- or lower-than-budgeted patient average daily census, higher or lower patient acuity, and staff replacement or overtime. Variances from the actual budgeted amount (above or below the budgeted amount) should be identified and closely examined and investigated by the manager to determine the cause of the variance. Identified variances can serve as signals in future months to steer the manager away from the cause of the variance. At this point, the manager will do a **gap analysis** to determine what caused the difference from the budget projections. In other words, the manager will investigate to find an explanation for the gap between planned and actual. An increase in patient days might require more staff and may explain why the total NHPPDs are over budget.

In planning a budget, past variances should be examined to determine any patterns of usage or any areas in which the budget should be adjusted. Figure 16-3 presents some examples of worked FTEs, flexed-budget worked FTEs, and the result-

Cost Center Description	Actual Worked FTEs	Flexed Budget Worked FTEs	Worked FTE Variance	Actual Paid FTEs	Flexed Budget Paid FTEs	Paid FTE Variance
ICU	37.25	35.41	1.84	44.80	40.03	4.77
ED	34.39	33.42	0.97	40.52	37.78	2.74
4 North	34.81	33.79	1.02	40.04	38.28	1.76
3 North	34.25	32.26	1.99	38.93	36.45	2.48
1 North	13.44	13.15	0.29	15.36	14.75	0.61
1 South	42.42	43.85	-1.43	48.28	49.63	-1.35
Respiratory	15.33	15.08	0.25	17.55	16.71	0.84
Administration	1.75	1.73	0.02	2.04	1.92	0.12
ER Holds	0.76	0.87	-0.11	0.76	0.94	-0.18
EKG Lab	5.94	6.17	-0.23	6.59	6.86	-0.27
Nursing Admin	7.15	8.00	-0.85	8.18	8.90	-0.72
	227.49	223.73	3.76	263.05	252.25	10.80

FIGURE 16-3 PSH Hospital salary expense summary.

ing variance. The manager in today's environment must explain why this variance occurred and what corrective action steps will be taken to bring the budget back on target. A solution might be beyond the manager's jurisdiction and may require a review group for re-adjusting.

Variances are experienced in three ways: price, outputs, or inputs. A price variance occurs when the price paid for the resource is different than what was budgeted. An example from a nursing budget is when an agency nurse is used for staffing with the resulting dollar per hour cost being higher. Output variances may be higher or lower than planned amounts and could be more or fewer patient days delivered or change up or down in planned surgical cases. The input variance would entail different resource use than the budget plan. This might be that the budgeted NHPPD was eight NHPPDs and the actual was 10 NHPPDs. Actual NHPPDs become FTEs and salary expense. Figure 16-3 illustrates actual worked FTEs and flexed-budget FTEs. The flexed budget responds to the difference in required FTEs and resulting variance.

Nurse managers control expenditures of a major portion of institutional resources. Those resources can be utilized most effectively when the manager takes an active role in preparing and administering the budget. The budget should be a perpetual cycle of examining what has been spent, determining variances within the budget, analyzing causes of variances, and making modifications to correct the causes of the variances.

Cost Containment

Cost containment refers to effective and efficient delivery of services while generating needed revenues for continued organizational productivity. The goal is to deliver the services with high quality at the lowest possible cost. Cost containment is the responsibility of every health-care provider. The viability of health-care organizations today depends on their ability to use their fiscal resources wisely.

"In a budget, expenses are classified as fixed or variable and either controllable or noncontrollable" (Marquis & Houston, 2006, p. 217). Fixed expenses do not vary with volume, whereas variable expenses will increase or decrease based on volume. Fixed expenses include a building's mortgage payment and the payroll of salary employees. Variable expenses

Practice Proof 16-1

Article: Struggling to find a balance: The paradox between caring & economics

Author: Turkel, M.C. *Source* Nursing Administration Quarterly, 2001, 26(1), 67–82.

[NOTE: Article is available as full text via libraries that have subscriptions to CINAHL or ProQuest.]

This research study focused on the nurse-patient relationship within a framework of benefit and cost parameters from the perspective of patients, nurses, and administrators. The author used grounded theory techniques to guide the data collection and to accommodate the complexity of the nurse-patient relationship. A 250-bed for-profit hospital was selected for the study. The participants were 10 patients, 10 nurses, and 8 administrators.

The results demonstrated that nurses are struggling to find a balance between caring and fewer dollars. Administrators in the study viewed "caring . . . as the cost of doing things right and . . .the cost of providing quality" (p.78). Patients in the study feared that a reduction in nurses might occur to save money and expressed that "care" was why they come to a hospital. The study reinforces the idea that nurses and management must work creatively together to maintain the caring environment in fiscally challenged times.

1. This study focused on the nurse-patient caring relationship within the context of cost and benefits as viewed by nurses, patients, and administrators. Did you find any common themes discussed by these participants.
2. What implications for nursing practice did the author present?

Practice to Strive For 16-1

Best Budget Practices
- *Based on mission and strategic plan*
- *Use conservative projections*
- *Accurate budget targets*
- *Monitoring variances and corrective action plans*
  Clark (2005)

might include supply costs and the payroll of hourly employees. Controllable expenses are those that can be managed or controlled. Controllable expenses include the number of employees working each shift or NHPPD. Uncontrollable expenses, such as equipment depreciation and supplies that are necessary to deliver care, cannot be managed or controlled.

In today's health-care market, the increasing costs of health-care delivery have resulted in a strained health-care system. It is essential for health-care organizations to operate at the highest level of efficiency and to be acutely aware of cost containment. Nurse managers need to become increasingly aware of the need for cost containment. The old "This is how we have always done it" will not work in today's health-care market. Cost containment does not have to be thought of in negative terms. It does not have to mean a deficiency of care; think of it as doing things differently while delivering the same high quality of care, to save money or, even better, so as not to waste money. See Figure 16-4.

All Good Things...

The budget as a plan and management control tool is a "guesstimate" at best. The historical trends, assessment of the environmental changes, projected patient days, and case mix index used to build the budget are not a perfect science. Hence, the management of the budget during its fiscal year is an ongoing activity. Understanding that resources are limited and that each of us is accountable for what we "consume" to provide our product of patient care is a key point for all providers in the health-care system.

Creativity and innovation are necessary to deliver our product of patient care within the fiscal limitations of our resources. Whether it's our own personal budget or that of the organization we work for, resources are finite and as such must always be monitored and carefully utilized. Dashboards as a management tool provide timely opportunities to recoup budget variances and plan new strategies to avoid them in the future.

The manager may be the facilitator and monitor of budget compliance, but all of us are the stewards of the financial resources available to provide our product, patient care.

Date 3/21/200X			
Budgeted Census	30	Budgeted NHPPD	8 hrs x 30 = 240
Actual Census	24	Actual NHPPD	260 hrs
Budgeted Case Mix Index	1.31	Budgeted Average LOS	3.6
Actual Case Mix Index	1.31	Actual Average LOS	3.7
Budgeted Supplies	$1256	Actual Supplies	$1160

Unusual Events: None in previous 24 hours

The newest tool to assist nurse managers and staff live within the budget plan and help in monitoring costs and variances is commonly called a Dashboard. In concept it presents information in one quick look, much like a car dashboard but instead of gas gauges, oil levels and so on, it has Daily Census, Nursing Hours Per Patient Day, Length of Stay, case mix and supplies. It also may have an area to comment on unusual events of the past 24 hours, such as a unit census of 120% or a weather related call-out rate. This tool facilitates problem solving early in the biweekly payroll and supply cycle and gives the manager and staff the opportunity to avoid future variances in the same area.

FIGURE 16-4 Dashboard calculation.

Let's Talk

1. *Think of a manager you have worked with in a recent job. How did the manager involve the staff in planning the budget? How would you like to have been involved?*

2. *This past week your unit has experienced a significant decrease in census. Knowing what the NHPPD standard is for your unit, how would you expect your manager to respond to this change?*

NCLEX Questions

1. Which of the following is a leadership role in fiscal planning?:
   A. Coordinates the monitoring aspects of budget control
   B. Accurately assesses personnel needs using agreed-on standards or an established patient classification system
   C. Assesses the internal and external environment of the organization in forecasting to identify driving forces and barriers to fiscal planning
   D. Is visionary in identifying short- and long-term unit fiscal needs

2. All department heads are required to rejustify their fiscal needs annually during the budget cycle. Budget allocations are made accordingly. This is a description of:
   A. Incremental budgeting
   B. Perpetual budgeting
   C. Zero-based budgeting
   D. Capital budget

3. When over budget, you should accommodate by:
   A. Spending less in another area
   B. Closely monitoring and managing future expenses
   C. Examining budget variances to determine the causes of excess spending
   D. All of the above

4. If unbudgeted money is spent:
   A. Money that was not budgeted has been expended
   B. There is an infinite supply of money that can be spent
   C. The category is over the projected budget
   D. A and C

5. The nurse manager has the following responsibility for the budget process:
   A. Should have a great deal of input into what is included in the unit budget
   B. Should be an inactive participant in the unit budget process

C. Should receive budget reports on a bimonthly basis

D. Should not be held accountable for the financial outcomes of the budget

6. All of the following are true about health care except:
   A. Health care is a business with limited financial resources
   B. Nurses are finding themselves delivering care in an environment where the cost of health care is not an issue
   C. Health care is undergoing a transformation that embraces business values while continuing to value the concept of caring
   D. The costs of health care are closely monitored

7. The goal of fiscal planning is:
   A. To control spending across the board
   B. To create a budget that will meet the needs of the nurse manager and the unit
   C. To plan for only controllable factors
   D. To implement a budget that does not require monitoring

8. The term "cost containment" means:
   A. Save money by not delivering all necessary services
   B. The health-care facility puts expenses back on the insurance companies and patients
   C. Delivery of effective and efficient health-care services while generating needed revenues
   D. Utilizing an excessive amount of supplies to deliver care

9. A tool that assists nurse managers to stay within the budget is called a dashboard. What is monitored by using the dashboard tool?:
   A. Daily census
   B. Nursing hours per patient day
   C. Length of stay
   D. All of the above

10. During the assessment phase of strategic planning:

A. The finance department should create this fiscal budget based solely on last year's budget

B. The department should be assessed to determine what should be included in the budget in order to meet the organizational goals

C. The standard of care hours or nursing hours per patient day should be validated

D. B and C

REFERENCES

Carruth, A.K., Carruth, P.J., & Noto, E.C. (2000). Nurse managers flex their budgetary might. *Nursing Management, 31*(2), 16–17.

Clark, J.J. (2005). Improving hospital budgeting and accountability: A best approach. *Healthcare Financial Management, 59*(7), 78–83.

Garretson, S. (2004). Nurse to patient ratios in American health care. *Nursing Standard, 15*(19), 33–37.

Marquis, B.L., & Houston, C.J. (2006) *Leadership roles and management functions in Nursing: Theory and application.* Philadelphia: Lippincott, Williams & Wilkins.

Rohloff, R.M. (2006). Full-time equivalents: What needs to be assessed to meet patient care and create realistic budgets. *Nurse Leader, 4*(11), 49–54.

Turkel, M.C. (2001). Struggling to find a balance: The paradox between caring and economics. *Nursing Administration Quarterly, 26*(1), 67–82.

BIBLIOGRAPHY

Brady, D.J., Cornett, E., & DeLetter, M. (1998). Cost reduction: What a staff nurse can do. *Nursing Economic$, 16*(5), 273–274, 276.

Brown, B. (1999). How to develop a unit personnel budget. *Nursing Management, 30*(6), 34–35.

Dowless, R.M. (1997). Using activity-based costing to guide strategic decision making. *Healthcare Financial Management, 51*(6), 87–90.

Eckhart, J. (1993). Costing out nursing services: Examining the research. *NursingEconomic$, 11*(2), 91–98.

Finkler, S.A. (2001). *Budgeting concepts for nurse managers.* Philadelphia: W.B. Saunders.

Finkler, S.A. (2004). Evidence-based financial management: What are we waiting for? *Research in Healthcare Financial Management, 9*(1), 1–3.

Schmidt, D.Y. (1999). Financial and operational skills for nurse managers. *Nursing Administration Quarterly, 23*(4), 16–28.

Staffing and Scheduling

BARBARA SHELDEN CZERWINSKI, PHD, RN, CNAA, BC, FAAN

CHAPTER MOTIVATION

"No system can endure that does not march."

Florence Nightingale (Ulrich, 1992)

CHAPTER MOTIVES

- Describe staffing as a process with a relationship to scheduling.
- Describe various care delivery models and staffing and scheduling systems utilized by nursing services.

The nurse manager's **staffing** and **scheduling** goals are to assure the presence of adequate, responsible, qualified, and competent personnel who will provide quality nursing care services in a timely manner and consistent with the Principles for Nurse Staffing of the American Nurses Association (ANA) (1999). Additional goals in staffing and scheduling include sustaining congruence with the mission, vision, values, philosophy, and strategic plan of the organization and its nursing services and maintaining compliance with regulatory guidelines. Overarching objectives in providing nursing care services include patient safety and patient satisfaction. This chapter will discuss the staffing process with relationship to staffing plan, care delivery models, staffing and scheduling systems, and scheduling outcomes.

Background

The late 1990s brought with them a nursing workforce shortage, which has had a significant effect on nursing care delivery systems. A widespread nursing shortage in the United States translated into demanding and less attractive work environments (Kimball & O'Neill, 2002). Compounding the nursing workforce shortage were the alarming findings by the Institute of Medicine (IOM) in 2000, 2001, and 2004. Based on the IOM quality chasm trilogy series, which provided strong evidence for the need for safer patient care environments in the health-care delivery system, a redesign of health-care processes became imperative (IOM, 2000, 2001, 2004). To redesign health-care processes, local, state, consumer, professional, and regulatory organizations joined to seek solutions. The redesign would include plans regarding nurse staffing.

The IOM reports identified nursing as a pillar of quality and patient safety that must be strengthened to keep patients safe and retain nurses. Transformation of the work environment of nurses requires improving staffing adequacy, administrative support, and good nurse-physician relations (IOM, 2004). Staffing and resource adequacy are system-centered measurements advocated by the National Quality Forum (NQF) in conjunction with other nurse-sensitive performance measures to achieve an environment of safety (Kurtzman & Kizer, 2005).

NQF is a unique public-private partnership of more than 170 organizations, including the ANA. Examples of measurable nursing-sensitive outcomes are satisfaction, burnout, intent to leave, and costs. Examples of patient-sensitive outcomes affected by nursing care are mortality, failure to rescue, complications, satisfaction, and costs. Nurse staffing influences nursing and patient-sensitive outcomes.

Staffing

In 1999, the ANA published *Principles for Nurse Staffing,* which emphasized the nursing work environment to provide safe patient care. Subsequently, the ANA advocated a work environment that supports nurses in providing the best possible patient care by budgeting enough positions, administrative support, good nurse-physician relations, career advancement options, work flexibility, and personal choice in scheduling (ANA, 1999).

Staffing, according to the Center for American Nurses (*The American Nurse*, 2006), refers to job assignments. Job assignments include the following: the volume of work assigned to individuals, the professional skills required for particular job assignments, the duration of experience in a particular job category, and work schedules.

The process of staffing begins with an assessment of the current staffing situation. The assessment includes the qualifications and competence of the staff available (ANA, 2004). The next step is to formulate a plan to meet future needs. The staffing process culminates with a schedule (organized plan) of personnel to provide patient care services. Scheduling variables are defined as:

1. The number of patients, complexity of patient condition, and nursing care required.
2. The physical environment in which nursing care is to be provided.
3. The nursing staff members' competency levels, qualifications, skill range, knowledge or ability, experience level.
4. The level of supervision required.
5. Availability of nursing staff members for the assignment of responsibilities.

Appropriate allocation of nursing staff for patient-focused care (American Association of Colleges of Nursing [AACN]-Critical Care, 2001) or patient-centered and essential patient safe care (Bleich & Hewlett, 2004) is the desired goal of nursing staffing levels.

The ANA *Principles for Nurse Staffing* (1999) offer standards to incorporate and balance the needs of patients, nurses, and organizations committed to positive patient outcomes. The principles recognize that providing nursing care services can be multivariate and complex. The ANCC Magnet Recognition Program (2004) is an example of a quality recognition organization that has incorporated the *ANA Principles for Nurse Staffing* as a program foundation.

The ANA patient care **unit-related** principle of "appropriate staffing levels for a patient care unit reflect analysis of individual and aggregate patient needs" (ANA, 1999) is aligned with current research findings. Appropriate staffing concentrates on a higher proportion of patient care hours provided by registered nurses as compared with patient care provided by licensed practical nurses or unlicensed personnel for better patient outcomes. An appropriate staffing system incorporates patient needs, staff member skill sets, and staff mixes (ANCC, 2004). The *2004 University HealthSystem Consortium Nursing Work Environment Benchmarking Survey* (2005) of 59 academic medical centers found better patient outcomes and improved nurse satisfaction when registered nurses deliver a higher proportion of care.

Another nursing quality recognition program, the Texas Nurses Association Nurse-Friendly Hospital Criteria (TNA, 2005), has incorporated the ANA principle of staff-related "clinical support from experienced RNs should be readily available to those RNs with less proficiency" (ANA, 1999). TNA Nurse-Friendly Hospital Criteria are 12 essential elements identified as an ideal practice environment for nurses. One of the essential elements is "nurse orientation." The facility must demonstrate that it has a nurse-specific orientation program that considers the education, experience, and identified strengths and weaknesses of the nurse being oriented (TNA, 2005).

The ANCC Magnet Recognition Program (2004), a quality-focused organization, advocates that the organization has a function and productive system of shared decision making among the nursing staff members. An example of a shared decision-making process is a decentralized nurse staffing and scheduling system that provides *staffing* throughout

Practice Proof 17-1

A University HealthSystem Consortium study consisted of eight performance issues that identified staffing targets using benchmark data (UHC, 2005). The measures used were as follows: worked hours at or near organization target, reduction in vacancy and turnover, reduction in agency use, and increased nurse satisfaction. Evidence suggests that better patient outcomes result when a higher proportion of care hours are provided by registered nurses as compared with care provided by licensed practical nurses or nursing assistants. Inadequate staffing also leads to nurse dissatisfaction, burnout, and turnover (Gallant & Lanning 2001).

Research suggests that patient safety is affected not only by nurse staffing levels but also by nurses' education levels (Aiken, et al., 2002). The UHC study looked at these elements:

1. How staffing effectiveness is monitored and reported
2. The retention and recruitment plans of Human Resources to decrease turnover and vacancy rates
3. The monitoring system in place for nurses working over 60 hours per week and the amount of overtime worked
4. How the centralized scheduling office obtains a broad overview of staffing needs
5. The type of supplemental staffing or flex pools used to reduce or eliminate agency use and manage behind-the-scenes staffing work (recordkeeping, calls for time off, etc.)

Question: what factors discussed in this chapter might affect staffing?

the nursing operations of the organization. The organization's personnel policies and programs need to reflect minimal rotating shifts and creative and flexible staffing models. The staffing system adapts and flexes internal and external factors such as staff illness, shift changes in workload, and other uncontrollable variables. Trending data are to be used to formulate the staffing plan and to acquire necessary resources to make staffing adjustments in response to fluctuating patient workload and acuity (e.g., agency staff, float pool staff, overtime).

In contrast to appropriate staffing is inadequate staffing. Inadequate staffing came to the forefront of the nursing profession in the early 21st century with such national published and publicized reports as the IOM (2000, 2001, and 2004). In response to the nursing shortage, nurse working condition studies reported nurses' dissatisfaction with inadequate staffing conditions (Unruh, 2005). For exam-

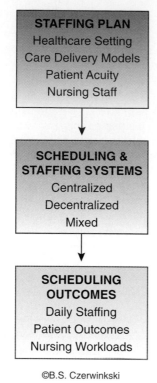

©B.S. Czerwinkski

FIGURE 17-1 Staffing process.

ple, inadequate staffing conditions are reported in acute-care (Aiken et. al., 2002) and long-stay nursing home (Horn et. al., 2005) studies as well as in national nursing (Stanton & Rutherford, 2004) and health-care standardization organization (JCAHO, 2004) studies.

The goal of nursing care is to provide patient-centered and essential patient-safe care (Bleich & Hewlett, 2004). The purpose of nurse staffing is to ensure patient care needs are met. The staffing process starts with a staffing plan and ends with positive patient outcomes and acceptable nursing workloads (Fig. 17-1).

STAFFING PROCESS

The staffing process is the linear incorporation of the staffing plan, the scheduling and staffing system, and the scheduling outcomes into a systematic flowing process. The following discussion describes the various components of each step of the process, beginning with the staffing plan.

Staffing Plan

The staffing plan consists of four different elements that must be addressed: the health-care setting, care delivery model, patient acuity, and nursing staff. They are then incorporated into the next step in the process, the scheduling and staffing system. A staffing plan can also be referred to as the staffing matrix.

Health-Care Setting

The health-care setting is where the patient care services are provided. It is the first consideration in developing the staffing plan. Geographical location and architectural design of the health-care facility will determine the accessibility of the nursing staff to the patient, which has ramifications regarding the work allocation and provision of the patient care services. Specific examples in the development of the staffing plan are the consideration of the location of the patient care supplies in relation to the point-of-use at the bedside and the walking distances between the patient bedside and the nursing station. The impact of the design of the health-care setting on system metrics was addressed by Gabow et. al. (2005). This study illustrated that nursing turnover and vacancy rates are influenced by efficiency, workforce development, and architectural effects on the work environment.

Care Delivery Models

Care delivery models, also referred to as nursing care delivery systems or patient care delivery models, can vary from one nursing unit to another, depending on the type of patients, the care requirements, and available resources. The focus of care delivery models is on the patient and how nursing care services are developed and provided. Nurse clinical decision making, work allocation (workload), communication, and management are included in care delivery models. The choice of model used is dependent on these factors, combined with the differing social and economic forces (Tiedeman & Lookinland, 2004). A care delivery model needs to address four components:

1. Patient needs
2. Patient population demographics
3. Number of nursing staff members
4. Ratio of nurses serving various roles and levels (ANCC Magnet, 2004, p. 46).

Care delivery models are classified into three main types: traditional, nontraditional, and emerging.

Traditional nursing care models are referred to as total patient care, functional, team, and primary nursing. Tiedeman and Lookinland (2004) found studies of traditional models of care delivery lacked the necessary methodological rigor. They were not able to draw conclusions about the impact of the model of care delivery on quality of care, cost, and satisfaction. Subsequently, nontraditional models of care delivery have been developed to address the changing needs of health care.

Nontraditional models of care delivery came about during the 1990s managed-care era. They reduced the professional staff in the skill mix and became a major cost-saving strategy in many organizations (Hall, 1998). Nontraditional models reviewed by Lookinland, Tiedeman, and Crosson (2005) used various combinations or skill mix of licensed nurses (registered nurses and licensed vocational nurses) and unlicensed assistive personnel (UAP). They found weak research evidence for the nontraditional models. They recommended that future studies must be rigorous and include nursing-sensitive outcomes such as nursing productivity; patient, staff, and physician satisfaction; and cost and quality indicators to allow comparisons across studies (Lookinland, Tiedeman, & Crosson, 2005, p. 79)

The traditional and nontraditional models are composed of division of labor, efficient use of time to perform nursing care tasks, cost, and training. These models use a mix of licensed and unlicensed personnel. Most traditional and nontraditional models are patient-centered. In specific patient populations such as adult critical-care and pediatrics, a family-centered care model is used. In the family-centered care model, family members with the patient are active participants in planning the care of their loved ones, including a role as direct caregivers. Nursing care activities are organizing care around the patient and the patient's family (Henneman & Cardin, 2002). In a redesigned model for providing professional nursing care for psychiatric patients, Allen et al. (2006) found the relationship-based nursing model provides an integrated network of relationships based on the values of caring: between nurses and patients, nurses and nurses, nurses and mental health workers, nurses and physicians, and nurses and the organization.

Hall and Doran (2004) studied three care delivery models in Canada: total patient care, team nursing, and primary nursing. The term "regulated nurse" is the Canadian equivalent of the U.S. RN, and in the total patient care model only regulated nurses provide patient care services. Their findings indicated that an all-regulated nurse staffing model has better quality outcomes for patients. They also determined that staffing models that include professional and unregulated staff may pose a challenge for unit-based communication and the coordination of care.

Donley (2005) advocates that care delivery models should emphasize radical redesign instead of incremental layering of tasks that are quickly becoming unmanageable. Summarily, the AACN-Critical-Care (2005) found that health-care organizations have systems in place that facilitate team members' use of staffing and outcomes data to develop more effective delivery models. Emerging models are concepts that are being developed and implemented. One emerging model of care delivery is the acuity-adapted room model. The acuity-adapted room model is patient-focused care that brings care to the patient rather than bringing the patient to the care. In this model, the room changes around the patient instead of the patient changing rooms. This is possible because each private patient room is equipped to treat all levels of care. From a joint research project conducted by a product manufacturer and a university health-care system, a cardiac universal bed was used in the acuity-adapted rooms (Johnson, Brown, & Neal, 2003). The acuity-adaptable rooms (also called universal bed or cardiac universal bed model) are appropriate for specific patient populations, such as coronary critical care and step-down units combined into acuity-adaptable rooms (Advocate Good Shepherd Hospital, 2005; AIA, 2001; Dunton et al., 2004; Hendrich, Fay, & Sorrells, 2004; Moody, 2005; and Pricewaterhouse Coopers, 2004). Thus, the time-consuming and costly patient transferring activities are eliminated. The nursing staff works as a team and is adaptable in scheduling to correspond to the patient acuities (personal correspondence with C. Gallaher, RN, MS, April 2005). The staffing plan is based on patient needs by patient classification level:

- Level 1 patient classification: one nurse for four to five patients
- Level 2 patient classification: one nurse for one to three patients
- Level 3 patient classification: one nurse for one patient

A new variation of the acuity-adapted room model has been developed. In this model, the acuity-adapted room within the health-care setting is designed for the patient to be physically closer to the nursing staff (Fig. 17-2). The diagram shows that well-designed units lead to increased efficiency,

elevate the quality of patient care. and improve the job satisfaction among the nursing staff. The objective of this model is to increase vigilance by the professional nursing staff, thereby enhancing patient safety (Meyer & Lavin, 2005). Each patient room is furnished with state-of-the-art medical equipment and a private bath. There is a nursing station for every two patient rooms. This arrangement allows the patient to be closely monitored without undue disturbance. Internet access is available in each of the rooms so the nursing staff can do their charting at the bedside. The rooms can accommodate family members who stay overnight.

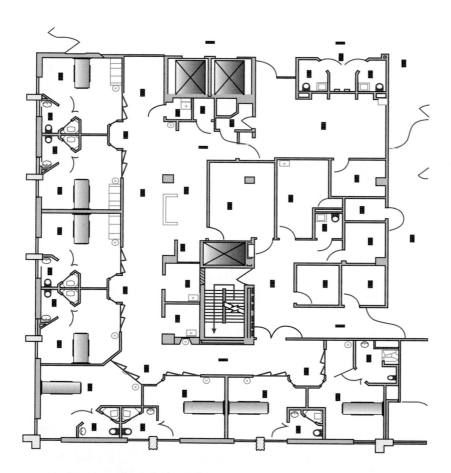

This architectural design provides a physical environment for nurses to be at patients' bedsides, the point of use.

The AACN-Critical-Care, the Society of Critical Care Medicine, and the American Institute of Architects Academy on Architecture for Health have recently cosponsored an ICU design award to recognize excellence in resolving both functional and humanitarian ICU design issues in a unique and complementary manner that focuses on planning and design. Criteria included a demonstrated commitment to creating a healing environment, promoting safety and security, efficiency, and attention to innovative, unique, aesthetic, and creative design features.

FIGURE 17-2 Cardiac Universal Beds (CUBs) floor plan at the Heart Center at La Porte Hospital, La Porte, Indiana (used with permission).

Acuity-adapted room models offer the following:

- Reduce the need to transfer patients to different hospital units as their status improves or worsens
- Assist with the continuity of care
- Increase patient satisfaction
- Provide isolation for infectious diseases
- Protect patient privacy
- Provide personal patient environment of comfort and reduced disturbances

Additionally, nursing satisfaction can be positive (Anderson, 2003).

Another emerging model is the Partnership Care Delivery Model. The AACN (AACN-Colleges, 2004) has advanced the role of clinical nurse leader, which requires the unit nurse leader to be prepared as a generalist at the master's level. The clinical nurse leader (CNL) provides care in the model. The CNL understands and interacts with the whole continuum and in partnership with all the disciplines (Tornabeni, Stanhope, & Wiggins, 2006). Smith, et al. (2006) reported a successful 6-month pilot using the model in an acute care setting.

Another emerging model example is the Transforming Care at the Bedside (T-CAB). T-CAB focuses on achieving outcomes associated with work reliability, patient centeredness, increased value (including reducing paper work), and work force vitality (Bleich and Hewlett, 2004). The T-CAB model pulls together an interdisciplinary team to assess problems, to develop, and to evaluate creative approaches for addressing the problems. The interdisciplinary team then disseminates solutions to other areas within the facility (Mason, 2006).

For critical care delivery in intensive care units, a practice model (Brilli et al., 2001) has emerged that is based on multidisciplinary group practice using the team approach. The team is led by a full-time critical care–trained physician in the intensive care unit 24 hours per day. This model is based on its ability to minimize mortality and to optimize efficiency while preserving dignity and compassion for patients. Nursing workloads in this model are defined by hours per patient day or the nurse-to-patient ratios.

Needleman et al. (2006) examined three approaches to increasing nursing staffing in hospitals and the cost of those approaches, without considering care delivery models. In an earlier study they analyzed data from 799 nonfederal acute care general hospitals in 11 states. In this study using the earlier data, they simulated the effect of three options to increase nurse staffing. They concluded that for hospitals using both RNs and LPNs, greater use of RNs appears to pay for itself in fewer patient deaths, reduced lengths of hospital stay, and decreased rates of hospital-linked complications, such as urinary tract infections, pneumonia, and cardiac arrest.

Regardless of what model of care is used, the nursing education and practice must be client- (patient)-centered, generate quality outcomes, and be cost-effective (AACN-Colleges, 2004). Outcome system-centered measures are skill mix (RN, LPN, UAP, and contract), nursing care hours per patient day (RN, LPN, and UAP), and practice environment measures that include staffing and resource adequacy (Kurtzman & Kizer, 2005). The quality and safety of the nursing services provided are tied to the professional nurse and patient ratios and/or the **nurse/patient index**.

Patient Acuity

Patient needs are summarized in patient acuity systems. Patient needs are specific to each patient, and conditions may change from hour to hour, shift to shift, day to day, and so on. Thus, staffing plans need to be modified constantly. In patient acuity or severity systems, patients are assigned a location in a hospital based on an acuity system and/or admitting diagnoses. For example, patients can be assigned to an intensive care, intermediate care, progressive care, medical-surgical, or obstetrical unit, and by age such as pediatrics versus adults. Medical-surgical unit patient assignments are often further refined into medical diagnoses or disease systems such as cardiac, oncology, and transplant. Patients are often transferred from one unit to another based on nursing skill levels and/or medical therapeutic and diagnostic procedures needed. Moving patients from one unit to another increases the nursing workload for admissions, transfers, and discharges during a 24-hour period. These activities are not usually accounted for in the **daily patient census** accountings. Daily patient census counts are done once during the 24 hours, most generally at midnight. The admission, transfer, and discharge activities of patient care add to the overall unit workload.

A benchmarking study of U.S. critical care units found the number of nurses needed for basic staffing plans involves expected patient census, specialized skills for patient-care technologies (e.g., balloon pumps, dialysis), and the skill mix of the staff (Kirchhoff & Dahl, 2006, p. 20). A formal patient acuity system has the lowest priority for staff planning. Patient activity is determined by services (nursing, medical, and pharmacy interventions) delivered and not by patient demographics. In a simulated model using actual data provided by Titler et al. (2005), the cost is related to the nurse staff using Nursing Interventions Classification (NIC) data captured in an electronic **documentation** system from 11,756 hospitalizations from 8988 patients. Titler, et al., analyzed the effects of staffing, treatment, pharmacy, and nursing intervention over cost. They found increased costs with higher nurse-to-patient ratios. The Titler study also found, however, that RN staffing below the unit's average (RN/patient dip proportion variable) also costs money. It is interesting to note that this finding (low RN staffing) had not been previously examined (p. 304).

Nursing Staff

The work activity of the nursing staff includes **direct care, indirect care, unit-related, personal time,** and **documentation** (Urden & Roode, 1997). Staff members refer to all personnel reporting to the nurse administrator (ANCC, 2004, p. 84). Staff nurse refers to an RN responsible for the direct and indirect care of patients in the hospital (McClure and Hinshaw, 2002, p. 7). Staff members, as defined by Mosby (2005), are people who work toward a common goal and are employed or supervised by someone of higher rank, such as the nurses in a hospital. Staffing is the process of assigning people to fill the roles designed for an organizational structure through recruitment, selection, and placement.

According to the ANCC 2004 Magnet Recognition Guidelines, direct patient care nurses (staff nurses) are responsible for patient-centered nursing activities carried out in a patient's presence (e.g., admission/transfer/discharge, patient teaching, patient communications). Nursing staff categories for direct patient care nurses include those counted in the staffing matrix or plan, assigned greater than 50% to direct care responsibilities, and replaced during a shift if they call in sick (ANCC, 2004, p. 118).

Staff competencies and qualifications are outlined in job or position descriptions and measured through continuing educational activities, manda-

tory education, and personnel evaluations. Those who require licensure or certifications to perform their job must keep up to date, with no lapse. Qualified nurses with disabilities *can be successful practitioners* with reasonable accommodations in the workplace (Gatens, 1972). Historically, nursing has been seen as a career requiring considerable physical function and strength. However, much of what the modern nurse accomplishes is done through cognitive function. Such cognitive functions are assessment, problem solving, deduction, counseling, and evaluation (Pischke-Winn, Andreoli, & Halstead, 2004).

A unit staffing plan needs to take into consideration specific patient dependency levels, high-risk patient handling tasks, and the nursing staffs' physical abilities. Nurses are working less in acute care settings as they get older, choosing instead employment in areas not as physically demanding (Norman et al., 2005). Work-site accommodations aimed to prevent potentially career-ending back, neck, and musculoskeletal injuries in nurses are considerations. Staffing for patient handling and nursing staff safety is determined by patient handling and lifting needs and institutional lifting policies and resources (Nelson & Baptiste, 2004). For example, the nurses face challenges in caring for morbidly obese patients in the acute care setting (Drake et al., 2005). A patient-handling resource example is the HoverMatt System for patient transfer using a lateral transfer and repositioning device (Barry, 2006).

SCHEDULING AND STAFFING SYSTEMS

Once the variables of health-care setting, care delivery models, patient acuity, and nursing staff have been determined, the staffing process continues into the development of the schedule. Scheduling is defined as the process of making the personnel work assignments for a specific period. Nursing schedules are communicated to the staff in a manual format (paper and pencil) or by computer. Computer software by traditional client server application is available. Online tools—partly or exclusively on the Internet—give personnel access to and responsibility for self-scheduling (Sabet, 2005). Automated nurse scheduling operational systems are commercially available. Using techno-solutions for staffing and scheduling systems will increase efficiency and improve patient care (Forte, 2004; Simpson, 2004). Technological advancements such as Flexestaff offer eShift and applications for computerized scheduling and staffing. Another, Per-Sé Technologies' ANSOS One-Staff, provides resource management capabilities that include enterprise scheduling with shift bidding and self-scheduling capabilities.

Depending on the organization, the period of the schedule can be determined from a matter of weeks up to a year in advance. Staffing refers to the filling of open shifts, or time periods, on the work schedule. A scheduling system pulls all of the variables together. The nurse manager's goal is to uphold standards to organize and schedule the nursing staff to provide quality patient care services.

Consideration and variables needed to plan and implement a nurse-staffing schedule are drawn from institutional policies, regulatory agencies, and professional organization standards. Legislatively mandated minimum staffing ratios, public postings, and collective bargaining agreements also help direct scheduling. In conjunction with budgetary guidelines and staff vacancies, the nurses' employment status of seniority, probationary, in-orientation, full- or part-time, and career ladder classification along with vacation, sick leave, and leave of absence benefits are also variables for consideration. Nurse-staffing schedules are multifaceted and complicated by seasonal changes, planned and unplanned life-changing events, and disasters.

Unlike manufacturing facilities where standard shifts and days off are the rule, hospitals and long-term health-care facilities operate 24 hours a day, 7 days a week, and face widely fluctuating demands. Hospitals primarily have five shifts: three 8-hour shifts (7 a.m. to 3 p.m., 3–11 p.m., 11 p.m. to 7 a.m.) and two 12-hour shifts (7 a.m. to 7 p.m.; 7 p.m. to 7 a.m.). Some hospitals utilize other shift times such as 4- and 10-hour shifts.

Work schedules can be 4-hour, 8-hour, 10-hour, 12-hour, longer than 12-hour, or a combination. The 40-hour work week typically constitutes full-time employment. However, a 36-hour work week is considered full-time in some organizations. Part-time employment status can vary by organization. Shift rotation systems vary by start time and have permanent designation or rotation combinations.

Actual time scheduled for a nurse to work centers around a normal working schedule of 40 hours to be worked in a 7-day period. Shift, weekend, and holiday rotations are considerations. For example, a nurse cannot be scheduled to rotate more than two different shifts in any 4-week scheduling period. Other considerations (Ohio Nurses Association, 2005) for scheduling nursing staff can be as follows:

- Staff should have at least two shifts off duty during the transition from the completion of working one shift or 8 hours to the starting time of a different shift (referred to as recovery time)
- 4-week schedules shall be posted at least 14 days prior to the beginning of the schedule
- Staff should be scheduled to be off duty two out of every four weekends
- No nurse will be required to work more than 6 consecutive days without a day off
- Flexible scheduling of 12 hours will be in agreement with affected nurses and on particular units
- Holiday time is rotated based on seniority

Scheduling and staffing models can be centralized, decentralized, or mixed (modified centralized staffing) (Lauw & Gares, 2006; Sabet, 2005). Centralized staffing involves a system whereby a master plan is developed as the top level of the organization in a centralized location, frequently the central nursing office. This system offers the opportunity to oversee the entire organization's nursing services activities. Decentralized staffing is a unit-based plan with corresponding schedules managed by the unit nurse manager. Mixed staffing combines centralized and decentralized to offer a comprehensive overview of a facility while offering individualization for unit and staff members.

Scheduling methodologies are rotational or cyclical scheduling, self-scheduling, and preference scheduling, which is a combination of the first two. Scheduling plans with various methodologies can be centralized, decentralized, and mixed, depending on management and staff nurse participation.

Centralized

Cyclical staffing is a centralized system in which workdays and time off for personnel are repeated in regular cycles, such as every 6 weeks (Howell, 1966). Centralized staffing involves a system whereby a master plan is developed at the top level of the organization. A centralized system works well in large organizations where management oversees strategy, budget, resources, and process (Sabet, 2005). A centralized system offers management a broader overview and closer control of the entire scheduling and staffing system. An obvious disadvantage of the centralized system is that individual considerations are minimized.

Decentralized

In decentralized staffing, the managers of individual nursing units have more control over the budget, resources, and process. For example, unit-based staffing and utilization committees can develop schedules. Membership consists of the nurse manager and staff members to oversee unit-specific staffing utilization, providing safe patient care on appropriate, efficient, and cost-effective bases. Staffing levels would be monitored on an ongoing basis (Texas Nursing, 2001). Under a decentralized scheduling and staffing system, a nursing unit can be accountable for outcomes and would be self-reliant for resources.

Mixed or Preference Scheduling

Mixed staffing combines centralized and decentralized staffing by offering individual units the ability to manage regular schedules with assistance from the central staffing office for shift coverage or other clinical resources for patient activity changes. Mixed staffing can accommodate nursing personnel's need for flexible or preference scheduling.

Flexible scheduling is one of the advantages of working in health care because many facilities are open 24 hours a day, but this also means some health-care professionals have to work on holidays. Flexible scheduling is a strategy aimed at improving retention and offers balance and enhancement between professional and personal-life activities. Flexible scheduling can be combined with **self-scheduling**. Self-scheduling offers increased autonomy and job satisfaction. Nursing staff is able to enjoy the ability to participate in self-scheduling as well as being able to work shifts that are in 4- to 12-hour increments. Many organizations now offer flexible schedules to accommodate the needs of both practicing nurses and students (Kimball & O'Neil, 2002), and have thereby improved the work environment.

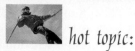

hot topic:
Shift Bidding

Because nursing is a 24/7 business, scheduling modalities are always a topic of discussion. In the past, hospitals tried the following: the 12-hour shift, work 32 hours and paid for 40 hours, weekend schedule composed only of two to three 12-hour shifts, and self-scheduling. Today with the growth of health-care informatics, shift bidding has become a popular scheduling modality.

Shift bidding is accomplished by the purchase of a software system. The system allows the nurse to access the software program via the Internet anywhere at any time and review available shifts. eShift is the trademark of one type of software. Shift bidding involves the use of the software system by the staff nurse to bid for extra shifts. Both part-time and full-time staff may choose their committed shifts for a month at a time. Shift bidding is similar to eBay, as the nurse can bid auction-style on available nursing shifts over the Internet. Shift-bidding software systems incorporate an overtime rate and a flat fee for the winning shift. Shift bidding allows not only part-time or registry nurses to bid for shifts but is also popular among health-care systems where a nurse may choose to work overtime at a system hospital other than the one where she normally works.

Shift bidding offers flexibility and control to the staff nurse over their schedule and higher rates of pay, which contribute to staff nurse satisfaction. The nurse has the opportunity to control her schedule, rate of pay, and in some cases commute to work. Shift bidding also affords the staff nurse the opportunity to reverse auction. After the self-schedule process, remaining shifts become available for auction. Shifts are posted with a maximum hourly rate. The lowest bidder wins the shift when the auction closes. Shift bidding automates the scheduling system because nurses are tapped from several pools. Hospitals save money in recruiting nurses to work overtime, pay less money in overtime costs due to the reduced use of agency nurses, and also reduce vacancy rates for hard-to-fill shifts. Times savings are another benefit for nursing management as shift bidding provides a 24-hour self-service process for staff nurses. Registry nurses do not have to share administrative costs with an agency and can make more money. Finally, shift bidding increases the quality of patient care as the system provides more continuity in staffing for units and hospitals.

SCHEDULING OUTCOMES

The implementation of the planned schedule culminates in the daily activities of the patient care team and the subsequent results of that care: the outcomes.

Daily Staffing

Daily staffing, or activation of schedule, is the outcome of the scheduling and staffing system for a specific date and time. It dictates who specifically will interact with which patient and when. Daily staffing, the implementation of the staffing schedule, is affected by the actual assigned nursing workload to the scheduled nursing staff. Daily staffing changes can be warranted for various reasons such as call-ins, patient care needs, patient census changes, and internal and external disasters. Often, staffing adjustments are needed hour-to-hour depending on the patient care activities and needs. Balancing the staff scheduled and the daily staffing workload is a major challenge to the nurse manager. Daily staffing adjustments can be managed by the following options: using other clinical resources and hiring overtime and temporary staffing. Examples of clinical resources for making staffing adjustments include STAT, float pool or admitting nurses, and a rapid response team.

STAT nurses are a pool of nurses, usually with critical-care experience, who respond to crisis situations such as sudden cardiac arrests ("codes") or traumas or who provide assistance with special procedures (e.g., conscious sedation, transport critically ill patients) (Scalise, 2005). STAT nurses may also be the skin and wound assessment team (Lancellot, 1996) to assist bedside nursing staff with prevention of hospital-acquired pressure ulcers.

Float pool nurses are experienced generalist or specialized staff available to be assigned as needed to any nursing unit. Often, these nurses can work 2 to 4 hours and move on to the next unit in need. Some providers have created in-house nursing agency pools to help meet seasonal demands.

Admitting nurses are an integral part of the patient throughput process in acute-care settings and intake process for home-health care. They complete databases, initiate consults (e.g., skin care and pain management) and falls protocols, initiate medical orders, and generally ease the patient's transition into hospital or home-care settings.

Rapid response team, also known as the medical emergency team, is a team of clinicians who bring clinical expertise to the patient bedside (Scholle & Mininni, 2006). Similarly, a multidisciplinary system-wide action team (SWAT) coordinated by nursing leadership in response to increasing patient census and acuity has been found to be effective for diagnostic testing and scheduling, expediting the admission process, reducing discharge delays, and staffing to hospital census demands (Tachibana & Hardy, 2001).

Temporary/supplemental staffing nurses come from agencies often referred to as "rent-a-nurse" providers, which, although not currently regulated, can apply voluntarily for JCAHO certification. Traditionally, these temporary nurses are paid per diem and are reimbursed for traveling expenses. Use of temporary staffing personnel has great patient safety implications because, often, credentials and experiences are not easily verified. The fatigue factor becomes an issue as, in some cases, agency nurses also work at another institution and do temporary staffing for extra income. There is a national trend to reduce dependency on temporary staffing options (Kovner et al., 2002; Morse et al., 2005).

Overtime

Overtime, or extended hours, is defined as continuing to work beyond or before one's scheduled hours. Nurses can work extended hours under mandatory and voluntary overtime scheduled conditions. Collective bargaining contracts often address the issue of overtime by setting the terms for mandating or requiring overtime work. An example contract (Ohio Nurses Association, 2005) defines mandatory overtime as no nurse will be required to work overtime for a period of more than 4 hours. No nurse may be mandated to work more than 16 hours of overtime in any 4-week schedule. A nurse will have a minimum of 8 hours off between shifts, when one such shift is a mandated shift. Overtime work can leave nurses fatigued and affect their ability to provide adequate clinical judgments and care.

Gaines and Carter (1989) offer a decision-making framework in which to analyze the overtime situation by examining individual rights and responsibilities as a professional nurse. Mandatory overtime should not be a "routine" staffing backup plan and should reflect staff nurse input (Shirey,

2005). Working long hours has caused nurse illness and injury, fatigue and safety problems, workplace violence, and depression (Mason and Kany, 2005). Major national and state efforts are under way to eliminate mandatory overtime (Unruh, 2005).

Currently, because there are no governmental regulations restricting overtime, nurse overtime is not federally limited. No state or federal regulations restrict the number of hours a nurse may voluntarily work in 24 hours or in a 7-day period (IOM, 2004, p. 388). Several states have laws that protect patients by limiting hospitals' use of forced overtime. In states with these laws, however, nurses can voluntarily work overtime, and the laws do not apply in the case of a government-declared state of emergency. Jacobsen et al. (2002) polled the nursing staff on their opinions about both voluntary and mandatory overtime and identified conditions that influence the nursing staffs' decisions and perceptions about overtime. This study enabled the nursing staff to develop strategies and policies to avoid mandatory overtime and improve staff satisfaction and quality patient care.

Patient Outcomes

The nurse staffing variables used to measure patient outcomes are daily average hours of care, ratio of RNs to **average patient census**, workload, and skill mix. Patient outcomes most generally are based on adverse occurrences such as unit rates of patient falls, pressure ulcers, respiratory and urinary tract infections, and family-patient complaints. Other nursing-sensitive indicators for outcomes are RN job satisfaction, RN education and certification, pediatric pain assessment cycle, pediatric intravenous infiltration rate, and patient assault rate. Since 1994, a national database program, the National Database of Nursing Quality Indicators (NDNQI), has been available to provide comparative information to health-care facilities for use in quality improvement activities and to develop national data on the relationship between nurse staffing and patient outcomes (NDNQI 7/m, 12/05, www.nursingquality.org). In the Commonwealth of Massachusetts for public disclosure, health-care consumers can go on line to access staffing plans for comparisons with actual staffing numbers when hospitalized (Scalise, 2006).

Nursing Workloads

Daily staffing is affected by the workload assigned to the scheduled nursing staff, as evident in research studies. Carayon and Gürses (2005) identified the assigned workload as the situation-level workload. Situation-level workloads are real-time performance obstacles and facilitators that contribute to daily workloads. For example, Tucker et al. (2002), in a qualitative study, observed 22 nurses in 8 hospitals for a total of 197 hours and documented 120 problems that prevented patient-care task completion. The problems ranged from missing or incorrect information, missing or broken equipment, waiting for a resource, and missing or incorrect medications. Similarly, Potter et al., (2005) found omissions in patient care due to interruptions in an ethnographic study involving seven staff registered nurses. Nurses were frequently interrupted during interventional work such as administrating medications, problem-solving intravenous infusions, and teaching patients. Interruptions pose risks for medical errors. Daily staffing continues to be influenced by workload predictor/tools. More extensive research and development of intensive care unit (ICU)–specific nursing workload predictor/tools are needed to determine the numbers of ICU nurses and their educational backgrounds (Robnett, 2006).

All Good Things...

The staffing and scheduling process incorporates professional nursing standards and accounts for the health-care setting, the care delivery model, patient acuity, and the nursing staff. Scheduling and staffing systems can be centralized, decentralized, or mixed. The outcomes of scheduling are the daily staffing, patient outcomes, and nursing workloads. The challenges faced by nurse managers in providing adequate staffing are the nurse shortage, the advances in patient care technology, the high patient acuity levels, and the health-care industry's continuous evolution. For the appropriate allocation of nursing staff for patient-focused care, staffing is both a process and an outcome (AACN-Critical Care, 2001).

Let's Talk

1. Describe staffing as a process with a relationship to scheduling.

2. Describe a care delivery model utilized by nursing services.

NCLEX Questions

1. The nurse manager's **staffing** and **scheduling** goals:
   A. Are consistent with the Principles for Nurse Staffing of the American Nurses Association and other regulatory guidelines
   B. Do not have to be congruent with the mission, vision, values, philosophy, and strategic plan of the organization and its nursing services
   C. Promote patient safety and patient satisfaction
   D. A and C

2. Staffing, according to the Center for American Nurses, refers to:
   A. The monthly work schedule produced for a unit or clinic
   B. The nursing hours per patient per day
   C. The professional skills required for particular job assignments
   D. A nurse's total years of experience

3. The process of staffing involves:
   A. Assessment of the qualifications and competence of the staff available
   B. Formulation of a strategic staffing plan to meet future needs
   C. Creation of a budget of personnel to provide patient care services
   D. Assigning nurses to the care of specific patients

4. Scheduling variables are defined as:
   A. The number of patients, complexity of patient condition, and nursing care required
   B. The nursing staff members' competency levels, qualifications, skill range, knowledge or ability, and experience level
   C. The level of supervision required
   D. All of the above

5. An appropriate staffing system incorporates:
   A. Patient needs
   B. Staff members' degrees and credentials
   C. A specific ratio of RNs to LPNs
   D. The personnel budget

6. Acuity-adapted room models offer the following:
   A. Transfer of patients to different hospital units as their status improves or worsens
   B. Assistance with the continuity of care
   C. Decreased patient satisfaction
   D. The use of patient room sharing

7. Nurse staff scheduling factors include:
   A. Staff may work one shift or 8 hours prior to the starting time of a different shift or 16 hours straight
   B. 4-week schedules will be posted at least 1 week prior to the beginning of the schedule
   C. Staff should be scheduled to be off duty one out of every four weekends
   D. No nurse will be required to work more than 6 consecutive days without a day off

8. The nurse staffing variables used to measure patient outcomes are:
   A. Nursing hours provided for a patient
   B. Ratios of RNs to nurse assistants
   C. Numbers of units to which a nurse may rotate
   D. Skill mixes

9. Centralized staffing is:
   A. Cyclical
   B. A system in which workdays and time off for personnel are changed monthly
   C. Loose management control of the entire scheduling and staffing system
   D. A system in which individual problems are always taken into consideration

10. Flexible scheduling is:
    A. Difficult to accomplish because health-care facilities are open 24 hours a day
    B. A schedule for health-care professionals that involves no work on holidays
    C. A means to improve staff retention by offering balance and enhancement between professional and personal life activities
    D. Not workable with self-scheduling

REFERENCES

Advocate Good Shepherd Hospital, Barrington, Illinois; http://www.advocatehealth.com/gshp/gshp/info/library/ham/win05/gshp1.htm; accessed February, 13, 2005.

Aiken, L.H., et al. (2002). Hospital nurse staffing and patient mortality, nurse burnout, and job dissatisfaction. *Journal of American Medical Association, 288*(16), 1987–1993.

Allen, D.E., et al. (2006). Relating outcomes to excellent nursing practice. *Journal of Nursing Administration, 36*(3), 140–147.

American Association of Colleges of Nursing (AACN-Colleges) (2004). *Working paper on the role of the clinical nurse leader* (white paper). http://www.aacn.nche.edu/publications/whitepapers/cnl.htm; accessed April 22, 2005.

American Association of Critical Care Nurses (2001). Maintaining patient-focused care in an environment of nursing staff shortages and financial constraints. Aliso Viejo, CA: Author.

American Association of Critical Care Nurses (2005). Standards for *Establishing and Sustaining Healthy Work Environments: A Journey to Excellence.* http://www.aacn.org/aacn/pubpolcy.nsf/Files/HWEStandards/$file/HWEStanda-rds.pdf, accessed April 22, 2005.

American Institute of Architects (2001). *Guidelines for design and construction of hospital and health facilities* (pp. 42–45). Washington, DC: Author.

The American Nurse (2006). A change will do you good. *The American Nurse, 38*(1), 9.

American Nurses Association (1999). *Principles for nurse staffing.* Washington, DC: Author. http://www.nursing-world.org/readroom/stffprnc.htm, accessed August 30, 2005.

American Nurses Association (2004). *Scope and standards for nurse administrators* (2nd ed.). Silver Spring, MD: Author.

American Nurses Credentialing Center (2004). *The magnet recognition program*® (2005 ed.). Silver Spring, MD: Author.

Anderson, P. (2003). Poster presentation: *The universal bed concept.* Quest for Excellence Nursing and Staff Development Conference, The Ohio State University Medical Center, Columbus, OH.

Artz, M. (2005). The politics of caring: solutions to RN staffing. *American Journal of Nursing, 105*(11), 35.

Barry, J. (2006). The HoverMatt system for patient transfer. *Journal of Nursing Administration, 36*(3), 114–117.

Bleich, M.R., & Hewlett, P.O. (2004). Dissipating the "perfect storm"-responses from nursing and the health care industry to protect the public's health. *Online Journal of Issues in Nursing, 9*(2), www.nursingworld.org/ojin/topic24/tpc24_4.htm

Bleich, M.R., et al. (2003). Analysis of the nursing workforce crisis: A call to action. *American Journal of Nursing, 103*(4), 66–74.

Brilli, R.J., et al. (2001). Critical care delivery in the intensive care unit: Defining clinical roles and the best practice model. *Critical Care Medicine, 29*(10), 2007–2019.

Donley, S.R. (2005). Challenges for nursing in the 21st century. *Nursing Economic$, 23*(6), 312–318.

Caryon, P., & Gürses, A.P. (2005). A human factors engineering conceptual framework of nursing workload and patient safety in intensive care units. *Intensive and Critical Care Nursing, 21*(5), 284–301.

Drake, D., et al. (2005). Challenges that nurses face in caring for morbidly obese patients in the acute care setting. *Surgery for Obesity and Related Diseases, 1*(5), 462–466.

Dunton, N., et al. (2004). Nurse staffing and patient falls on acute care hospital units. *Nursing Outlook, 52*(1), 53–59.

Forte, J. (2004). Tap techno-solutions to workload measurement. *IT Solutions, 34,* 12–14.

Gabow, P., et al. (2005). *A toolkit for redesign in health care.* Washington, DC: Agency for Healthcare Research and Quality (AHRQ Publication No. 05-0108-EF).

Gaines, C., & Carter, D. (1989). Overtime: A professional responsibility? *Focus on Critical Care, 16*(4), 270–273.

Gallant, D., & Lanning, K. (2001). Streamlining patient care processes through flexible room and equipment design. *Critical Care Nursing Quarterly, 24*(3), 59–76.

Gatens, C.G. (1972). Who's handicapped? *ANA Clinical Sessions, 17*(4), 176–178.

Hall, L.M. (1998). Policy implications when changing staff mix. *Nursing Economic$, 16*(6), 291–312.

Hall, L.M., & Doran, D. (2004). Nurse staffing, care delivery model and patient care quality. *Journal of Nursing Care Quality, 19*(1), 27–33.

Hendrich, A.L., Fay, J., & Sorrells, A.K., (2004). Effects of acuity-adaptable rooms on flow of patients and delivery of care. *American Journal of Critical Care, 13*(1), 35–45.

Henneman, E.A., & Cardin, S. (2002). Family-centered critical care: A practical approach to making it happen. *Critical Care Nurse, 22*(6), 12–19.

Horn, S.D., et al. (2005). RN staffing time and outcomes of long-stay nursing home residents. *American Journal of Nursing, 105*(11), 58–71.

Howell, J.P. (1966). Cyclical scheduling of nursing personnel. *Hospitals, 40*(2), 77–85.

Institute of Medicine (2001). *Assessing the quality chasm: A new health system for the 21st century.* Washington, DC: National Academy Press.

Institute of Medicine (2004). *Keeping patients safe: Transforming the work environment of nurses.* Washington, DC: National Academy Press.

Institute of Medicine (2000). *To err is human: Building a safer health system.* Washington, DC: National Academy Press.

Jacobsen, C., et al. (2002). Surviving the perfect storm: Staff perceptions of mandatory overtime. *JONA's Healthcare Law, Ethics, and Regulation, 4*(3), 57–66.

Johnson, J., Brown, K.K., & Neal, K. (2003). Designs that make a difference: the Cardiac Universal Bed model. *Journal of Cardiovascular Management, 14*(5), 16–20.

Joint Commission on Accreditation of Healthcare Organizations (2004). *JCAHO 2004 accreditation manual for hospitals (AMH) standards.* Chicago, IL: Author.

Kimball, B., & O'Neil, E. (2002). *Health care's human crisis: the American nursing shortage.* Princeton: The Robert Wood Johnson Foundation.

Kirchhoff, K.T., & Dahl, N. (2006). American Association of Critical Care Nurses' National survey of facilities and units providing critical care. *American Journal of Critical Care, 15*(1), 13–28.

Kovner, C., et al. (2002). Acute care: Nurse staffing and postsurgical events: An analysis of administrative data from a sample of U.S. hospital, 1990–1996. *Health Services Research, 37*(3), 611.

Krail, K.A. (2005). Retaining the retiring nurse: Keeping the nursing shortage at bay. *Nurse Leader*, April, 33–36.

Kramer, M., & Schmalenberg, C. (2005). Revising the essentials of magnetism tool: There is more to adequate staffing than numbers. *Journal of Nursing Administration, 35*(4), 188–198.

Kurtzman, E.T., & Kizer, K.W. (2005). Evaluating the performance and contribution of nurses to achieve an environment of safety. *Nursing Administration Quarterly, 29*(1), 14–23.

Lancellot, M. (1996). CNS combats pressure ulcers with skin and wound assessment team (SWAT). *Clinical Nurse Specialist, 10*(3), 154–160.

Lauw, C., & Gares, D. (2005). Resource management: What's right for you? *Nursing Management, 36*(12), 46–49.

Lookinland, S., Tiedeman, M.E., & Crosson, A.E.T. (2005). Nontraditional models of care delivery: Have they solved the problems? *Journal of Nursing Administration, 35*(2), 74–80.

Mason, D.J. (2006). Do the right thing: Advocate change, or find a workplace where you can do so. *American Journal of Nursing, 106*(4), 11.

Mason, D.J., & Kany, K.A. (2005). The state of the science: Focus on work environments. *American Journal of Nursing, 105*(3), 33–34.

McClure, M.L., & Hinshaw, A.S. (2002). *Magnet hospitals revisited: Attraction and retention of professional nurses.* Washington, DC: American Academy of Nursing.

Meyer, G., & Lavin, M.A. (2005). Vigilance: The essence of nursing. *Online Journal of Issues in Nursing, 23*(10), 8. http://www.nursingworld.org/topic22/tpc22_6news.htm, accessed June 29, 2005.

Moody, R.A. (2005). Patient delivery model: CUB (cardiac universal bed). (La Porte Hospital and Health Services, La Porte, Indiana). Presentation at Sigma Theta Tau Annual Meeting, Indianapolis, IN; http://stti.confex.com/stti/bcclinical38/techprogram/paper_21066.htm, accessed April 27, 2005.

Morse, E.L, et al. (2005). One hospital's strategic initiative to eliminate agency staffing. *Nurse Leader*, April, 49–51.

Mosby's Dictionary of Medical, Nursing and Health Professions (7th ed.) (2005). St. Louis: Author.

National Database of Nursing Quality Indicators (2006). Kansas City, KS: The National Center for Nursing Quality Indicators. http://www.nursingworld.org/quality/database.htm or http://www.nursingquality.org/; accessed April 22, 2005.

Needleman, J., et al. (2006). Nurse staffing in hospitals: Is there a business case for quality? *Health Affairs, 25*(1), 204–211.

Nelson, A., & Baptiste, A.S. (2004). Evidence-based practices for safe patient handling and movement. *Online Journal of Issues in Nursing, 9*(3), www.nursingworld.org/ojin/topic25_3.htm, accessed March 15, 2006.

Norman, L.D., et al. (2005). The older nurse in the workplace: does age matter? *Nursing Economic$, 23*(6), 282–289.

Ohio Nurses Association (2005). *Agreement between the Ohio Nurses Association and the Ohio State University, April 29, 2005 through July 1, 2007.* Columbus, OH: Author.

Pischke-Winn, K.A., Andreoli, K.G., & Halstead, L.K. (2004). *Students with disabilities: Nursing education and practice.* Chicago: Rush University College of Nursing; http://www.rushu.rush.edu/nursing/disable/fulldoc.pdf, accessed September 24, 2005.

Potter, P., et al. (2005). Understanding the cognitive work of nursing in the acute care environment. *Journal of Nursing Administration, 35*(7/8), 327–335.

Price Waterhouse Coopers, LLP (2004). *The role of hospital design in the recruitment, retention and performance of NHS nurses in England.* www.cabe.org.uk (2004-healthyhospitals.org.uk-sykehusplan.no-cabe.org.uk-sykehusplan.org), accessed April 29, 2005.

Robnett, M.K. (2006). Critical care nursing: Workforce issues and potential solutions. *Critical Care Medicine, 34*(3), (suppl) S25–S31.

Sabet, L. (2005). *Adopting online nurse scheduling and staffing systems.* Oakland, CA: California HealthCare Foundation.

Scalise, D. (2005). Clinical staffing: SWAT nurses. *Hospitals & Heath Networks, 79*(9), 28, 30.

Scalise, D. (2006). Staffing: public disclosure. *Hospitals & Heath Networks, 80*(3), 20.

Scholle, C.C., & Mininni, N.C. (2006). Best-practice interventions: How a rapid response team saves lives. *Nursing 2006, 36*(1), 36–40.

Shirey, M.R. (2005). Ethical climate in nursing practice: the leader's role. *JONA's Healthcare Law, Ethics, and Regulation, 7*(2), 59–67.

Simpson, R.L. (2004). Where will we be in 2015? *Nursing Management, 35*(12): 38–44.

Smith, A., & Chalker, N.J. (2005). Preceptor continuity in the nurse internship program: The nurse intern's perception. *Journal of Nurses Staff Development, 21*(2), 47–52.

Smith, S.L, et al. (2006). Application of the clinical nurse leader role in an acute care delivery model. *Journal of Nursing Administration, 36*(1), 29–33.

Stanton, M.W., & Rutherford, M.K. (2004). Hospital nurse staffing and quality of care. *Research in Action*, 14. AHRQ Publication No. 04-0029, March 2004. Agency for Healthcare Research and Quality, Rockville, MD; http://www.ahrq.gov/research/nursestaffing/nursestaff.htm, accessed April 19, 2005.

Tachibana, C., & Hardy, D. (2001). System-wide action team (SWAT): A new level of collaboration. *Seminars for Nurse Managers, 9*(2), 98–101.

Texas Nurses Association (2005). TNA Nurse-Friendly Criteria, media release May 3, 2005, Austin, TX: Author. http://www.texasnurses.org, accessed April 10, 2006.

Texas Nursing (2001). Rules proposal intended to clarify nurse staffing. *Texas Nursing, 76*(March), 1–2.

Tiedeman, M.E., & Lookinland, S. (2004). Traditional models of care delivery. *Journal of Nursing Administration, 34*(6), 291–297.

Titler, M., et al. (2005). Cost of hospital care for elderly at risk of falling. *Nursing Economic$, 23*(6), 290–306.

Tornabeni, J., Stanhope, M., & Wiggins, M. (2006). The CNL vision. *Journal of Nursing Administration, 36*(3), 103–108.

Tucker, A.L., Edmondson, A.C., & Spear, S. (2002). When problem solving prevents organizational learning. *Journal of Organizational Change Management, 15*(2), 122–137.

Ulrich, B.T. (1992). *Leadership and management according to Florence Nightingale.* Norwalk, CT: Appleton & Lange.

University HealthSystem Consortium (UHC) (2005). *Nursing work environment benchmarking project.* Chicago, IL: Author.

Unruh, L.Y. (2005). Employment conditions at the bedside: A cause of and solution to the RN shortage. *Journal of Nursing Administration, 35*(1), 11–14.

Urden, L.D., & Roode, J.L. (1997). Work sampling: a decision-making tool for determining resources and work redesign. *Journal of Nursing Administration, 27*(9), 34–41.

BIBLIOGRAPHY

Baggs, J.G., et al. (1999). Association between nurse-physician collaboration and patient outcomes in three intensive care units. *Critical Care Medicine, 27*(9), 1991–1998.

Baggot, D.M., et al. (2005). The new hire preceptor experience: Cost-benefit analysis of one retention strategy. *Journal of Nursing Administration, 35*(3), 138–145.

Ballard, K.S. (2003). Patient safety: A shared responsibility. *Online Journal of Issues in Nursing, 8*(3); http://www.nursingworld.org/ojin/topic22/tpc22_4.htm, accessed May 04, 2005.

Barrett, J. (1962). *The head nurse.* New York: Appleton-Century-Crofts.

Beard, E. L. (2003). The Internet as an "essential function" during an emergency. *JONA's Healthcare Law, Ethics, and Regulation, 5*(1), 2.

Benner, P. (1984/2001). *From novice to expert: Excellence and power in clinical nursing practice.* Menlo Park, CA: Addison-Wesley.

Berney, B., Needleman, J., & Kovner, C. (2005). Factors influencing the use of registered nurse overtime in hospitals, 1995–2000. *Journal of Nursing Scholarship, 37*(2), 165–172.

Bolton, L.B., et al. (2003). Nurse staffing and patient perceptions of nursing care. *Journal of Nursing Administration, 33*(11), 607–614.

Budd, K.W., Warino, L.S., & Patton, M.E. (2004). Traditional and non-traditional collective bargaining: Strategies to improve the patient care environment. *Online Journal of Issues in Nursing, 9*(1), http://www.nursingworld.org/ojin/topic23/tpc23_5.htm, accessed May 5, 2005.

Buerhaus, P.I. (2004). Lucian Leape on patient safety in U.S. hospitals. *Journal of Nursing Scholarship, 36*(4), 366–370.

Buerhaus, P.I. (2005). Six-part series on the state of the RN workforce in the United States. *Nursing Economic$, 23*(2), 58–60.

Carayon, P., & Gürses, A.P. (2005). A human factors engineering conceptual framework of nursing workload and patient safety in intensive care units. *Intensive and Critical Care Nursing, 21*(5), 284–301.

Cheng, D.C., et al. (March). Randomized assessment of resource use in fast-track cardiac surgery 1-year after hospital discharge. *Anesthesiology, 98*(3), 651–657.

Choi, J., et al. (2004). Perceived nursing work environment of critical care nurses. *Nursing Research, 53*(6), 370–378.

Cimiotti, J.P., et al. (2005). The magnet process and the perceived work environment of nurses. *Nursing Research, 54*(6), 384–390.

Clarke, S.P. (2005). The policy implications of staffing-outcomes research. *Journal of Nursing Administration, 35*(1), 17–19.

Clarke, S.P., & Aiken, L.H. (2003). Registered nurse staffing and patient and nurse outcomes in hospitals: a commentary. *Policy, Politics, & Nursing Practice, 4*(2), 104–111.

Coffman, J.M., Seago, J.A., & Spetz, J. (2002). Minimum nurse-to patient ratios in acute care hospitals in California. *Health Affairs, 21*(5), 53–64.

Colias, M. (2005). The disaster after the disaster. *Hospitals & Health Networks, 79*(10), 36–38, 40, 42, 44.

Collins, M.L., & Thomas, T. L. (2005). Creation of a step-down nurse internship program. *Journal of Nurses Staff Development, 21*(3), 115–119.

Connelly, L.M. (2005). Welcoming new employees. *Journal of Nursing Scholarship, 37*(2), 163–164.

Cowan, D.T., Norman, I., & Coopamah, V.P. (2005). Competence in nursing practice: A controversial concept: A focused review of literature. *Nurse Education Today, 25*(5), 355–362.

Curtin, L.L. (2003). An integrated analysis of nurse staffing and related variables: Effects on patient outcomes. *Online Journal of Issues in Nursing.* http://nursingworld.org/ojin/topic22/tpc22_5.htm, accessed April 22, 2005.

Diers, D. (2005). Reflections: Am I a nurse? I'm old but never former. *American Journal of Nursing, 105*(10), 39.

Donovan, L. (2004). Mapping a staffing blueprint to match competencies. *Nursing Management, 35*(Supplement 5), 14.

Eriksen, W., Bruusgaard, D., & Knardahl, S. (2003). Work factors as predictors of sickness absence: A three-month prospective study of nurses' aides. *Occupational and Environmental Medicine, 60*(4), 271–278.

Estabrooks, C.A., et al. (2005). The impact of hospital nursing characteristics on 30-day mortality. *Nursing Research, 54*(2), 74–84.

Flynn, M., et al. (2004). Fast-tracking revisited: Routine cardiac surgical patients need minimal intensive care. *European Journal of Cardiothoracic Surgery, 25*(1), 116–122.

Forman, H. (2004). Do we really practice relationship-based care? *Journal of Nursing Administration, 34*(1), 9.

Goode, C.J., & Williams, C.A. (2004). Post-baccalaureate nurse residency program. *Journal of Nursing Administration, 34*(2), 771–777.

Haberfelde, M, Bedecarré, D., & Buffum, M. (2005). Nurse-sensitive patient outcomes: An annotated bibliography. *Journal of Nursing Administration, 35*(6), 293–299.

Heinz, D. (2004). Hospital nurse staffing and patient outcomes: A review of current literature. *Dimensions of Critical Care Nursing, 23*(1), 44–50.

Hendrich, A.L., Bender, P.S., & Nyhuis, A., (2003). Validation of the Hendrich II fall risk model: A large concurrent case/control study of hospitalized patients. *Applied Nursing Research, 16*(1), 9–21.

Hess, A.K. (2005). Ensure a long and safe career. *American Journal of Nursing, 105*(6), 96.

Hiser, B., et al. (2006). Implementing a pressure ulcer prevention program and enhancing the role of the CWOCN: Impact on outcomes. *Ostomy Wound Management, 52*(2), 48–59.

Hoban, V. (2004). Nurses taking second jobs. *Nursing Times, 100*(28), 20–22.

Hodge, M.B., et al. (2002). Developing indicators of nursing quality to evaluate nurse staffing ratios. *Journal of Nursing Administration, 32*(6), 338–345.

Hodge, M.B., et al. (2004). Licensed caregiver characteristics and staffing in California acute care hospital units. *Journal of Nursing Administration, 34*(3), 125–133.

Hu, J., Herrick, C., & Hodgin, K.A. (2004). Managing the multi-generational nursing team. *Health Care Management, 23*(4), 334–340.

Jennings, B.M. (2001). The role of research in the policy puzzle: Nurse staffing research as a case in point. *Research in Nursing & Health, 24,* 443–445.

Joseph, A.J. (2004). The chest pain center as an operational model. *Critical Pathways in Cardiology, 3*(1), 14–17.

Josten, E.J.C., Ng-A-Tham, J.E.E., & Thierry, H. (2003). The effects of extended workdays on fatigue, health, performance and satisfaction in nursing. *Journal of Advanced Nursing, 44*(6), 643–652.

Kaestner, R. (2005). An overview of public policy and the nursing shortage. *Journal of Nursing Administration, 35*(1), 8–9.

Kirkby, M., et al. (1998). Improving staffing with a resource management plan. *Journal of Nursing Administration, 28*(11), 25–29.

Koviack, P. (2004). A review of the effect of an accommodation program to support nurses with functional limitations. *Nursing Economic$, 22*(6), 320–324, 355.

Krail, K.A. (2005). Retaining the retiring nurse: Keeping the nursing shortage at bay. *Nurse Leader*, April, 33–36.

Kramer, M., & Schmalenberg, C. (2005). Revising the essentials of magnetism tool: There is more to adequate staffing than numbers. *Journal of Nursing Administration, 35*(4), 188–198.

Manojlovich, M. (2005). Predictors of professional nursing practice behaviors in hospital setting. *Nursing Research, 54*(1), 41–47.

Manthey, M. (2001). A core incremental staffing plan. *Journal of Nursing Administration, 31*(9), 424–425.

Manthey, M. (2003). AKA primary nursing. *Journal of Nursing Administration, 33*(7/8), 369–370.

Massachusetts Nurse. (1999). Nurses hail California staffing law mandating staffing levels. *Massachusetts Nurse, 69*(10), 11.

McCabe, P.J., & Kalpin, P. (2005). Using shared decision making to implement evidence-based practice in progressive care. *Critical Care Nurse, 25*(2), 76–87.

McCartney, P. (2005). Online bidding for open nursing shifts. *MCN American Journal of Maternal Child Nursing, 30*(5), 335.

Miller, J.G. (1978). *Living systems.* New York: McGraw-Hill.

Murray, M.K., & Matchulat, J.J. (2005). Hospital charity care and billing practices: The labor movement pans for gold. *Journal of Nursing Administration, 35*(6), 286–292.

Naughton, C., Cheek, L., & O'Hara, K. (2005). Rapid recovery following cardiac surgery: A nursing perspective. *British Journal of Nursing, 14*(4), 214–219.

Needleman, J., et al. (2002). Nurse-staffing levels and the quality of care in hospitals. *New England Journal of Medicine, 346*(22), 1715–1722.

Nelson, R. (2005). AJN reports: nurses with disabilities. *American Journal of Nursing, 105*(6), 25–26.

Osborne, S. (2004). The art of rewarding and retaining staff: Part 2. *Nurse Leader*, August, 43–45.

Potter, P., et al. (2003). Identifying nurse staffing and patient outcome relationships: A guide for change in care delivery. *Nursing Economic$, 21*(4), 158–166.

Robb, E.A., et al. (2003). Self-scheduling: Satisfaction guaranteed? *Nursing Management, 34*(7), 16–18.

Rogers, A.E., et al. (2004). The working hours of hospital staff nurses and patient safety. *Health Affairs, 23*(4), 202–212.

Rosenfeld, P., et al. (2004). Nurse residency programs: A 5-year evaluation from the participants' perspective. *Journal of Nursing Administration, 34*(4), 188–194.

Saba, J.L., & Bardwell, P.L. (2004). Universal design concepts in the emergency department. *Journal of Ambulatory Care Management, 27*(3), 224–236.

Schmidt, L. (1996). A seasonal staffing model. *Journal of Nursing Administration, 26*(4), 52–55.

Schmidt, L.A. (2004). Patients' perceptions of nursing staffing, nursing care, adverse events, and overall satisfaction with the hospital experience. *Nursing Economic$, 22*(6), 295–306.

Seago, J.A. (2002). A comparison of two patient classification instruments in an acute care hospital. *Journal of Nursing Administration, 32*(5), 243–249.

Seago, J.A., Spetz, J., & Mitchell, S. (2004). Nurse staffing and hospital ownership in California. *Journal of Nursing Administration, 34*(5), 228–237.

Smith, L.N. (2003). Maximizing hospital capacity. *Healthcare Executive, 18*(1), 58–59.

Spetz, J. (2005). Public policy and nurse staffing: What approach is best? *Journal of Nursing Administration, 35*(1), 14–16.

Stone, P.W., et al. (2003). Evidence of nurse working conditions: A global perspective. *Policy, Politics, & Nursing Practice, 4*(2), 120–130.

Stone, P.W., et al. (2004). Nurses' working conditions: Implications for infectious disease. *Emerging Infectious Diseases, 10*(11), 1984–1989, www.cdc.gov/eid; accessed April 22, 2005.

Sugrue, N.M. (2005). Public policy initiatives and the nursing shortage. *Journal of Nursing Administration, 35*(1), 19–22.

Texas State Board of Nursing Examiners (2005). Charge nurse concerns for patient safety and an overworked staff nurse. *Texas Board of Nursing Bulletin, 36*(2), 5–6.

Thomas, L. (1983). *The youngest science: Notes of a medicine-watcher.* New York: The Viking Press.

Thorgrimson, D.H., & Robinson, N.C. (2005). Building and sustaining an adequate RN workforce. *Journal of Nursing Administration, 35*(11), 474–477.

Waters, T. (2004). Fourth annual safe patient handling & movement conference speech: State of the science in ergonomics. *Online Journal of Issues in Nursing, 10*(2), 4. http://www.nursingworld.org/ojin/keynotes/speech4.htm, accessed April 4, 2005.

Weinstein, S.M. (2002). A nursing portfolio: Documenting your professional journey. *Journal of Infusion Nursing, 25*(6), 357–362

Whitman, G.R., et al. (2002). The impact of staffing on patient outcomes across specialty units. *Journal of Nursing Administration, 32*(12), 633–639.

Wilson, J.L. (2002). The impact of shift patterns on healthcare professionals. *Journal of Nursing Management, 10*(4), 211–219.

Youngblut, J.M., & Brooten, D. (2001). Evidence-based nursing practice: Why is it important? *AACN Clinical Issues, 12*(4), 468–476.

chapter 18

Maximizing Employee Performance

EMILY HARMAN, MSN, RN

CHAPTER MOTIVATION

"Sandwich every bit of criticism between two layers of praise."

Mary Kay Ash

CHAPTER MOTIVES

- Define the terms: coaching, counseling, and discipline.
- Discuss the purpose of performance appraisals.
- Describe the relationship between management by objectives (MBO) and performance appraisals.
- Identify common types of performance appraisal tools.
- Characterize common rater errors.

Providing safe, high-quality patient care is the goal of health-care organizations. To accomplish this goal, the organization depends on the teamwork of its personnel. The nursing administrator is responsible for planning, organizing, directing, and coordinating the activities of the nursing personnel. Team building is a critical part of this process. The objective of team building is to develop a group that is committed to the work and each other (Creasia & Parker, 2001, p. 171).

Another important responsibility of the nurse manager and the focus of this chapter is monitoring and evaluating the performance of personnel, a function called controlling. According to Creasia & Parker (2001), controlling includes personnel evaluation, discipline, and behavior modification. For nurse managers, this function requires interactive contact with employees that is unlike any of their other responsibilities. Successful nurse managers require knowledge and skill in interpersonal relationships to enhance the performance of employees. This chapter will focus on the role of the nurse manager in motivating employees to achieve their professional performance goals within the organization.

Performance Appraisal

Performance appraisal, as the term implies, is a formal evaluation of an employee's performance. The Joint Commission on Accreditation of Healthcare Organizations (JCAHO) requires regular performance appraisals, and most health-care organizations offer them annually. Regular oversight and evaluation of performance are the responsibilities of nursing administration, whether or not they are required annually. The purpose of a performance appraisal is to provide opportunities for personal and professional growth and to ensure the quality of nursing care (Creasia & Parker, 2001, p. 172).

Generally, the process is intended to clarify how well the employee is performing the requirements of the job. A job description often provides the baseline or minimal performance criteria. Additional standards may be used to evaluate employees, depending on the setting. For example, nurse educators in a university setting would be held to university standards for annual merit and/or promotion. These standards generally include guidelines for performance in instruction or teaching; scholarly pursuits, such as research; and service activities to the community and the university. In a clinical setting, the standards or benchmarks for job performance often include the American Nurses Association (ANA) clinical standards and the JCAHO patient safety guidelines.

Typically, upon hire, the individual will receive a copy of the appraisal tool and the criteria that will be used in the evaluation process. The type of tool used will vary from organization to organization. Yoder-Wise (1999, p. 273) described some of the most commonly used tools for performance assessment as either structured or flexible. The most commonly used structured tools are the forced distribution scales and the rating scales. The low and high values found on these types of scales may lead to problems in evaluation.

Forced distribution scales are one of several comparative methods that can be used alone or in conjunction with other tools to evaluate employees. A common practice in many organizations requires the evaluator to place a certain percentage of employees into equally divided categories. For example, each employee would be placed into one of three categories. In a forced distribution scale, these three categories might be labeled: (a) above average, (b) average, and (c) below average. To many employees this seems unfair as any comparative differences in their overall performance may be ever so slight. When this method is used to determine merit raises, it frequently lowers the morale of employees who were found to be average or below (Fig. 18-1).

Most rating scales are constructed to evaluate the performance of employees. They usually include a

After reviewing the performance of the RN Staff on your unit, rank order them as follows: 10% (Excellent), 15% (Above Average), 50% (Average), 15% (Below Average-Need Improvement), and 10% (Poor Performance-Need Assistance). On a unit with 40 employees, the result should be similar to the example below:

10%	Excellent	4 employees
15%	Above Average	6 employees
50%	Average	20 employees
15%	Below Average	6 employees
10%	Poor Performance	4 employees

FIGURE 18-1 Sample directions for a forced distribution scale.

Directions: Complete this form by circling the number that most closely corresponds to your observations of the employee. Do this on at least two different occasions.

Scale:

1=Poor 2=Below Average   3=Average   4=Above Average   5=Excellent

---

Quality of Work:	1	2	3	4	5
Knowledge of Job:	1	2	3	4	5
Communication Skills:	1	2	3	4	5
Interpersonal Skills:	1	2	3	4	5
Concern for Patient Safety*:	1	2	3	4	5
Concern for Patient Comfort^^:	1	2	3	4	5

Total: _____

* e.g. Observing universal precautions
    Washing hands between patients

**e.g. Administering pain medication as needed
    according to prescribed guidelines

Date: _____ **Name of Employee:** _____

Supervisor's Signature: _____

FIGURE 18-2 Sample performance evaluation tool.

variety of measures that are common to nursing practice in general. The biggest problem with these scales is that the behavior to be evaluated may not actually be observed by the evaluators, leaving them to make assumptions about the individual's behavior. For example, an item like "provides safe nursing care" is rather ambiguous and perhaps even circumstance-specific. The individual may be rated low or high on that item depending on when she is evaluated and whether previous evaluations were low or high. Figure 18-2 is an example of a rating scale.

Flexible tools like the behaviorally anchored rating scale (BARS), management by objectives (MBO), and peer review give a better picture of the individual's performance and are less open to bias. A variety of tools will be discussed later in this chapter.

For staff members, the performance appraisal process provides feedback about their progress toward career goals and changes in performance and provides an opportunity to review their last evaluation. For the nursing administrator, the performance appraisal process provides opportunities to review the quality of patient care, identify those staff members with the potential for advancement, identify problem employees, and make decisions about the overall operation of various units within the facility. For example, when a number of employees are not performing at optimum, this may indicate problems within the organization, such as high acuity rates and low staffing numbers. If only one or two individuals are having problems, it could indicate a need for further training, coaching, or counseling.

In most organizations, individuals will be evaluated using both formal and informal procedures. Formal evaluations may occur only once or twice a year (Tappen, 2001, p. 273). In most cases, formal evaluation is required by accrediting agencies or is part of the organization's policy. With a formal evaluation, there is usually a written procedure or timetable to be followed. Forms that must be completed by the nursing supervisor and/or administrator are also part of the typical process. All employees should be aware of the procedure, the timetable, the tools, and their own role in the process.

According to Tappen (2001, p. 274), informal evaluation is commonly thought of as individual feedback or information regarding one's performance. The organization may or may not have a procedure for conducting informal evaluations. In most cases, the individual collects data from various sources to document her performance during the year. The wise administrator and/or supervisor should being doing the same with each staff member. For example, the supervisor should make a point of observing staff members in action and keep anecdotal records, noting the date, time, circumstances, and employee performance. During these periods, feedback should be honest so that any employee who is not performing as expected can take corrective action. Conversely, those employees who are doing well should be told so.

According to Barnum and Kerfoot (1995, p. 256), feedback and correction should be ongoing, spontaneous, and to the point. The employee should not be made to wait for an official evaluation date to receive this type of feedback. Ongoing feedback can help motivate the employee toward outstanding performance.

BASELINES FOR PERFORMANCE APPRAISAL

Federal guidelines have stipulated that performance appraisal of employees be based on a valid job analysis. Because a job analysis is used for recruiting purposes as well as for evaluation and promotion guidelines, it should be current. A job analysis generally describes the tasks, characteristics, skills, knowledge, and abilities required to perform a specific job. As such, it serves as a basis for career development, in-service training, job forecasting, and performance appraisals. In most cases, the job analysis helps determine the value of a job in terms of compensation while ensuring that pay equity is maintained. A job analysis includes a job description and the job specifications. Job specifications generally describe the qualities and characteristics of the person needed to perform the job. A job description specifies the duties and responsibilities of a particular role. The job analysis is often used by

administration to determine recruitment needs and to make forecasting decisions for staffing within the organization.

Employees are generally given a job description when they are hired or promoted. Job descriptions are not as comprehensive as a job analysis because they list only the basic requirements of the job (Fig. 18-3).

Job Description

The employee's job description details the basic skills and abilities needed to fulfill the job's responsibilities; it serves as the starting point for a performance appraisal. Ellis and Hartley (2004, p. 461) defined job descriptions as written statements stipulating the duties and functions of various jobs within the organization and the scope of authority, responsibility, and accountability involved in each position. Job descriptions should define minimum standards for effective job performance and employment and should not be too detailed (Swansburg & Swansburg, 2002, p. 600). A comprehensive job description should describe what is to be done, not how to do it. For example, each nurse would be expected to use aseptic technique when doing a dressing change, but the dressing Nurse A applies may not look like the dressing Nurse B applies, even though both have maintained a sterile field while doing the procedure.

Most organizations have written job descriptions in their policy manuals. As job responsibilities and performance requirements for employees are constantly changing, job descriptions should be reviewed and updated on a regular basis. Employees should have an opportunity to provide input with regard to their job descriptions.

ANA Standards and Guidelines

Contributing to job descriptions and to performance evaluation criteria for nurses are the standards of clinical practice established by the ANA and the guidelines for patient safety established by JCAHO. The standards and guidelines proffer the measurements to be used by hospitals and a variety of healthcare agencies when evaluating their employees. They can also provide additional information about job requirements for the nursing staff. Nursing is guided by these ANA standards of practice and standards of professional performance (ANA, 2004, p. 12). The ANA standards provide a framework for the evaluation and improvement of nursing practice.

Position Type: Full Time

Education: BSN preferred

Experience: 2–5 years as a medical-surgical staff nurse, previous experience in an Emergency Department desirable, experience with telemetry monitoring desirable

Other: RN licensure, ACLS certification

Knowledge and Skills Required*:

- Assessing patient status
- Planning and implementing emergency care
- Evaluating responses to care
- Documenting nursing activities for individual clients
- Operating a variety of technical equipment
- Rapidly responding to trauma and disaster situations
- Participating as a team member with other nurses and physicians
- Coordinating activities related to the care of emergency and trauma patients
- Communicating effectively with patients and family members
- Educating the public as needed in the following areas:
  - Reducing preventable injuries
  - Promoting health and safety

* The above list only covers basic responsibilities

FIGURE 18-3 Sample job description; emergency department nurse.

It makes sense, therefore, to include these standards developed by the profession when evaluating the performance of the practicing nurse. Most agencies will incorporate many or all of these standards as part of their performance appraisal process.

For instance, the first six standards articulated by the ANA are directly related to the practice of nursing. These standards should be quite familiar to nurses and are more commonly known as the nursing process. Beginning with the assessment of clients, the nurse is expected to proceed through a series of steps that include diagnosis, outcomes identification, planning, implementation, and evaluation. The nursing process is based on a critical thinking process and provides the foundation for evidence-based nursing practice.

The standards of professional performance, on the other hand, reflect the commitment of nurses to the profession and the clientele they serve. These standards include:

- Quality of practice
- Education
- Professional practice evaluation
- Collegiality
- Ethics
- Research
- Resource utilization
- Leadership

These standards are also included as part of most performance appraisal tools. Quality of practice typically means that the nurse engages in activities to improve nursing care and nursing practice. This might include serving on committees to update or improve policies and procedures or documenting outcomes of practice. Continuing education can be formal or informal. Most state boards require periodic continuing education for relicensing. Ideally, nurses will seek educational opportunities to enhance or improve the knowledge and skills needed for their practice area. Lifelong learning is a professional commitment.

Professional practice evaluation is a process. It implies that nurses should seek feedback actively on their performance as it relates to standards, guidelines, and job descriptions. Feedback can come from a variety of sources such as patients, peers, and superiors. Nurses have a responsibility to evaluate the care they give. Soliciting input from others is one way to determine the effectiveness of care given. For example, nurses understand the importance of checking the patient's response to medications and treatments. This can either be by observing the response of the patient or asking the patient how he is doing after receiving the said medication or treatment. Today's nurses must continually assess their strengths as well as areas needing improvement. Peer evaluation, for example, is one means for ongoing self-assessment. Peers generally have similar goals and experience. New nurse graduates often seek advice from their superiors with experience when they take on new responsibilities. Ongoing self-evaluation by nurses makes the performance appraisal process seem less threatening. Periodic informal feedback should prepare nurses for the more formal process when it occurs.

Nurses constantly interact with other health team members. Collegial relationships serve several purposes. For one, they provide a learning forum for the nurse and enhance the outcome of the patient's situation. During the course of patient care, the nurse collaborates with patients, families, and colleagues. Collaboration through communication and documentation is one way to ensure continuity of care for the patient.

Patients and their families have a right to expect nurses to engage in ethical practice, which is why it has become a component of performance evaluation. Patients expect confidential handling of information about them and to be treated with dignity and respect. Today's nurse is also expected to participate in research at some level. This may include helping to collect data, implementing new procedures based on research, sharing research findings, or serving on research committees. This type of activity may be new to many nurses, but it can often be very rewarding. Many of the practice guidelines that nurses take for granted are based on research findings.

The term "resource utilization" may be somewhat misleading but refers to keeping patients (as consumers) informed about their options. Many nurses have been doing this for some time. If there is a less costly but safer treatment available, nurses have usually discussed it with their clients. For example, soap and water might work as well as an expensive hand cleanser.

An additional component here is delegation of patient care to unlicensed personnel. Delegation requires finding the right person for the right job. The five rights of delegation identified by the National Council of State Boards of Nursing are:

- Right task
- Right circumstance
- Right person
- Right direction
- Right supervision

In short, using nursing judgment and following these standards of delegation, nurses are able to assign tasks to other caregivers safely. This is often difficult for new nurses, who may not be familiar with the job responsibilities of other health team members. It is critical, however, that nurses use delegation appropriately to save themselves time and energy and to distribute the workload better.

Leadership implies that the nurse assumes a larger role in the community or outside of the practice setting. This may mean, for instance, teaching first-graders about hand washing or spreading germs. Nurses are expected to participate in committees within the practice setting either as a member or a leader. They are also expected to take an active role in advancing their profession, usually by joining a professional organization.

One purpose of performance appraisal is to make good employees better. According to Ash (1984), good employees are a company's number one asset. Management usually describes a good employee as one who is loyal to the organization and/or one with good work ethics. Additionally, management has indicated that these individuals seem satisfied with their work and have low rates of absenteeism. Ash believes that one way to make good employees better is for management to help them reach their potential.

MANAGEMENT BY OBJECTIVES

Management by objectives (MBO) systems indicate a two-way communication process of evaluation (Houston, 1995). This implies that both management and employee establish goals to be discussed during the evaluation process. Encouraging employees to set their own goals is often a good way to enhance performance and behavior. Whereas there is a sense of self-satisfaction derived from achieving goals, there may also be some extrinsic reward as well. Achieving one's goals could result in a salary increase or a promotion. This idea for setting one's own goals is based on McGregor's theory of management and is often referred to as MBO.

Many health-care organizations have included MBO as part of the performance appraisal process. For the nursing staff, MBO offers an opportunity to do a self-assessment and set goals that are realistic and meaningful to career aspirations. Some details on developing goals as part of the MBO process follow:

- The staff should limit their goals to two or three.
- Goals should be meaningful and realistic.
- Strategies for achieving the goals should be included as well.
- An in-service session on writing goals and strategies may be helpful when introducing the idea of MBO.
- The nurse manager and nursing supervisor should review goals with staff members.
- Before the goals are submitted, all parties should agree on them.

Working with the nursing supervisor and/or administrator, the performance appraisal process can become a meaningful and rewarding experience. When one's superior shows an interest in his or her career goals and aspirations, the employee may be motivated to reach his potential. This is a win-win for both parties because the success of the administrator is often measured by the success of her subordinates.

The job description and standards of performance provide the starting point for assessing employees. Performance appraisal, however, should make use of additional data sources depending on the requirements of the organization. Standardized tools may be used to evaluate employees in some organizations, while others may opt for the use of tools developed in-house. In any case, the responsibility for data collection rests with the nursing supervisor.

DATA COLLECTION

The employees' immediate supervisor usually carries out data collection for evaluations at various points during the review period. The employee should be aware of the methods and have a copy of the tool or tools that will be used to evaluate performance. Data collection methods might include: (a) making notations on the tool based on observations, (b) keeping anecdotal notes, (c) reviewing charting, (d) interviewing patients, (e) attending staff meetings, (f) talking with the employee's coworkers, and/or (g) reviewing the employee's skills or competency evaluations. Any or all of these may be used.

Performance Appraisal Tools

Input from nurses working in different settings suggested that organizations are using a wide variety of tools. Sophisticated, standardized tools are used in some organizations while others use simple checklists. There seemed to be little consistency in the type of tool used from area to area. Checklists, ratings, rankings, anecdotal records, peer reviews, and self-appraisals have their place in health-care organizations. Several of these methods are described below in detail.

Peer Reviews

Peer reviews are one means of evaluating staff, especially in a decentralized organization. Peer review is a process of assessing, monitoring, and evaluating the quality of patient care provided. Acceptable standards of practice are often used to determine the quality of care. The process of peer review may vary from organization to organization. Each institution should establish guidelines for conducting peer reviews. These guidelines should describe who, what, when, how often, and under what circumstances. A method that is commonly used in many institutions is critiquing patient records.

Generally, this involves a group of peer reviewers. One or more of those individuals might randomly review patient records with attention to specific criteria. The same criteria should be used when reviewing any patient records. Because patient records are legal documents, certain criteria should apply from institution to institution, such as assessing the patient's level of pain and documenting the patient's response to any pain medication that may have been administered. Other methods of peer review may require one or more of the peer reviewers to observe an employee giving patient care. Here again, the criteria should be specified and the same for each person being observed. Despite its increasing popularity, employees may see peer review as intimidating.

Parks and Lindstrom (1995) reported that the potential rewards for instituting unit-based peer review included increased trust, communication, and job satisfaction. In the situation they described, performance appraisal was one of three reasons for instituting peer review. Quality assurance and professional development were the other reasons given. The peer review groups consisted of senior nurses who were experienced in mentoring and adept at group process skills.

Peer reviews can provide informal feedback to the nursing staff. If used properly, peer evaluation can provide a powerful incentive for personal and professional development. According to Marquis and Huston (2000, p. 427), peer review has the potential to increase the accuracy of performance appraisal. The idea of having colleagues or peers evaluate each other makes sense from the standpoint of similarity of experiences, knowledge, and familiarity with skill requirements. This practice is becoming more widely accepted in health care and lends more credence to the overall performance evaluation of employees. Although peer review offers some benefits, it cannot be entered into lightly, and it is unrealistic to think peers can be involved with evaluations without extensive training (Barnum & Kerfoot, 1995, p. 256).

Checklists

Kelly-Heidenthal (2003, p. 558) described checklists as the most commonly used type of performance evaluation tool. Checklists are easy to use and only require the rater to determine whether the person being evaluated falls below the standards, meets the standards, or exceeds the standards of the organization. The problem with checklists is that they often lead to rater errors, especially central tendency. Central tendency occurs when the evaluator rates nearly everyone the same. Most often this happens when the evaluator is not familiar with the persons she is evaluating or because she has not actually observed them in the performance of certain activities. In organizations where this type of tool is used, employees often complain that they really have no idea of whether they are doing well or improving because their evaluations vary little year after year.

Rating Scales

Rating scales are also used to evaluate performance. The rater selects a number (usually between 1 and 5) that best describes the individual's perfor-mance (see Fig. 18-2). While rating scales are only slightly more illuminating than a checklist, the rater does have more options from which to choose. Although ratings and rankings are intended to be applied subjectively, any rating or ranking could reflect the rater's bias (Houston, 1995).

Ranking Employees

Rankings are sometimes used to determine how an individual performs in relation to others in a similar situation. Nursing administrators are sometimes required to rank subordinates based on a variety of criteria. This method is one that is often used when decisions have to be made about promotion or merit raises. Typically, ranking requires assigning numerical points rather than narrative descriptors when totaling data.

When ranking systems are used, the performance of individual employees is compared with those of other employees, usually those at the same level. Rankings should not be used alone, however, because they do not address the quality of the performance. A ranking system is generally used in organizations where performance is used to determine merit increases or promotions.

For example, in a recent merger at Central Hospital, two staff nurses were being considered for a newly created position in pediatrics. The nurse manager was unable to determine which nurse, Janet or Joyce, should be given the position. Both of them had worked on the pediatric unit for 5 years, and both of them had earned a bachelor's degree in nursing. Using the outcomes from the performance appraisal data, the supervisor was able to differentiate between the two individuals in terms of their overall performance for the past 3 years. On the 10 items listed on a rating scale similar to the one in Figure 18-2, Janet had scored 35, 43, and 45, respectively, for the past 3 years. Joyce, on the other hand, had scored 35, 40, and 40 during the past 3 years. Their scores on several other tools also reflected a similar pattern. As a result, Janet received the job offer.

Anecdotal Records

Anecdotal records are generally written records of observations. If used to evaluate performance, criteria should be established for the evaluator. For example, the evaluator might observe the individual's behavior in a given situation to ascertain whether or not he has explained the side effects of a client's medications. When the behaviors to be observed are clearly defined, the evaluator knows what to look for, and the individual knows the criteria by which he is being evaluated.

Skill Testing

Many organizations are now evaluating the skills of their employees. Testing skills in working with specialized equipment or performing specific procedures is one way to evaluate the employee's performance in areas that are unlikely to be observed in all situations. Skill testing may be part of the orientation of new nurses in a given agency to bridge the gap between education and practice.

When skill testing is involved, nurses are often required to demonstrate expertise in such areas as cardiopulmonary-resuscitation, handling the crash cart, preparing and/or starting intravenous medications, isolation techniques, tracheostomy care, dressing changes, removing staples (sutures), and other skills as deemed necessary by the agency. Some agencies have ongoing in-service programs whereby the staff are tested on a regular basis to maintain their expertise. Brykczynski (1998) recommends identifying and describing levels of nursing skills into the performance evaluation. Those demonstrating exemplary skills or the expert nurses could then serve as role models for the staff.

Patient Surveys

Most health-care agencies use some form of patient survey. Whereas supervisors often depend on patient surveys to evaluate the productivity and performance of the agency itself, they may also be used to assess patient satisfaction with care received. Unfortunately, it is difficult to collect information about individual employees in an acute care setting using a patient survey form. There are some rehabilitation centers and nursing care facilities that do provide opportunities for the residents and family members to evaluate the staff. In some cases, employees may be given a bonus for positive comments on these surveys.

Reviewing patient satisfaction data is part of the administrator's responsibility. Client care is the focus; when clients are dissatisfied, something is amiss. Consumer satisfaction continues to be a major concern of health-care agencies. Several tools have been used, most of which only describe the patient's overall satisfaction or dissatisfaction with the experience. For example, patients may be asked if someone explained the treatments and medications they received and then how satisfied they were with the explanations they received. Because most patients are not required to give their names, there may be no way of knowing who took care of them or perhaps even when they were hospitalized. This kind of general information serves as a starting point, but the current thinking is that more relevant patient satisfaction measures should be used, based on patient outcomes or evidence-based practice.

EVALUATOR BIAS

The more examples of behavior that the nursing administrator has to work with, the less biased the appraisal will be. Performance appraisal is an interpersonal process containing an element of subjectivity (Huber, 2000, p. 335). Regardless of the tool used, someone must evaluate the employee. In most instances, the employee's immediate supervisor is the person who does this. To guard against subjective attitudes and values influencing the appraisal, the appraiser should develop an awareness of her own biases and prejudices, according to Marquis and Huston (2000). How can this be accomplished? The nurse manager could consult with other managers when questions of personal bias exist, gather data appropriately, and keep notes on observations, others' comments, chart reviews, and care plans (p. 417).

Try as they might, raters are likely to be less objective than the ideal. This could result in one or more evaluator rating errors (Nauright, 1987). Some of the most common rater errors include: (a) central tendency, (b) "halo effect," and (c) "horn effect." Central tendency occurs when the rater, unsure of how persons are performing, ends up rating them as good or average on most items listed. The "halo effect" occurs when the employee has recently shown exceptional performance in one or more areas. If this behavior is apparent to the rater during the last few observations, the rater may rate the employee as above average in most areas listed, regardless of the actual performance in some of those areas. The "horn effect" is the opposite of the "halo effect." In other words, an employee who has recently displayed less than satisfactory behavior in one or more performance areas may be rated as per-

TABLE 18-1　Rater Errors

- **Halo effect:** Trait carryover; person whose performance is good in several known areas is assumed to be good in other perhaps unknown areas
- **Recency effect:** Recent events (good or bad) could bias the rater
- **Horn effect/problem distortion:** One poor performance may weigh heavier with the rater than many good performances
- **Sunflower effect:** Rater may grade all employees high if she thinks her team is great
- **Central tendency:** Rater may mark everyone as average, especially if she is unsure how certain people performed
- **Rater temperament effect:** Different raters will be stricter or more lenient than others
- **Strict ratings:** The rater may score the person lower than he deserves in an effort to motivate him
- **Lenient ratings:** The rater may score the person higher than he deserves so the person will think kindly of the rater
- **Guessing error:** "Guesstimates" by the rater about a particular performance she did not really observe
- **Initial impression:** Rater judges the person on appearance or some personal attribute and therefore assumes the person is doing a good job if she made a favorable impression, or perhaps the rater assumes the performance is less than satisfactory if the initial impression was less than favorable.
- **Status:** Rater judges the person according to position, education, or other criteria rather than on actual performance

Nauright, L. (1987). Toward a comprehensive personnel system: Performance appraisal part IV. *Nursing Management, 18*(8) 67–77.

forming below average in many other areas. This may not be a fair reflection of the individual's usual behavior (Table 18-1)

The Appraisal Meeting

Once all the data are compiled, the nurse manager sets aside time on her calendar for employee appraisal meetings. As a rule, these are conducted at about the same time each year for all employees. The purpose of the meeting is to discuss the employee's performance for the year. At the conclusion of the meeting, both parties should reach an agreement as to the employee's overall performance status, areas for improvement, and plans for maximizing performance.

THE ROLE OF THE EMPLOYEE

In preparation for performance appraisals, employees should collect their own data. They can begin by listing their strengths, especially contributions to the organization, as well as to patient safety and welfare. In addition, they will want to identify any accomplishments since their last review that indicate progress toward their stated goals. If little or no progress was made, they should be able to explain why. In most organizations, employees would have been required to submit goals for the upcoming appraisal meeting well in advance, perhaps at the last meeting. The employee should be prepared to address the goals they established at the time of their performance appraisal meeting.

Some of the long-term goals may be ongoing, while short-term goals may be completed or nearing completion by the time of the meeting. Employees should identify any problems encountered with reaching their goals and ascertain why. For example, an employee may have determined that she would have become a certified nurse midwife this year. The employee might first look at the needed resources and/or strategies she identified in relation to the stated goal. Next, the employee needs to ask herself a series of questions about failure to meet the goal. Was it due to time constraints? Was it a matter of finances, or was it a lack of adequate experiences or preparation? Was there anything the organization or the supervisor could have done to assist the employee? The employee should be as honest as possible when identifying the reasons the goal was not accomplished.

Self-Appraisals

Self-appraisals are commonly used to address whether or not employees have met established goals and if not, why not. Self-appraisals can also be used in conjunction with any of the other tools as can anecdotal records. In fact, self-appraisals should relate to performance of the job as defined by the job description, according to Swansburg and Swansburg (2002). When all parties are using like criteria or standards, there ought to be no surprises at the time of the appraisal interview. The goals established by the employee should therefore have relevance to the goals and mission of the organizations as well as to her own career goals. For example, a staff nurse who would someday like to be the team leader would need to determine what that job entails. Her goals should be defined clearly with that idea in mind. When meeting with her supervisor, the discussion should center on her career goals as well as on her capabilities as a staff nurse.

Before the performance appraisal meeting, the employee would be expected to submit self-appraisal materials to the nurse manager, including the goals developed for the coming year. This information will be added to the data that have already been compiled by the nurse manager.

THE ROLE OF THE NURSE MANAGER

Prior to meeting with her subordinates, the nurse manager should organize materials for the upcoming meeting. This begins with reviewing the employee's past performance and goals established for the past year. Next, the manager would review data from tools, peer evaluations, self-evaluations, and any anecdotal records. The benefits of prior planning cannot be overemphasized. The manager should be in charge and prepared for all contingencies. According to Rondeau (1992), successful performance appraisal sessions require a well-conceived and well-executed plan of action.

To evaluate subordinates better, the manager needs to know as much about the person being evaluated as possible. For example, knowing the current position held by the employee and how long she has held that position could make a difference in terms of how the person is evaluated. When looking at records of any critical incidents, the manager should remember that a single critical incident might not represent a true picture of the individual.

A date and time for the meeting should be established well in advance, and the manager should make certain the date and time for the meeting are satisfactory for both parties. It is important that the meeting be free of interruptions. The employee should believe that the manager considers this time to be important.

When employees are performing well, the meeting should go fairly smoothly for both parties. The purpose of planning for the meeting is to review the employee's job-related behaviors and the available evaluation materials. The focus of the meeting is always on the performance level of the individual past and present and the progress she has made toward the established goals. The manager should also review and be prepared to discuss any positive comments from peers, patients, or the person's immediate supervisor. Anecdotal records can be discussed if needed, but the employee deserves an opportunity to discuss his self-analysis and career aspirations as well.

When evaluating others, the nurse manager engages in active listening and assertive communication. Assertive communication means being open and honest but treating others fairly and with respect. This means giving criticism when needed and handing out praise when deserved. The focus of performance appraisal should be on the individual's performance, not on personal characteristics or problems. The manager needs to think through what he needs to discuss with the employee while making every effort to put the person at ease.

According to Ash (1984), there is a gender difference in responses to criticism. Although many societal changes have occurred for working women in general, nursing has always consisted primarily of women. In general, women are much more sensitive to criticism than men. In other words, women take it much more personally and tend to react more negatively to criticism.

Difficult as it may be, the nurse manager must decide how to approach an employee who has demonstrated an unsatisfactory performance. The nurse manager's role is to encourage and motivate employees toward excellence in performance. None of the manager's roles is as personal as appraising the work performance of others (Marquis & Huston, 2000, p. 414). This aspect of the process is considered extrinsic motivation. Because most employees are sensitive to comments about their performance, good interpersonal skills are as important as good leadership and managerial skills. At the beginning of this chapter was a quote from Ash (1984), "Sandwich every bit of criticism between two layers of praise." In short, this means that managers should start by focusing on the person's good points, then bring up the problems identified, and end by discussing how these can be resolved. Rondeau (1992) advocates using criticism sparingly as it tends to build up individual resistance and shut down communication.

Leaming (1998) described several improvement pointers for academic leaders engaged in evaluation of their subordinates. Many of these pointers would work well for the nursing administrator in any setting. In general terms, it is important to:

- Keep channels of communication open
- Let people know they are appreciated for their contributions to the organization
- Involve your subordinates in departmental governance
- Be positive and encourage an attitude of cooperativeness
- Treat people fairly and with respect
- Spread the workload around
- Create a supportive culture in the workplace
- Tolerate differences among subordinates (pp. 131–134).

THE MEETING

Once all the data are collected, the nursing manager or supervisor can begin to summarize the findings. A good rule of thumb is to list the strengths first and then to list the areas in need of improvement. If the employee submitted goals for the year and provided documentation, assess these as well. Although the nursing manager can list a few strategies for improving performance, the employee should take the major responsibility for this. According to Smith (2003), the appraisal meeting should be scheduled at a convenient time for the employee so the meeting can proceed uninterrupted for at least 45 minutes. She also recommends that the environment be nonthreatening and relaxed and that managers be prepared for the meeting. Lack of preparation is a time-waster and sets a poor example for subordinates. It may also display a lack of concern or interest in the employee. The meeting is a very personal, face-to-face interaction and should not be taken lightly by either party (Box 18-1).

The focus of the meeting should be to review the employee's performance and explore with him ideas for being successful within the organization. The manager sets the tone for the meeting by first explaining the purpose for the evaluation, which may vary from organization to organization. When merit raises or promotions are dependent on the outcome of the appraisal, the employees are likely to be somewhat nervous, so the manager should make every effort to put the employee at ease.

The nurse manager should initiate the evaluation process by reviewing with employees their goals for the year. From there she should proceed to discuss her findings based on data collection. Next,

---

Box 18-1

Tips for a Successful Performance Appraisal Meeting

- Conduct the meeting in a nonthreatening or neutral environment.
- Allow 45–60 minutes per person.
- Remember that information discussed during the meeting is confidential and should be shared only with committee members and the appropriate administrators.

According to Hecht, et al., (pp. 109–110), the administrator should:

- Maintain the focus of the meeting on the individual's performance, not his personality.
- Give specific suggestions for improving performance.
- Establish a time frame for achieving the goals, and review progress at that time.
- Recognize and reward positive achievement following unsatisfactory performance. If the employee has been unsatisfactory but has turned around, be sure to make note of improved behavior.

---

the manager can move on to the periodic observations or input from others, such as patients or peers. Employees should have an opportunity to respond to these findings and to discuss their performance and accomplishments.

By the conclusion of the meeting, the manager and the employee should mutually agree on a plan of action for the professional or career development of the individual. Both long-term and short-term goals should be addressed. A preprinted form can be used for this purpose. Such a form should include a space for a narrative summary and dated signatures of both the supervisor and employee. This plan of action might also include the employee's future goals with the organization.

FOLLOW-UP

Implementing the plan of action may require long-term intervention by the supervisor, such as motivating, coaching, or counseling the employee. If, at the conclusion of the meeting, the manager is convinced that none of those approaches would be beneficial to the employee, she may need to resort to disciplinary measures.

Motivating

The nursing manager/leader is in the best position to motivate employees to achieve their goals because managers set the tone for an environment that encourages productivity and success. When the employees look good and perform well, the nursing manager/leader looks good and, in turn, the organization looks good. A large part of motivation involves feelings related to self-worth and satisfaction. According to Swansburg and Swansburg (2002), a motivating environment is one in which the nurse leader/manager:

- Establishes a career development program
- Helps employees to meet their career goals
- Communicates the organization's goals and priorities
- Involves the staff in the development of department and organizational mission and goals
- Encourages teamwork
- Rewards teamwork, innovation, and creativity

While the above list does not cover all aspects of motivation, the list specifies those environmental factors that would encourage excellence in employee performance.

Coaching

In assisting employees to reach their goals and develop professionally, the nurse manager often assumes the role of a coach. According to Donner, Wheeler, and Waddell (1997), coaching is an ongoing, face-to-face, collaborative process. The purpose of coaching is to assist the employee in carrying out job responsibilities or gaining knowledge and skills required for the job. The immediate supervisor often has ongoing contact with the employee and is in the best position to evaluate progress and identify areas for improvement. Coaching might be likened to on-the-job training or teaching. The employee on the receiving end of the coaching has the advantage of immediate application of learning in the real world. This is a common practice in many organizations when new hires or individuals being considered for promotion have no educational experience related to the requisite knowledge or skills the job requires. Loveridge and Cummings (1996, p. 368) described coaching as informal counseling that can be used for the short term or over the

chapter star:
The Performance Appraisal Meeting

July is staff appraisal time for Unit X. Nurse Manger J (NMJ) has scheduled her 30 staff nurses over the first two weeks of July for performance review. Some appointments will occur on the weekends for the weekend staff and at the beginning of the evening shift and end of the night shift to cover employees on those permanent rotations. Thus, employees will not have to come in on an off day or off-duty time.

All staff nurses set goals at last year's appraisal meeting and have submitted their progress reports in advance of the meeting. In addition to meeting standard staff nurse competencies, Staff Nurse A (SNA), who is scheduled for the first meeting, sets the following goals:

1. Participation on one continuous quality improvement (CQI) project.
2. Attend a continuing education session on cardiac arrhythmias.
3. Develop skills in reading EKGs.

NMJ has approved SNA's attendance at the cardiac arrhythmia workshop, noted that she participated in the CQI project concerning reduction of length of stay for cardiac pacemaker patients, and reviews her chart notes, which state that SNA included notation of rhythm strips on her assigned patients.

The performance appraisal meeting begins. NMJ offers SNA a beverage of her choice. While the secretary is bringing them, she inquires about SNA's family to set a friendly, concerned tone for the meeting. NMJ reviews all of the staff nurse competencies, which are rated "met" or "above or exceeds expectations." She commends NMA on her performance. Then she reviews her documentation on PRN pain medication and explains and coaches SNA on how she might improve her notation of the patient's response by focusing on the following key factors, i.e., pain scale rating after receipt of medication, location of pain, and duration of pain, etc., at 2 hours and 4 hours after receiving the PRN medication. Together they plan to include objectives for the next year to improve SNA's documentation with milestones three, six, and nine months out. SNA is informed that she will receive an "exceeds expectations" for her overall rating and therefore will receive a 3.5% pay raise. The meeting concludes in 45 minutes. SNA will forward her finalized goals for the next year within the next 2 weeks.

long term. Short-term coaching is generally sponta-neous, brief, and open. Long-term coaching can be used to correct performance deficiencies. This type of coaching is usually planned and behavior-specific (Loveridge & Cummings, 1996, p. 200). Coaching also might involve providing opportunities for the employee to attend workshops or conferences or serve on committees.

Counseling

The nurse managers may also find themselves counseling employees. According to Hecht, et al. (1999, p. 111), this process provides the nursing administrator with an opportunity to demonstrate genuine interest in subordinates. Deciding if an employee would benefit from counseling requires interpersonal contact between the nurse manager and the employee. Counseling is one of the most pro-ductive functions to improve employee performance (Loveridge & Cummings, 1996, p. 368). Counsel-ing generally occurs in a private session where the focus is on helping the employee solve a problem. Generally, these are personal problems that may be interfering with the employee's performance. Frequent absenteeism is a good example. While fre-quent absenteeism can be due to many other factors, it is a common symptom of substance abuse.

Other problems that require counseling might include disputes or conflicts with other employees. In counseling sessions, the nurse manager should help employees get to the bottom of problems and adjust their attitude if necessary. Sometimes this means separating the employees, putting them on different shifts or on different units. If the problem is potentially life-threatening or requires therapeu-tic intervention, the employee should be directed where to seek help. Because nurses are not always equipped or trained as therapists, the problem employee may need referral to another agency or a professional counselor for support.

Disciplining

Managers may also be required to mete out disci-pline. Although discipline is generally thought of as some form of punishment for negative behavior, Gillies (1994, p. 557) stated that its purpose is to improve job performance. According to *Webster's Dictionary* (1995), disciplining can mean taking

corrective action or bringing about self-control through instruction or training. The definition also includes conformity to rules and regulations. Marquis and Huston (2000, p. 442) stated that when employees continue undesirable conduct, either in breaking rules or in not performing their job duties adequately, disciplinary action must be taken. This approach may seem a little extreme, but in any organization there are standards and guiding principles. Employees are expected to conform and perform accordingly. In health-care systems, many of these standards exist to protect the patients and others. One good example is universal precautions. JCAHO (2005) published its list of disease-specific care national patient safety goals, one of which was to reduce the risk of health-care–associated infections. One of the strategies listed was com-pliance with the Centers for Disease Control and Prevention (CDC) hand hygiene guidelines.

Nurses learn early on that aseptic technique is essential to preventing the spread of organisms from person to person. But how often have nurses been observed rushing from one situation to another without taking the time to wash their hands between patients? Most health-care agencies have begun to post signs in plain sight in every patient room and anywhere that hand washing is considered essential. Some nurses might view this as a form of discipline simply because somewhere, someone did not take the time to wash his hands. When considered in a broader perspective, how-ever, most nurses realize that this is a reminder for everyone who might transmit organisms: nursing staff members, physicians, other health-care work-ers, family members, and even the patients.

Few responsibilities of the nursing manager are as personal and time-consuming as performance appraisal. The manager's job includes a number of other personnel responsibilities, including work-ing with new employees, probationary employees, and problem employees. Although most health-care organizations have personnel departments, the nursing manager is generally involved whenever the nursing staff is the focus of attention.

New Employees and Probationary Employees

In this era of nursing shortages, new employees and probationary employees rarely have the luxury of a long orientation period. Agencies should take care with new employees and develop an evaluation procedure for determining their ability to succeed. When the organization shows an interest in the employee and is willing to spend time teaching him, he may be more likely to stay. Metcalf (2001) stated that it is crucial for newly graduated nurses that the process of staff development begin at the commencement of and continue throughout their employment. A collaborative environment is a motivating environment where the nursing administration provides ongoing support and encourages the professional development of each employee.

Conversely, any new or probationary employee who demonstrates problematic behavior in one department is likely to have difficulty on other units in the same facility. Documenting behavior and evaluating abilities from the beginning of employment provides the agency with information about performance in general. New hires and probationary employees who do not measure up, especially with coaching and counseling efforts, may need to be terminated.

THE PROBLEM EMPLOYEE

Once an employee is a part of the organization, the administration has a responsibility to assist that person. A variety of personal difficulties can lead to poor performance in the workplace. Most notable would be problems related to chemical impairment. Chemical impairment refers to impairment due to drug or alcohol addiction (Marquis & Huston, 2000, p. 459). Some common problems resulting from these impairments are excessive absenteeism, decreased quality of work, errors in judgment, work-related accidents, and high rates of turnover. When evaluating employees, the manager should note when these problems occur with regularity. Excessive absenteeism, tardiness, and sick leave can create a serious staffing deficiency unless guidelines or policies exist. Most unionized settings address these problems, and nonunionized settings would do well to address them as well (Box 18-2).

In many states, nursing organizations or boards of nursing sponsor programs for the impaired nurse. Many agencies and health insurance plans also cover the cost of such programs. The nurse manager needs to be familiar with the policies existing in the organization and in the state. For example, in Ohio, employers are required to report employees for con-

> ### Box 18-2
> ### Developing Organizational Policies for Absenteeism, Tardiness, and Sick Leave
>
> 1. Recognize the existence of employee problems
> 2. Take a proactive approach for dealing with the problem
> 3. Review existing policies
> 4. Solicit employee input
> 5. Determine how many absences per year are considered excessive
> 6. Determine how many successive sick days are permitted within a given period
> 7. Decide what action should be taken for violations of the policy
> 8. Develop a staffing protocol to be instituted when absenteeism and sick leaves occur
> 9. Distribute policy to all employees, post policy on each unit, and add it to the policy manual

duct requiring disciplinary action, such as a positive drug screen, even if that employee has been referred to an employee assistance program. Ohio sponsors two programs for problem employees: a program for nurses with substance abuse problems and a program that requires nurses to obtain additional education to improve their practice skills. Nurses in these programs are monitored by the state board of nursing and are able to remain employable with minimal threat to the public. Other states as well as most professional organizations and many health-care organizations offer similar programs.

Although most organizations have a personnel department to deal with all kinds of issues that develop during corporate changes such as reorganization and downsizing, the nurse manager may find herself called upon for input when the nursing staff is involved. Nurse managers may also be involved at the decision-making level when it comes to transferring or terminating nursing staff.

Transfers and Termination

Transfers and termination within an organization can lead to increased productivity and success. Good employees may be transferred to other areas within an organization as part of a promotion package or to make better use of their potential. In some instances problem employees may be transferred to other areas where they may be more successful.

When an employee exhibits problem behavior that is unlikely to change and may be detrimental to the organization, she should be terminated. Restructuring within an organization may result in the termination of employees, even those with good performance records.

Transfers

Transfers are common in the corporate world; they often involve moving an employee to a new location, often with a promotion and an increase in salary. In health-care organizations, this may not be the case. Many employees, especially the nursing staff, are place-bound and unwilling or unable to move to another location. When mergers or acquisitions occur in the health-care industry, it is often necessary to eliminate positions. Mergers occur when two or more organizations join together to form a single new organization (Lancaster, 1999, p. 99). When one organization buys another, the acquired organization no longer carries its original identity (Lancaster, 1999, p. 99). In either of these situations, for example, there may be no need to have two evening supervisors for the intensive care unit (ICU). One of them could, if willing, be transferred to another unit as a supervisor, if they were unwilling to take a staff position in the ICU. One type of transfer is the *lateral transfer,* meaning the individual would be moved to a position with a similar scope of responsibilities within the same organization (Marquis & Huston, 2000). Another type of transfer is the *downward transfer,* which occurs when someone takes a position within the organization that is below his or her previous level (p. 539). If the transfer is unrelated to performance, the individual may be able to select a position that best relates to her career goals. A person who eventually wants to be a nurse educator may opt to switch to the education department. If this is not in her future, she may decide to take the open position as relief supervisor for the emergency department.

Downsizing refers to reducing the number of positions within an organization, normally done to reduce organizational costs and often accompanied by changes in job design to enhance the productivity of the remaining staff (Lancaster, 1999, p. 93). Two personnel issues related to downsizing are transfers and termination of employees. Usually, a transfer is no reflection on the employee's performance because the person's salary often remains the same. With downsizing, this is becoming a fairly common practice.

Termination

While termination is certainly possible with restructuring, the shortage of nurses makes it unlikely that nursing personnel would be let go. More often, it is the unlicensed personnel whose jobs are in jeopardy. Termination should be the final step in the performance appraisal process, when other measures have failed to bring about improvement of the employee's performance. As with other policies in the organization, it is critical that a well-defined procedure for termination be in place. The guidelines should be followed strictly by the nursing administrator, after efforts at coaching, counseling, and disciplining have proved unsuccessful. When an employee is a member of a collective bargaining unit, the contract delineates the steps leading to termination. In many organizations, outplacement services are available for employees who have been terminated. This might be a comprehensive program that helps individuals to prepare résumés and applications and work with counselors as they search for another job. This type of program may also be instituted when an organization is going through a major transition, such as downsizing or closing. When valued employees must be terminated, they may be recommended to other facilities within the corporate system.

All Good Things...

The purpose of performance appraisal is to improve the quality and productivity of the employee and enhance career aspirations. The nursing administrator has the responsibility for overseeing the performance appraisal and motivating the employee toward excellence in practice. When employees appear to need support or assistance in reaching goals, their supervisors may be able to work with them, coaching and counseling as needed. Performance appraisal should be an ongoing process, which has both informal and formal components. Employees should take an active role in the process by establishing meaningful career goals for themselves and working toward those goals. The outcome of the process should be satisfied employees who realize their aspirations with the support of the nursing administration.

NCLEX Questions

1. In most organizations, a current, valid job description should do all of the following except:
   A. Outline the duties, skills, and knowledge required for the job
   B. Describe how the person is to carry out basic responsibilities
   C. Be used as the baseline for a performance appraisal
   D. Identify the department or unit for the work assignment

2. Performance appraisals are primarily done for which purpose?
   A. Comparing the performance of employees on the unit
   B. Identifying employees with personal problems
   C. Recruiting new employees into the organization
   D. Improving the performance of individual employees

3. A peer review may be done as part of the performance appraisal to:
   A. Compare the employee's past and present performance
   B. Document a single outstanding observation
   C. Assess the level of a colleague's performance
   D. Make a list of desirable employee behaviors

4. The following statements about management by objectives are all true except:
   A. Employees have an opportunity to appraise their own performance
   B. The employee's supervisor establishes the performance standards
   C. Performance is compared with goals established by the employee
   D. The end result is usually a more realistic appraisal of performance

5. Which of the following methods is likely to be most effective in motivating a new employee with poor performance?
   A. Coaching
   B. Counseling
   C. Disciplining
   D. Supervisor praise
   E. Additional training

6. In preparing for the yearly performance appraisal meetings, Ellen Jones' new supervisor noted that Ellen had an unusual increase in the number of absences and reported late to work on at least six occasions during the previous year. Up until this point, Ellen, an employee at the organization for 3 years, had received good, but not outstanding, evaluations. What should the supervisor do?
   A. Talk to Ellen as soon as possible and determine if this was due to some temporary problem or one that is likely to continue
   B. Talk with Ellen's previous supervisor and/or her peers see if they are aware of any problems
   C. Talk with Ellen about this when she comes in for her performance appraisal next month
   D. Talk to Ellen about seeing a counselor as her attitude toward work seems to have taken a turn for the worse

7. Janet Smith is a new employee at the hospital. She graduated from nursing school 5 years ago, passed the NCLEX, and worked part time in a skilled care facility for a year. Janet since married and had twin girls 2 years ago. As her supervisor, you have noticed some knowledge and skill deficiencies. For example, she has not started an IV recently and is unfamiliar with many of the medications being given to patients on her unit. Which of the following are most likely to be helpful?
   1) Give her a book on pharmacology
   2) Tell her to contact the local nursing program and sign up for a pharmacology course
   3) Have her spend time in the hospital pharmacy
   4) Make arrangements for her to spend additional time with one of the preceptors
   5) Arrange practice time for her in the hospital skills laboratory
   A. 1 and 2
   B. 3 and 4
   C. 2, 4, and 5
   D. 1, 2, and 3
   E. 4 only

8. During a performance appraisal report, the supervisor should focus on all of the following except:
   A. The employee's current level of performance
   B. The employee's career development plans
   C. Determining why the employee may be performing poorly
   D. Discussing the employee's contributions to the organization

9. It is difficult for most supervisors to avoid bias when evaluating their subordinates, mainly because many of the tools lead to rater errors like the halo effect, which can best be defined as:
   A. Rating someone based on her education or position
   B. Giving someone an average rating because the supervisor is unsure of the actual performance
   C. Rating someone based on his most recent positive behavior, not his overall performance
   D. Giving someone a high rating because she is popular with her peers

10. Which of the following is the last step in a progressive disciplinary procedure?
    A. Reprimand
    B. Counseling
    C. Transfer
    D. Termination

REFERENCES

American Nurses Association. (2004). *Nursing: Scope and standards of practice.* Washington, D.C.: ANA.

Ash, M.K. (1984). *Mary Kay on people management.* NY: Warner.

Barnum, B.S., & Kerfoot, K.M. (1995). *The nurse as executive* (4th ed.). Gaithersburg, MD: Aspen.

Brykczynski, K.A. (1998). Clinical exemplars describing expert staff nursing practices. *Journal of Nursing Management, 6*(6):351–360.

Creasia, J.L., & Parker, B. (2001). *Conceptual foundations: The bridge to professional nursing practice* (3rd ed.). St. Louis: Mosby.

Donner, G.J., Wheeler, M.M., & Waddell, J. (1997). The nurse manager as a career coach. *Journal of Nursing Administration, 21*(12), 14–18.

Ellis, J.R., & Hartley, C.L. (2000). *Managing and coordinating nursing care* (3rd ed.). Philadelphia: Lippincott.

Ellis, J.R., & Hartley, C.L. (2004). *Nursing in today's world: Trends, issues, and management* (8th ed.). Philadelphia: Lippincott, Williams & Wilkins.

Gillies, D.A. (1994). *Nursing management: A systems approach* (3rd ed.). Philadelphia: Saunders.

Hecht, I.W.D., et al. (1999). *The department chair as academic leader.* Phoenix, AZ: Oryx Press.

Houston, R. (1995). Integrating CQI into performance appraisals. *Nursing Management, 26*(3):48A-C.

Huber, D. (2000). *Leadership and nursing care* (2nd ed.). Philadelphia: Saunders.

Joint Commission on Accreditation of Healthcare Organizations (JCAHO). (2005). 2005 Hospitals' national patient safety goals. Retrieved May 16, 2005, from http://www.jcaho.org/accredited+organizations/patient+safety/05+npsg/05_npsg_hap.htm

Joint Commission on Accreditation of Healthcare Organizations (JCAHO). (2005). National patient safety goals for 2005. Retrieved May 16, 2005, from http://www.jcaho.org/accredited+organizations/patient+safety/npsg.htm

Kelly-Heidenthal, P. (2003). *Nursing leadership & management.* Clifton Park, NY: Delmar.

Lancaster, J. (1999). *Nursing issues in leading and managing change.* St. Louis: Mosby.

Leaming, D.R. (1998). *Academic leadership: A practical guide to chairing the department.* Bolton, MA: Anker.

Loveridge, C.E., & Cummings, S.H. (1996). *Nursing management in the new paradigm.* Gaithersburg, MD: Aspen.

Marquis, B.L., & Huston, C.J. (2000). *Leadership roles and management functions in nursing: Theory & application* (3rd ed.). Philadelphia: Lippincott.

Merriam-Webster's desk dictionary. (1995). Springfield, MA: Merriam-Webster.

Metcalf, C. (2001). The importance of performance appraisal and staff development: A graduating nurse's perspective. *International Journal of Nursing Practice, 7*(1): 54–57.

Nauright, L. (1987). Toward a comprehensive personnel system: Performance appraisal part IV. *Nursing Management, 18*(8), 67–77.

Parks, J., & Lindstrom, C.W. (1995). Taking the fear out of peer review. *Nursing Management, 26*(3), 48–49.

Peterson, J.V., & Nisenholz, B. (1995). *Orientation to counseling* (3rd ed.). Boston: Allyn & Bacon.

Rondeau, K.V. (1992). Constructive performance appraisal feedback for healthcare employees. *Hospital Topics, 70*(2): 27-33.

Smith, M.H. (2003). Empower staff with praiseworthy appraisals. *Nursing Management, 34*(1): 16–18.

Swansburg, R.C., & Swansburg, R.J. (2002). *Introduction to management and leadership for nurse managers* (3rd ed.). Boston: Jones & Bartlett.

Tappen, R.M. (2001). *Nursing leadership and management: Concepts and practice* (4th ed.). Philadelphia: Davis.

Yoder-Wise, P.S. (1999). *Leading and managing in nursing* (2nd ed.). St. Louis: Mosby.

chapter 19

Nursing Celebrates Cultural Diversity

JOSEPHINE A. KAHLER, EDD, RN, CS

"Cultural diversity is not an obstacle, it's a gift."

Anonymous

CHAPTER MOTIVES

- Define and explain the concept of culture.
- Explain the foundational impact of culture on nursing practice
- Discuss models describing cultural competence.
- Describe the characteristics of some prominent cultures.
- Analyze transcultural nursing perspectives as they pertain to the work environment.
- Evaluate the challenges of managing a culturally diverse workforce.

The minority population in the United States is expected to make up more than 40% of the total population by 2035 (Giger & Davidhizer, 1995). Addressing the needs of an increasingly diverse population has become a major challenge to all health-care providers, especially nurse leaders and managers. Cultural diversity concerns can be viewed from two perspectives: caring both physically and spiritually for a diverse client population and providing a culturally diverse workforce with positive work experiences (Dreher, 1996). With the present-day nursing shortage, recruitment of foreign nurses will result in a new workforce of individuals who bring with them an understanding of other cultures but also different values and beliefs. This chapter explores the concept of cultural diversity, along with the theories used to explain cultural differences. It offers guidance to nurses who are providing leadership and care in an increasingly more diverse health-care system, with increasing diversity of team members. See Box 19-1 on terms commonly used when discussing cultural diversity.

Foundations of Cultural Study

The swell in the ethnic diversity of the United States has put new demands on health-care systems to provide health care that is culturally acceptable. In order to achieve this, practitioners need to increase their knowledge of the health-care practices of people from different sociocultural groups and recognize the differences in perspectives between themselves and their clients (Anderson, 1990).

CULTURAL CONCEPTS

Culture encompasses shared values, behaviors, and beliefs that are reinforced through social interactions, shared by members of a particular group, and transmitted from one generation to the next. Culture exerts considerable influence over most of an individual's life experiences, including illness. It can be perceived as a form of tradition for a group, which is based on beliefs about survival of group mores and customs. These concepts make culture very distinct from external managerial control, such as policies and procedures (Coeling & Simms, 1993). Culture is deeply rooted within the group and within the human interpersonal dynamics that occur naturally within the groups—brought about by child rearing, language, and religious beliefs—as a natural result of people in the groups. Dochterman and Kennedy-Grace (2001) describe culture as being a system of learned patterns unique to members of a group. Spector (2000) has specified that one's cultural background is a fundamental component of one's ethnic heritage and should have a vast impact on the type of nursing care that is rendered to patients. Culture has also been described as differences and variety in customs and practices of defined social groups (Poss, 1999). Three levels of culture have been identified by Schein (1985):

1. The visible level: this includes physical space and social environment. What image is projected at first encounter? Does the nurse use sensitivity when admitting a client from another culture? Are respect and understanding demonstrated by the nurse who is questioning the new client?
2. The values: this includes elements of what ought to be; for example, nurses value caring and high quality of care. Whose values should predominate? Is there awareness of the values within the culture of the client being cared for, or is the client treated like any other within the general population?

Box 19-1

Cultural Terms

To ensure that there is an understanding of terms commonly used to describe culture, some definitions follow:

Culture: Shared values, beliefs, and practices of a particular group of people that are transmitted from one generation to the next and are identified as patterns that guide thinking and action.

Cultural competence: Providing effective nursing care to patients from many cultures in a respectful and knowing way.

Cultural diversity: Differences in race, ethnicity, religion, national origin, gender, and economic status.

Stereotyping: Assigning certain beliefs and behaviors to groups without recognizing individuality.

Values: Abstract standards that give a person a sense of what is right or wrong and establish a code of conduct for living.

3. The basic underlying assumptions: this includes the actual guides to behavior that are deeply held and not open to challenge or debate, such as the influence that our own cultural inheritance has on our personal health beliefs (Betancourt, Green, & Carrillo, 2002).

Without an understanding of cultural differences, U.S. health-care providers tend to impose Western ideas on individuals from other cultures, which infringe on their values. Nurses tend to respond to sick people based on their own socialization, culture, and education. For instance, because the U.S. culture is an informal one, nurses may be inclined to call patients by their first names. People who grew up in another culture, however, may consider it disrespectful to address others by their first names, especially when there is an age difference between the client and caregiver. The caregiver should ask clients how they wish to be addressed so as to not seem disrespectful. Moreover, nurses are trained to respect patient autonomy and decisions. Yet some Asian clients may expect nurses to provide directives, be authoritative, and be expert practitioners who take charge. Out of respect for this authority, they may nod, smile, verbally agree to anything that the nurse proposes, and may not speak until spoken to (Giger & Davidhizar, 1999). Nurses may also find their perceptions of appropriate personal space called into question. Many people from South America and the Middle East stand close to the person with whom they are conversing. Many Americans feel very uncomfortable if someone is standing closer than 3 feet while conversing. Hispanic patients expect the health-care provider to shake hands with them at the beginning of the conversation, whereas most Japanese clients would feel uncomfortable with shaking hands, preferring to bow instead (Salimbene, 1998).

Most immigrants to the United States appear to be fully acculturated and speak without a trace of a foreign accent, such as those who immigrated from Western Europe and other English-speaking countries. Values change as new generations adopt the new country's views over time. It is easy for health-care practitioners to overlook the impact that cultural inheritance has had on both conscious and subconscious health beliefs, however.

In the United States, individuals are classified into five ethnic groups: African-Americans, Asian-Americans and Pacific Islanders, Hispanic-Americans, Native Americans, and Caucasian Americans. This tendency, however, does little to promote understanding of the health beliefs, practices, needs, and diversity that are represented within each of these population classifications. It may, in fact, impose stereotypical judgments on persons within these groups because they are viewed by the health-care providers in traditional ways. But nurses should keep in mind, as Benner and Wrubel (1998) observe, "changes in lifestyles and health habits work best when they are integrated into the person's own cultural patterns and traditions, for it is hard to sustain new patterns if they go against the grain of one's social patterns" (p. 155).

IMPACT OF CULTURE ON NURSING PRACTICE

Nurses today are recognizing that awareness of cultural differences in their health-care delivery is imperative for their practice. The role expectations of nurses may even vary from culture to culture. A common Anglo-American view of nurses is that they treat people as equals, tend to be passive, and take direction from physicians. These patients feel free to ask questions of their nurses that they may not ask of physicians.

Despite the fact that awareness of cultural diversity directly affects diagnosis, assessment, and intervention strategies, cultural diversity is often not seen as an essential variable in how nurses mediate conflict, communicate, or interpret different behaviors.

For instance, in the Navajo culture, great value is placed on keeping pain and discomfort to oneself. Therefore, the nurse who expects clients from the Navajo nation to request medication for pain may make a false assumption on the client's comfort level, when the opposite is true (Kirkpatrick & Deloughery, 1995).

Communication is a vital part of the cultural interaction that takes place between the health-care provider and client. Patterns of communication are strongly influenced by culture and include not only language differences but verbal and nonverbal behaviors as well. Without a sense of their own cultural values, nurses fail to provide culturally competent care to patients. Nurses must culturally assess each patient individually while keeping in mind that differences can occur not only between cultures but also within cultures. Culture directly affects client care. Often, culture affects a client's compliance with medication directives, or culture can affect who makes the health-care decisions within a family. Differences such as these need to be learned by nurses, who can be educated into being culturally competent caregivers.

Models of Cultural Competence

Cultural competence models serve as frameworks for providing effective nursing care to patients from many cultures in a respectful and knowing way (Bartol & Richardson, 1998). Cultural competence is a vital component for practicing effective com-

Practice Proof 19-1

Article: Improving health outcomes in diverse populations: Competency in cross-cultural research with indigenous Pacific Islander populations.

Authors and Journal: Palafox, N.A., et al. (2002). *Journal of Ethnicity and Health, 7*(4), 270–285.

Abstract: The disparity in health status between the indigenous Pacific Island populations and the United States–associated Pacific Island populations was examined in order to acquire an understanding of their unique paradigms of health knowledge and address their disparate health issues. The researchers recognized that U.S. institutions and federal agencies had been limited in their ability to develop competency in cross-cultural research in the past with these populations. A descriptive review was used of the investigators' experience in Hawaii and other Pacific Island locations. The results confirmed the researchers' views that in order to conduct successful culturally competent research, they need to recruit Pacific Islanders from indigenous backgrounds. These Pacific Island researchers with the skills and knowledge of Western scientific inquiry were found to understand the complex health situation of their own population and determine the changes in health-care delivery that could make a difference. Once this was accomplished, the researchers felt that positive changes in health-care disparity could be effected in the Pacific Island population.

QUESTIONS:
1. Why is cultural research important in determining access to health care?
2. How does cultural awareness impact treatment of Western Pacific nations?
3. Why is it important to include cultural competence when studying other cultures?

munication, valuing, understanding, and caring in health care (Poss, 1999).

The following models are frequently used in health-care settings.

Purnell and Paulanka's (1998) model for cultural competence has been found useful in any setting (Fig. 19-1). The outer zone of the model's circle represents global society; the second zone depicts community; the third zone represents the family; and the inner zone symbolizes the individual. The interior of the circle is divided into 12 pie-shaped wedges depicting cultural domains and their concepts, i.e., family organization, workplace issues, and health-care practices.

The innermost center circle is dark, depicting unknown phenomena. Cultural consciousness is expressed in behaviors from "unconsciously incompetent-consciously incompetent-consciously competent to unconsciously competent" (p. 9). This model can be used in any health-care setting because of its concise structure. Once the cultural data have been analyzed, this model allows the nurse to determine whether to adopt, modify, or reject health-care treatment regimens according to the needs of the client. Ultimately, it can determine whether these treatment protocols improve the quality of health-care delivery and the client's own personal well-being (p. 9). This model allows the nurse to use culturally competent care for the client by analyzing the client's care plan and adapting treatment modalities to the client's cultural needs.

Another model of culturally competent care was developed by Campinha-Bacote in 1994. She identified four constructs: (1) awareness (including biases and sensitivity); (2) skills (including use of assessment tools); (3) knowledge (including worldview and frameworks); and (4) encounters (including exposure and practice). In 1999, Campinha-Bacote used this model to illustrate how cultural competence concepts could be used in nursing:

Cultural awareness should be a deliberate process that assists the nurse in becoming aware of and more sensitive to the client's cultural differences while at the same time making caregivers more conscious of their own cultural values so as not to impose them on the client. This awareness focus can be achieved by experiential exercises and critical incidents.

Cultural knowledge can be obtained by education on different cultures and accumulating a knowledge base of transcultural nursing. Cultural

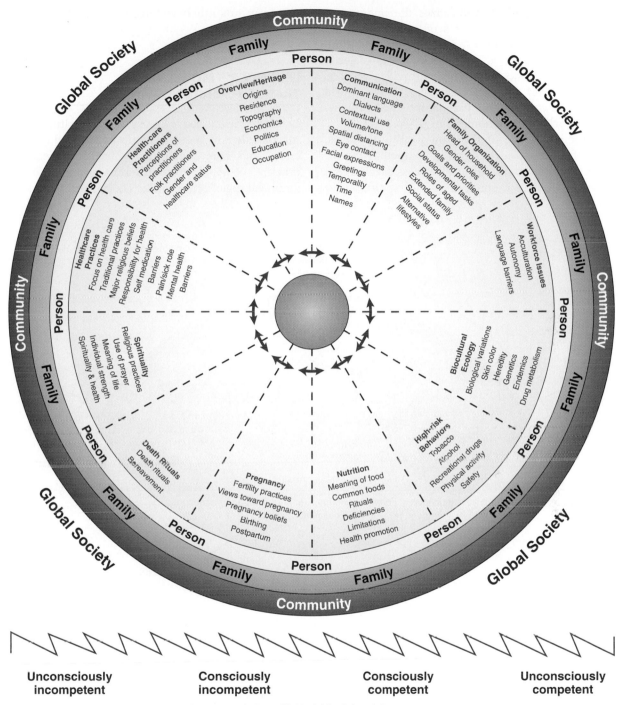

FIGURE 19-1 Purnell's Model for Cultural Competence

skill is achieved by the nurse learning how to do a cultural assessment and identifying the client's beliefs, practices, and perceptions of health. Cultural encounters are the actual face-to-face encounters and interactions with the client.

Campinha-Bacote (1999) also defines cultural competence as "the process in which the health-care provider continuously strives to achieve the ability to effectively work within the cultural context of the client (i.e., individual, family or community)"

(p. 203). This author emphasizes the importance during the awareness process of examining one's own biases and prejudices. She states that cultural knowledge is gathered from receiving an eclectic educational foundation, which provides various global views of different cultures. "One's world view can be considered a paradigm or way of viewing the world and phenomena in it" (p. 204).

Without a sense of their own cultural values, nurses fail to provide culturally competent care to patients. Nurses must culturally assess each patient individually while keeping in mind that differences can occur not only between cultures but also within cultures.

LEININGER'S MODEL OF TRANSCULTURAL NURSING

Leininger developed a theory of transcultural nursing that depicts a relationship between the differences and commonalities in health beliefs and practices of people from different countries or geographical regions (Fig. 19-2) (Leininger, 1991).

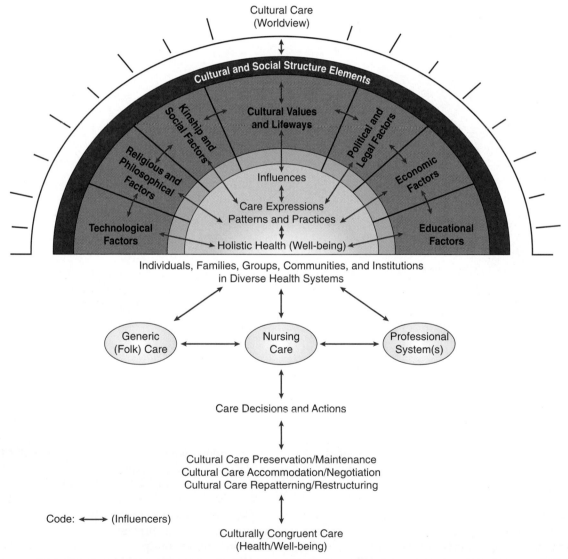

FIGURE 19-2 Leininger's Model of Transcultural Nursing. (Redrawn by Leininger, M. [1991]. *Cultural care diversity and universality: A theory of nursing.* New York: National League of Nursing.)

Leininger (1991) is credited with developing a theory of culture care. The theoretical framework, depicted as "The Sunrise Model," embraces the idea that cultural constructs are embedded in each other and their application is both broad and holistic. The arrows on the model indicate "influencers" but are not causal or linear relationships. The arrows flow in different areas and cross major factors to depict the interrelatedness of factors and the fluidity of influencers. The dotted lines indicate an open world or an open system of living reflective of the natural world of most humans. Leininger (1990) describes the upper part of the model as being extremely important but often challenging to nurses because it often leads to the discovery of embedded, deeply valued, and meaningful data about human care and well-being. Transculturism describes a nurse who is grounded in one's own culture but has the skills to be able to work in a multicultural environment.

Leininger (1997) emphasizes that there is a greater need for cultural awareness because of increased global mobility, the importance of cultural identity, migration, and role change. Care, she states, should be viewed as culturally defined, with predictors defining health or illness. It should be assumed that when persons are given "human caring" the person's cultural characteristics will be addressed and incorporated into the overall plan of care. Leininger (2002) defined cultural care as the "synthesized and culturally constituted assistive, supportive, and facilitated caring acts toward self or others focused on evident or anticipated needs for the client's health or well-being or to face disabilities, death or other human conditions" (p. 83). Leininger emphasizes that an important step in providing care to diverse clients is cultural assessment. To demystify the process, it may be helpful to think of cultural assessment as "merely asking people their preferences, what they think, who we should talk to in order to make a decision" (Villaire, 1994, p. 138). Culturally competent nurses take cultural differences into consideration when doing assessments. This assessment helps them to interpret patient behavior accurately and recognize the necessity for developing a culturally congruent plan of care and to achieve outcomes. Leininger (1978) identified the basic domains to review when conducting a cultural assessment:

1. Lifestyle patterns
2. Cultural norms and values
3. Cultural taboos and myths
4. Ethnocentric tendencies and worldviews
5. Health and life care rituals
6. Caring behaviors
7. Degree of cultural change
8. General features that the client perceives as different from or similar to other cultures
9. Folk and professional health-illness systems used

The Cultural Assessment Checklist (Box 19-2) was originally designed for home health nurses but is easily adapted for use in other settings. Its concise yet comprehensive nature takes into account the limited amount of time nurses may have to get to know new patients.

Cultural Competence in Practice

Caring for culturally diverse clients presents the nurse with many challenges. The nurse must be sensitive to differences such as language, interpretation of communication, eye-contact norms, gender issues, touching and physical contact, food practices, and caregiver acceptability issues (Galanti, 1999).

For instance, a Native American man who is 22 years of age has been involved in a severe automobile accident and is in the intensive care unit in a comatose state. Being aware of the culture involved may make a difference between life and death issues for this young man. An understanding of his tribal customs and beliefs is an imperative part of his care. The hospital staff in this case demonstrated that they understood the tribal customs and beliefs of this client. They were able to accommodate the family's wishes and individual needs in a meaningful way. By using transcultural concepts and principles, the staff prevented any cultural conflicts or clashes and were able to meet the needs of the family with what proved to be the inevitable death of their relative. Later, the staff was able to evaluate the outcome of the intervention in a constructive way. This incident became a classic teaching tool for both medical and nursing students.

Attention to the spiritual domain in providing holistic care to the above client depends on the beliefs and values of both the client and nurse (Oldnall, 1996). Watson (1985 and 1988) specifically advocates that nurses have an obligation to identify the spiritual and religious beliefs in their

BOX 19-2

Cultural Assessment Checklist

Patient-identified cultural/ethnic group _____

Religion _____

Typical greeting. Form of address: Handshake appropriate? Shoes worn in home?

Social customs before "business." Social exchanges? Refreshment?

Direct or indirect communication patterns?

Eye contact. Is eye contact considered polite or rude?

Tone of voice. What does a soft voice or a loud voice mean in this culture?

Personal space. Is personal space wider or narrower than in the American culture?

Facial expressions, gestures. What do smiles, nods, and hand gestures mean?

Touch. When, where, and by whom can a patient be touched?

Diagnosis. What do you call this illness? How would you describe this problem?

Cause. What caused the problem? What might other people think is wrong with you?

Course. How does the illness work? What does it do to you? What do you fear most about this problem?

Treatment. How have you treated the illness? What treatment should you receive? Who in your family or community can help?

Prognosis. How long will the problem last? Is it serious?

Expectations. What are you hoping the nurses will do for you when we come?

Pattern of meals. What is eaten? When are meals eaten?

Sick [comfort] foods.

Food intolerance and taboos.

Cultural responses to pain.

Patient's perception of pain response.

Patient's perception of Western medications.

Possible pharmacogenetic variations.

Decision maker.

Sick role.

Language barriers, translators.

Cultural/ethnic community resources.

From Narayan, M.C. (1997). Cultural assessment in home health care. *Home Health Care Nurse 15*(10), 663–672.

---

clients and respect them, no matter how unusual they may seem. In some cultures, illness may be deemed a punishment for some sinful action. At times, clients may make decisions that conflict with the beliefs of their religious communities or even their caregivers. These decisions often affect the physical, mental, and spiritual well-being of the client. It must be recognized that spirituality is an integral part of culture. The following is a classic example of a client dealing with a religious dilemma that leads to spiritual distress.

A patient is considering aborting a severely handicapped child, knowing that it would go against the teachings of her church. A visit from the patient's pastor has left her very upset and angry. He told her that God may not forgive her for having this abortion. Because of the patient's high level of distress, the nurse asked the hospital chaplain to visit with the patient. This action resulted in both prayer and discussion and eventual peace of mind for the patient, who proceeded to have the planned procedure.

Two cultural trends that have become prevalent since the middle 1970s support the movement toward spirituality in health care. First, managed

care consumers and clients complain that their health needs are not being met. More than one-third of American adults are seeking alternative solutions to health and illness problems from various non-mainstream sources, including spiritual practices (Eisenberg, et al., 1992). The second trend is the growth of well-designed and controlled research that examines the relationship between spiritual practices and health outcomes of both the clients and providers of care (Byrd, 1988; Kass, et al., 1991). In a study conducted (Byrd, 1988) on patients in a coronary care unit, the group that received regular intercessory prayer had fewer episodes of cardiac arrest, congestive heart failure, and pneumonia. The group also required fewer antibiotics and diuretics and less ventilator assistance than the control group, which received no prayer interventions (Box 19-3).

Clients often make cultural choices that are difficult for nurses to understand and accept. For instance, based on religious beliefs, clients may refuse commonplace treatments such as blood transfusions, medications, or even minor surgery. When patients' wishes are contrary to the nurse's with respect to spirituality and religion, nurses

Sociocultural Self Assessment

Directions: Use your answers to help yourself have a better understanding of your own cultural and social beliefs.

1. What is my cultural heritage? Which ethnic groups do I belong to? My age group? My religious affiliation? My socioeconomic status?
2. Do I assume that others have the same values and beliefs that I have?
3. What type of contact have I had with persons from different backgrounds? Do I assume that other people have the same values and beliefs that I have?
4. What group affiliations am I proud of? Are my attitudes and behavior ethnocentric? What would I change about my group affiliations, if I could? Why?
5. Have I ever felt rejected by another group? Did this experience make me more sensitive to other cultures or cause me to vilify others who were different from myself?
6. Did I get messages about people who were different from me from family and friends? Have these attitudes influenced my opinions today?
7. What are the main biases I have about individuals from different cultures? Do these stereotypes impede me from developing cultural sensitivity?
8. What attitudes do I need to change within myself in order to work effectively with individuals from other cultures?

Chitty, K.K. Illness and culture: Impact on patients, families and nurses. (2005). In *Professional Nursing: Concepts & Challenges*, St. Louis: Elsevier, p. 468.

personal religious beliefs and the desire to placate the wishes of the family. This can occur even though the patient has a living will on file in his chart. The physician's values in turn may create an ethical dilemma, which could result in stressful working conditions for the nursing staff. Subsequently, this creates a conflict between the nursing staff's value system and the institution's practices in honoring the patient's advance directives.

In the face of any conflict, however, Leininger (1997) describes a culturally competent nurse as one who demonstrates the following skills and attributes:

1. Uses nursing concepts, principles, and available research findings to assess and guide practices
2. Understands and values the cultural beliefs and practices of designated cultures so that nursing care is adapted to meet that individual client's needs in a meaningful way
3. Knows how to avoid and prevent major cultural conflicts, clashes, or hurtful care practices
4. Demonstrates the confidence to be able to work effectively and knowingly with clients from different cultures and is also able to evaluate transcultural nursing care outcomes

When clients have received culturally based nursing care, they exhibit signs of satisfaction, are pleased with the cultural accommodations that have been made for them, and praise their overall care.

should pose their responses to such situations in a holistic way. Effective nursing practice recognizes that there is a need to adopt nonjudgmental attitudes toward patients' religious beliefs in order to avoid conflicts and confrontation. It is important for caregivers to diffuse any emotions by providing respect, support, and understanding for the family's religious beliefs, even if they are contrary to their own (Grube, et al., 1994)

In considering end-of-life decision making, cultural values and spirituality may be even more important. Elderly clients who are dying may find their values in direct conflict with those of hospital staff. Collaboration and cooperation are key components to ensure that patients receive optimal health care. When end-of-life issues arise, there may be a conflict between the physician's and/or nurse's own

Managing a Culturally Diverse Workforce

It is important for nurse managers to approach every staff person as an individual when directing a diverse team of health-care workers. Staff members, like clients, may be diverse in values, beliefs, and mannerisms. But they do have many things in common. They want to succeed in their jobs and be accepted by others (Blank & Slipp, 1994). Nurse managers hold the key to expose the full potential of each person on the staff and should openly support the contributions and competencies of staff members from all cultural groups. Husting (1995) believes that management has a responsibility to address cultural issues because of the rapidly chang-

hot topic:
Recruitment of Foreign Nurses

Delivery of high-quality health care in our multicultural society will continue to be a challenge for many hospitals, especially with the present nursing shortage in the United States. Due to the inability of the workforce to keep pace with the demands for more health-care providers, many health-care facilities are recruiting nurses from other countries such as Canada, Ireland, Great Britain, and the Philippines. The U.S. Bureau of Labor Statistics (BLS) (1998) has projected that nursing, the largest health-care occupation, will grow faster than average for all occupations in the next decade. Already, the U.S. government has relaxed rules allowing temporary work visas for Canadian and Mexican nurses who qualify. There are also provisions for allowing nurses educated in other English-speaking countries to work in the United States without taking the licensing examination. Some countries, such as the Philippines, train more nurses than they can use, so some believe that hospitals in this country should be permitted to recruit them. The nursing shortage dilemma will continue to generate many arguments both for and against importing foreign nurses. Meanwhile, as the United States continues to be a melting pot of many nations, a culturally diverse nursing workforce is a reality despite being intentionally ignored in many parts of the United States or being given rhetorical "lip service." Nursing will need to implement strategies to reflect the cultural mix of society more closely. Recommendations from the American Academy of Nursing expert panel on cultural competence include recruitment and retention of a diverse workforce (Meleis et al, 1995). Strategies include mentoring by same-culture minorities together with workshops, continuing education programs, and the use of consultants who are trained to promote culturally competent care.

ing health-care workforce. Diversity of values and beliefs can create conflict and result in a work environment that is not conducive to worker effectiveness and quality client care. One alternative Husting proposes is to create equal worker partnerships that capitalize on the best aspects of all cultures for an effective, harmonious work setting. She suggests that this can be accomplished by discussing cultural viewpoints as a part of decision making and acknowledging and respecting differing cultures, such as rotating the chairing of staff meetings to ensure equal participation and access to the agenda. This approach, Husting states, eliminates one-way communication within the work group and encourages alternative points of view and group discussion while enhancing the concept of shared governance.

Managing one's own personal thinking and assisting coworkers to think in innovative ways are part of the leading and management role in cultural diversity. Management of issues that involve culture, whether gender, religious, ethnic, or any other kind, requires patience, persistence, and a great deal of understanding. When the workforce includes nurses who speak English as a second language, the nurse manager needs to carefully evaluate the communication systems that are in use along with the manner in which messages are communicated. Slowly repeating instructions may be necessary to ensure comprehension and understanding of what is required. Culturally skilled nurse managers can provide cultural safety to patients by making sure that messages about patient care are received and understood. This might be accomplished by sitting down with the staff nurse and analyzing the situation to make sure that understanding has occurred. In addition, the nurse manager might use a communication notebook that allows the nurse to slowly "understand" information by writing down ideas that may appear to be unclear. By addressing cultural diversity directly, the nurse manager is offsetting future negative effects on performance and staff interactions (Meleis, et al., 1995).

Sullivan and Decker (2001) described the importance of communication and how cultural beliefs, attitudes, and behavior affect communication. Gestures, verbal tone, body movements, and physical closeness when communicating are all part of a person's culture. For the nurse manager, understanding these cultural behaviors is imperative in accomplishing effective communication within the workforce population. Tappen (2001) addressed differences across cultures that the nurse manager needs to monitor. These differences include spatial differences, relationships to people in authority, eye contact, expressions of feelings, thinking modes, meanings in different languages, evidence-based decision making, and preferred leadership/management style. Nurses need to ensure that effective communication by staff with clients and others does not lead to misunderstandings and eventual alienation. Nurse managers must also work with their staff to foster respect for different lifestyles.

The complexities of culture strongly influence opinions, perceptions, and generalizations.

Mancini (1997) wrote about the need for supervisors and nurse managers to be vigilant about attitudes and behaviors that encourage ethnic or racial stereotypes and that inhibit trust and communication. Managers can help eliminate stereotyping by presenting alternative views or referring to lists of commonalities among the staff. Mancini believes that a culturally skilled manager who understands and values differences can build trust and enhance communication, motivation, and production in a team. Ultimately, experience working with a diverse staff may be the best educational environment for learning about different cultures.

Lowenstein and Glanville (1996) challenge nurse managers to use their leadership positions to address communication and motivational issues when working with nurses from other cultures. They recommend that cultural conflicts be confronted and effective resolutions be reached. One example is that staff members may be reluctant to admit language problems that hamper their written communication. Unit-oriented workshops arranged by the nurse manager, together with effective mentoring by nurses trained in cross-cultural care, can result in quality care outcomes.

Andrews (1998) reported on the increasingly more diverse workforce in the United States. She advocated development of a transcultural nursing administration. She advocated that if nursing administrators are committed to transcultural management, they should actively promote recruitment of diverse staff members and be alert to any signs of prejudice in their organization. Likewise, mission statements and policies should be reviewed to reflect workforce diversity.

All Good Things...

One must remember that in a multicultural society as diverse as the United States, health care cannot come in one form only to fit the needs of everyone. Culture has a powerful influence on the type of health care that is both delivered and sought by clients. Population demographic projections in the United States show dramatic changes in ethnicity and age groups. All individuals have the need to be accepted by their health-care providers and have

Practice to Strive For 19-1

The nurse manager needs to employ strong cultural competence initiatives in order to be an effective leader in today's workplace environment. Cultural competence is illustrated by cultural assessment, planning, and familiarity with and respect for various traditional healing systems and beliefs. Time should be taken to get to know and understand one's colleagues, which facilitates learning about their ethnic and cultural heritages and assists in building trust and confidence in the leadership and management of the unit. Planning workshops in cultural sensitivity to discuss issues on cultural diversity can motivate others toward culturally competent communication and ultimately leads others toward cultural competence in their own nursing practice. Integrating cultural diversity into the workplace and successfully organizing teams that include culturally diverse workers are key to providing effective role models and mentors on the unit. Treating all staff members equally and with patience can provide them with a feeling of value, respect, and dignity. All of these techniques are essential for enhancing, maintaining, and retaining culturally diverse professionals in today's workforce (Office of Minority Health, 2000).

their cultural interpretations of health acknowledged and respected. Nurses have always accepted the concept of holistic health care, more than any other group in the health profession. Transcultural nursing provides a theoretical base for nursing regarding cultural competence. Nursing also needs to implement effective strategies to reflect the cultural mix of society within the workforce. Thus, with increased knowledge, sensitivity, respect, and understanding, nurses can provide the highest quality of health care for clients in our multicultural society.

This chapter has presented several models, tools, and techniques for meeting the health-care needs of an increasingly diverse population. Understanding cultural diversity and its impact on effective health-care delivery requires a commitment on the part of all health-care providers. The chapter has also provided information to assist nurse leaders in providing effective management of a culturally diverse workforce. It emphasized the importance of creating a culturally sensitive work environment. Nurses need to stay abreast of major population shifts in the United States and be prepared to manage diversity effectively in order to be competent health-care providers.

Let's Talk

1. *Think of a patient you have cared for from another culture. Did you perceive you were able to communicate effectively with the patient? Did you believe the patient understood all aspects of the care being provided? What did you do to facilitate the care of your patient?*

2. *Think of a foreign nurse with whom you have worked. Did you and your coworkers accept this nurse? Was this nurse incorporated into the "team" willingly? Did you have trouble understanding the nurse's accent?*

3. *Think of the nurse manager on this unit. How did the manager help the foreign nurse assimilate into the unit's culture? Were workshops conducted to assist the staff in understanding some of the cultural differences? How did the manager promote acceptance of this foreign nurse by the other team members?*

NCLEX Questions

1. Culture is:
   A. Shared values, behaviors, and beliefs that are reinforced through social interactions
   B. Specific only to the individual
   C. Transmitted from one generation to the next
   D. A and C

2. Levels of culture that have been identified by Schein (1985) include:
   A. The visible level; this includes physical space and social environment; for example, the image that is projected at first encounter
   B. The values; this includes the nurse's personal value system
   C. Traditions; this includes behavior based on ones' ethnicity
   D. B and C

3. Leininger (1991) is credited with developing a theory of culture care that includes:
   A. The ideas that cultural constructs are embedded in each other and that their application is both broad and holistic
   B. Influencers that are not causal or linear relationships

C. An open world or an open system of living reflective of the natural world of most humans
   D. All of the above

4. Transculturism describes a nurse who:
   A. Is grounded in his or her own culture
   B. Has the skills to be able to work in a multicultural environment
   C. Works with more than one culture
   D. A and B

5. A cultural assessment involves:
   A. Asking people their preferences
   B. A detailed description of the patient's ethnicity
   C. A description of the traditions to which a patient ascribes
   D. All of the above

6. Leininger's domains to review when conducting a cultural assessment include all of the following EXCEPT:
   A. Bowel and bladder patterns
   B. Cultural norms and values
   C. Cultural taboos and myths
   D. Ethnocentric tendencies and worldviews

7. Leininger describes a culturally competent nurse as one who demonstrates all of the following skills and attributes EXCEPT:
   A. Uses nursing concepts, principles, and available research findings to assess and guide practices
   B. Understands and values the cultural beliefs and practices of designated cultures so that nursing care is adapted to meet that individual client's needs in a meaningful way
   C. Knows how to avoid and prevent major cultural conflicts, clashes, or hurtful care practices
   D. Demonstrates use of the nursing process to work effectively and knowingly with the client

8. Spirituality is defined as:
   A. One's religious preference
   B. Each person's unique life experience and one's personal effort to find purpose and meaning in life
   C. Believing in a supreme being
   D. All of the above

9. Cultural diversity is defined as:
   A. When a nurse cares for patients from different backgrounds
   B. A hospital with patient demographics from different ethnicities
   C. Differences in race, ethnicity, religion, national origin, gender, and economic status
   D. A and B

10. Taboos and beliefs are:
   A. Truths held by some cultures to be actual or true, based on specific rationale
   B. Beliefs that are morally wrong
   C. Taboos that describe what one should not do
   D. Beliefs about what is right and taboos about what is wrong

REFERENCES

Anderson, Y. (1990). Health care across cultures, *Nursing Outlook, 38*(3), 136–139.

Andrews, M. (1998). Transcultural perspectives in nursing administration. *Journal of Nursing Administration, 28*(11), 30–38.

Bartol, G., & Richardson, L. (1998). Using literature to create cultural competence. *Image, 301*(1), 75–79.

Benner, P., & Wrubel, I. (1989). *The primacy of caring: Stress and caring in health and illness.* Menlo Park, CA: Addison-Wesley.

Betancourt, J., Green, A., & Carrillo, J. (2002). *Cultural competence in health care: Emerging frameworks and practical approaches* (Field Report Publication No 576). New York: The Commonwealth Fund.

Blank, R., & Slipp, S. (1994). *Voices of diversity: Real people talk about problems and solutions in a workplace where everyone is not alike.* New York: AMACON (American Management Association).

Byrd, R. (1988). Positive therapeutic effects of intercessory prayer in coronary care unit population. *Southern Medical Journal, 81*(7), 826–829.

Campinha-Bacote, J. (1999). A model and instrument for addressing cultural competence in health care. *Journal of Nursing Education, 38*(5), 203–207.

Campinha-Bacote, J.(1994). Cultural competence in psychiatric nursing: A conceptual model. *Nursing Clinics of North America, 29*(1), 1–8.

Coeling, H., & Simms, L. (1993). Facilitating innovation at the nursing unit level through cultural assessment, part 1: How to keep management ideas from falling on deaf ears. *Journal of Nursing Administration, 23*(4), 46–53.

Dochterman, Y., & Kennedy-Grace, H. (2001). *Current issues in nursing* (6th ed.). St. Louis: Mosby.

Dreher, M. (1996). Nursing: A cultural phenomenon. *Reflections, 22*(4), 4.

Eisenberg, D., et al. (1992). Religion and spirituality defined according to current use in nursing literature. *Journal of Professional Nursing, 8*(1), 41–47.

Galanti, G. (1999). Caring for culturally diverse patients at home. *Home Health Care Consultant, 6*(1), 33–34.

Giger, J., & Davidhizer, R. (1995). *Transcultural nursing* (2nd ed.). St. Louis: Mosby.

Giger, J., & Davidhizer, R. (1999). *Transcultural nursing* (3rd ed.). St. Louis: Mosby.

Grube, J., et al. (1994). Inducing change in values, attitudes, and behaviors: Belief system theory. *Journal of Sociological Issues, 50*(4), 153–173.

Husting, P. (1995). Managing a culturally diverse workforce. *Nursing Management, 26*(8), 26, 28–29.

Kass, Y., et al. (1991). Health outcomes and a new index of spiritual experience. *Journal for the Scientific Study of Religion, 30*, 203–211.

Kirkpatrick, S. & Deloughery, G. (1995). Cultural influences on nursing. In Deloughery, G.L. (ed.). *Issues and trends in nursing,* St. Louis, Mosby.

Leininger, M. (1990). Culture: The conspicuous missing link to understanding ethical and moral dimensions of human care. In Leininger, M. (ed.). *Ethical and moral dimensions of care.* Detroit: Wayne State University.

Leininger, M. (2002). The theory of culture care and ethno-nursing research method. In Leininger, M. (1997). Transcultural nursing research to transform nursing education and practice: 40 years. *Image, 29*(4), 341–347.

Leininger, M. (1978). *Transcultural nursing: Theories, concepts and practices.* New York: John Wiley & Sons.

Leininger, M., & McFarland, M. *Transcultural nursing: Concepts, theories, research and practice* (3rd ed., pp 71–98). New York: McGraw.

Leininger, M.M. (ed.). *Culture care diversity and universality. A theory of nursing.* (NLN Publication No. 15 2402, 5-68). New York: National League for Nursing.

Lowenstein, A., & Glanville, C. (1996). Cultural diversity and conflict in the health care workplace. *Nursing Economics, 13*(4), 203–209, 247.

Mancini, M. (1997). Managing cultural diversity. In Vestal, K.W. (ed.). *Nursing management: Concepts and issues* (2nd ed). Philadelphia: Lippincott.

Meleis, A., Isenberg, M., Koerner, Y., Lacey, B., & Stern, P. (1995). *Diversity, marginalization, and culturally competent health care issues in knowledge development.* Washington, DC: American Academy of Nursing.

Office of Minority Health (OMH). (2000). Assuring cultural competence in health care: Recommendations for national standards and an outcomes-focused research agenda. *Federal Register, 65*(247), 80865–80879.

Oldnall, A. (1996). A critical analysis of nursing: Meeting the spiritual needs of patients. *Journal of Advanced Nursing, 23*, 138–144.

Poss, Y. (1999). Providing culturally competent care: Is there a role for health promoters? *Nursing Outlook, 47*(1), 30–36.

Purnell, L., & Paulanka, B. (1998). *Transcultural health care: A culturally competent approach.* Philadelphia: F.A. Davis.

Salimbene, S. (1998). Multicultural health care tips. http://www.wcbofculture.com/edu/multicul.html

Schein, E., (1985). *Organizational culture and leadership.* San Francisco: Jossey-Bass.

Spector, R.E. (2000). *Cultural diversity in health & illness* (5th ed.). Upper Saddle River, NJ: Prentice Hall Health.

Sullivan, E., & Decker, P. (2001). *Effective leadership and management in nursing* (5th ed.). Upper Saddle River, NJ: Prentice Hall.

Tappen, R. (2001). *Nursing leadership and management: Concepts and practice* (4th ed.). Philadelphia: F.A. Davis.

Watson, Y. (1988). *Human science and human theory of care: Theory of nursing.* New York: National League for Nursing.

Watson, Y. (1985). *Nursing: The philosophy and science of caring.* Boulder, CO: Colorado Associated University Press.

BIBLIOGRAPHY

Andrews, M., & Boyle, J. (1999). *Transcultural concepts in nursing care* (3rd ed.). Philadelphia: J.B. Lippincott.

Health Resources and Services Administration, Bureau of Health Professions. (2000). *A national agenda for nursing workforce racial/ethnic diversity,* Washington, DC: Author.

Huff, R.M. (1999). *Promoting health in multicultural populations: A handbook for practitioners,* Thousand Oaks, CA: Sage.

Kelley, M.L., & Fitzsimons, V.M. (1999). *Understanding cultural diversity: Culture, curriculum, and community in nursing.* Boston: Jones & Bartlett/NLN.

Leininger, M. (1994). Transcultural nursing education: a worldwide imperative. *Nursing Health Care, 15*(5), 254–257.

Munro, B.H. (2003). Caring for the Hispanic populations: The state of the science. *Journal of Transcultural Nursing, 14,* 174–176.

Purnell, L.D., & Paulanka, B.J. (1998). *Transcultural health care: A culturally competent approach.* Philadelphia: F.A. Davis.

Rundle, A.K., Carvalho, M., & Robinson, M. (1999). *Honoring patient preferences: A guide to complying with multicultural patient requirements.* San Francisco: Jossey-Bass.

Snyder, M., & Lindquist, R. (2002). *Complementary/alternative therapies in nursing* (4th ed.). New York: Springer.

Tate, D.M. (2003). Cultural awareness: Bridging the gap between caregivers and Hispanic patients. *Journal of Continuing Education in Nursing, 34,* 213–217.

Villaire, M. (1994). Toni Tripp-Reimer: Crossing over the boundaries. *Critical Care Nurse, 14*(3), 134–141.

Constructive Conflict Management

SUSAN SPORTSMAN, RN, PHD

CHAPTER MOTIVATION

"Conflict happens."
Wilmot and Hocker

CHAPTER MOTIVES

- Discuss the concept of conflict in health-care organizations.
- Make a complete and accurate assessment of a conflict situation, using the Parties, Events, Power, Regulation of Conflict, and Style of Conflict (PEPRS) framework.
- Choose appropriate management strategies to deal with conflict.
- Develop a negotiation plan designed to resolve conflict constructively.
- Consider the effect of collective bargaining in managing conflict in health care.

When two or more people interact, there is the potential for conflict. The way conflict is managed has a major impact on its outcome. The stereotypical response to a conflict is to prepare to "win." However, "beating your opponent" may not be possible, or it may not provide the most positive outcome to the conflict. In fact, depending on the circumstances, the methods chosen to resolve the conflict may have harmful consequences.

Since 2000, patient safety and the work environment have received major emphasis in health care. Nearly three in four errors in health care are caused by human factors associated with interpersonal interactions (Maxfield, et al., 2005). A recently released study, "Silence Kills," a joint project of the American Association of Critical Care Nurses (AACN) and VitalSmarts, highlsights specific "difficult to discuss" issues, which may contribute to avoidable errors and other chronic communication problems in health care (Maxfield, et.al, 2005). Accompanying this report are new AACN Standards to establish and sustain a healthy work environment. The first of these standards is: "Nurses must be as proficient in communication skills as they are in clinical skills" (AACN, 2005). One of the communication skills that improves the work environment is the ability to manage conflict constructively.

This chapter explores the concept of conflict in health care and considers ways to deal constructively with interpersonal and professional conflicts to reach a positive outcome. The chapter also considers strategies to assess conflict situations as well as to use negotiation in constructive conflict management. A topic such as conflict management cannot be learned in a vacuum; it is discussed best by using everyday examples. Consider the following three conflict scenarios, which will be used throughout the chapter to illustrate specific points under discussion.

A. The nurse manager and the physician:

A nurse manager and a physician are having a conflict over a protocol for teaching newly diagnosed diabetic patients. The nurse manager has developed a protocol for teaching foot care based on recently released nursing research. The physician is not convinced that this approach is effective and wants to use a protocol that has been endorsed by the hospital for a number of years.

B. The nursing director of ICU and the director of respiratory care:

The nursing director of an intensive care unit (ICU) and the director of respiratory care in a 500-bed tertiary hospital, both of whom report to the vice president of patient care services (VPPCS), have an ongoing conflict over financial resources available for nursing and respiratory care staff. Both disciplines believe they are short-staffed. The VPPCS is a registered nurse, active in professional nursing activities, and many believe she is partial to nurses under her supervision. The conflict has escalated because there is a rumored plan to revise the administrative organization from a traditional discipline-specific departmental structure to an interdisciplinary model.

C. A pediatric surgical service:

The nurse manager of a pediatric surgical service and the night charge nurse on the unit are having a conflict about timing for surgery preparation. The nurse manager has asked that all children scheduled for surgery on any given day be ready for their preoperative mcdication when the day shift arrives. The nurse manager's rationale is that the surgeries are minor elective surgeries, and there is little lag time between each surgery. If the day shift staff has to do preoperative preparation, in addition to giving preoperative medication, patients scheduled for surgeries later in the morning may not be ready when the operating room (OR) staff arrives to transport the children to the OR. As a result, the surgical schedule is disrupted. The night charge nurse contends that waking children up early enough for the night staff to complete all the preparation for all children going to surgery that day means that some of the children will be awakened earlier than necessary. Not only will the children not get sufficient sleep but the resulting wait may increase the anxiety for the children and their families.

Dimensions of Conflict

In order to use conflict constructively, it is critical first to understand the concept of conflict. Traditionally, conflict has been viewed negatively as a power struggle, with the intent to neutralize, injure, or eliminate rivals. Several assumptions drive the perception of conflict as negative:

- Harmony is normal and conflict is abnormal.
- Conflict occurs because of personal problems.
- Conflict should never be forced, because anger, the predominant emotion, will escalate the conflict.
- Management of conflict should be polite and orderly.
- There is only one right way to resolve differences (Wilmot & Hocker, 2001, pp. 11–13).

In the 1960s, however, scholars began to suggest that properly managed conflict could facilitate organizational and/or personal growth (Valentine, 1995). When conflict is viewed from a positive perspective, there are a number of benefits to be gained. Assumptions underlying a positive perception of conflict include:

- Conflict is inevitable; learning to manage it effectively is necessary.
- Conflict brings problems to the surface.
- Conflict helps people discuss their goals.
- Managing conflict can help to resolve resentments and increase understanding (Wilmot & Hocker, 2001, pp. 15–16).

Many different types of conflicts arise in organizations. Conflicts often instigate positive change in organizations, but the parties involved must learn to manage them constructively. Understanding what conflict is and its potential outcome is a prerequisite to creating growth-producing experiences.

CONFLICT DEFINED

Conflict can be defined as an **expressed struggle** between at least two **interdependent** parties who **perceive** that **incompatible goals, scarce resources, or interference from others** are preventing them from achieving their goals (Wilmot & Hocker, 2001, p. 41). The words highlighted emphasize the key ingredients of a conflict. Identifying these ingredients in a particular situation is the first step in addressing the conflict situation.

The conflict in situation A easily illustrates this definition. The difference of opinion in this situation rises to the level of expressed struggle when the nurse manager and the physician cannot agree how to move forward in teaching foot care. The difference in opinion impedes progress because of the interdependence of the manager and the physician.

The physician depends upon nurses to provide education for her diabetic patients; the nurses are dependent upon the physician to admit patients to their unit. Although both share the goal of ensuring that patients are competent to deal with the effects of their disease, the methods to reach the goal are in conflict.

CONFLICTS CATEGORIZED BY UNDERLYING ISSUES

Applying the definition of a conflict in a particular situation is only the first step in understanding a conflict. Constructive conflict management also requires an understanding of the underlying issues. Classifying issues according to categories helps to explain the subtleties of the conflict. Categories of issues underlying conflict typically include: relationship, value, data, interest, and structural. **Relationship conflicts** occur when those in a relationship hold different views, beliefs, or values that negatively affect the functioning of the relationship because of poor communication, strong negative emotions, and/or misperceptions. Conflicts that arise because of opposing values that have an impact beyond a single relationship are often referred to as **value conflicts. Data conflicts** result when parties do not have sufficient information to make a decision or when the data required for decision making are interpreted differently by the various parties. Data conflicts may also occur when participants disagree about the relevance or interpretation of the data. **Interest conflicts** result from perceived incompatible needs. External forces, such as limited physical resources, time, geographical constraints, or organizational changes, often result in **structural conflicts** (Wilmot & Hocker, 2001).

The conflict between the nursing director of the ICU and the director of respiratory care services (situation B) illustrates several categories of conflict. The directors are in conflict because both need additional staff to care for patients with increasingly complex conditions. This conflict could be considered an **interest conflict,** because there is competition over perceived incompatible needs. The reorganization at the director level aimed at consolidating the number of departments into fewer interdisciplinary teams represents a situation in which one of the directors may lose power if her position is eliminated. This results in a potential **structural conflict,** which could escalate the conflict over resources. In addition, the **relationship** the directors have with their supervisor may also contribute to the conflict. For example, if the director of respiratory care believes that the vice president will favor the nursing director of the ICU because they are both nurses, this perception may escalate the conflict.

TYPES OF ORGANIZATIONAL CONFLICT

In addition to classifying conflicts by the underlying interest, other frameworks have been used to categorize conflicts within organizations. For example, Rowland and Rowland (1997, p. 381) identify seven types of organizational-specific conflicts that occur when there is disagreement over work issues: **goal**, **affective**, **cognitive**, **vertical**, **horizontal**, **line/staff,** and **role conflicts**. At first glance, some of these categories may seem to be interpersonal; in fact, they are organizational. The individuals involved represent organizational units or levels that are in conflict over resources, authority, or power.

Goal conflict occurs when preferred goals are incompatible, such as in the situation between the director of respiratory care and the nursing director of the ICU (situation B). Both of the directors want to hire new staff to work in the ICU and are competing for the limited available funding to do so. **Affective** conflict occurs when feelings or emotions are incompatible. The feelings of injustice that the director of respiratory care may harbor from reporting to a nurse illustrate an affective conflict. **Cognitive** conflict occurs when ideas or opinions are believed to be incompatible. For example, the conflict between the physician and the nurse manager over the proposed teaching protocol (situation A) illustrates cognitive conflict.

Vertical conflict occurs between levels of authority when superiors try to exert their authority over subordinates. The conflict between the pediatric surgical service nurse manager and the night charge nurse (situation C) illustrates such a conflict. **Horizontal conflict** takes place between those in the same hierarchical level. The conflict between the nursing director of the ICU and the director of respiratory care represents horizontal conflict.

Role conflict occurs when there is inconsistency or misunderstanding about the way a job should be performed. **Line-staff conflict** occurs when line managers believe that staff members use their technical knowledge to intrude on the line manager's area of legitimate authority. This sort of conflict often erupts in the hospital setting, for example, when the quality management staff dictates changes in practice without the supervisor's commitment to the process. An awareness of the various categories of conflict assists in a complete assessment of the circumstances. As will be discussed later in the chapter, these categories suggest what direction the assessment should take. The ability to assess factors influencing the conflict at its beginning and through the resolution process is crucial to constructive conflict management.

Practice Proof 20-1

Article: Seago, J., & Ash, M. (2002) Registered nurse unions and patient outcomes. *JONA, 2*(3), 143–151.

Organizational characteristics in hospitals have been shown to influence patient outcomes; however, the association between RN unions and patient outcomes is unclear. This study examined the relationship between the presence of a bargaining unit for RNs and the acute myocardial infarction (MI) mortality rate for acute care hospitals in California. In California, 35% of hospitals had unions. The signficant finding in the study is that California hospitals with RN unions had a 5.7% lower mortality rates for acute MIs after accounting for patient age, gender, type of MI, other chronic diseases, and several organizational characteristics. A causal relationship between RN unions and patient outcomes could not be determined.

QUESTIONS:

1. In the review of the literature, Seago and Ash (2002) discuss various organizational characteristics that are known to influence patient outcomes. What were some of these variables?
2. The authors discussed some limitations to the study. What were they and how did the authors address these limitations? Do you see additional limitations to this study?
3. What are the implications of the results for practice in hospitals that have RN unions?
4. What are the implications of the results for practice in hospitals that do not have RN unions?
5. What additional research questions do the results of this study suggest?

Assessment of the Conflict Situation

A constructive conflict resolution is one that reaches an agreement and enhances future interaction. Wilmot and Hocker (2001, p. 93) note that the outcome of a conflict can be considered positive when agreements are made that are fair and durable and that consider the interests of both parties. Such an outcome cannot be achieved without an accurate intial assessment of the conflict. In the same way that a physical assessment can inform the diagnosis of a physical problem, an assessment of the conflict situation can direct the resolution of a conflict.

Sportsman (2005) described a framework, adapted from Weber's Conflict Map and the Wilmot-Hocker Conflict Assessment Guide (Wilmot & Hocker, 2001), for use in assessing conflict within the health-care environment. The major components of the framework are reflected in the acronym **PEPRS,** which stands for:

- **P**arties involved
- **E**vents/issues
- **P**ower
- **R**egulation of conflict
- **S**tyle of conflicts

A description of each of the components will help in applying the framework.

PARTIES INVOLVED

Assessment of the conflict situation begins with identification of all involved participants. Conflict participants may include primary, secondary, or interested third parties. All have some level of interest in the conflict, although their distance from the conflict situation dilutes the intensity of their concern (Sportsman, 2004).

In situation A, the physican and the nurse manager are the primary parties. Secondary parties include diabetic patients on that unit, the nurses on the unit who will implement the teaching protocol, other physicians who admit to that unit, and the nurse manager's supervisors. Interested third parties might include nursing and medical staff members on other units.

Identification of the parties involved is also important to determine the type of organizational conflict. For example, when the primary participants are involved in a vertical conflict between supervisor and staff, as in situation C, the dynamics are different than if there was a horizontal conflict as described in situation B.

EVENTS/ISSUES

In an effort to determine the events or issues involved in the conflict, it is important to outline the triggering event, historical context, the level of interdependence among the participants, the "named" issues, available resources, and previously considered solutions. Underpinning these elements are communication behaviors of each party and their perceptions of these behaviors. Because behaviors do not occur in a relational vacuum, the relationship between the conflict participants and the meanings ascribed to their relationship(s) are also important. In other words, if the relationship is very important to all participants, the conflict will have much more meaning than if the relationship is a transient one. This is particularly true if participants define themselves through the relationship. The perceptions of these relationships are influenced by gender, culture, and socioeconomic status (Sportsman, 2005). For example, the attempt to introduce the new teaching protocol was the triggering event in situation A. The historical relationship of nurses being "handmaidens" of physicians, based in part on traditional male-female roles, may also influence this conflict. Despite this historical background, as previously noted, the physician and nurses are interdependent in their ability to care for diabetic patients.

In situation B, if the respiratory care director believes that nothing he can do to demonstrate the needs of his department will outweigh the professional relationship of two nurses, he reduces the variety of behaviors he might use to resolve the issue. Having the mindset that the vice president will always give the majority of the resources to the nursing director may reduce the energy he is willing to expend to advocate for resources for his department. The financial, human, and/or emotional resources available to resolve the conflict also provide important information about the situation. In situation B, if the hospital is experiencing financial difficulties, the options for resolving the need for respiratory and nursing staff may be very different than if the hospital is strong financially.

DIVERGENT GOALS

The most significant factors to assess in order to define the event/issues are the divergent goals of the various parties involved in the conflict. Goals inherent in a conflict are typically referred to as CRIP because they fall into one or more of these types: Content, Relational, Identity, and Process. **Content goals** can be determined by asking "What do I want?" **Relational goals** involve answering the question, "Who are we to each other, and how does this affect what I want?" **Identity, or face-saving, goals** can be determined by answering "Who am I in this interaction, and how does this affect what I want?" **Process goals** involve asking "What processes will be used in this interaction" (Wilmot & Hocker, 2001).

In situation C, both the pediatric surgical-service nurse manager and the night charge nurse have a **content goal** of ensuring that children and their families get appropriate preoperative care. The nurse manager also has the content goal of maintaining the flow of surgery. Her **relationship goal** may be for her subordinate to follow her order. The night charge nurse may also recognize that she is subordinate to the nurse manager; therefore, her **relationship goal** may be to maintain a positive relationship with her supervisor. The **identity goals** of these two nurses are influenced by the difference in their roles in the hierarchy. For example, the nurse manager may be committed to demonstrating her power as a supervisor. On the other hand, the night charge nurse, while recognizing her subordinate role, may see herself as the main advocate for the children preparing for surgery and their families. The **process goals** in situation C may direct how the situation is resolved. If the nurse manager's process goal is to resolve the conflict by exerting her authority, she will be less likely to negotiate alternative outcomes, such as consulting the nursing literature or requesting feedback from other practice experts.

All types of goals are not present in all disputes, and they may vary in importance in any given situation. Identity and relational goals typically underlie the content and process issues, which are more likely to be named as the goals in dispute (Wilmot &

Hocker, 2001). For example, in the physician–nurse manager conflict in situation A, implementing the teaching protocol based on nursing research may be the content goal for the nurse manager. His need, however, to have the worth of nursing research, and more importantly the worth of his own practice, recognized is an underlying identity goal in this conflict. If only the content goals are achieved, the conflict is likely to remain (Wilmot & Hocker, 2001). For example, if the physician agrees to use the teaching protocol suggested by the nurse manager but continues to belittle the underlying research, the conflict has not been truly resolved.

As part of issue identification in the conflict assessment, goals must be clarified. It may be difficult to define effective resolutions for vague goals because such goals cannot be quantified (Wilmot & Hocker, 2001, pp. 91–92) For example, in situation A, if the nurse manager has the goal that " the physicians in this hospital will respect nursing research," it will be difficult to know whether that goal has been achieved. Instead, if the goal is to implement the teaching protocol for diabetic patients based on specific nursing research, its achievement can be more easily determined.

POWER

All conflicts are based, in part, on attempts to protect participants' self-esteem or alter perceived inequities in power (Boule, 2001; Wilmot & Hocker, 2001). Therefore, examining the influence of power related to conflict participants is central to assessing and understanding the conflict. Boule (2001, p. 224) describes some assumptions about power in conflict that may be helpful in this examination:

- There are many different contexts in which there might be varying levels of power. Some of these are easy to observe, and some are not.
- All participants in a conflict have some power. This may come from money, knowledge, or the ability to damage or reward. It may also be derived from rules, standards and principles, the morality of the situation, and/or the need to maintain or improve a reputation.
- The perception of power may be more important than power itself.

The perception of power is fueled by certain assumptions about what constitutes power. Kritek, in Marcus, et al. (1995), outlines assumptions about power as translated into privilege in the United States:

- The wealthy are more privileged than the poor.
- Men are more privileged than women.
- Professional people are more privileged than laborers.
- Healthy people are more privileged than the ill.
- Strong people are more privileged than the weak.
- Management is more privileged than employees.
- People who act in a rational manner are more privileged than those who are emotional.

In addition to power drawn from societal influences, assumptions can also be drawn about power in organizations. Wilmot and Hocker (2001, p. 11), synthesizing research on organizational power, indicate that people have power in organizations when they:

- Are required to deal with important problems
- Control valuable resources
- Are closely connected to the work flow of the organization
- Are not easily replaced
- Have a history of using their power effectively

These characteristics are built on the "bases of power" work of French and Raven (1960), which describes power as coming from reward, coercive, legitimate, referent, and expert power bases.

All told, the powerful in work or personal conflict are those who have the advantage of physical and psychological strength by virtue of gender, education, health, or resources. The extent to which this power is actualized contributes to the resolution of the conflict. Therefore, it is important to assess the power base of each participant in a conflict.

The bases of power should be used as a starting point to assess the power of individuals. Nonetheless, Wilmot and Hocker (2001, p. 11) suggest that in a conflict assessment, power is typically defined too narrowly, and too much emphasis is put on the source of the influence. They recommend including an assessment of the use of power within the relationship in conflict rather than simply the amount of power one participant potentially has over another. For example, evaluating the decision-making process within the relationship (who typically makes the decisions?) and the extent to which each participant attempts to control conversation can provide helpful information about the use of power in a relationship. Identifying other methods of using covert power, such as passive-aggressive behavior or "submitting but resisting," can also be instructive (Wilmot & Hocker, 2001, p. 113).

The conflict in situation A between the nurse manager and the physician illustrates principles regarding power. From an organizational perspective, both parties hold significant power. Both deal with important relationships, control valuable resources, and would be difficult to replace. Both are central to the work flow related to the care of patients. To determine any inequities of power, one must analyze the specific relationship. Questions that might help in this analysis include: "What are signs of dominance or passivity in their conversations?" and "What decision-making strategies have been used in past conflicts?"

A broad assessment of power is critical to a constructive resolution of conflict because the relative power of each party and the power within the specific relationship can be used to generate possible solutions. If the possible solutions to the conflict are only based on the power of each party in general, the range of possible solutions will not reflect the power distribution in their intimate relationship. This narrow assessment will reduce the range of possible solutions to the conflict. For example, observing the way the physician and the nurse manager in situation A relate to each other can give additional information about the power distribution in their relationship beyond what is assumed from their relative positions in the organization.

REGULATING RESOURCES

The resources for constructive conflict management are available in every conflict situation. These resources might include internal or external limiting factors, interested or neutral third parties, and various styles used to manage conflict. Internal factors include common values of participants or the value of the relationship to each of them. External factors might include an authority with the ability to intervene and force a settlement. Third parties would include those trusted by both sides that can facilitate a resolution acceptable to all. Possible conflict management styles used by the participants, which will be discussed in the next section of the chapter, also have the potential for regulating the conflict (Wilmot & Hocker, 2001, p. 204).

Situation C illustrates various internal and external resources likely to regulate this conflict. The nurse manager and the night charge nurse share the desire for patients to be prepared for surgery. In addition, they recognize the interrelatedness of their work. They also are both aware that others in the hospital hierarchy could intervene if necessary, providing an external regulator to this conflict. Both participants value the need for adequate patient preparation; however, the nurse manager may value smooth collaboration between the operating room and the patient unit more than the night charge nurse. The effectiveness with which the conflict is managed may be related to the extent to which regulating resources that support resolution rather than continued conflict are available.

Some conflicts are relatively easy to resolve; others are more difficult. Lewicki, et al. (2001, p. 21) suggest that the ease of resolution depends, in large measure, upon the issue in conflict. An accurate assessment, driven by identification of the conflict category, can help participants evaluate, in advance, the possible ease of resolution. The size of "the prize" to be won or lost, the level of interdependence of the participants, and the extent to which participants must continue to work together influence the likelihood of a constructive resolution. The extent to which the resolution process seems fair to each participant also contributes to a constructive resolution. Similarly, the structure that is in place to encourage or discourage participant interaction and conflict resolution also influences the ease of resolution (Lewicki, et al., 2001, p. 21).

STYLE OF CONFLICT MANAGEMENT

Conflict management styles are behavioral approaches used to regulate or resolve the conflict. When these behaviors are used together over time, they become patterned responses. These patterns develop over a lifetime, influenced by genetics, life experiences, and personal philosophy. People tend to use the same patterns over and over in a wide range of conflicts. In some situations, these patterned responses may effectively resolve the conflict. In other circumstances, however, the same

pattern of behavior may only escalate the conflict. To be effective in conflict management, one must be able to choose consciously the behaviors that best fit the circumstances of the conflict.

There has been signficant research on conflict management styles in an effort to understand what behavior is most appropriate in various situations. For example, three groups of researchers, Blake and Mouton (1964), Thomas and Kilmann (1974), and Rahin (1990), have described five styles or behavioral patterns that might be used in a conflict. The styles identified by the three groups of researchers, although differently named, describe the same phenomena. **Competing, forcing,** or **dominating** refer to a behavior pattern of being uncooperative and demanding one's own way. The results of such an approach are often categorized as a win-lose situation. Sports analogies in conflict management usually refer to competitive situations in which achieving a goal takes place by blocking the opponent's goal. In these situations, only one goal can be met, resulting in a "winner take all" scenario. **Avoiding** or **withdrawing** refers to avoiding the conflict so that it cannot be resolved. The result may be categorized as a lose-lose situation. **Accommodating, smoothing,** or **obliging/capitulation** refers to being cooperative yet unassertive so that only the other person's needs are met. The result may be considered a lose-win outcome. **Compromise** or **sharing** suggests that each party relinquishes something, which might be described as a no-win no-loss resolution, because no one gains or loses everything she or he wanted. **Collaboration** or **problem solving,** which is the most time-consuming process, may be considered a win-win situation, in which new ideas are generated that resolve most of the issues in the conflict. The important point to understand is that each of these styles has some merit; there is *no one right way* to manage conflict. The style that is most effective in reaching a constructive outcome to the conflict depends on the participants and the context of the conflict.

Effective collaboration or problem solving results in the greatest benefit (win-win) for all involved in a conflict, so logically this should be the conflict management style most often used. In reality, other styles are frequently chosen over collaboration. In some cases, particularly for short-term gain, it may even be appropriate to choose avoiding (lose-lose) as a solution. This choice may be made intentionally, after comparing the time required for collaboration with the impact of the problem being resolved. In situation C, for example, if the nurse manager knows that the night charge nurse will be resigning in a short time, it might be in everyone's best interest, including the patients', to avoid a confrontation about this schedule.

Table 20-1 reviews the five conflict management styles outlined by Thomas and Kilmann (1974) and gives examples of circumstances in health care in which each of the five styles might be appropriate.

CONFLICT STYLES IN NURSING AND HEALTH CARE

No place is the need to use various conflict management styles more important than in the complex world of health care. Health-care organizations are

particularly vulnerable to the negative effects of conflict among providers because of multiple stakeholders with competing interests and values (Marcus, et al., 2001). There is some evidence to suggest that increased positive interaction among health-care disciplines positively influences outcomes of care for patients (Bartol, Parrish, & McSweeney, 2001). Conversely, according to data from the Joint Commission on Accreditation of Healthcare Organizations (JCAHO), breakdown in team communications is a top contributor to sentinel events (AACN, 2005). Poor communication is often the result of unresolved or poorly managed conflict. Constructive conflict management is an effective strategy in improving communication and, in effect, improving patient safety.

Despite the recognition that use of a variety of conflict management styles is necessary for constructive conflict resolution, many people uncon-

TABLE 20-1	Conflict Management Styles
STYLE	**SITUATION**
Competition (win-lose)	■ When patients' well-being is clearly at stake and the opposing position would harm it ■ When working with a peer who would take advantage of you if you did not compete
Accommodation (lose-win)	■ When other staff members care about the results of the monthly schedule more than you do ■ To counteract previous negative feelings, you agree to adopt a treatment protocol that is not your first choice but appears to have positive patient results
Avoiding (lose-lose)	■ When you know that an employee wants to discuss the promotion that you are not prepared to give, you cancel a scheduled appointment with the employee. The employee loses because she is unable to ask about the promotion, and you may also lose the support of the employee, who sees you as unresponsive ■ When staff wants to buy a new piece of equipment, but administration has indicated that no new equipment will be purchased for the next 6 months
Compromise (no-win no-loss)	■ When two hospital units need a new staff member but there is only sufficient funding for one new employee and a 0.5 FTE position is assigned to each unit ■ When a new electronic charting system is scheduled to be implemented in 6 months but accreditation processes require a change in documentation of a particular instance immediately
Collaboration (win-win)	■ When a new 23-hour unit is being opened as a cost-reduction strategy and the opinions of multiple stakeholders are in conflict about how to proceed; the support of all the stakeholders is needed to make the unit successful ■ When the discharge planning process is being revised and there has been long-term animosity between the social workers and nurses; when representatives from the two groups interact to revise the process, positive relationships may be forged

Adapted from Thomas and Kilmann (1974)

sciously use a predominant style regardless of the circumstances. In numerous studies, staff nurses have been found to use avoidance as their predominant style of conflict management (Cavanagh, 1991; Eason & Brown, 1999; Hightower, 1986; and Marriner, 1982). Operationally, this means that nurses choose to avoid a conflict rather than use other conflict management styles.

In two studies, nurses in supervisory positions were found to use compromising most frequently as a conflict management style (Barton, 1991; Woodtli, 1987). Eason and Brown (1999), however, found that both supervisors and staff nurses used avoidance as their primary style, followed by accommodation. Despite the fact that these studies identified different prevalent conflict management styles of nurses, it is significant that competition and, more important, collaboration were used less often.

Because 92 % of the nurses in the United States are female (ANA, 2004), gender, professional socialization, or both probably influence choice of conflict management styles. Research in non–health-care environments suggests that gender influences the choice of conflict management styles (Wilmot & Hocker, 2001). But because of the small number of men in nursing, it has been difficult to weigh gender differences as a factor in conflict management style in nursing. Further research in this area may prove instructive in determining whether it is gender or other factors associated with choosing a career in nursing that influence the choice of conflict management styles.

To update findings regarding nurses and allied health-care professionals' use of various conflict management styles, Sportsman and Hamilton (2007) studied the predominant conflict management style(s) of nurses and allied health professionals enrolled in professional programs at a comprehensive university. Researchers identified some trends when comparing different groups. In a change from some of the earlier studies, nurses tended to use compromise most often. Allied health professionals tended to choose avoidance. Females in all of the health professions tended to choose compromise, and males tended to choose avoidance. Each group used collaboration more often than competition but less often than the other styles. Although competition was the least prevalent style for both, males chose it more frequently than females, and nurses chose it the least. All groups tended to choose more than one style.

The changes in the findings of the research on conflict styles among health-care providers over the last 15 years suggest that nurses may slowly be increasing the variety of conflict management styles they use. They seem reluctant, however, to use styles such as collaboration and competition. Given that collaboration is often recommended in the literature as the best strategy to accomplish systematic changes in an organization, nurses must learn collaborative skills to effect change in the health-care delivery system (Sportsman & Hamilton, 2005).

Destructive Conflict Resolution

The outcome of any conflict may be positive or negative, depending upon the skill with which the issues are managed. Unfortunately, it is easier for an outcome of a conflict to be destructive than for it to be positive. Conflict may be considered destructive if participants are dissatisfied with the outcome and believe that they have "lost." This feeling of loss often results in anger and the desire to get even. While it is difficult to predict whether the conflict will be constructive or destructive during the process, Gottmann in Wilmot and Hocker (2001, p. 49) identified four communication behaviors that portend a destructive outcome. These include: criticism at the beginning of the interaction, defensiveness, stonewalling, and contempt. Individually, these behaviors are destructive; in addition, the use of one of the behaviors will often encourage the use of others. Consider how these behaviors might influence several of the situations under discussion.

Criticism of one party by another will set a negative tone for the conflict. Moreover, if one party becomes defensive, the conflict will continue along a destructive path. Stonewalling occurs when one person "withdraws" from the interaction, even though the person continues to be involved in the conflict (Wilmot & Hocker, 2001, p. 51).

The identification of these behaviors as they occur is important as the first step in moving from a destructive to a constructive conflict resolution. If participants recognize these behaviors in their own communication, they can make efforts to adopt a more neutral position, perhaps apologizing to the opponent for unhelpful behavior. It is important to avoid responding negatively when others exhibit destructive behavior in a conflict. In an emotionally charged issue, listening as a means of learning will reduce defensiveness and turn the conflict around onto a more constructive course (Wilmot & Hocker, 2001, p. 50).

The Role of Negotiation in Constructive Conflict Management

Negotiation, also known as bargaining, is the process by which a conflict is resolved between opposing parties. Negotiation occurs every day when participants would rather reach an agreement together than have another person resolve the issue for them (Lewicki, et al., 2001).

Wilmot and Hocker (2001, p. 211) describe negotiation as the active phase of conflict resolution when participants generate options and brainstorm in an effort to get their needs met. This process is helped or hindered by the choice of conflict management styles used during the negotiation. Negotiations are most successful when the parties:

- Recognize their interdependence
- Have been able to clarify their issues
- Are willing to work on both incompatible and overlapping goals
- Have sufficient power to be able to participate in the negotiation
- Have formal and informal procedures to be able to interact in problem solving

COMPETITIVE VERSUS COLLABORATIVE NEGOTIATION

There are two different approaches to negotiation: the competitive (distributive) approach and the collaborative (integrative) approach. The choice of approach depends upon the negotiator's philosophy about conflict and the outcome desired, which may then determine the specific conflict styles chosen. Competitive negotiation results in a win-lose outcome. A competitive conflict management style is the style most often used by the "winners" in a distributive negotiation. Avoidance and accommodation are more likely to have been used by the "losers." The negotiator taking this approach is typically not concerned about an ongoing relationship with the other party and is trying to maximize gain/minimize loss. The goal is to win as much as possible, especially more than the other side (Wilmot & Hocker, 2001, p. 222.). Behaviors that are typical of a competitive negotiation include:

- Making high opening demands and moving downward slowly
- Hiding information and using confrontation and argument to make points
- Being unwilling to respond to persuasion by the other side
- Exaggerating one's own concession (Wilmot & Hocker, 2001, p. 222).

On the other hand, collaborative negotiation assumes that people have both diverse and common interests and that the negotiation can result in both parties gaining something. This type of negotiation is based upon the assumptions that interdependence is important and common interests can be identified, even if there are some competing interests. Limited resources do exist, but they can usually be expanded through cooperation (Wilmot & Hocker, 2001, p. 226). In a collaborative negotiation, both sides use collaboration and/or compromise most frequently.

In situation B, if the nursing director of the intensive care unit and the director of respiratory care use a collaborative approach to negotiating, they may be able to expand the resources available to their staff. For example, they might be able to share the time of unlicensed assistive personnel to allow the professional staff in both departments more time for patient care. On the other hand, if the nursing director uses a competitive approach to negotiation, she may have sufficient power to capture most of the resources for her staff. In actual practice, the two types of negotiation are not nearly so well delineated, and many negotiations have elements of both competition and collaboration.

NEGOTIATION PROCESS

Once the parties have decided to negotiate, six negotiation phases in three specific stages guide the process. Based upon the work of Lewicki, et al., (2001), the stages incorporate the previously discussed assessment of the conflict, the development of relationships, and the development of the negotiation plan. The negotiation model can be used in either a competitive or collaborative interaction. Table 20-2 outlines this negotiation model and identifies questions to be answered in order to move through each stage and phase.

hot topic:
Collective Bargaining: An Example of Competitive Negotiation

The process of collective bargaining is built upon the notion of competitive negotiation. Management and labor are conceptualized as opposing forces where the collective action of labor is necessary to overcome the greater power of management.

Union activity in health care has been most common in states with deep union penetration in other industries. The growth in collective bargaining in health care in the last 15 years, even in less unionized states, has been stimulated by the health-care reorganization movement of the 1990s.

The collective bargaining model requires that representatives of the designated union negotiate work contracts on behalf of the membership. Nursing issues likely to be negotiated as part of a contract include not only wages and benefits but also workplace issues such as staffing ratios that affect patients and nurses. The process of negotiation provides an opportunity for union representatives to articulate the needs of staff nurses. Competitive negotiation typically provides the framework for collective bargaining; however, most successful collective bargaining negotiators also use elements of the collaborative approach. In addition, administration may also use collaborative negotiation strategies at times other than formal collective bargaining as a means of improving staff-management relationships and/or preventing unionization of their facility. For example, when hospital representatives know that, because of poor profit margins, they are limited in the range of compensation they can offer, they may focus the negotiation on the development of self-governance councils for nurses.

ASSESSMENT STAGE

The assessment stage in the negotiation process requires implementation of the conflict assessment previously discussed. Data from the assessment can help each party determine whether they will take a competitive or collaborative approach to negotiation or a mixed approach that uses both some time during the negotiation.

RELATIONSHIP DEVELOPMENT STAGE

The relationship development stage of negotiation involves framing the results of the assessment to understand the other party. Determining the similarities and differences in the history, experience, values, and expectations of the other party will provide a context for the negotiation plan, including whether competition or collaboration is most valued by the parties. For example, in situation A, if the physician values being "right at all cost," the nurse manager may have to use competition in order to have any chance of his protocol being accepted.

NEGOTIATION PLAN DEVELOPMENT STAGE

Four phases make up the final stage of negotiation plan development: information synthesis, bidding, closing the deal, and implementing the agreement. In the information synthesis phase, the divergent goals of each party will be clarified from the events/issues of the conflict. For purposes of the negotiation process, these goals can be expressed either as **positions** or **interests. Positions** involve identification of the specific outcome of the conflict as the participant wishes it would be. **Interests** are factors underlying participants' claims and include issues that are actually motivating the participants in the conflict (Lewicki, et al., 2001, p. 62). If the negotiation is centered on positions, the negotiation is likely to be distributive. Conversely, if interests guide the negotiation, collaborative negotiation is more likely to result, because a variety of interests are underlying the two positions in the conflict.

In situation A, for instance, the nurse manager's position is to implement the teaching protocol based on nursing research. Negotiating with the nurse manager's narrow, specific position in mind may prove difficult because the parties will either adopt the protocol or they will not; his position does not allow for compromise or collaboration. If the negotiation centers on the underlying interest of the nurse manager (the need to integrate nursing research into practice) however, it opens up the negotiation to many more avenues of exploration and resolution.

In the information synthesis phase, there is often an opportunity to provide participants with infor-

TABLE 20-2	Negotiation Model

PHASE	DATA TO BE COLLECTED
Assessment Stage of Conflict	
Preparation	■ Use a conflict assessment guide, such as PEPRS.
Relationship Development Stage	
Information framing	■ How are the opposing parties alike? ■ How are they different? ■ Can they accept value differences? ■ Are they committed to a positive outcome for both sides?
Negotiation Plan Development Stage	
Information synthesis	■ Will the negotiation focus on positions or interests? (Will it be a competitive or collaborative negotiation?) ■ What is the Best Alternative to a Negotiated Agreement (BATNA) for each party? ■ How likely are the various options to succeed? ■ What happens if negotiation fails? ■ What conflict management style(s) should be used? ■ What pieces of information can be used to support the negotiators' case? ■ What clarifications can be made to resolve areas of conflict? ■ What options for resolution might be available?
Bidding	■ If negotiators cannot have exactly what they want, what outcomes are they willing to accept? ■ What steps should be taken to get there?
Closing the deal	■ What components must be in place for the negotiators to agree?
Implementing the agreement	■ What are the next steps? ■ Who needs to take responsibility for various parts of the agreement? ■ Should there be a written contract, and what should it include?

Adapted from Lewicki, et al. (2001), pp. 52–53.

mation that might resolve some areas of conflict. For example, if a data conflict exists, this stage may provide an opportunity to clarify the data or provide new information that adds understanding to the situation. In situation A, the nurse manager might have an opportunity to bring additional published information to the physician regarding the new teaching protocol. If a relationship conflict is involved, this phase provides an opportunity to clarify misperceptions and stereotypes and perhaps improve communication skills needed for the interaction.

Also as part of the information synthesis phase, Ury, Patton, and Fisher (1991) suggest that each participant should determine the Best Alternative

To the Negotiated Agreement (BATNA) from his/her own perspective. Table 20-3 outlines the steps to using the BATNA in negotiation.

In situation A, the nurse manager might decide that the best alternative would be implementation of the teaching protocol over a trial period with a subset of patients, using evaluation data from mutually agreed-upon outcome markers to decide if the new teaching protocol would be fully implemented on the unit. This alternative does not ensure immediate acceptance of the new protocol, but it does provide an opportunity for a trial while recognizing the physician's concerns.

An important part of the information synthesis is to consider what happens if the conflict is not

TABLE 20-3	Uses of BATNA in Negotiation

1. Determine the best alternative to the negotiated agreement from your perspective.
2. Using information from the conflict assessment, hypothesize what might be the best alternative to the negotiated agreement from the viewpoint of the other party.
3. Consider ways in which the other party's BATNA can be amended to meet your own goals while satisfying the other party.

Adapted from Ury, Patton, and Fisher (1991).

Practice to Strive For 20-1

Analysis of a possible interaction between the nursing director of the intensive care unit (ICU) and the director of respiratory care in situation B can be instructive in applying the negotiation model. Assume that the vice president of patient care services has allotted $100,000 to increase the nursing and respiratory staff assigned to the ICU. She has indicated that the two directors must work together to develop a plan to use this money. This strategy encourages the two directors to negotiate on the basis of issues rather than principles. Before meeting to develop a plan, each director should assess the conflict situation. Each should also analyze the assessment data independently, determining the BATNA for themselves as well as what they believe the BATNA to be for the other party. In this situation, the directors' initial desire may be to hire several professional staff members in each discipline to work in the ICU. The limit of $100,000 may reduce the number of professional staff members they can hire. As they begin to negotiate and address what they are willing to take if they cannot have what they want, however, they may find that hiring support/nonprofessional staff or reorganizing the way the ICU nurses and respiratory care staff interact may be part of the plan they develop.

resolved. Recognizing the consequences of a failure in the negotiation may serve as a stimulus to continue to negotiate, even when a stalemate looms ahead. Of equal importance is considering possible options for resolution. This prepares each negotiator for the brainstorming that occurs as part of the bidding process.

In the bidding phase, the negotiators work together to determine options that might resolve the conflict. If participants are clear about what they are willing to accept, they can more easily reach a desired outcome. This will allow them to outline the components that must be in place for the negotiators to agree and close the deal. Depending upon the formality of the negotiation, the implementation of the agreement phase may include development of a contract. In the most formal negotiation, a contract is written to be legally enforceable. Even if the negotiation does not lead to a legally binding contract, an informal written agreement at the end of negotiation increases the likelihood that the agreement will be kept. This agreement should outline all agreed-upon points.

All Good Things…

Conflict is inevitable and, in the high stakes of health care, patient care can be negatively affected by destructive conflict. As a result, nurses and other health-care providers must use constructive conflict management skills to resolve these issues.

A negotiation process model can be used to effect a resolution. A complete and accurate assessment of the conflict is the first stage of the negotiation model. Such an assessment includes the use of an assessment framework, such as PEPRS, which identifies the parties involved, events and issues of the situation, power underlying the conflict, regulating resources, and conflict management styles typically used by the participants.

The second stage of the negotiation process involves development of the relationships among parties. The information gathered in the assessment stage can be used to explore the similarities and differences of the parties in conflict and can determine the context in which the parties will negotiate.

The third stage, the development of the negotiation plan, involves synthesis of the information obtained from the first two steps, bidding, closing the deal, and implementing the agreement. In health care, using a structured approach to conflict management not only improves the working conditions for employees but also improves the outcomes of patient care.

Let's Talk

1. *How does your personal and professional background influence the ways in which you deal with conflict?*

2. *What conflict management style(s) do you use most frequently? How has this affected the outcomes of conflicts you have been involved in?*

3. *What are the advantages and disadvantages of competitive negotiation and collaborative negotiation? In what health-care situations might each be useful?*

4. *Consider a conflict you have observed in a clinical setting. What was its impact on the primary participants of the conflict? the patients being cared for by these participants? the work environment? What strategies would you recommend using to resolve this conflict?*

NCLEX Questions

1. Factors that influence the ease with which a conflict is resolved include all of the following EXCEPT:
   A. The level of interdependence of the parties
   B. The importance of the outcome
   C. The perceived fairness of the process of resolution
   D. The extent to which support systems that encourage resolution are in place
   E. All of the above

2. An example of a role conflict is:
   A. When the director of respiratory care and the nursing director of the ICU both want to hire a new employee in their discipline to work in the ICU
   B. When the director of respiratory care believes she does not receive as many resources as the nursing director of the ICU
   C. When two secretaries are hired to help with excess work load but the job expectations for each of them is not clear
   D. When line managers believe that support staff use their technical knowledge to intrude on the line manager's legitimate authority

3. Which of the following is true regarding power in conflict?
   A. Some participants have no power in the conflict
   B. An individual's power in a conflict tends to remain constant
   C. The perception of power may be more important than the actual power
   D. All of these are true
   E. None of these is true

4. Value conflicts are likely to occur when:
   A. Parties in conflict share values not held by the general population
   B. Parties in conflict hold opposing values
   C. Parties in a conflict disagree about the facts in a situation
   D. Issues occur because of incompatible emotions
   E. All of these are true

5. Which of the following questions assist in the identification of identity or face-saving goals in a conflict?
   A. What do I want?
   B. Who are we in this relationship, and how does this affect what I want?
   C. What processes should be used in the resolution?
   D. Who am I in this interaction, and how does it affect what I want?

6. The most effective conflict management style:
   A. Is collaboration
   B. Is competition
   C. Is compromise
   D. Depends on the situation
   E. Depends upon the participant's core personality traits.

7. Research over the last 15 years suggests that nurses are most likely to use which of the conflict management styles?
   A. Competition, compromise
   B. Avoidance, accommodation, compromise
   C. Competition, collaboration
   D. All styles

8. Which of the following communication behaviors used in a conflict do NOT point to a destructive outcome?
   A. Criticism
   B. Defensiveness

C. Stonewalling
D. Anger
E. Contempt

9. Which of the following is likely to be found in integrative (collaborative) negotiation?
A. Hiding information
B. Exaggerating one's concessions
C. Compromising
D. Using confrontation to make points
E. Moving slowly toward the other's point of view

10. Which of the following is true of distributive (competitive) negotiation?
A. Competition is typically used by the "winner"
B. The ongoing relationship between the two parties is an important element in the negotiation
C. Making a modest opening bid and moving down slowly
D. All of these are true
E. None of these is true

REFERENCES

American Association of Critical-Care Nurses (2005). *AACN standards for establishing and sustaining healthy work environments: A journey to excellence.* www.aacn.org; accessed February 2005.

American Nurses Association. www.nursingworld.org; accessed March 2004.

Bartol, G.M., et al. (2001) Effective conflict management begins with knowing your style. *Journal for Nurses in Staff Development, 17*(1), 34–40.

Barton, A. (1991). Conflict resolution by nurse managers. *Nursing Management, 22*(5), 83–86.

Blake, R., & Mouton, J. (1964). *Managerial grid.* Houston: Gulf Publishing.

Boule, L. (2001). *Mediation: Skills and techniques.* Australia: Butterworths Skill Series.

Cavanagh, S.L. (1991). The conflict management styles of staff nurses and nurse managers. *Journal of Advanced Nursing, 16*(10), 1254–1260.

Eason, F.R., & Brown, S.T. (1999). Conflict management: Assessing educational needs. *Journal for Nurses in Staff Development, 15*(3) 92–96.

French, J. & Raven, B. (1960) *Bases of social power.* http://www.valuebasedmanagement.net/methods_french_raven_bases_social_power.htm. Accessed November, 2006.

JCAHO. (2005). *Sentinel event resource index.* www.jcaho.org; accessed April 2005.

Ury, W., Patton, B., & Fisher, R. (1991). *Getting to yes.* (2nd ed.). New York: Penguin Books.

Hightower, T. (1986). Subordinate choice of conflict-handling modes. *Nursing Administration Quarterly, 11*(1), 29–34.

Kritek, P. (2002) *Negotiating at an uneven table: Developing moral courage in resolving our conflicts.* (2nd ed.). San Francisco: Jossey-Bass Publishing.

Lewicki, R., et al. (2001). *Negotiation.* (4th ed.). Boston: McGraw Hill.

Marcus, L., et al. (2001). Renegotiating health care: Resolving conflict to build collaboration. San Francisco: Jossey-Bass Publishing.

Marriner, A. (1982). Managing conflict. *Nursing Management, 13*(6), 29–31.

Maxfield, D., et al. (2005). *Silence kills: The seven crucial conversations for health care.* American Association of Critical-Care Nurses & VitalSmarts. www.rxforbettercare.org; accessed February 2005.

Rahim, M.A. (1990). *Theory and research in conflict management.* NY: Praeger Publishers.

Rowland, H., & Rowland, B. (1997). *Nursing administration handbook.* Gaitherburg: MD: Aspen Publications.

Sportsman, S. (2005). Build a framework for conflict assessment. *Nursing Management,* 2005, 32–40.

Sportsman, S., & Hamilton, P. (2007). Conflict management styes in nursing and allied health professionals. *Journal of Professional Nursing.* January-February, 2007.

Thomas, K.W., & Kilmann, R. (1974). *Thomas-Kilmann conflict mode instrument.* Tuxedo, NY: XICOM.

Valentine, P. (1995). Management of conflict: Do nurses/women handle it differently? *Journal of Advanced Nursing, 22*(1), 142–149.

Warner, C. (1992). *Treasury of women's quotations.* Englewood Cliffs, NJ: Prentice Hall.

Wilmot, W., & Hocker, J. (2001). *Interpersonal conflict.* (6th ed.). Boston: McGraw-Hill.

Woodtli, A. (1987). Deans of nursing: Perceived sources of conflict and conflict-handling modes. *Journal of Nursing Education, 26*(7), 272–277.

Delegation: An Art of Professional Practice

CAROLE A. MUTZEBAUGH, EDD, CNP, CNS, MS

CHAPTER MOTIVATION

*"It is neither to do everything yourself nor to appoint
a number of people to each duty, but to ensure
that each does that duty to which he [sic] is appointed."*

F. Nightingale, 1859

CHAPTER MOTIVES

- Identify universal "rights" for delegation.
- Define "delegation" as discussed in state/province nurse practice acts.
- Review key elements of successful delegation, along with problems associated with task delegation.

Nursing management is truly an art. Whether an experienced manager or newly hired for the first professional position, the registered nurse (RN) seldom works alone. The interdisciplinary and interactive nature of nursing calls for juggling creative applications of the art of nursing. Skills for interdependent health-care delivery begin with direct patient care and can culminate in directing large groups or organizations. Financial pressures inside and outside the health-care agency, Medicare reimbursement reductions, managed care, and professional salaries create a greater need for increased delegation.

The ideal nursing practice incorporates many skill levels of health-care personnel with goals for patient care, yet within legal definitions and fiscal awareness. To achieve both patient care goals and goals of employers, the RN plans to extend his or her scope of practice through task delegation. Delegation is seen not only as a management skill but also as an ethical issue for nurses. The Code of Ethics for Nurses (American Nurses Association, 2001) endorses delegation where, "[t]he nurse is responsible and accountable for individual nursing practice and determines the appropriate delegation of tasks consistent with the nurse's obligation to provide optimum patient care."

Within health-care systems, the nurse may delegate to a technician, an orderly, a management assistant, or another nurse. The National Council of State Boards of Nursing (NCSBN, 1995) views delegation as "transferring to a competent individual, the authority to perform a selected nursing task in a selected situation. The nurse retains accountability for the delegation." The importance of delegation in the delivery of nursing care is emphasized on the NCLEX-RN study guide within the topics of leadership, staffing, and communication (NCSBN, 2004).

Although delegation is the skill most used to extend and expand the nurse's sphere of influence, certain aspects of the nursing process cannot be delegated. For instance, the practice-defining functions of assessment and evaluation, which require nursing judgment, can never be delegated. Implementation of nursing care, even delegated care, still remains the responsibility of the nurse.

Components of Delegation

Delegation to others in the workplace involves four principal components: delegator, delegatee, task, and client/situation.

DELEGATOR

The delegator possesses the **authority** to delegate by virtue of both position in the agency and state government license to do certain tasks. The license defines the **scope of practice** within a profession, whereas agency policy describes the role of employees. The RN degree, license, and policy create the authority to delegate to another individual in the workplace. Finally, delegation does not change the delegator's **accountability** or **responsibility** for task completion. These two concepts mean that the delegator can only delegate tasks within his or her scope of practice and that the responsibility for the skillful completion of the task remains with the delegator.

DELEGATEE

A delegatee receives direction for what to do from the delegator. The relationship between the two individuals exists within the workplace environment or through agency policy. The delegatee has the obligation to refuse to accept tasks that are outside of his or her training, ability, or job description. Although the delegatee may be registered or certified for certain skill sets, that is not always the case. In fact, even when assistive persons holds a permit to work as **unlicensed assistive personnel (UAP)**, that permit stipulates that performance of activities occur under the direction or supervision of a licensed nurse. A trained delegatee should have skills that relate to the work setting, but the delegator is responsible for knowing the performance level of each delegatee.

TASK

The task is the delegated activity. The delegated activity generally should be a routine task. Routine tasks have predictable outcomes, and a step-by-step method exists to complete the task. Decision making on the part of the delegatee for delegated tasks is limited to how to organize time and complete the task with different patients or variations in equipment. The procedure for the task is found in training manuals for teaching skills.

CLIENT/SITUATION

Identification of a specific client or situation for delegated nursing care is necessary to ensure that goals for patient care can be met by the delegatee. Familiar situations and environments enhance client safety and competent performance of any task. Situations include client care, such as direct care, responding to client calls for assistance, and distributing meals, or involve other tasks such as data entry, cleaning areas, stocking supplies, or phoning to confirm appointments. New situations require orientation, even if the client and task are familiar. Client-specific care fosters success with delegated task performance.

Delegation is not easy and not simple. Delegation is about getting other people to perform activities to meet specific client and organizational goals. Successful delegation means that the nurse understands nursing practice, knows UAP skills, identifies tasks, clarifies goals for client care, reinforces delegation, provides authority, fosters communication, and gives feedback.

Client care goals range from daily personal hygiene to treatment or recovery from a health problem. Organizational goals, on the other hand, relate to providing cost-effective services to help meet client care goals. Awareness of the rights, benefits, and pitfalls of delegation helps you recognize how to work through others with greater trust and confidence.

Rights of Delegation

Delegation is a precursor to the management functions of coordination and supervision. Without a delegatee, there is no one to supervise and no activities to coordinate. The NCSBN developed Rights of Delegation to guide the nurse in safe delegation in

---

Practice to Strive For 21-1

Without delegation, your work will not be done.

DO:

Select the right person for the task(s).

Communicate directions clearly.

Provide sufficient authority and independence to complete tasks.

Remain available and approachable.

Supervise and give feedback on performance.

Recognize efforts by others.

Use nursing staff for nursing decisions.

Know the scope of your practice and agency policy on delegation.

DON'T:

Think that you can delegate accountability.

Expect good results from poor delegation

---

response to an increasing number of nurse assistants or UAP in the workplace. The delegator nurse assigns the Right Person to perform the Right Task under the Right Circumstances and provides the delegatee with the Right Direction and the Right Supervision.

THE RIGHT PERSON

Delegation involves the nurse as either delegator or delegatee. Matching the specific client care goals and activities with the person to entrust with the appropriate responsibility and authority is a challenge. Do you delegate care for an aging patient to new UAP enrolled in a nursing program or to more experienced employees? Do you focus on the benefits of staff development or needs of the individual client? Do you plan time to offer support or only anticipate the outcome? How do you plan to supervise?

Delegating to UAP

The RN delegates client care to UAP in order to provide nursing care to more patients. Knowing the training of UAP can help make better delegation decisions. Both RNs and licensed practical/vocational nurses (LPN/LVN) are licensed nurses within federal and state statutes unless specifically differentiated. Both RNs and LPNs might have authority to delegate care in circumstances defined by law and agency policy.

UAP can be a certified nursing assistant or home health aide or hold a different work title within almost any health-care setting. UAP refers to "any unlicensed personnel, regardless of title, to whom nursing tasks are delegated" (NCSBN, 1997). ANA (1997) refers to UAP as an "unlicensed individual who is trained to function in an assistive role to the licensed registered nurse in the provision of patient/client care activities as delegated by the nurse." Although states maintain registries and titling of trained UAP and provide certificates or registrations from the board of nursing, the most inclusive title is UAP. See Box 21-1 for different titles that fall under the umbrella of UAP.

The operative phrase for UAP is "assist the nurse." Assessment of the skills and strengths of UAP is essential to obtain the benefits of their assistance in the setting. UAP have always worked in health care in some capacity, but the evolution toward formalizing training of UAP is fairly recent. The Nursing Home Reform Act, adopted by Congress in 1987 as part of the Omnibus Budget Reconciliation Act, defined training and evaluation standards for UAP working in long-term health-care facilities. Other health agencies developed similar policies for a variety of care settings.

It is important for delegators to understand the scope and limitations of UAP based on training. Content and duration of training are defined further by the Centers for Medicare and Medicaid

Services—§484.36 (a)(1)—and includes observation, reporting, documentation skills, basic infection control, recognition of emergencies, and skills for personal hygiene and grooming (Box 21-2). Training, instruction, and testing for manual skills and written knowledge are conducted by public and private contractors with approval of state nursing boards. The National Nurse Aide Assessment Program (NNAAP), developed by the NCSBN, operates in many states as a competency certification process. Results are then reported to a board of nursing. Students enrolled in basic nursing programs (associate and baccalaureate degree) often present as candidates for NNAAP testing. Successful completion of the test means that students can be employed as UAP until graduating and passing the NCLEX.

Generally, UAP work to assist licensed nurses in caring for clients in hospitals, nursing homes, patient residences, long-term care facilities, and clinics. Physician offices, schools, day-care centers, public health centers, and offices of other licensed professionals also employ UAP. Because of the wide range of employment settings, the nurse should be cognizant of the training of UAP in his or her specific work setting.

"I can do this or that faster/better/more skillfully by myself" is an attitude that prevents the nurse from taking full advantage of UAP skills. Of course, the nurse has more overall knowledge, but UAP may have more experience with a particular type or age of client. Care based on the knowledge of team members helps the nurse to take full advantage of strengths of other workers and promotes working relationships. Working in a unit with other nurses

---

Box 21-1

Names for UAP

Attendant	Assistive Personnel
Certified Nurse Assistant (CNA.)	Dietary Assistant
Home Health Aide	Medication Technician
Nurse Aide	Nursing Assistant
Orderly (PCA)	Patient Care Assistant
Health-Care Assistant Personnel	Unlicensed Assistive
Registered Nurse Assistant (RNA.)	Technician

Box 21-2

Training for Home Health Aides (42 CFR §484.36)

Duration: 75 hours classroom; 16 hours supervised practice

Content: Reporting, documentation observation of patient, and reading and recording of temperature, pulse and respiration; basic infection control; basic body function; clean and safe environment; respect for privacy and property; personal hygiene and grooming; transfer techniques; range of motion and position; nutrition and fluid intake; and any other task that the HHA may choose to have the. . . aide perform.

and UAP teams requires respect and judgment to avoid delegation to UAP who are already assisting other nurses. The UAP can receive conflicting instructions or overlapping information, both of which can serve to confuse and disorganize. Similarly, do not expect the same kind of skill from UAP unfamiliar with the patient population in your area.

Delegating to Nurses

To be promoted, a nurse manager must have competent personnel to step into her position. In health care, advancement in the workplace often starts in the same work area. Here, supervisors have an opportunity to select from among the staff for promotion to management levels within their supervisory sphere. Selecting the right person requires creative thinking: Who is reliable? Who has the most appropriate experience? Who will take acceptable risks? Who understands the workload? Who wants to succeed? Delegation can help the manager to assess the ability and potential of staff nurses, provide motivation through new challenges, and contribute to development of other skills on the team. As you become comfortable in an employment position, discuss your interest and willingness to accept management tasks with your supervisor.

As a new employee, you might be the delegatee for many activities, especially during the orientation period. Accepting delegated tasks assumes that you have the time, authority, knowledge, and skill to complete the job, but the delegator may not transfer the responsibility to get something done. Accepting delegated activities can leave you with little time left for your own workload; consequently, delegated jobs may require that you negotiate performance requirements. If you are delegated the job of "Arrange for a meeting of all staff on the unit," what does that mean? Do you set the time? The location? The agenda? Do you provide substitute staff during the meeting time? Do you order refreshments? Understanding the anticipated outcomes and possessing adequate information and authority for successful completion are crucial considerations.

Physicians, too, might choose to delegate a medical task to an RN without consideration of the skills, education, and experience of that nurse. This situation can create communication problems and a risk to client safety if the nurse is not clear about practice limitations to the physician. Physicians who delegate to advance practice nurses (APNs) retain responsibility for the task, whereas APNs who function independently within the state nurse practice act are responsible for the outcomes of their decisions. During surgical procedures, a nurse might function as a first assistant with definitive education and experience or perform a delegated task usually assigned to a second physician.

Physician Assistant Delegation

Where delegation of patient orders or treatment plans becomes less clear is when a physician assistant (PA) is the delegator. A PA works in collaboration with an MD or DO and generally evaluates and treats patients in clinics, medical offices, and sometimes in hospitals. When the PA delegates orders to an RN, what is the responsibility of the RN to carry out the order? Does he treat PA verbal and written orders as if those directives came from the physician? Does he contact the physician to validate the order? Does he do nothing because the order is not given and signed by the physician? The answer to the nurse's response to a PA delegator is based on the medical, nursing, and PA practice acts in the state/province. In any event, the response is to do something and not ignore the order for patient treatment. Lack of response to a patient treatment order can result in issues of negligence or malpractice. Questions about the authority of a prescribing professional can be referred to a unit supervisor until clear guidelines exist for the work setting. If you happen to be the supervisor, the physician of record can be contacted for clarification.

APN Delegation

Delegation is clearly an empowerment issue. The nurse is empowered, by statute and often by agency policy, to give direction to others. However, along with the power to direct others remain the authority and responsibility to see that the delegated activity is safely and correctly performed. This principle exists for nurses who delegate to UAP or for APNs who give verbal or written orders for other nurses to perform such activities as treatment or medication administration. The authority of the APN to delegate medical orders depends upon the state/provincial regulations. In Minnesota, for example, a Memorandum of Understanding between an APN and a physician defines delegated responsibilities related to the prescription of drugs, related devices, and activities (MN Statutes 2005, 148.171, subd.6, 13, 15). The relationship of the hospital or nursing home to an APN determines the extent to which patients can be admitted and treated independent of a physician order. If you are working in a setting where APNs routinely manage care for patients, that information will be part of the unit orientation. Again, when you are unclear about assuming a delegated task, refer the issue to the supervisor.

Student Delegation

Can a student nurse accept delegation from an RN who is not a faculty member? What are the consequences of refusing to complete a delegated task? The student role is fraught with ambiguities: the student wants a variety of clinical experiences but might not have covered the content in class, or a long time might have elapsed since learning academic content relative to the clinical practice.

Before entering the clinical setting, faculty members should provide clear guidelines to students on accepting delegated tasks not yet addressed in the curriculum. Guidelines might include options for the student: contact the faculty to ask permission to proceed with the task; ask the delegator to observe the student doing the task; ask if the task can be delayed until the faculty is present; assist task completion with the staff person. Each situation will vary.

RIGHT TASK

One reason to delegate is that each nurse has finite time and energy to care for clients, maintain the environment, and communicate with other health professionals. Tappen (2001) uses a framework of time management to explain delegation. When a nurse has responsibility for 5, 8, or 20 patients, routine and repetitive aspects of care can be assigned to "a competent individual with the authority to perform in a selected situation a selected nursing task included in the practice of professional nursing as defined by state statute in the Nurse Practice Act" (Colorado Revised Statutes, 2004). Inappropriate delegation or otherwise unauthorized performance of nursing tasks by UAP could lead to legal action against the licensed nurse and the UAP by the board of nursing and employer.

Appropriate tasks for delegation to UAP must fall within the delegator's scope of practice unless otherwise prohibited and should meet all five criteria: Standardized procedure, Technical in nature, Routine task, Unlikely risk, and Predictable results (**STRUP**).

- Standardized procedure: A standardized procedure is taught in training classes, written in an agency manual in a "how to" approach, and performed the same way by persons with similar training. Often, one standardized procedure, such as Bed Bath, is coupled with another, such as Changing Bed Sheets, to become a series of standardized procedures that comprise Personal Hygiene. Standardization does not mean that UAP cannot vary procedures, sequence, or combination for the individual client.
- Technical in nature: Technical tasks require little decision making about performance of the task. However, the ability to recognize normal from abnormal condition of the client and usual from unusual response to the task is part of UAP-tested competency. UAP need to recognize client response, determine if the task can be safely completed, and seek clarification as to how to continue if there is a question about safe care. Examples of technical tasks are listed as Personal Hygiene training (Box 21-3).
- Routine task: Routine implies that the task is recurring for both the client and the UAP. UAP are experienced in completing the task; the client has experienced the task previously. There is no task that is routine the first time

---

Box 21-3

Personal Hygiene Training for Home Health Aides

Home Health Services General Provisions: 42 Code of Federal Regulations §484.36 (2004).
Bed bath
Sponge, tub, or shower bath
Shampoo, sink, tub, or bed
Nail and skin care
Oral hygiene
Toileting and elimination
Safe transfer techniques and ambulating
Normal range of motion and positioning
Adequate nutrition and fluid intake

that you perform it. Even Measuring Intake and Output becomes routine only after the training is completed, competency is tested, and accuracy is established. Even the most routine tasks become "new" when the equipment changes.

- Unlikely risk: The stability of the client's condition predicts risk. Here, focus is on delegator knowledge of the person and the task. Unlikely risk of adverse or unexpected events during the task also relates to safety. An unlikely risk does not mean that a bad event never happens, only that the delegator considers the likelihood of an unusual event. The nurse delegates Personal Hygiene to UAP and does not expect the client to fall from the bed, incur an infection, or choke on candy. Similarly, UAP are not expected to incur low back strain, fall on a water spill, or be assaulted by the client. Problems happen. Conscientious supervision and active listening to UAP concerns can aid in delegating situations that pose an unlikely risk to client and worker.

- Predictable results: Before delegation of any activity, the nurse anticipates the result of the activity. Outcomes of tasks assigned to UAP need to be predictable. Assignment of Personal Hygiene for a group of clients can be predicted and easily assessed. Are the clients clean? Is there an odor about anyone? Is hair combed? Is the area clean and orderly? Are clients safe in their environment?

Review all tasks for delegation to ensure that personnel receive the appropriate level of delegation. The delegation decision model (Fig. 21-1) can serve as a guide. Delegate, do not "dump." Dumping can be a perceptual or a real issue. Clarification of roles and open discussions of dumping less desirable assignments can promote understanding (Cohen, 2004). Repeated assignment of difficult clients or boring, unchallenging, nonclient duties to the same UAP can result in frustration.

Refusing Delegated Task

Refusal to administer an inappropriate medicine or to carry out a procedure that may place the patient at risk or cause harm are common occurrences. Medication orders that create risk for patient wel-fare include routes, dosage, frequency, and the drug itself. A Dutch study by di Bie and others cited refusal of orders by nurses because the nurses did not perceive that they had the authority needed to do a risky procedure (2005, p. 765). Interestingly, although fewer than 30% of the survey nurses experienced problems, most of the refusals, both actual and contemplated, involved medication policy.

RIGHT CIRCUMSTANCES

When one nurse cares for one client, there is little need to delegate care. True or false? False. Complexities of science and technology have changed the concept of "private duty" nursing except in the realm of home care. Even nurses in critical care units require assistance with the multiplicity of client, housekeeping, and non-nursing tasks. Delegating tasks that do not require decision making, assessment, or evaluation allows the nurse to concentrate on complex interventions.

What are the right circumstances in which to designate other care providers? The right circumstance for delegation is whenever a task can be appropriately completed by UAP or whenever an opportunity arises for education of another nurse in clinical or managerial experiences. Often, a delegating situation permits on-site observations of staff and the opportunity to answer questions and improve performance.

Often, the ultimate goal of health care is cost containment. The nurse can extend practice influence to more clients through delegation, thereby reducing the cost of routine client care to the agency. Experienced nurses seem able to delegate through emergencies in client care or staffing. Minute-to-minute "on-the-fly" delegation is not innate; it is learned through experiences during previous circumstances and knowledge of the capabilities of personnel in the setting (Hoban, 2003). Failure to delegate prevents the recent graduate or nurse who has changed jobs from having the opportunity to participate in a variety of situations and events that translate into experience.

Failure to delegate results in expensive overtime and fatigue on the part of employees. As the RN delegator in the role of managing client care or managing all unit activities for a shift, consistent inability of staff to complete workload on time

Assessment completed by Licensed Nurse for client nursing needs			
YES	**NO**	**DELEGATE**	**DO NOT DELEGATE**

Tasks for care needs within Nurse Scope of Practice			
YES	**NO**	**DELEGATE**	**DO NOT DELEGATE**

Delegating Nurse directly responsible for client care			
YES	**NO**	**DELEGATE**	**DO NOT DELEGATE**

Task **DOES NOT** require nursing judgment, evaluation, or decision making			
YES	**NO**	**DELEGATE**	**DO NOT DELEGATE**

Task technical, routine, and written procedure states predictable results with unlikely client risk			
YES	**NO**	**DELEGATE**	**DO NOT DELEGATE**

Client stable in familiar setting			
YES	**NO**	**DELEGATE**	**DO NOT DELEGATE**

UAP has appropriate training and documented competency			
YES	**NO**	**DELEGATE**	**DO NOT DELEGATE**

UAP willing and able to accept delegation			
YES	**NO**	**DELEGATE**	**DO NOT DELEGATE**

Nurse delegator available for supervision			
YES	**NO**	**DELEGATE**	**DO NOT DELEGATE**

FIGURE 21-1 Delegation decision model. (Adapted from Arkansas State Board of Nursing [1996]. *Delegation Model*. Arkansas State Board of Nursing, Rules and Regulations.)

can be a symptom of lack of delegation or poor delegation.

Cost factors are apparent when valued employees look for other health-care jobs that are more "challenging" with "greater opportunity." Additionally, work that is not challenging leads to complacency and boredom; opportunities are missed to sharpen professional decision-making skills, and mistakes

hot topic:
Institutional License or Delegation?

Can any worker in a health-care setting legally give medications? The answer may be "yes" using the concept of delegation. Physicians and nurses can delegate tasks and that includes medication. However, as Dr. Starr, JD, writes, "Delegation is a high-risk activity because there are many things that can go wrong" (2005).

"Pill pushing" or medication administration has long been the domain of the RN in the hospital setting. Schools, occupational and community health clinics, medical offices, and nursing care centers once identified the RN as the health worker with sufficient education and knowledge to select and give the correct medicine to the right person. Currently, the responsibility of maintaining prescribed medical treatment through medication administration varies widely.

Many state statutes and regulations as well as federal rules already contain wording that permits delegation of medication administration to UAP—42 CFR §484.36(a)(xiii). One caveat to delegated medication administration is clear in the Colorado Nurse Practice Act—12-38-132(1); for example, where a specific prohibition is given for PRN type of time or dosing schedules: "In no event may a registered nurse delegate to another person the authority to select medications if such person is not, independent of such delegation, authorized by law to select medications." Consider the range of situations where "selection of medication" might be encountered. One such example may be providing acetaminophen for joint pain to an assisted living resident. At the other end of the spectrum might be a variable narcotic dose.

Prisons, boarding homes, assisted living residences, schools, and other settings already have short-term training programs that "qualify" employees with no health training to administer a variety of scheduled oral prescription drugs and medications taken for specific problems. Over-the-counter analgesics are often given upon request or upon a description of symptoms by that person. Agency or institutional employees are trained by a nurse working for the system or a contracted trainer. In-house training programs offer an institutional certificate to the employee to perform the tasks.

are made. Finally, failure to delegate is not efficient use of professional expertise. Use nursing staff for nursing decisions.

RIGHT DIRECTION

Clear, accurate, written directions convey the best direction for delegation. When that information is both written and verbal, chances are even greater that communication is understood.

Communication that provides more information or direction in delegation is preferred to too little detail. Directions should include what is to be done, where or to whom it is to be done, how it should be done, when it should be done, and what criteria will judge completeness. Consider the difference between the following two directives: "Provide a bath to the woman in Room 2314" and "Provide a shower with this antibacterial soap to Ms. Lee in Room 2314 before 7:30 a.m. as she will be going surgery at 8:00. Remind her to soap twice and to dress in surgery garb afterwards."

The manner of delegation is important as well. Directions can be defined verbally, in writing, or both. Written client assignment(s) reinforced with up-to-date verbal information is superior to a single communication method. Distraction or inattention can cause the delegatee to miss a piece of information or a detail. Written details and time frames serve as a guide to assigned tasks; follow-up through oral report provides timely information and reinforces the assignment. Additionally, using both methods allows for questions or negotiation of the assignment. Again, assignment making takes time, but using written and verbal delegation reduces misinterpretation and, as a consequence, mistakes.

Provide time to confer briefly with each delegatee at least twice during the shift to collect information about clients and evaluate the progress of UAP performance. Planned communication helps predict and anticipate changes during the shift and avoid surprises. Finally, provide feedback about performance to UAP. Recognize individual contributions to team functions. Public recognition and private corrective actions encourage team relationships.

Any delegated direction should provide the opportunity to ask questions or clarify information. To achieve clarity, the delegator must be available. Availability is sometimes a specific board of nursing criterion for delegation to UAP. Availability may be direct or indirect and is defined by the agency and board of nursing. For example, a pager may constitute availability for groups of delegatees, whereas physical presence may be required for other situations. In either event, it is important to communicate how you can be reached and under what circumstances. UAP discover availability quickly and the reception that questions receive.

RIGHT SUPERVISION

Just as training is a critical component of the delegation decision, supervision of personnel is essential to ensure safety and completeness of client care. Pairing experienced UAP with a less experienced supervisor does not eliminate the need for supervision. Recall your own experiences as faculty, nurse

Practice Proof 21-1

Article: McLaughlin, F.E., et al. (2000). Perceptions of registered nurses working with assistive personnel in the United Kingdom and the United States. *International Journal of Nursing Practice, 6*(1), 46–57.

The use of UAP to expand and augment the scope of nursing practice is an international concern. Articles that study UAP and their relationship to nurses have been published in nursing journals representing the United States, Canada, United Kingdom, Ireland, Italy, Australia, and New Zealand. Perceptions of individual nurses, UAP, managers, and clients have, for the most part, examined attitudes, satisfaction, preferences, and working conditions among various groups. This study compares perceptions of RN role change when working with different types of UAP. Another variable in the study examined perceptions between U.S. and U.K. nurses about UAP performance of delegated tasks, communication of important client information, and increasing time for professional nursing activities. U.K. nurses perceived less role change when working with UAP and showed more satisfaction with their use than U.S. nurses.

QUESTIONS:

1. What are the independent and dependent variables in the study?
2. Speculate as to how your workplace might compare with the study group variables.
3. The theoretical framework for this study was based on role theory; that is, the norms, behaviors, and values of the RN in the nursing role of delegator of patient care or "team leader." Discuss other frameworks that might have been used in a cross-cultural nursing study.
4. What impact would Project 2000 have if the study were repeated today?
5. Evaluate the study, citing both shortcomings and useful findings.

managers, and other employers have supervised your performance. What was helpful for professional growth, and what situations created distress, anger, or resentment?

NCSBN (1997) defined **supervision** as "provision of guidance and direction, evaluation and follow-up by the licensed nurse for the accomplishment of a nursing task delegated to UAP." Onsite supervision becomes a strong tool for gathering information for personnel evaluation or corrective action. Also, personal contact through supervision gives the delegatee an opportunity to ask questions and learn skills.

The amount of supervision depends upon the **competency** of the delegatee for nursing care or other duties. The key to delegation is to understand how your board of nursing defines nursing practice and the skills required by UAP that define competence. The NCSBN (1997) describes competence of the licensed nurse as "applying knowledge and interpersonal, decision-making, and psychomotor skills expected in the practice role within the context of public health, safety and welfare." Competency is performance judged by others in the profession or occupation that exhibits requisite knowledge, skill, and judgment for appropriate certification or license by virtue of completed education, training, and/or experience. UAP competence is summarized as the ability to use effective communication, collect basic objective and subjective data, perform simple nursing activities safely and according to standard procedures, and to seek direction when appropriate.

How does a nurse determine UAP or even another nurse's competence? It is not sufficient to simply ask UAP, "Are you able to do this task?"

Begin by reviewing a list of UAP competencies for the work area; then locate the procedure manual for your agency, and compare the two sources. Competencies should include skills comparable to Training for Home Health Aides (see Box 21-2) and personal hygiene tasks included in Personal Hygiene Training for Home Health Aides (see Box 21-3). A look at UAP certifications, hire dates, and completed in-service education programs will provide more background to keep supervision appropriate and expectations of performance realistic.

Temporary staff members from other units or staffing companies create concern about skill level during initial assignment in a work setting. In this circumstance, asking about skill level and experience is the only option until direct observation of performance has occurred. The delegator RN is still responsible for direct knowledge that UAP can, in fact, perform the skills assigned.

All Good Things...

Delegation is a primary function of management and includes both tasks delegated *to* the RN from other RNs and physicians as well as tasks delegated *by* the RN to others involved in the delivery of health care. State nurse practice acts specify RN delegator functions within designated environments. Agency policies offer guidance for delegating appropriately and lawfully, and job descriptions further guide the functions of practical nurses and UAP. Accountability and responsibility are part of a licensed position and cannot be delegated. Tips for appropriate delegation are based on the four components and five Rights of Delegation.

The NCSBN offers many resources about the process of delegation. Outcomes of thoughtful, appropriate delegation reflect partnership with UAP and safe, satisfied clients. Inappropriate delegation carries the risk of professional censure, legal action, and possible loss of license.

Let's Talk

1. *Obtain the nurse practice act for your state, including the sections on RN, LPN, LVN, and nurse aide/HHA. Compare the sections on scope of practice and delegation. Discuss the tasks and level of performance for the three groups.*

2. *Obtain a copy of the manual used to teach nurse aide/HHA candidates in your community. List the skills that are taught in a recognized program. Select 10 skills, and explain how these skills are considered to be standard procedure, technical in nature, routine, unlikely to carry risk, and have predictable results.*

3. *Discuss the implications for the nurse of the directive pertaining to UAP delegation "any other task that the HHA may choose to have the home health aide perform."*

NCLEX Questions

1. Delegation is a primary function of:
   A. Evaluation
   B. Management
   C. Mentoring
   D. Training

2. Aspects of professional nursing practice that CANNOT be delegated are:
   A. Monitoring and recording
   B. Implementation and planning
   C. Assessment and evaluation
   D. Reporting and recording

3. Effective delegation:
   A. Gets something done by someone else
   B. Permits an agency to operate with fewer RN staff
   C. Provides licensed nurses with recognition for heavy patient loads
   D. Uses skills of less educated employees in nursing homes

4. The transfer of authority to perform a selected nursing task in a selected situation to a competent individual is called:
   A. Assignment
   B. Buck passing
   C. Delegation
   D. Transference

5. Nancy Nurse, RN, completes an assessment on Patti Patient and delegates bathing, mobility, and nutrition care to a newly hired certified nurse assistant. Nancy Nurse, RN, is then able to admit another patient to the agency. The principle of delegation that Nancy must remember here is:
   A. Implementation of nursing care, including delegated care, remains the responsibility of the nurse
   B. New employees have completed an orientation program to ascertain skill levels
   C. Certified nursing assistants are licensed by a national testing agency
   D. Skills involved in this scenario are common, and completion can be expected

6. The licensed nurse delegator can delegate only tasks:
   A. Approved by the nursing standards committee in each state or province
   B. That were included in training programs for assistive personnel

C. Within his or her area of responsibility and scope of practice

D. When an appropriate licensed person is not available to complete those tasks

7. With each task delegated, accountability and responsibility for the skillful completion of the task remain
   A. Part of the physician's oversight
   B. With the delegator
   C. With the delegatee
   D. With the nurse supervisor

8. The Right Person to receive a delegated task is:
   A. A licensed or unlicensed delegatee with training in the delegated tasks
   B. Always UAP
   C. Available with sufficient time to complete the task
   D. One who has done the task before

9. The Right Circumstance for delegation by the licensed nurse:
   A. Is a routine and recurring event for a specific client
   B. May change from situation to situation
   C. Occurs with the patient approval and assent
   D. Occurs on the evening and night schedule rotations

10. The agency that determines the scope of practice for a licensed nurse, and therefore determines what can and cannot be delegated, is:
    A. American Nurses Association
    B. Council of State Boards of Nursing
    C. State/Provincial Board of Nursing
    D. National League of Nursing

REFERENCES

American Nurses Association (1997). Five rights of delegation: Unlicensed assistive personal legislation, 1997. Washington, DC: American Nurses Publishing.

American Nurses Association. (2001). *Code for nurses with interpretive statements*. Washington, DC: American Nurses Association.

Cohen, S. (2004). Delegating vs. dumping: Teach the difference. *Nursing Management, 35*(10), 14,18.

di Bie, J., et al. (2005). Risky procedures by nurses in hospitals: problems and (contemplated) refusals of orders by physicians, and views of physicians and nurses, *International Journal of Nursing Studies, 42*(7), 759–771.

Hoban, V. (2003). How to enhance your delegation skills. *Nursing Times, 99*(13), 37–38.

Home Health Services General Provisions. *42 Code of Federal Regulations.* §484 (2004).

Hospice Care. *42 Code of Federal Regulations.* §418 (2004).

National Council of State Boards of Nursing (1995). *Delegation: Concepts and decision-making process.* December, 1–4.

National Council of State Boards of Nursing (1998). National Council position paper. *Delegation: Concepts and decision-making process.* The Delegation Resource Folder. Chicago: National Council of State Boards of Nursing, Inc.

National Council of Boards of Nursing (2004). Working with others: A position paper. Chicago: Author.

National Council of State Boards of Nursing (1997). Delegation concepts and decision making process. Chicago: Author.

Nightingale, F. (1859). *Notes on nursing: What it is and what it is not.* London: Harrison and Sons. (Reprinted 1992). Philadelphia: Lippincott.

Nurse Practice Act 17, Arkansas Code of 1987, Replacement Acts 1995. Chapter 86. (1996)

Nurse Practice Act, 12, *Colorado Revised Statutes.* §38 (2004).

Registered Nursed Association of British Columbia. (2004). Assignment between nurses. *Nursing Practice Guideline.* Vancouver, BC: Registered Nurses Association of British Columbia.

Regulations relating to training of certified nursing assistants. 32 M.R.S.A. §2102-380 Chapter 5 (2003). Augusta, ME.

Starr, D.S. (2005). The art of effective delegation. *The Clinical Advisor.* April, 86.

Tappen, R.M. (2001). *Nursing leadership and management: concepts and practice* (4th ed.). Philadelphia: F.A. Davis.

Virginia Department of Health. (2001). Delegation of nursing tasks to unlicensed personnel, Retrieved July 9, 2004, from http://www.vahealth.org/wih/Perinatal%20Guidelines/SECTION%203.pdf

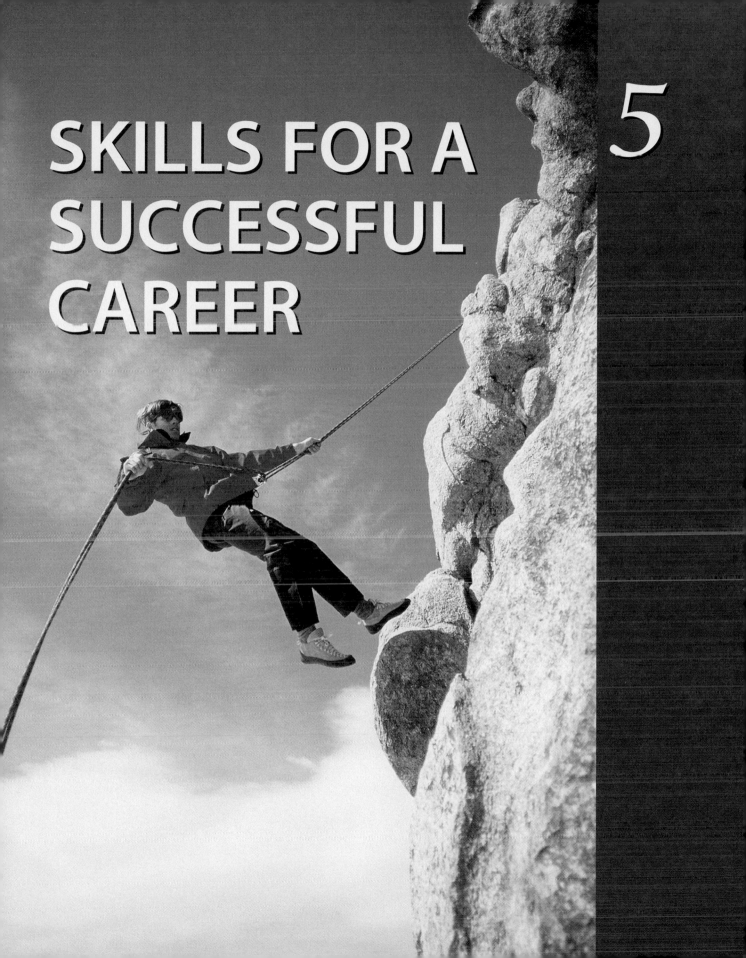

SKILLS FOR A SUCCESSFUL CAREER

chapter 22

Manage Yourself for a More Fulfilling Career

THERESA L. CARROLL, PHD, RN, CNAA

"Destiny is not a matter of chance, it is a matter of choice;
it is not a thing to be waited for, it is a thing to be achieved."

William Jennings Bryan

CHAPTER MOTIVES

- Critically reflect on who you are as a person and a professional nurse.
- Determine what you want and where you want to go.
- Take charge of the process of meeting the challenges of balancing personal and professional goals.
- Transition successfully from student to professional nurse.

*S*elf-management is all about knowing who you are, what you want, and where you want to go, and then taking charge of the process of gathering the resources and positioning yourself to get there. Self-management is the focused drive that enables us to achieve our goals (Goleman, Boyatis, & McKee, 2002). Self-management is important because it enables you to maximize experiences and achieve goals that ultimately lead to personal happiness and fulfillment. Learning the skills of self-management can help individuals to cope with personal and professional challenges that occur naturally in life's journey. When planning a nursing career, self-management becomes critical to achieving happiness because of the many challenges inherent in balancing personal responsibilities, like family life, and professional demands such as finding time for continuing education. This chapter will talk about the skills that are necessary to be successful at self-management. Specifically, the chapter will challenge you to:

1. Critically reflect on who you are as a person and a professional nurse.
2. Determine what you want/where you want to go in terms of your career.
3. Take charge of the process of meeting the challenges of balancing personal and professional goals.
4. Transition successfully from the student to the professional nurse role.

Who Am I?

The first step to self-management is discovering who you are. This is the psychological process of developing a self-concept. Self-concept is an overall term that is used to describe:

- Our thoughts and evaluations regarding specific aspects of self, such as gender, racial identity, and social class membership
- The ideal self, which includes hopes and dreams about personal attributes such as being scholastically able, having a sense of humor, and forming plans for the future, like becoming well-educated or achieving a leadership position in a career

- Overall self-esteem and self-acceptance, which includes how we evaluate our own abilities in relationship to others and learn to accept what we can and cannot do (Wylie, 1979).
- Self-concept evolves from a self-awareness of one's place in the world. From such awareness, self-concept becomes personalized as "a picture of one's self within a role, situation or position, performing a set of functions, or in some web of relationships" (Super, in Niles & Harris-Bowlsbey, 2002, p. 36).
- Self-concept is constantly evolving and requires a lifelong process of making decisions and adjusting to these choices. The person that you are now is a result of all the choices you have made to date (Luciani, 2004). For example, several years ago you made a decision to become a nurse. That decision led to other choices such as what school you would attend, when you would start, how you would pay for this education, and how much time you were willing to devote to your studies. Your self-concept is expanding to include becoming employed as a professional nurse.
- Many of the choices that affect self-concept reflect our needs and values. Needs vary from the most basic, such as food, clothing, shelter, and safety, to more complex needs like acceptance, belonging, and love. Once our needs are clearly identified, we can make a conscious effort to manage our behaviors to get these needs met. In order to understand how we go about meeting these needs and in what order we choose to meet them involves identifying and clarifying our **personal values**. Values determine what we care about the most. Values also provide a compass to keep our life and career on course and allow us to make wise decisions that move us forward rather than backward or off course entirely (Borgatti, 2004). For example, think about why you decided to enter a nursing program at this particular time. Some answers might include any or all of the following: the need for a steadily paying job to support yourself and family, a desire to work with a special population such as the elderly or childbearing families, or because you or a family member experienced care from a special nurse who impressed you with her knowledge and understanding of

your problems. Examining why you decided to enter the nursing profession is an exercise in identifying and understanding personal values. Examining our values also contributes to the self-concept by providing us with an understanding of what "feeds our soul and makes us happy" (Borgatti, 2004, p. 1).

- Personal values form the basis for recognizing and developing professional values. Professional values are the beliefs that provide a guide for how we practice professional nursing. A constant awareness of both personal and professional values helps us to set goals and make choices that move our career in directions that help to create and sustain personal happiness and professional satisfaction.

- One strategy that can help us articulate our personal and professional values is to write a personal mission statement. A personal mission statement should focus on "what you want to be (character) and to do (contributions and achievements) and on the values and principles upon which being and doing are based" (Covey, 1990, p. 106). You could call the personal mission statement your personal constitution; like the U.S. Constitution, it can provide the fundamental standard by which you set priorities and make personal and professional decisions. When this personal mission statement is based on an honest assessment and clear articulation of personal and professional values, it can provide a compass for steering these decisions in times of rapid and turbulent change.

- Self-management is about being proactive, taking charge, and making conscious decisions that are consistent with self-concept and personal and professional values about issues, such as "What do I want, and where do I want to go?"

"WHAT DO I WANT, AND WHERE DO I WANT TO GO"

Effective self-management behaviors require developing a plan that encompasses a personal and professional perspective and goals. One way of managing both personal and professional perspec-

tives is to view life as a journey. Successfully managing life's journey involves learning from the past, handling the challenges of the present, and preparing for the future. There are two different ways of viewing the journey of life. The first perspective focuses on external goals like achieving a leadership position, establishing a happy family, completing an academic program, and becoming a professional nurse. Life events are stepping stones, hurdles, or crossroads in the journey. This journey has a recognizable destination that is so desirable that people are willing to withstand hardships along the way. The downside of viewing life's journey as a means to a destination is the risk of feeling, "Is that all there is?" after achieving the goal. This revelation leads to the need to re-evaluate the destination when the journey is complete (Bridges, 1994).

The second kind of journey focuses on becoming the person we are meant to be. This metaphor of life as a journey toward "becoming" frames difficulties along the way not so much as hurdles to be cleared but as signals to be attended to or even lessons to be learned. It views our experiences as messages. The traveler on the journey to "becoming" finds the whole world full of guides, and events become the guideposts that indicate whether the path is correct (Bridges, 1994, pp. 132–133). These two views of life's journey as a destination and "becoming" are not necessarily mutually exclusive. Probably the most holistic view incorporates elements of both destinations in the same journey. For example, our destination may be to become employed as a professional registered nurse, and we can also view this job as a way of becoming a better, more fulfilled, and happier person. Both the successes and challenges we encounter in the process of becoming a professional nurse are viewed as ways to learn about ourselves and provide guides for future decision making. Happiness and satisfaction occur when we make choices that are consistent with our self-concept and values.

Whatever metaphor a person chooses to use to interpret life events, one thing is certain: self-management requires taking charge of both personal and professional destinations. In order to live meaningfully in a changing world, individuals need a skill set so that they can adapt to change but at the same time stay true to the values that are integral to the self-concept.

Achieving Goals

Goal setting is an important self-management tool. **Long-term goals** provide a more abstract direction for what needs to be done to achieve the preferred future. **Short-term goals** describe what needs to be done daily, weekly, or monthly in order to achieve the preferred future. During times of change and uncertainty, goals can provide a framework for setting priorities, judging progress, and maintaining focus. Goals provide structure and organization to daily life and help with maintaining a sense of control and organization. In order to be useful, goals need to follow the SMART guidelines: goals should be **Specific, Measurable, Attainable, Realistic,** and **Time-oriented**. The more specific the goal, the easier it is to determine what needs to be done to accomplish it. Goals need to be measurable in order to chart progress and to be able to know when replanning may be necessary. In order for goals to be attainable, they need to be realistic and time-oriented. If goals are not attainable, then instead of providing a benchmark that can motivate, they become frustrations and lead to feelings of defeat. For example, you may set a goal to walk a minimum of 10 miles per week. This goal is specific, measurable, and time-oriented. But if you are working full-time, going to school part-time, and have three active children who require transportation to multiple after-school activities, the 10-mile-per-week goal may be unrealistic and probably unattainable. It might be more realistic to walk 1 mile each time you drop one of the children at soccer practice, for a total of 3 miles/week. This goal may fit the SMART formula of Specific, Measurable, Attainable, Realistic, and Time-oriented better than the original 10 miles/week goal.

Another factor to consider when setting goals is a **realistic** understanding of whether something is within or outside of our control to change. Stephen Covey (1990) uses two circles to depict the **sphere of concern** and the sphere of influence. Within the sphere of concern are the things over which we have no control, such as the weather, the availability of funds for a raise, or the price of gasoline. The sphere of influence includes the things that we can do something about. For example, we cannot change the weather but we can be prepared for the kind of weather that is predicted; we cannot affect whether our employer will have funds available for a raise, but we can be sure that our performance is at a level that would merit a raise if money is available; and we cannot control the price of gasoline, but we can affect how much money we spend on gasoline by organizing a car pool, taking public transportation, or driving a more fuel-efficient vehicle.

Understanding what is controllable and what is not can eliminate the huge frustration of setting goals that are inherently unattainable because realistically the situation is beyond our ability to change. In addition, understanding what is within one's control can help the individual to avoid the **victim mentality.** The victim mentality arises when an individual feels helpless to change a situation that is interpreted to affect him negatively. Differentiating the sphere of concern from the sphere of influence allows individuals to realize that they are accountable only for their own choices, responses, and happiness. While they may be able to influence what other people think and do, they cannot control others.

STRATEGIES FOR ACHIEVING SMART GOALS

Establishing SMART goals is just the beginning of self-management. There are potentially many challenges to achieving these goals. Some of these challenges include encountering seemingly insurmountable obstacles like managing relationships with difficult people; coping with stress or sleep deprivation; and never having enough time to do the things life and living require. Some strategies for dealing with these challenges include positive self-talk; developing emotional intelligence; and stress, sleep, and time management.

Positive Self-Talk

Even though you establish goals using the SMART formula, challenges can occur between goal planning and achievement. Positive self-talk, or positive self-affirmation, can help with moving forward toward goal achievement. An affirmation is simply a sentence spoken in the present tense that reflects what you want to happen or want to be. The successful use of affirmation is based upon a belief that the power of words can create reality. Repeated affirmations help to develop a positive mind-set about the ability to achieve desired goals (Borgatti, 2004, p. 61). The positive mind-set translates into the actions that make the words reality. For example, a person who establishes a goal of being able to give 5-minute presentations before professional groups might engage in positive self-talk by repeating the phrases "I am prepared. I have rehearsed this speech. I know the material. I have something important to say. I know that I can deliver my message to this group." The assumption inherent in positive self-talk is that the capacity to do anything resides within the individual. This includes creating the experience and life that you want (Luciani, 2004).

Emotional Intelligence

Self-management requires that we have an understanding of what factors contribute to our behavior. Both intellectual capacity and emotions contribute to how we act toward and interact with others. Much of the time spent in formal academic experiences focuses on developing intellectual capacity, which leads to such skills as knowledge synthesis and critical thinking. Little attention is paid to developing emotional intelligence. Research has demonstrated that intellectual capacity alone cannot account for success and goal achievement. **Emotional intelligence** has been identified and described as at least as important as intellectual capacity in managing life's journey (Goleman, 1995). Intellectual capacity and emotional intelligence provide two fundamentally different ways of knowing and learning about the world. The **emotional** and **rational minds** are semi-independent parts that have physiological and neural connections to each other. The emotional and rational minds are distinguished in folklore as the dichotomy between "heart" and "head" (Goleman, 1995, p.8).

The intellectual, or rational, mind focuses on comprehension, allowing a person to interpret thoughts, ponder, and reflect. The emotional mind promotes knowing from feelings. "Ordinarily there is balance between the emotional and rational minds, with emotion feeding into and informing the operations of the rational mind and the rational mind refining and sometimes vetoing the inputs of the emotions" (Goleman, 1995, p. 9). This exquisite coordination allows thought to contribute to feeling and feeling to contribute to thought. "But when passions surge, the balance tips" (p. 9). It is the emotional mind that highjacks and controls the decision to act. Behavior that results from this emotional highjacking can be destructive to both personal and professional relationships. Learning to control this emotional highjacking is at the heart of emotional intelligence. Acquiring emotional intelligence can lead to healthier interaction with family, friends, and colleagues.

The first step in gaining emotional intelligence is developing self-awareness. Self-awareness entails paying attention to one's inner state and includes attention both to our moods and thoughts about our moods. Self-awareness contributes to emotional intelligence because it allows individuals effectively to turn that self-awareness into actions that translate into positive self- and social management. Enhancing our emotional intelligence can have many benefits in the work environment because emotional intelligence is a key component to being a successful professional nurse. An employee who is attuned to the feelings of others and is able to handle disagreements so they do not escalate is recognized as a valuable asset. In terms of our own careers, "there is nothing more essential than recognizing our deepest feelings about what we do—and what changes might make us more truly satisfied with our work" (Goleman, 1995, p. 149). For example, you may really want to work with children, yet you take a position working on an adult medical-surgical unit because you have been told that "everyone needs at least 1 year of medical-surgical experience" before working in a specialty area. Nine months into your first job you begin to find the patient requests annoying, the other staff demanding, and your enthusiasm for nursing decreasing. Emotional reactions and feelings are very complex, and there can be many reasons for these feelings. But as a beginning action, it may be time to reflect and reconnect with your original values and motivations for becoming a nurse and your original desire to work with children. In this case, your emotional reaction to the work situation may be based at least in part on not being able to work with the children. It may be time to negotiate a change in job setting and population. Box 22-1 describes the competencies and skills that will help you to increase your emotional intelligence.

Stress Management

Along the journey toward achieving your goals, there may be barriers. Some of these barriers include stress; sleep deprivation, especially when transitioning to shift work; and the challenges of time management while juggling multiple personal and professional roles. Self-management involves not just recognizing these challenges but proactively planning ways to avoid, cope with, and/or overcome these barriers.

In the 1950s, Hans Selye coined the term **stress** to mean "the nonspecific response of the organism to any pressure or demand" (Selye, in Kabat-Zinn, 1990, p. 236). "Stressor" is used to describe the stimulus or event that produced the stress response. The stress response is nonspecific because it involves both mind and body and may yield physiological, psychological, and/or social outcomes. Stress is a natural part of life and cannot be avoided. Therefore, the stress response needs to be managed. Research has demonstrated that it is not the stressor itself that causes a stress response but how it is perceived and handled that determines what, whether, or how much stress it causes (Kabat-Zinn, 1990). Some common sources of stress include:

1. Problems with weight management
2. Substance abuse issues, such as alcohol, drugs, cigarette smoking
3. Mental disorders such as untreated depression or anxiety
4. Dysfunctional relationships
5. Lack of exercise
6. Shift work
7. Inability to manage time effectively

Strategies to resolve these stressors involve a personal commitment to lifestyle changes and sometimes interventions planned with professional help. Tips for stress management, adapted from the National Chronic Pain Society Facilitators Training Manual, are in Box 22-2. A discussion of how to cope with the common stressors sleep deprivation, clutter, and time management follows.

Sleep Deprivation

A major source of stress for nurses and others who rotate shifts even when working a steady tour is sleep deprivation. More than 22 million Americans work evening, night, rotating, or on-call shifts. Shift work has the potential to cause social, psychologi-

Box 22-2

Tips for Stress Management

*1. **Get enough sleep.** "Sleep isn't just 'time out' from daily life. It is an active state important for renewing our mental and physical health each day. Yet more than 100 million Americans of all ages . . . fail to get a good night's sleep" (American Academy of Sleep Medicine, 2000, p. 1)

2. **Prepare ahead for the morning the night before.** Think about everything you will need for the morning, and organize the items where they can be easily accessed.

3. **Simplify your life.** Clutter is a stressor. Get rid of clothes you do not wear, things that collect dust, furniture you hate. Do not put up with things that do not work properly. If something is an aggravation, get rid of it or replace it.

*4. **Schedule more fun.** Do at least one thing that you like every day. Schedule time for solitude like taking a brisk walk, practicing low-impact yoga, or meditation. Do not give up seeing friends and doing things you enjoy because you "do not have time."

*5. **Practice preventive maintenance** on your car, home, health, and relationships. Preventive maintenance saves time and frustration (and health!).

*6. **Anticipate your needs, and plan ahead.** Do not let the gas tank get below half full, especially when traveling at night. Keep a well-stocked first aid kit in your home and vehicle. Buy postage stamps when you get halfway through the booklet.

*7. **Schedule a realistic day.** Allow ample time between appointments so you do not have to rush, worry, apologize for being late, or get a speeding ticket. Take advantage of your body rhythms. If you are a morning person, then schedule complicated tasks that require concentration in the morning. If you do not reach your peak until later in the day, start with easier things first that do not require much thought. Keep reading material with you to help cope with long waits in line or for appointments.

8. **Make contingency plans.** Make alternate plans "just in case" the primary plan does not work

9. **Rearrange work hours if possible.** A 30-minute change in arrival or departure time can make a big difference in traffic, crowds, and other stress producers. When traveling, allow extra time to arrive well ahead of schedule. It is better to arrive well ahead of schedule than to fret over every stop light or traffic jam along the way. Use red traffic lights to remind yourself to breathe.

10. **Choose friends wisely.** Choose to spend time with people who are positive, upbeat, and nonworriers. Spending time with friends gives us time to share problems, explore solutions, and unwind.

11. **Change your outlook.** For everything that goes wrong, there are 50 more things that go right. Count them. Maintain a sense of humor.

12. **Write thoughts and feelings in a journal to help clarify things and put them in perspective.**

13. **Do not over-extend yourself.** Learn to say "No, thank you" to extra projects when you do not have the time or energy to complete the tasks to which you have already committed. Make promises sparingly, and keep them faithfully when you do commit.

14. **Ask for help with the jobs you hate.** If you find that certain chores always make you tense, such as paying bills, grocery shopping, defrosting the freezer, or scrubbing tubs, get someone else to do them for you or with you. Relax your standards. Life is a lot easier if you ignore a little dirt.

*15. **Do not rely on your memory.** Take time out to make lists. Write down addresses and phone numbers in an organized place. Ask questions. You are less likely to make mistakes or get lost if you make sure to get detailed directions first.

*16. **Take time out.** Breathe deeply, stretch your muscles when tense, nap, meditate, and take a long soak in the tub. Unplug the telephone, or take a walk. Ten-second "breathers" at work can help.

17. **Think . . . think . . . think.** Use this list to get started in creating your own de-stressors.

*Relate need for time management skills

Earl, R. (2004). Stress management: De-stress your life. *Chronic Pain Report* 4(4), 3, 5.

cal, and physical problems. The reason that shift work is detrimental to health is because the body is so sensitive to changes in **circadian rhythms.** A circadian rhythm is the body's alternating cycle of sleep and waking. Predictions about how long it takes to adjust circadian rhythms to a shift-work schedule range from 3 years to never. Yet whether sleep issues become a stressor is very dependent on the individual. Some people are more naturally suited to working one kind of shift or another. "Night people" adjust to the night shift better than "morning people." Older workers in general find it harder to work nights or rotate shifts. For example, one person who rotates to the night shift may adapt well and enjoy the quiet time during the day when family members are at school and at work to sleep. Another person may have difficulty sleeping, which may lead to difficulty with family and peer relationships because of constant fatigue and resulting ill temper. Left unmanaged, the stress response can result in profound physical and/or psychological strain and even illness. Making sleep a priority can reduce stress levels and enhance the effectiveness of your behavior. Suggestions for managing sleep are in Box 22-3.

Box 22-3

How to Sleep Well

- Maintain a regular waking time, even on days off work and on weekends.
- Try to go to bed only when you are drowsy.
- If you are not drowsy and are unable to fall asleep for about 20 minutes, leave your bedroom, and engage in quiet activity elsewhere. Return to bed when, and only when, you are sleepy. Repeat this process as often as necessary throughout the night.
- Use your bedroom only for sleep, sex, and times of illness.
- Avoid napping during the daytime. If you nap, try to do so at the same time every day and for no more than 1 hour. Mid-afternoon (no later than 3 p.m.) is best for most people.
- Establish relaxing presleep rituals such as a warm bath, a light bedtime snack, or 10 minutes of reading.
- Keep a regular schedule. Regular times for meals, medications, chores, and other activities help the inner clock run smoothly.
- A light snack before bedtime can help promote sound sleep; avoid large meals.
- Avoid ingestion of caffeine within 6 hours of bedtime.
- Do not drink alcohol when sleepy. Even a small dose of alcohol can have a potent effect when combined with tiredness
- Sleeping pills should be used only conservatively. Most doctors avoid prescribing sleeping pills for periods longer than 3 weeks
- Do not drink alcohol when taking sleeping pills and other medication.

American Academy of Sleep Medicine. (2000). *Coping with shift work.* Rochester, MN: American Academy of Sleep Medicine, pp. 10–12.

In addition to managing sleep issues, other strategies for managing fatigue include eliminating surreptitious energy drains (Borgatti, 2004). Surreptitious energy drains are those things in life that, by their mere existence, sap away at our vigor a little at a time, which in turn drains away energy needed to deal with daily tasks. Clutter is an example of a surreptitious energy drain because it reminds us that we really do not have things under control. Eliminating clutter provides immediate rewards of both physical and psychological space (Borgatti, 2004). Some suggestions (Bryce, 2004) for dealing with clutter include:

- When sorting the clutter, e.g., piles of paper or clothing, start small, and go through one stack at a time.
- When deciding what to throw away, ask yourself "Have I ever used it? Will I ever use it? Can I find it somewhere else?"
- On your desk, keep one tray for reading and one tray for filing.
- Periodically schedule yourself to take care of the clutter, e.g., organize, file, or hang up discarded clothing.

Time Management

Time management is another common potential stressor. Unfinished tasks represent another surreptitious drain on energy. Unfinished tasks can include such things as an overdue writing assignment, a stack of unpaid bills, or an unfinished academic program. Unfinished tasks drain energy because they are always present in either conscious or unconscious awareness. Whatever the task, recognizing and making a firm commitment to act can help to stop the surreptitious energy drain (Borgatti, 2004). Some suggestions for managing time and getting to unfinished tasks include:

- Use a planner or electronic calendar for your appointments and "to do's"
- Block off time in your planner to work on projects
- On your "to do" list, do the worst or oldest task first
- Learn to say "no." Being aware of your own limitations, priorities, and boundaries is important.

Some additional strategies for more effectively managing time are included in Box 22-4.

Box 22-4

Time Management

- Do two things at one time but only if neither requires special concentration, e.g., listen to the news while preparing meals; combine exercising with socializing: walk or jog with a friend.
- Go low-maintenance, e.g., buy low-maintenance clothing, get a wash-and-wear hairstyle, and select food that requires little preparation; eating raw or plain food is healthier anyway.
- Keep lists for all regular or routine activities, e. g., avoid extra trips to the store by putting items on your list as soon as they are used; maintain a weekly errand list; combine as many trips as possible, and plan an efficient route to minimize time and mileage.
- Always carry your daily schedule book with you. Attach a post-it notepad to the inside cover to make temporary notes. Clip a pen on the inside cover.
- Organize a filing system. Keep a "pending" file and sort through it once a month. Keep unanswered letters or e-mails filed, and schedule a regular time to respond. Keep a file of unpaid bills, and review this every 2 weeks. Keep a "health" file with all medical, pharmacy, dental, and optometry records.
- Keep a current alphabetical directory of all people and businesses important in your life.
- Have a regular assigned place for everything. This applies especially to small articles like keys, pagers, cell phone, watches, wallets, and pens.
- Do things when other people do not do them: go to the movies at 5 p.m. and eat afterward; avoid the grocery store at 6 p.m.

Adapted from Kelman, E., & Straker, K. (2000) *Study without stress.* Thousand Oaks, CA: Sage Publishing Inc., pp. 36–37.

Transitioning From Student to Professional Nurse

Self-management involves understanding and balancing multiple roles with all of their inherent changes and transitions. As you give up the role of student, you are also giving up your dependency on the presence of a clinical instructor and/or a preceptor. You are giving up the uniform of a student for that of a professional nurse and employee. These are external signs of the changes you are experiencing. There are also more subtle transitions taking place, such as the way you think about yourself, including the full weight of responsibility that you assume for your behavior as a nurse.

Sociologists have studied these times of transition and formulated several theories about the transition from student to employee and professional. Role theory provides the underpinnings for interpretation of roles in society. Symbolic interaction and social structural role theory are the two major branches of role theory. Although they vary on a number of parameters, both theories have in common such concepts as role, role behavior, norms, sanctions, and status. These concepts are defined in Box 22-5.

An example of a role behavior is the systematic way a nurse approaches an initial assessment of a patient. Within the employment settings there are policies and procedures and probably a form to guide the assessment process. The policy defines the expected role behavior, e.g., the initial assessment must be completed within 8 hours of the patient's admission to the hospital. If the nurse consistently fails to follow policy regarding completing the assessment, the nurse may be reprimanded by the manager for this failure. The reprimand represents a negative sanction. The status of the nurse manager is determined by the official designation within the hospital structure as one who is in

Box 22-5

Definitions for Role Theory

Role: Term commonly used to refer to both the expected and actual behaviors associated with a position (Hardy & Conway, 1988, p. 165)

Role behaviors: Position-specific norms that identify attitudes, expectations, behaviors, and cognitions required and anticipated for a role occupant (Hardy & Conway, 1988, p. 165).

Norms: Rules, standards, or guidelines that suggest what role occupants should and should not do (Hardy & Conway, 1988, p. 164).

Sanctions: Incentives or disincentives used to modify behavior and maximize adherence to prevailing group norms or prescriptions. Sanctions may be either negative or positive (Hardy & Conway, 1988, p. 164).

Status: The official location of a role in the social structure (Hardy & Conway, 1988, p. 164).

charge of supervising other nurses in the provision of care to patients.

Normal human development follows a pattern of transitions that have their own set of unique characteristics and tasks. For example, an infant transitions to the toddler period. Both the infancy and toddler stages have a distinct set of developmental tasks. Yet each individual child experiences the infancy and toddler stages in a unique way. The transition from student to professional nurse is not unlike the transition from infancy to toddler. There are predictable developmental tasks and skills to be achieved. Yet each transition is unique to the experience of each nurse. One of the developmental tasks of adulthood involves a recognition of responsibility for our reaction to circumstances and any resulting behavior. Self-management skills empower the student to proactively transition from the student role to that of professional nurse.

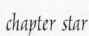 *chapter star*

John M. is a staff nurse in a critical care unit of a medical center hospital. John is working 12-hour shifts and is frequently called upon to work extra shifts to cover unit staffing. John's goal has always been to become a nurse anesthetist. He has delayed enrollment because anesthesia programs require students to be full-time, which allows little time for part-time work. He is married to Kira, who is a nurse manager in the same institution and is on permanent call to assist with unit decision making; e.g., she frequently works a 10-hour day and receives calls at home about unit problems. In addition to working full-time, Kira is pursuing an MSN on a part-time basis. When Kira becomes pregnant, John and Kira are excited about becoming parents but realize that their lifestyle will need to adjust with the birth of their first child. They discuss their personal goals for school and career and consider their mutual goals for family lifestyle, home life, and their relationship. After carefully assessing their economic situation, they decide that they can afford for Kira to resign her position when the baby is born and to continue to attend school and finish her MSN as a full-time student. Meanwhile, John will continue to work at his job as a staff nurse. When Kira is near finishing her MSN, they agree to reassess their personal and mutual goals as a family and determine when it might be feasible for John to enroll in a program to become a nurse anesthetist.

ADJUSTING TO THE ROLE OF PROFESSIONAL NURSE

The nursing student, new graduate nurse, and staff nurse roles each have role behaviors, norms, sanctions, and status dimensions that are unique to their specific designation. When a person changes roles, the process of learning the new role is called **socialization.** Professional socialization is a term used to describe the social processes that occur between the time a student enters a nursing program and graduates. The professional socialization that goes on during education in a professional nursing program is designed to shape attitudes, values, self-identity, role skills, role knowledge, and role behavior (Hardy & Conway, 1988). As intense as the socialization is during the nursing program, there is still need for socialization to the nursing role within the employment setting. During the orientation to the employment setting, the new graduate nurse must reconcile the values and expectations of the educational program with the values and expectations of the job. For example, while a student, the usual assignment may be one or two patients. This allows the student time to provide total patient care, including a bath and all treatments. The expectation is the student is learning skills and gaining in-depth knowledge of all aspects of the patient's condition. As a nurse, the assignment may increase to six to eight patients, and the bath and treatments may be delegated to a nurse aide. It may take new nurses time to adjust to the idea that while they alone are not giving total patient care, they are responsible for all care for the patient whether they physically supply that care or delegate it to another employee. The transition from student to professional nurse employed in an organization frequently involves giving up the practice of personally providing total patient care to being sure that patient care is accomplished according to the model of care delivery that is adopted by the hospital or other organization.

Making a successful transition from student to new graduate to professional nurse is affected by past experience with transitions as well as the socialization to the profession that went on in the educational program. The transition to an employment setting is particularly important because this experience can establish precedents and patterns for dealing with the many future transitions that can be anticipated in the rapidly changing healthcare delivery system. The transition from student to professional nurse involves unplugging from the world of student and plugging into the values and expectations of becoming an employee and staff nurse. In general, all role transitions involve:

1. Letting go of old ways and old identities
2. An "in-between time" when the old is gone but the new identity is not fully operational, which involves psychological realignments and repatterning of behavior
3. Emerging from transition when the new identity is established and a new sense of purpose arises (Bridges, 1980; Bridges, 2003).

Moreover, role transitions may elicit a sense of loss and/or anxiety as old roles fade and new roles—and accompanying expectations—demand attention. For example, as the role of professional nurse demands more time and attention, the days of being able to call the instructor when a new procedure must be done are being replaced with locating the procedure manual or co-opting the assistance of an experienced nurse to help with the learning process. The realization that you are totally responsible for patient care can produce much anxiety until you can gain confidence through experience and successfully access the resources of the workplace to provide help and support for your professional practice.

REALITY SHOCK

Role transition from student to new graduate to registered professional nurse is a process that has been studied from a variety of perspectives and disciplinary orientations.

In the 1970s and 1980s, Marlene Kramer studied the new graduate adjustment to the hospital work world. She concluded that during the process of adjusting to the professional nurse role in the hospital, the new graduate may recognize that there are differences in the values and expectations between school and workplace. Dr. Kramer called this phenomenon **reality shock**. Reality shock is a universal phenomenon used primarily to describe newcomers' reactions when they move into an occupation, after years of arduous preparation, only to find that many of the professional ideals and values learned in school are not operational and go unrewarded in the work setting. They end up feeling less than competent and uncomfortable. Resolving reality shock occurs when the new nurse learns to live comfortably with the values and expectations of the work world and the profession (Kramer & Schmalenberg, 1977).

Reality shock has several phases, including the honeymoon, shock, recovery, and resolution. The honeymoon phase occurs early after hire when only the best aspects of the job are apparent. During the honeymoon phase, nurses believe that the good things they experience far outweigh any negative experiences. Shock occurs when the full extent of the differences in expectations between being a student and being a graduate nurse becomes apparent. The recovery stage involves the new graduate regaining a balanced and modified view of the work world. For example, the new graduate may continue the commitment to learning but recognize that the kind of learning involved in the work setting will be focused primarily on the task at hand and the procedure as dictated by the agency. Resolution takes place when the conflicts become resolved, new expectations are met, and the new graduate becomes assimilated into the culture of the work world and able to position professional values within the work environment (Kramer, 1974). Resolution takes place as new nurses realize that they can handle a patient assignment and complete tasks within the given shift. New nurses begins to hear from peers, managers and, most important, the patients that they are doing a good job. Resolution comes as new nurses experience a sense of accomplishment and purpose.

Experience has demonstrated that many new graduates experience this phenomenon to some extent. In order to ease the transition from school to work, nursing programs have initiated role transition experiences like partnering with a preceptor and working the preceptor's schedule. This provides experiences that are closer to the reality of the work world while still in school. These experiences are aimed at easing the transition from school to work.

TRANSITIONING TO ROLE OF SKILLED CLINICIAN

Embedded within the transition from school to work is the process of becoming a skilled clinician.

Dr. Patricia Benner studied the process of new nurse skill acquisition and critical thinking and concluded that new graduates' perceptions of complex clinical situations were significantly different from those of nurses with more experience and skill (Benner, 1984; Benner, Tanner, & Chesla, 1996). Benner (1984) identified the stages of skill acquisition as novice, advanced beginner, competent, proficient, and expert. Knowing about the characteristics of these stages allows an individual to increase his awareness of what he is experiencing. This awareness is the first step of learning to manage the transition from new graduate to skilled clinician.

Dreyfus and Dreyfus (1996), whose work with chess players provided the basis for Benner's work, offer the following descriptions of this process of skill acquisition. The **novice stage** is a time of using the theory and translating the lessons of the nursing program into the real-life patient care environment. This is a time for learning the rules and rule-based reasoning. The beginnings of intuition related to patient care start developing during this stage. The new graduate begins the professional nursing career as a novice. After experiencing a variety of real patient care settings, the novice progresses to the **advanced beginner** stage, during which professional performance improves to become marginally acceptable. During this stage, the nurse is beginning to discern the situational elements to clinical decision making. The nurse knows the rules that govern care in a situation but begins to understand how and when the rules can be applied based upon the patient's condition, desire, and needs. Both rules and skills become more complex, and it is not unusual for the advanced beginner to feel overwhelmed "by the effort required to notice all relevant elements and to remember an increasing number of more and more complicated rules" (Dreyfus & Dreyfus, 1996, p. 38). During the **competence stage**, the number of elements that the nurse is able to recognize as relevant in a clinical care situation may still be overwhelming. But during this stage the nurse begins to understand and adopt a hierarchical perspective, i.e., to categorize the rules according to relevance and set priorities. Nurses at this stage must devise a plan to determine which elements in a situation are deemed to be important enough to require action or

intervention. These new rules cannot be taught by lecture or come from a textbook. Another characteristic of this stage is recognition that by making decisions that affect the outcome, the competent nurse becomes emotionally involved in the outcome. The competent nurse begins to assume and feel responsibility. This emotional involvement marks the end to the detached rule-following stance of the advanced beginner and the beginning of the rather frightening acceptance of risk and responsibility that sets the stage for further advancement.

The hallmark of the **proficient stage** of performance involves approaching a care situation with both concern and involvement and knowing intuitively what the priorities are and being able to perform the required procedures with proficiency, speed, and confidence. Action becomes easier and less stressful as the nurse simply sees what needs to be achieved and does it (Dreyfus & Dreyfus, 1996, p. 41).

The **expert** nurse can handle complex and unique situations. Achieving the expert level requires the ability to discriminate and set priorities among situations all seen as important and to know how to achieve goals once a decision has been made. This ability to discriminate and choose one priority over another requires both maturity and practice (Dreyfus & Dreyfus, 1996). Not every nurse achieves the expert stage of practice. Furthermore, when a nurse transfers from one specialty area to another, a proficient nurse may return for a time to the competence stage while he learns and gains experience in the new specialty.

Results from Kramer's and Benner's work have been applied by employers to design new graduate orientations, internships, and residencies: these reflect the nursing profession's concern with actively managing the transition from student to employee and to professional nurse. These efforts are also a response to the high turnover rate of new graduates within the first year of employment (Goode & Williams, 2004).

Part of self-management is finding an organization where you can meet your professional goals. Within the job search and interview process for that first job, you need to assess whether a potential employer offers a special orientation, internship, or residency for new graduates and whether this is something that will be available to you.

Practice to Strive For 22-1

In order to ease the transition from nursing student to graduate nurse and to decrease attrition, many health-care organizations have initiated nurse internship programs. These programs extend the period of traditional orientation from several weeks to as long as a year. When this period is extended to a year, it is frequently referred to as a nurse residency program. Both the duration and content of the program are determined by a variety of factors, including but not limited to financial and human resources of the organization, type of specialty unit, number of new graduates hired, and type of academic program attended by the majority of new graduates. Whatever the duration of the program, the goals in general are to:

- *Help the new graduate develop clinical knowledge and skill to function as an independent professional nurse.*
- *Provide support for the new graduate during the transition from student to nurse employee.*
- *Help the new graduate gain increased awareness of the patient/family needs and how to access the resources of the system to meet these needs.*

The format for most internship programs includes experiences in the classroom, skills and computer laboratories, and on the clinical units. While classroom and laboratory experiences are directed by instructors from the education department, experience on the clinical units is directed by a preceptor who is an experienced RN who works closely with the new nurse to supervise patient care and introduce her to the culture of the clinical unit and the nursing organization. Some organizations predetermine how long the new nurse must work with the preceptor; other organizations establish an expected time frame for the relationship. Usually, the new nurse works the same schedule as the preceptor until the new nurse has achieved self-confidence and the trust of the preceptor. (Blanzola, Linderman, & King, 2004; Bowes & Candela, 2005; Casey, et al., 2004; Ihlenfeld, 2005; Rosenfeld, et al., 2005).

BALANCING CAREER/LIFE LINKAGES

Adjustment to the role of professional nurse does not occur in a vacuum, away from the expectations of other life roles and transitions. "Recognizing ties between one's personal well-being and work life is what is called '**career life linkages**.' It is impossible to segregate work and personal life" (Miller, 2003). Being able to balance the interaction of professional and personal life roles results in "life sat-

isfaction, which differs from the sum total of the marital, job, leisure and other role indices taken separately. High-functioning people have well-developed and prioritized values" (Brown & Crace, in Niles & Harris-Bowlsbey, 2002, p. 81). People who are happy and satisfied know what they want and have a plan for achieving their goals that are consistent with their personal and professional values. Achieving and balancing personal and professional goals require self-management. Balancing career/life linkages involves timing and pacing. Timing involves deciding when to begin a new project or approach a new goal. Pacing is about how quickly one proceeds with implementing the project or achieving the goal. An example of timing involves a decision about when to start the next educational program. Pacing relates to the decision whether one will attend full- or part-time and, if part-time, whether one will enroll in one or two courses a term. Balancing career/life linkages adds the dimension of personal to this professional decision. For example, the decision to enroll part-time may be affected by the need to work full-time and use employer-provided tuition benefits or the need for quality time with school-age children. There are no hard and fast rules about achieving a career/life balance for everyone. The best strategy is to approach goal setting and planning with a realistic understanding about what is possible for you and those who are important in your life. Any potential decisions about plans, including timing and pacing, need to take into account your personal and professional values and the values and preferences of the important others in your life.

All Good Things...

People who are happy and satisfied know what they want and have a plan for achieving their goals that are consistent with their personal and professional values. They proactively take charge and make conscious decisions to act in ways that lead to goal achievement, i.e., they are skilled in self-management. Self-management is built upon a clear differentiation between what is within our power to control and what we can only influence. With this understanding, goal setting can be specific, measurable, attainable, realistic, and time-oriented. Strategies that help with goal achievement include positive self-talk and developing emotional intelligence.

Managing life to achieve goals involves dealing with the barriers along the way. One of the biggest barriers is stress. Stress is a natural part of life and cannot be avoided, but the stress response can be managed and controlled. The first step in managing stress is identifying sources of stress. Some examples of stressors that frequently affect the lives of nurses are sleep deprivation, surreptitious energy drains, and lack of time to manage all the competing demands of our fast-paced lives with their multiple roles. There are many strategies for dealing with each of these stressors.

A stressor that has received attention from the nursing profession is the process of transitioning from student role to the role of professional nurse to expert clinician. Two nurse researchers have studied this process. Evidence-based programs can help you with these transitions in many employment settings. Dr. Marlene Kramer has identified this process as reality shock. Many employers have programs in the form of orientations, internships, and residencies aimed at helping you to cope with this transition and the resulting reality shock. Dr. Patricia Benner studied the process of acquiring nursing skill and outlined a series of stages that nurses pass through on the journey from novice to expert. Many hospitals have adopted a novice-to-expert model for progression within a clinical career ladder.

Decisions that you make in your career will affect your personal life, and what goes on in your personal life affects your professional development. These career/life linkages must also be managed to achieve personal happiness and professional fulfillment. Having a clear understanding of personal and professional values helps to provide the compass for decisions about timing and pacing related to both personal and professional issues and these linkages.

Let's Talk

1. *Write a personal mission statement to meet the following criteria: What you want to be (character); what you want to do (contributions and achievements); what values and principles you will use to accomplish "being" and "doing."*

2. *Based on the mission statement, develop a long-term goal (something that will take more than a year to achieve), and then develop some short-term goals to operationalize the long-term goal. Evaluate the goals using the SMART criteria.*

3. *Develop a list of things that are within your control, that are outside of your control, and the things that you may be able to influence. How does this realization of the ability to control, have no control, and possibly influence affect the kinds of goals that we set for ourselves?*

4. *Review the characteristics of emotional intelligence. Identify someone you think is emotionally intelligent. Describe the behaviors that this person exhibits that demonstrate emotional intelligence. How does your behavior compare with the behavior of the person? How would you go about developing your own emotional intelligence?*

5. *Identify a time when you experienced a great amount of stress, but others around you did not perceive the situation as stressful. What factors made the situation stressful for you? Why did other people respond in different ways to the same experience?*

6. *As this chapter is about self-management, what stressors do you anticipate, and how do you plan to manage your stress response?*

NCLEX Questions

1. Self-management is all of the following EXCEPT:
   A. Knowing who you are
   B. Knowing what you want and where you want to go
   C. Taking charge of the process of gathering the resources and positioning yourself to achieve your goals
   D. Developing a time line for activities of daily living

2. Self-concept is an overall term that is used to describe all of the following EXCEPT:
   A. Thoughts and evaluations regarding specific aspects of self, such as gender, racial identity, and social class membership
   B. The ideal self, which includes hopes and dreams about personal attributes

C. Overall self-esteem and self-acceptance

D. One's position in the job hierarchy of an organization

3. In order to be useful, goals need to follow the following guidelines:
   A. Be broad and cover a 10-year period
   B. Be measurable
   C. Be attainable within 30 days
   D. Cover the social and work aspects of one's life

4. Strategies for dealing with challenges to achieving personal goals include all of the following EXCEPT:
   A. Positive self-talk
   B. Developing emotional intelligence
   C. Stress, sleep, and time management
   D. Working longer hours to achieve the goal

5. Some common sources of stress include:
   A. Problems with weight management
   B. Substance abuse issues such as alcohol, drugs, and cigarette smoking
   C. Mental disorders such as untreated depression or anxiety
   D. All of the above

6. Strategies for time management include all of the following EXCEPT:
   A. Use a planner or electronic calendar for your appointments
   B. Always schedule projects for completion as the last thing on your "to do" list
   C. Complete the worst or oldest task first
   D. Be aware of your own limitations, priorities, and boundaries

7. Role transition from student nurse to staff nurse involves:
   A. Letting go of old ways and old identities
   B. Psychological realignments and repatterning of behavior
   C. Emerging from transition when the new identity is established and a new sense of purpose arises
   D. All of the above

8. Social competence involves the following social awareness capability that determines how one manages relationships:
   A. Sympathy: showing sorrow for another's losses
   B. Organizational awareness: reading decision networks and politics at the organizational level

C. Service: belonging to one's professional organizations

D. Developing interpersonal relationships

9. Social competence involves the following relationship management capability:
   A. Transformational leadership: guiding and motivating by transforming followers
   B. Influence others via monetary rewards
   C. Developing others through continuing education
   D. Teamwork and collaboration

10. Strategies to promote a good night's sleep include:
    A. Maintain a regular waking time, even on days off work and weekends
    B. Try to go to bed only when you are drowsy
    C. Establish pre-sleep rituals that energize you, such as physical activity
    D. A and B

REFERENCES

American Academy of Sleep Medicine. (2000). *Coping with shift work.* Rochester, MN: American Academy of Sleep Medicine.

Benner, P. (1984). *From novice to expert.* Menlo Park, CA: Addison-Wesley Publishing Company.

Benner, P., Tanner, C., & Chesla, C. (1996). *Expertise in nursing practice: Caring, clinical judgment, and ethics.* New York: Springer Publishing.

Blanzola, C., Linderman, R., & King, M. (2004). Nurse internship pathway to clinical comfort, confidence, and competency. *Journal for Nurses in Staff Development, 20*(1), 27–37.

Borgatti, J. (2004). *Frazzled, fried . . . finished?* Boston: Borgatti Communications.

Bowles, C., & Candela, L. (2005). First job experiences of recent RN graduates. *Journal of Nursing Administration, 35*(3), 130–137.

Bridges, W. (1994) *Jobshift.* Reading, MA: Perseus Books.

Bridges, W. (2003) *Managing transitions.* (2nd ed). Cambridge, MA: DaCapo Press.

Bridges, W. (1980). *Transitions.* Cambridge, MA: Perseus Books.

Bryce, C. (2004). Stress on the job: Beating it before it beats you. *MD Anderson Cancer Center Messenger, 33*(6), 4–6.

Casey, K., et al. (2004). The graduate nurse experience. *Journal of Nursing Administration, 34*(6), 303–311.

Covey, S. (1990). *The 7 habits of highly successful people.* New York: Simon & Schuster.

Dreyfus, S., & Dreyfus, H. The relationship of theory and practice in the acquisition of skill. In Benner, P., Tanner, C. & Chesla, C. (1996). *Expertise in nursing practice: Caring, clinical judgment, and ethics.* New York: Springer Publishing.

Earl, R. (2004). Stress management: De-stress your life. *Chronic Pain Report, 4*(4), 3, 5.

Goleman, D. (1995). *Emotional intelligence.* New York: Bantam Books.

Goleman, D., Boyatis, R., & McKee, A. (2002). *Primal leadership.* Boston: Harvard Business School Press.

Goode, C., & Williams, C. (2004). Post-baccalaureate nurse residency program. *Journal of Nursing Administration, 34*(2), 71–77.

Hardy, M., & Conway, M. (1988). *Role theory: Perspectives for health professionals.* (2nd ed.). Norwalk, CN: Appleton & Lange.

Ihlenfeld, J. (2005). Hiring and mentoring graduate nurses in intensive care units. *Dimensions of Critical Care Nursing, 24*(4), 175–178.

Kabat-Zinn, J. (1990). *Full catastrophe living.* New York: Delta.

Kelman, E., & Straker, K. (2000). *Study without stress.* Thousand Oaks, CA: Sage Publishing.

Kramer, M. (1974). *Reality shock.* St. Louis: Mosby.

Kramer, M., & Schmalenberg, C. (1977). *Path to biculturalism.* Wakefield, MA: Contemporary Publishing.

Luciani, J. (2004). *The power of self-coaching: The five essential steps to creating the life you want.* Hoboken, NJ: John Wiley & Sons.

Miller, T. (2003). *Building and managing a career in nursing.* New York: Nurse Week Publishing.

Niles, S.G., & Harris-Bowlsbey, J. (2002) *Career development interventions in the 21st century.* Columbus, OH: Merrill–Prentice Hall.

Rosenfeld, P., et al. Nurse residency program: A five-year evaluation from the participants' perspective. *Journal of Nursing Administration, 34*(4), 188–194.

Wylie, R. (1979). *The self concept: Theory and research on selected topics.* (Rev. ed.). Lincoln, NE: University of Nebraska Press.

Getting Your First Job

SHARON WALKER, MA

SHARON BATOR, MSN, RN, ABD

JACQUELINE J. HILL, PHD, RN, CRRN

CHAPTER MOTIVATION

"Very few people ever make it alone. We all need someone to lead the way, to show us the ropes, to tell us the norms, to encourage, support, and make it a little easier for us."

N. Josefowitz, 1980, p. 93.

CHAPTER MOTIVES

- Use an organized process for developing your résumé, succeeding at interviewing, and finding your first job in nursing.

- Capitalize on your critical thinking, "soft" skills (caring), and technological savvy as a basis for your résumé, interview, and correspondence processing.

- Use networking opportunities to facilitate obtaining your first job in nursing.

- Avoid procrastination, a major barrier to a successful career path.

- Understand how the Hallmarks of the Professional Nursing Practice Environment, the Core Competencies for Health Professionals, and the Pew Foundation's Twenty-One Competencies for the 21st Century provide guidance to your career journey.

The purpose of this chapter is to show you how to approach getting your first job in nursing by creating a résumé and interviewing successfully. The uninformed view of landing your first job is that it is something you should be able to do naturally; however, this is not always the case. In some situations, career development requires the guidance of someone who is experienced in that area, such as a career planning specialist. In this chapter, you will be given the essential guidelines to assist you in securing the best job for you. Upon obtaining employment as a registered nurse, you alone will have to take the responsibility for understanding how the Hallmarks of the Professional Nursing Practice Environment and Core Competencies for Health Professionals undergird the integrity of your choice of where to work. Using the exercises and suggestions integrated throughout the chapter, you will be able to write your résumé with scrupulous accuracy. Additionally, you will be prepared to interview as appealingly as possible by being able to articulate your nursing skills, related experiences, and potential as a new graduate. Hiring a novice registered nurse (RN) is appealing to employers because they have the opportunity to more easily integrate you as a member of their institution, training you in its values and mission. In order to select your first job successfully, you will need to strike a balance between selling yourself and carefully scrutinizing the intricacies of the professional environment where you believe you would like to work.

Getting Your First Job

Getting that first job as an RN can be both exciting and scary. It is exciting finally to get an opportunity to work as an RN. You have worked hard to complete nursing school and pass the NCLEX-RN examination, and you will now get to reap some of the benefits of being a nurse. The scary aspect of transitioning from student to RN is that you are on your own; your professors will not be there to guide you anymore. It is at this juncture that having a mentor is important (Box 23-1).

SELECTING A WORK ENVIRONMENT

With a serious nursing shortage projected far into the 21st century, you will face challenges to main-

---

Box 23-1

Mentors

A mentor is an experienced person who can "show you the ropes" of the profession. Specifically, a mentor is "a person who oversees the career and development of another person, usually a junior, through teaching, counseling, providing psychological support, protecting, and at times promoting or sponsoring" (Zey, 1984, p. 7). Some of the attributes that mentees look for in a mentor are experience, personality, reputation, and common interests (Hill, 2004). The benefits noted by mentees from being in a mentoring relationship include self-confidence, self-awareness, and enhanced productivity (Hill, 2004). One of the outcomes of mentoring can be summed up in the following quote by a nurse leader: "I learned to believe in myself. My confidence grew and once realizing I had abilities, I was able to recognize where I could go with them. My mentor made me feel more comfortable and competent in my skills and knowledge. I knew I had something to offer and subsequently I could not be as easily intimidated when the challenges came and they did come" (Hill, 2004, p. 79).

---

tain the integrity of your practice (Billings & Halstead, 2005; Catalano, 2003). For now, however, new graduates will reap the benefits of the law of supply and demand. Accordingly, better salaries will emerge as well as the availability of health benefits and educational and career ladder opportunities. For this reason, prospecting for your first job in nursing will offer many possibilities. It is up to you to align your job options with your personal and professional strengths (Catalano, 2003; Nunnery, 2005). The downside of the supply and demand principle regarding the nursing shortage is that poor staffing ratios may emerge, which risks your own health as well as that of your patients (Nunnery, 2005). It is therefore very important to search for your job with care and to analyze your potential working environment. The environment "greatly affects how the nurse can meet the role obligations" (Catalano, 2003, p. 209).

The American Association of Colleges of Nursing (AACN) provides direction in the selection of a working environment that fosters growth as an RN and better outcomes for the patients. The AACN has published information online that can provide guidance to "What Every Nursing School Graduate Should Consider When Seeking Employment." This AACN literature outlines Hallmarks of the Professional Nursing Practice Setting, which you can access through www.aacn.nche.edu for more details.

More specifically, AACN has identified key characteristics to look for in a potential employer and suggested interview questions of the future employer you are researching. There are eight key characteristics with action suggestions that are briefly summarized as follows:

1. Manifest a philosophy of clinical care emphasizing quality, safety, interdisciplinary collaboration, continuity of care, and professional accountability. (Check the published mission statement to confirm that nurses have input; check nurse/patient ratios; and confirm an organization's commitment to its published philosophy.)

2. Recognize the value of nurses' expertise on clinical care quality and patient outcomes. (Are nurses working in areas that fit their expertise?)

3. Promote executive-level nursing leadership. (Are nurses represented in governance? Does the top nurse executive have an appropriate position and influence?)

4. Empower nurses' participation in clinical decision making and organization of clinical care systems. (Do nurses control decisions related to nursing practice and care delivery? Staffing? Quality control?)

5. Demonstrate professional development support for nurses. (What resources are made available? Mentors? Internships? Educational assistance?)

6. Maintain clinical advancement programs based on education, certification, and advanced preparation. (What rewards are available for professional and educational development?)

7. Create collaborative relationships among members of the health-care team. (Are there interdisciplinary leadership, quality, peer review, and patient care models?)

8. Utilize technological advances in clinical care and information systems. (Do nurses have electronic access to clinical and health-care research results? Is there an integrated information system?)

AACN also suggests other statistics and information to request from a potential employer, such as, "RN vacancy rate and RN turnover rate, patient satisfaction scores, employee satisfaction scores, average tenure of nursing staff, education mix of nursing staff, percentage of registry/travelers used, key human resource policies, copy of the most recent JCAHO report, whether nurses are unionized, and a copy of a contract" (p. 18). AACN also illuminates the advantage of a health-care facility having **magnet status**. Knowledge of this information can help you choose a job where your health as well as the health of your patients has greater potential for a positive outcome.

The Institute of Medicine (IOM) also indirectly reinforces the importance of acquiring these statistics when it writes about risk factors for patient safety in the nursing work environment. The risk factors germane to AACN's suggested statistics and other information are "high staff turnover, long working hours, rapid increase in new knowledge and technology, and increased interruptions and demands in nurse's time" (Page, 2004, pp. 37–40). Having such high risks threatens patient care and increases the potential for legal interventions. From both legal and ethical perspectives, the choice of where you work deeply affects your health, the patients, and the community in which you decide to provide nursing care.

In conjunction with understanding the choice of the environment you choose to work in, you also need to understand the expectations of all health-care professionals that were outlined by the Institute of Medicine (IOM, 2003). These expectations provide insight into attributes that you want to develop as a new RN and that employers will want to foster in order to provide the best possible collaboration with other health-care professionals in the delivery of patient care. These attributes are fostered in the type of work environment outlined by IOM and are as follows:

- Individual clinical competence
- Mutual trust and respect
- Shared understanding of goals and roles
- Effective communication
- Shared decision making
- Conflict management (Nunnery, 2005)

Your relationships with the multidisciplinary health-care teams of which you are a part will be successful and rewarding as you continue to take responsibility for developing these attributes over time.

Finally, concomitant with AACN's position on selecting the right work environment to develop

Box 23-2

Pew Foundation's Twenty-One Competencies for the 21st Century

1. Embrace a personal ethic of social responsibility and service.
2. Exhibit ethical behavior in all professional activities.
3. Provide evidence-based clinically competent care.
4. Incorporate the multiple determinants of health in clinical care.
5. Apply knowledge of the new sciences.
6. Demonstrate critical thinking, reflection, and problem-solving skills.
7. Understand the role of primary care.
8. Rigorously practice preventive health care.
9. Integrate population-based care and services into practice.
10. Improve access to health care for those with unmet health needs.
11. Practice relationship-centered care with individuals and families.
12. Provide culturally sensitive care to a diverse society.
13. Partner with communities in health-care decisions.
14. Use communication and information technology effectively and appropriately.
15. Work in interdisciplinary teams.
16. Ensure care that balances individual, professional, system, and societal needs.
17. Practice leadership.
18. Take responsibility for quality of care and health outcomes at all levels.
19. Contribute to continuous improvement of the health-care system.
20. Advocate for public policy that promotes and protects the health of the public.
21. Continue to learn and help others learn (Nunnery, p. 509)

IOM's professional attributes for all health-care workers is the Pew Foundation's Twenty-One Competencies for the 21st Century (Box 23-2).

These competencies reflect the reality that "pursuing a career involves life-long learning" (Tappen, 2001, p. 138). Your first job selection is just the beginning of a portfolio of experiences and ongoing education you will need to develop and integrate into your résumé as you go from being a "novice to an expert" (Benner, 1984). As you develop your résumé over time in your career, look toward polishing these 21 competencies through formal and informal educational opportunities. First, you need to understand the nuts and bolts of prospecting for a job (Box 23-3).

Practice What You Preach and Teach: Use an Organized Process for Job Prospecting

Most nurses are excellent at applying standard protocols to provide patient-centered care but often seem "unable to do the same for themselves" (Catalano, 2003, pp. 220–221). In light of Catalano's criticism, the résumé, interview, and hiring aspects of this chapter are described using an organized process. In this case, the specific purpose is finding a first job in nursing that is truly a healthy fit between you and the organization to which you are applying.

STEP I: SELF-APPRAISAL

Self-appraisal is the first step of the organizing process. It incorporates an evaluation of one's goals and prospects. In the case of landing your first job, it involves creating an objective to maximize your career satisfaction and foster your own health. This means you are assessing what is best for you in light of your own strengths and limitations as well as

Box 23-3

Using the Internet to Search for a Job

On a practical level, landing your first job can be facilitated by having Internet savvy. Using an Internet search engine and inputting "RN" or "Nurse" as the search criterion, you will have access to 300,000 sites and online job application features for suitable positions. You can also list a university site with an associated health science center and enter into the postings of nursing positions at that center.

Here is a list of popular Internet sites for nursing positions:
www.nursingjobs.com
www.allnurses.com
www.greatnurse.com
www.hoovers.com
www.hospitalsoup.com
www.idealist.org
www.miracleworkers.com
www.monster.com
www.nursejobs.com
www.nursing jobs.org
www.careers.yahoo.com
www.degreehunter.com

future patients and future team members with whom you will work. Throughout your student career and now as you work toward landing your first job, you will have worked with a **career planning specialist** who can help you with this self-appraisal. The appraisal phase always takes the longest; if not done properly, the remaining steps will not be on target. For example, a new graduate may want to work in a coronary intensive care unit, but in looking at her strengths she discovers some physical limitations that would preclude the hectic physical pace of such a unit.

STEP II: DISCERNMENT

Discern and deal with potential issues that might arise in your job-prospecting process. For example, literature suggests that there are generational issues and generational expectations of potential employees. Generation X expects to be able to have a balanced work schedule so that family and personal time are not lost. Hiring agencies that expect new employees from Generation X to work 12–20 hours per week of overtime will have a problem with covering the unit when there is short (inadequate) staffing (Greene, 2005).

STEP III: CREATE A PLAN

Planning involves the creation of the sequence of actions that will lead to the desired outcome. The job seeker's plan must include the creation of a cogent and compelling résumé of his/her skills and experience. Box 23-4 outlines how to write a résumé, and Box 23-5 is a sample résumé. Subsequent planning must include the determination of recipient organizations or persons and how to obtain the attention and approval of hiring decision makers.

Résumé Writing

As you actually begin to write your **résumé** and prepare for an interview, you need to ask yourself the following questions:

- What am I prepared to do?
- What do I really want to do?
- What type of positions are available? (Tappen, 2001, p. 492)

A résumé is a "reflection of your professional persona" (Prasad, 2004, p. 57). Your résumé needs to show your current state of knowledge and

chapter star

Clara Adams-Ender retired from the Army as a Brigadier General. She started out as a staff nurse and eventually became chief executive officer of 22,000 nurses. One of the very first nurses to attain that rank, she ascribes her success to doing the best job possible in positions with visibility. Along with her skills and work ethic, she also took time to build relationships with **mentors** and colleagues who could give advice on how to manage her career.

One of 10 children in a black sharecropper family, she credits her parents' work ethic, moral training, and high expectations for much of her success. She is a dynamic leader who has 10 honorary doctoral degrees in law, public service, humane letters, and science. She models through her career accomplishments the path that new graduates need to follow in landing their first job and continuing on through decades of professional nursing.

Adams-Ender cultivated mentor relationships, clearly communicated her professional goals, and always earned her next job with an enthusiastic and excellent performance in the one that preceded it. Her moral principles, personal integrity, expertise, future planning, and mentoring are qualities that undergird an outstanding résumé and successful career over time. Her aphorisms are helpful to the new graduate nurse in landing a first job and building one's career over time. "Clara's Aphorisms" are as follows (Adams-Ender, p. 243):

1. Whatever you do, do it with enthusiasm.
2. In all relationships with people, relate to them so that they will speak kindly of you, especially when you are not present.
3. There is only one thing in life over which you have total control, and that is your attitude.
4. Always encourage others, especially youngsters.
5. Taking action will cure most fears.
6. Keep your body tuned.
7. Only to the extent that you love yourself can you ever love another person.
8. Possess high expectations of yourself. After all, it is what you expect of you that really counts.
9. You have choices in all situations—whether you like them or not.
10. To not decide is also to make a decision.
11. Giving service makes you feel better about yourself that you made a difference in someone's life.
12. It is not what happens to you in life that is important—it's how you react to what happens to you.
13. A good sense of humor will help you over many rough spots.
14. Take your work seriously, but never take yourself too seriously.
15. Above all else, be kind.

www.claracares.com

BOX 23-4

Tips for Résumé Writing

- Résumés should be one page long, unless you have extensive experience in the position for which you are applying
- Light blue, ivory, white, or beige paper (if you mail your résumé, the envelope must be same color)
- Use Times Roman or similar font; no fancy fonts; do not use underline or italics because they do not scan correctly
- Margins should be 1 inch top, bottom, and sides
- Use 12-point font if possible, no smaller than 10-point font
- Do not use pronouns

Name and Address Section: May be centered on page or split on each margin; name should be in a slightly larger font than the rest of résumé; name should be **bold**; list phone number where you can be reached: list home and/or cell number and make sure you have an answering machine or message capability so a message can be left for you (ensure that greeting on answering machine is appropriate for a potential employer to hear); use e-mail address, and check it several times a day.

Objective: Be very **specific,** even if you have to list more than one job title; if not specific, omit this section.

Education: List college, city, and state (not street address), years attended
- List graduation date or anticipated graduation date
- List degree, major, or program
- Give your grade point average (GPA) (if your overall GPA is not good, give your GPA in your major if it is better; e.g., Nursing GPA 3.5)
- Once you have graduated, you can list your degree first, then the school and date
- If you have graduated from a college or university, you do not need to list your high school

Relevant Skills and Experience or Accomplishments: Use bullet format for clinical rotations, volunteer experiences, accomplishments at other jobs if relevant, computer skills

Job History:
- List jobs **starting with the most recent**, and work back from there
- List name of company, city, state (not street address), years you worked (not months)
- Give your job title
- Use bullets to state your accomplishments
- Begin each bullet statement with an **ACTION VERB;** use present tense for current job only, past tense for all previous jobs
- Do not use "responsible for" or "duties include"; list accomplishments in each job
- If you have had jobs in the health-care field or experience relevant to the job you are now seeking, give it more space on your résumé; jobs that are unrelated to what you are seeking can be given minimal space

Professional Affiliations and Honors:
- List any organizations as a student and/or other jobs you have had; honors; honor societies
- **Do not** put References Available on Request at the bottom of the résumé
- References are always listed on a separate page that you can take with you to an interview
- **Do not** list personal information (age, marital status, height, weight, etc.)
- Debated issue: hobbies (some experts say this is not appropriate; some say it humanizes the candidate)

Proofread! Proofread! and Proofread Again!

Have someone else proofread your résumé. Do not rely on computer software.

---

expertise so that employers can hire the best nurse who can help their patients achieve the best possible outcomes for patient health in mind, body, and spirit. Résumés reflect professional achievements and abilities and minimize weaknesses.

As you work on your résumé, you may see references about a "curriculum vitae" (CV). The CV is a form of résumé, mostly used in educational environments for teaching and administrative level positions. Like a résumé, it summarizes educational, professional, and scholarly experience. Therefore, keep a journal of all that you do as you build your repertoire of career experiences so that you can be a

successful candidate for any job for which you decide to apply in the future.

Note that the human resources person may devote only 15–30 seconds to looking at your résumé on the first pass, so it is important that it be error-free and have the appropriate "buzz" words that identify your résumé as one that merits further scrutiny (Kelly-Heidenthal, 2003). Employers want graduates who can function "independently, require little retraining or orientation, and can supervise a variety of less educated and unlicensed employees" (Catalano, 2003, p. 210). They look for *preceptorships* and *internships* in the heart of the résumé that

Box 23-5

Sample Résumé

NAME (ALL CAPS, BOLD)

Street Address

City, State, Zip

Phone Number

e-mail address

Objective: To obtain a position as a Registered Nurse

Education

Caring College, Baton Rouge, LA, 2002–Present

Anticipated date of graduation: May 2007

Nursing Program GPA: 3.8

List other colleges or universities you have attended, years attended, major while there

Relevant Skills and Experience

- List clinical rotations you have had and/or related courses
- List experience you have had as a volunteer
- List specific experience you have had in a job that pertains to the one you are applying for or that demonstrates desirable qualities (teamwork, organizational skills, communication skills, attention to details, etc)
- Computer skills

Job History

Best Hospital, Baton Rouge, LA, 2003–Present

Volunteer

- Assist patients in filling out paperwork and locating physicians' offices
- Document arrival and departure times of patients
- Provide directions and instructions

XYZ Hospital, Baton Rouge, LA, 2001–2003

Nursing Assistant

- Scheduled appointments for four physicians
- Accompanied patients to rooms and took vital signs
- Assisted patients with meals

ABC Clinic, Baton Rouge, LA, 1999–2000

Office Assistant

- Directed patients to appropriate physician's office
- Received co-pays and other payments
- Answered questions from patients regarding insurance

Professional Affiliations and Honors

Student Nursing Association

Student Government Association

Dean's List 2002-2005

---

give clues to having a more independent new graduate (Dunham & Smith, 2005). Important words that reflect the independent abilities that employers are looking for on the résumé are referred to as **buzzwords.** For those individuals who are using an online computer program, there are **informatic words** programmed into a computer that will pull out your résumé over others if it has the proper words. Box 23-6 lists the common buzzwords needed for a human resources person to select your résumé from among many. It also lists the common "informatic" words that would cause a computer program to select your résumé and arrange for human resources to have an interview with you.

STEP IV: ACTIONS TO CARRY OUT THE PLAN

After creating the plan—the résumé and where to send it—it is time to put the plan into action. Putting the plan into action entails sending out a cover letter with each résumé to the selected targets, gaining an interview, and carrying out strategies for an effective interview.

Cover Letter

Cover letters are very important. They reveal:

- How well you communicate
- What your experience and qualifications are in brief
- Your level of professionalism
- Clues to your personality
- How detail-oriented you are (i.e., are there typos or other errors?)

Box 23-7 summarizes qualities of effective cover letters; Box 23-8 is an example of a cover letter.

Interview Preparation

The key to a successful interview is preparation. Have you researched the company where you are

Practice to Strive For 23-1

Your résumé is both a subjective and objective self-portrait that reflects a professional and empowered attitude. The purpose of the résumé is to get you the right job at the right time in the right place on the right team at the right salary. Résumés can be written in a **chronological** *or* **functional** *format. The chronological résumé lists information in order, beginning with the most recent, whereas the functional résumé focuses on the strengths that align best with the position being sought. The following are some of the major do's and don't's to consider when preparing your résumé:*

DO:

- *Remember that your résumé is your first introduction to a prospective employer, so be careful in how you present yourself*
- *"Know thyself" so that you can communicate your value to a prospective employer*
- *Work as hard at getting the right job as you did getting into school*
- *Write as though the job market is tight even if it isn't*
- *Have a plan where you want to be now and in 4 to 5 years (your next job target)*
- *Consult a career planning specialist or online source to assist with résumé writing*
- *Limit cover letters to one page*
- *Type cover letter and résumé on visually appealing cotton paper*
- *Write a concise, interesting, and error-free résumé that is truly worthy of you*
- *Get someone to proofread your résumé several times before mailing it*
- *Send your résumé with a cover letter addressed to a specific person, showing knowledge of the company*
- *Remember: 80% of positions are gained through networking*
- *Remember to write a thank-you note within 48 hours after an interview*

DON'T:

- *Use white copy paper (less appealing)*
- *Procrastinate*
- *Exaggerate or fabricate; be honest*

Box 23-6

Action Words and Phrases for Health-Care Résumés and Cover Letters

Assessed
Diagnosed
Directed
Educated
Prepared treatment plans
Provided follow-up care
Implemented
Quality assurance
Safe environment
Compliance
Managed
Variety
Teamwork
Self-motivated
Time management
Organizational skills
Accuracy
Flexibility
Professionalism
Dedicated
Detail-oriented
Volunteerism
Insertion and maintenance of invasive lines
Committed to quality patient care
Compassion
Ensuring continuity of patient care
Absolutely reliable and punctual
Total patient care
Determined needs of patients
Initiated beneficial changes
Established nursing care plans
Developed comprehensive patient histories
Maintained strict confidentiality in compliance with all
    federal, state, and institutional policies
Proactive approach to patient care
Fulfilled basic patient assistance
Coordinated patient care
Ordered laboratory studies
Ordered referrals
Contacted insurance companies
Liaison between provider and patient
Performed direct patient care
Presented in-services
Planned, organized, and managed nursing care
Carried out detailed assessments
Taught proper high-tech care to patients and families
Communicated findings to physicians and other health
    professionals
Gave case presentations
Participated in treatment planning and family conferences

interviewing? Do you know the approximate industry standard salary for the position you are seeking? Have you written out answers to the typical, most frequently asked interview questions? Have you practiced answering questions with family, friends,

Box 23-7

Qualities of an Effective Cover Letter

- Brief, neat, without errors
- In business format
- Name and title of person to whom the letter is addressed
- Why interested and what position would like to apply for
- Appointed time for taking NCLEX-RN
- Express appreciation for consideration and eagerness to be part of team
- How can be reached (telephone number)
- Use 9- by 12-inch envelope to send résumé and cover letter (first-class mail)
- Expect response to letter in 2 weeks
- If not, call after 3 weeks; check with Human Resources

Box 23-8

Example of an Effective Cover Letter

May 1, 2006

Elizabeth B. Wise, PhD, RN

Director of Nurse Recruitment and Hiring

Caring Hospital USA

Joy City, LA 70777

RE: Nursing Position on Medical-Surgical Unit

Dear Dr. Wise:

I have just graduated from Caring College and would like to apply for a new graduate nurse position on Medical-Surgical Unit II at Caring Hospital. I served there as a nurse technician while going through nursing school. I will take the NCLEX-RN exam on June 7, 2005, and will be available to start work by June 21, 2005.

Having worked as a nurse technician on Medical-Surgical Unit II for 3 years, I developed positive interpersonal and professional relationships with the team. Furthermore, I am well organized, have effective time-management skills, and am enthusiastic about the prospect of returning to the unit. I am proud to have worked at Caring Hospital for 3 years in light of its high rating and Magnet status. The mission of Caring Hospital is congruent with my values.

Thank you very much for your consideration. You may reach me any time on my cell phone at (999) 709-2525. I look forward to hearing from you to schedule an interview at your convenience.

Sincerely,

Scelitta Source

or professionals? Do you have the appropriate clothes to go on a moment's notice? These are steps you should be taking in preparation for your job interview. See Boxes 23-9 through 23-12 for further interview preparation.

What are employers looking for in an interview? Of course, they are looking for the basic educational requirements for an entry-level nurse. After that requirement, what are they seeking? Many human resources managers have found that employers are looking for nurses who exhibit excitement and enthusiasm and who are a "good fit" with the people who are already working there. When the Divisional Director of People Services at a large regional medical center was recently asked, "What do you look for in an interview to convince you to hire that person?" she was quoted as saying "Are you a job fit? 'Fit' means do you have the qualifications, and do you have the attitude? We hire for attitude and train for skills. If you do it the other way, you're usually not that successful. You can train someone what to do, but you can't usually train 'attitude' " (personal communication, Lulu Ford, Our Lady of the Lake Regional Medical Center, 2005).

The interview process begins when you are called to schedule your interview. Keep your schedule handy, and speak professionally. Ask where the interview will be conducted—the address and directions if you are not familiar with the facility—and who you will be interviewing with. Write this information down, and take it with you. Research the institution. Go online, conduct a search, and read all available information.

It is always helpful to anticipate possible interview questions. Categories of potential questions include:

1. Self-assessment
2. Career goals
3. General information
4. Behavioral
5. Professional

While going through the interview, you also may have questions you want to ask. It is helpful to have these questions written down ahead of time so that you do not forget or get distracted from what you want to know. Do not ask about salary or benefits unless the interviewer initiates this conversation; the best time to discuss these issues is after you have been offered the job. Review the questions in Box 23-12.

Box 23-9

Essentials to Know for Interview Preparation

What to Take to the Interview

- A simple portfolio or a new, clean, file folder
- Pen/pencil and paper to make brief notes if necessary
- Extra copies of your résumé
- Your reference sheet
- List of questions you want to ask
- Copy of your license, certifications, and any special training you have had

What to Wear to the Interview

- Dress in business or business-casual attire; suit, nice dress, or pants suit and appropriate hose and shoes in good condition; no jeans, tight clothes, or low-cut blouses (see Box 23-10)
- Clean hair, nails, and clothes; simple jewelry; no excess rings, dangling earrings; only ear piercings noticeable
- Avoid perfume or cologne—many medical institutions are fragrance-free

Manners

- Be courteous and friendly to all personnel you encounter—parking attendant, information desk personnel, secretaries
- Arrive about 10 minutes early; do not be late

First Impressions With Interview

- First impressions are lasting and occur in the first 20–30 seconds
- Walk in confidently; introduce yourself if necessary, give the interviewer a firm handshake, make direct eye contact, acknowledge other people in the room
- Do not be surprised if there is more than one person present to interview you; often there will be a human resources staff member and possibly the immediate supervisor and/or department manager
- Smile and try to relax; smiling will relax you as well as the interviewer

After the Interview

- Thank everyone present for the interview
- Offer your reference sheet
- Ask when a decision is expected
- Ask the next step in the interview process
- When you get home, immediately write a short thank-you note/letter to everyone who interviewed you
- If you have not heard from them by the time they indicated a decision would be made, call and talk to the person who interviewed you and ask the status of the position

Box 23-10

Appropriate Dress

This person is dressed appropriately for a job interview. She is wearing a conservative suit, minimal and tasteful jewelry, and she projects a confident and professional appearance. Her smile shows a relaxed, comfortable demeanor that would put others at ease (Fig. 23-1).

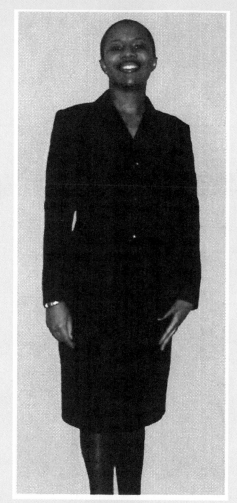

FIGURE 23-1 Photo of woman dressed for an interview.

STEP V: FOLLOW UP

After the interview, the candidate must determine whether the goals/outcomes were met and, if not, what follow-up needs to be done. Box 23-13 offers questions you may want to ask once you are offered the job.

Box 23-11

Possible Self-Assessment Interview Questions

Self-Assessment Questions

1. Tell me about yourself.
2. Briefly summarize your educational and work history for me.
3. What clinical rotations did you have in your nursing program?
4. Which clinical rotation did you like the least? Why?
5. What do you think are the most important characteristics and abilities a person must have to be a successful nurse?
6. What do you consider your greatest strength?
7. What do you consider your greatest weakness?
8. What personal characteristics are your greatest assets?
9. What personal characteristics cause you the most difficulty?
10. Give me three adjectives you think describe you.
11. What types of situations frustrate you the most? How do you usually cope with them?
12. Tell me about a time when you had difficulty with a supervisor or coworker and how you resolved the conflict.
13. Why do you want to be a nurse?
14. How do you work under pressure? Give me an example.
15. Is there any reason why you might not be able to work as regularly scheduled?
16. Tell me about a time when you had to adapt to a new situation.
17. What makes you the best person for this job, and why should we hire you?

Career Goals Questions

1. What are your career goals?
2. Where do you see yourself 5 years from now?
3. How does this job fit in with your overall career goals?
4. What can you offer this company/organization?
5. What would you most like to accomplish if you had this job? What future educational endeavors do you plan?

General Questions

1. What criteria are you using to evaluate this job?
2. What is most important to you in this job?
3. What are your expectations regarding promotions and salary increases?
4. Nursing can be a very stressful job. What do you do to relieve your stress outside the job?
5. What do you know about our organization? Do you have any questions?

Behavioral Questions

1. Tell me about a time in which you had to handle an irate physician or patient/family member. How did you handle the individual, and what were the results? What would you do differently next time?
2. What has been the most difficult decision you have ever had to make? Are you satisfied with the outcome?
3. Have you ever been asked to do something that was unethical, illegal, or against your own personal belief or integrity standards? What did you do? If not, what would you do in such a case?
4. Tell me about a situation in which you disagreed with instructions given to you by a physician, supervisor, or instructor. What did you do?

Professional Questions

1. What nursing organizations do you belong to?
2. What journals do you read?
3. How do you plan to stay current in your profession?
4. What continuing education areas are of interest to you?

Box 23-12

Possible Questions You May Want To Ask

1. What unit will I be placed in?
2. Who will be my immediate supervisor?
3. What is the nurse-patient ratio in that unit?
4. What kind of orientation is available? How long is orientation?
5. What are the goals of the unit?
6. What is the length of service of other nurses in this unit?
7. Can I have a tour of the unit in which I will be working?
8. Will I have a preceptor?
9. What is the turnover rate for nurses?

Box 23-13

Possible Questions to Ask When You Are Offered the Job

1. What is the salary?
2. What is the shift or hours I will work?
3. What are the benefits?
4. Is there any mandatory overtime?
5. Do you offer tuition reimbursement, loan repayment, or sign-on bonus?
6. When is orientation?
7. When and where do I report for work?

VI. RESTART THE PROCESS

Suppose you discover that you have chosen the wrong job, or you begin to feel that you are suffering "burnout." Suppose that the organization in which you have invested your career violates its promises. In nursing, as in any relationship, there is a predictable pattern. Usually, and ideally first, is the honeymoon phase when you are accepted and your work is enthusiastic and productive. Then comes the period where only experience can give you skills, and you are working the extra hours, sometimes the long shifts, and enjoying a sense of success. As in a long marriage, you evolve into the maintenance period. This is often the most difficult time as there are not a lot of new, exciting developments. It is up to you to build on educational opportunities, maintain good personal health, and make the maintenance phase more productive. Then one day, you may begin to feel that you have overstayed your welcome and exhausted the learning opportunities at that workplace. Then it is time to leave. It is actually better to leave and find a new job before feeling burnout and to be at the top of the cycle of your energy, positive patient outcomes, and interdisciplinary collaborative relationships. When you leave, there are happy memories for both you and the employers. Move on. Creating your career is an ongoing process during which it may be healthy to seek a change of scene (Sullivan, 2004).

All Good Things...

You have done a great deal of work to get to this point. You are ready to enter the job market to start a career in nursing. Applying some of the talents that have helped you up to this time should ease the transition from school into a new position.

Gather trusted advisors to help you form a career plan. Then try to target a position that will move you in the right direction toward that plan's attainment. Having a mentor during the job-seeking process can be as helpful as having one after landing the job.

Prepare a résumé that accurately represents your achievements, talents, and potential, and then work hard to present yourself well in the interview process. After getting the job, do the best you can to make your colleagues, your department, and your entire organization a success.

Finally, as your career progresses, remember to re-evaluate your goals, your plans for their achievement, and take action to realign when necessary. Remember that you are entering nursing in the 21st century when there is an actual nursing shortage that will continue for decades. Use AACN's Hallmarks of the Professional Nursing Environment to help guide you into selecting the best position for you.

Let's Talk

1. *What are your priorities regarding your career?*

2. *What do you believe is most important to accomplish immediately upon completing nursing school?*

3. *As a new graduate, who or what do you consider to be your greatest resource as you start your journey into the workforce?*

4. *How important is it to gain technical skills that become second nature on your first job?*

5. *What professional organizations would be most helpful for you to join and where perhaps you could meet a mentor?*

6. *What are your beliefs about returning to school for an advanced degree? Do you believe it is necessary?*

NCLEX Questions

1. The chronological résumé includes:
   A. Education section
   B. Listing of jobs starting with most recent job
   C. Objective statement
   D. All of the above

2. A functional résumé is:
   A. Used only in the nursing profession
   B. Used when you want to emphasize skills and abilities
   C. Used when you are changing careers
   D. B and C

3. A career planning specialist can help you:
   A. Determine the jobs for which you are a good fit
   B. Develop a winning résumé
   C. Prepare for an interview
   D. All of the above

4. You need a two-page resume when:
   A. You have extensive experience in the job for which you are applying
   B. You have had more than four jobs
   C. You are older than 40 years
   D. You have a master's degree or above

5. Each bullet statement in your résumé should begin with:
   A. The pronoun "I"
   B. An action verb
   C. The words "responsible for"
   D. None of the above

6. The key to a successful interview is:
   A. Who you know
   B. Preparation
   C. Wearing a black suit
   D. A cordial relationship between you and the interviewer

7. Your references should:
   A. Be included on your résumé
   B. Call the employer before the interview
   C. Be listed on a separate page
   D. Be provided only if you are asked

8. You should take the following to an interview:
   A. Extra copies of your résumé
   B. A list of questions to ask the interviewer
   C. Pen and paper to take notes
   D. All of the above

9. You prepare for an interview by:
   A. Researching the company
   B. Knowing industry standard salary for the position
   C. Writing out and practicing answers to typical interview questions
   D. All of the above

10. According to experts, what percentage of jobs are gained through networking?
    A. 50%
    B. 80%
    C. 10%
    D. 100%

REFERENCES

Adams-Ender, C. (2001). *My rise to the stars.* Lake Ridge, VA: CAPE Associates.

American Association of Colleges of Nursing (AACN) (2002). *Hallmarks of the professional nursing practice environment.* Washington, DC: Author. http://www.aacn.nche. edu/Publications/positions/cerreg.htm.

Benner, P. (1984). *From novice to expert: Excellence and power in clinical nursing practice.* Menlo Park, CA: Addison Wesley.

Billings, D.M., & Halstead, J. (2005). *Teaching in nursing: A guide for faculty.* St. Louis: Elsevier/Saunders.

Catalano, J.T. (2003). *Nursing now!* (3rd ed.). Philadelphia: F.A. Davis.

Dunham, K.S., & Smith, S.J. (2005). *How to survive and maybe even love your life as a nurse.* Philadelphia: F.A. Davis.

Greene, J. (2005). Different generations different expectations, *Hospitals & Health Networks Research, (3)*34–42.

Hill, J.J. (2004). *The role of mentoring in the development of African American nurse leaders.* Dissertation Abstracts International (UMI No. 3136177).

Institute of Medicine. (2003). Keeping patients safe: Transforming the work environment of nurses. http://www.ion.edu/report.asp? id = 16173.

Josefowitz, N. (1980). *Paths to top power: A working woman's guide from 1st job to top executive.* Reading, MA: Addison-Wesley.

Kelly-Heidenthal, P. (2003). *Nursing leadership & management.* Clifton Park, NY: Thomson/Delmar Learning.

Nunnery, R.K. (2005). *Advancing your career: Concepts of professional nursing.* Philadelphia: F.A. Davis.

Page, A. (2004). Keeping patients safe: Transforming the work of nurses. Washington, D.C.: National Academy Press.

PEW Health Professions Commission. (1995). *Critical challenges: Revitalizing the health professions for the 21st century.* San Fancisco: UCSF Center for the Health Professions.

Prasad, C. (2004). *Outwitting the job market.* Guilford, CT: The Lyons Press.

Sullivan, E.J. (2004). *Becoming influential: A guide for nurses.* NJ: Pearson/Prentice Hall.

Tappen, R.M. (2001). *Nursing leadership and management: Concepts and practice.* Philadelphia: F.A. Davis.

Zey, Michael G. (1984). *The mentor connection.* Homewood, IL: Dow Jones-Irvin.

Career Development

DENISE TOP RHINE, MED, RN, CEN
JUDY A. DAVIS, MS, MPH, APN, CNP

CHAPTER MOTIVATION

"There is no security on this earth, only opportunity."

Douglas MacArthur

CHAPTER MOTIVES

- Identify and differentiate among the three career models.
- Describe nursing as a profession and career.
- Identify key innovative opportunities: entrepreneurship and intrapreneurship.
- Differentiate between nurse intrapreneur and nurse entrepreneur.
- Identify the career planning and development phases.
- Describe the dynamic environmental forces that promote nursing career growth.
- Describe qualities, roles, options, and benefits of the nurse intrapreneur and entrepreneur.
- Describe organization characteristics that support intrapreneurship.
- Define marketing, mentoring, and networking, and relate them to the roles of nurse intrapreneur and entrepreneur.

In nursing, even more so than in other fields, leaders will need to think creatively to conceive new ways of working in today's cyberworld. It is critical to recognize one's personal joys and to take advantage of (and to seek) opportunities as they develop during the course of your **career**. Developing a nursing career extends through a lifetime and is not limited to the institution in which you work; be in tune with opportunities that arise within a changing environment.

Opportunities emerge while one assesses future health-care needs. Equally important is for the nurse to be ready to take action when opportunity knocks by positioning herself educationally and experientially to meet health-care needs. Selecting **mentors**, seeking a supportive working environment, **networking** successfully, and positioning yourself strategically will require having people skills. Whether the goal is to become a valued member within the organization as an **intrapreneur** or to branch out as an **entrepreneur**, the nurse will need the skills to predict people's reactions and needs and the ability to interact with different populations and personalities. Thus begins the process of building or rejuvenating oneself, recognizing what gives joy, breaking away from old beliefs and assumptions, reassessing strengths, networking to open new doors, seeking mentors to learn new skills and, most important, taking a risk. Opportunities arise outside and inside the organizations and outside and within one's position. So tailoring or refining personal career goals requires the nurse to keep abreast of the world's economic and political forces while keeping attuned to the health-care organization.

This chapter focuses on nurses, from early career to later. The aim is to help guide nurses who desire to take charge of career development and shape their careers and themselves more intentionally within the dynamic world in which they live.

Building a Nursing Career: A Chance to Grow

Given today's health-care environment, what does an individual nurse do to continue in nursing, yet manage job frustrations and achieve satisfaction at the end of the day? Building a career of enduring depth, breadth, and growth is a lifelong process, not unlike growth in one's personal intellectual development. With the advent of advanced practice, higher education in nursing, and the economic necessity of full-time employment, most nurses have come to realize that nursing is a career and **profession**, not just a job. The evolution of your career should not be left to chance; when you do not plan a direction for job movement, the stage is set for stagnation and inertia. Haphazardly moving from one position to another based on intangibles and whims negates the ability to achieve career goals. Although nursing positions are still plentiful and the need for nurses promises to increase, today's nurse wants more than a paycheck. For too long, nursing placed importance on the *way* nurses worked and the tasks they completed, not on what they do to bring about successful patient outcomes. In reality, satisfaction with the employment environment, commitment to patient care needs, and enjoyment of pertinent activities and patient-nurse interactions are requisites for career enhancement and stability.

NURSING AS CAREER DEVELOPMENT

Nursing, as a profession and a career, is founded upon principles of science, arts, and the humanities (Chinn & Kramer, 1999). Its education and practice are accredited by the various nursing education organizations and accrediting bodies that ensure the quality and integrity of the profession and its educational curriculum (Bellack & O'Neil, 2000). Characteristics of a profession are described by the American Nurses Association (ANA, 1975, 1991) as attaining a common body of knowledge, practicing with agreed performance standards and a code of ethics, having an agreed certification procedure, having a representative professional organization, and having an external perception as a profession. Nursing's core value is centered on people and serving the good of society (Strader & Decker, 1999); these values are timeless, but the nature of the nursing practice evolves with the times and environment. ANA (1975) described nurses as having "specialized skills essential to the performance of a unique professional role" (p. 3). The specialized skills, unique to the professional, are sensitive and responsive to the dynamic environmental forces and to the future advancements (Williams-Evans & Carnegie, 2002). Hence, the profession of nursing melds its timeless core values with its ability to adapt to the needs of the dynamic environment.

Career development is a dynamic, growing, and continuous process requiring ongoing contemplation and planning. Not unlike a development of a life skill, it involves sets of steps or phases of development whereby there are markers to ensure achievement to its maximum potential. There are various permutations of the career developing or building process. It can be viewed from a perspective of mapping (Ellis & Hartley, 2005); mobility (Hall, 2002; Riverin-Simard, 2000); staging (Broscio, Paulick, & Scherer, 2005); patterns (Super, 1980); and styles (Coombs, 1987; Driver, 1979a; Gardner, 1992; Orr, 1991).

Current literature on career models has moved away from static views; whereas earlier career models, such as career mapping, helped to keep the vision of a career alive, this merely provided a snapshot of what direction to go in terms of career goals. It did not provide a road map that reflects changing environmental conditions, such as "detours ahead" or "alternate routes" to take "due to inclement conditions." Likewise, linear career mobility, which once had natural "up the ladder" promotions, does not reflect today's careers, which are more fluid and unstable.

Today's career development tends to be more fluid, dynamic, and sensitive to socioeconomic forces and requirements of family household needs. Therefore, careers reflect more complex trajectories and work patterns, typical of today's two-career family households (Hall, 2002). When it comes to career trajectory, it is more apt to appear jagged with erratic turns rather than linear. Brown and associates (cited in Hall, 2002) found in their interviews of career experts that an average person will change careers (not jobs) five to seven times within his or her lifetime. In nursing, although there does not seem to be such a dramatic exiting of the profession, there does appear to be greater "entrance and exit" mobility to parallel family needs and commitments (Gardner, 1992; McLees, 1988). Nurses have become more accustomed to tailoring their career mobility to their family stage and personal needs (Gardner, 1992; Hall, 2002; McLees, 1988; Moen, 1998). Nicholson (1996) noted that careers that do not follow a steady pattern of continuous service and regular and steady promotion are likely to be considered "imperfect," when in fact they can be a creative way of negotiating the potentially incongruent goals of a successful career and a successful family life. Typical of a two-career family with children, nurses may enter, exit, and reenter the job market multiple times within their career development, thus maintaining a fluid, flexible work schedule. Even later in their careers, as a prelude to retirement preparation, nurses are apt to reenter the job market, not solely for financial supplement but purportedly due to career identity and career satisfaction (Riverin-Simard, 2000) and personal and family needs (Gardner, 1992; Hall, 2002, McLees, 1988; Moen, 1998).

Berg (2004) noted that, after retiring, many nurses either remain in the workforce or later return to it and/or return to society what Erikson (1997) termed "generativity." Quietly advocating for patients/families as they provide care, retired nurses find a variety of job opportunities to fit their needs of retirement, financial situations, and interests. Part-time work is becoming increasingly common among retirees, with a third working part-time for "interest and enjoyment" (Roper, 2002). The flexible hours, no commitment to grown family, and unique jobs across country and abroad are opening up virtually all possibilities. Many retired nurses, viewing their personal values as integral to their professional values, find creative means to share this with the community. There are numerous stories about retired nurses, with a wealth of lifetime experience, who use their integrated knowledge and skills to volunteer and work part-time in various settings: teaching in classrooms and hospitals, being involved in ministries abroad, leading community groups, recruiting new nursing students, lobbying for political causes, and helping professional organizations. Some take leadership positions, volunteering for a local hospital board of trustees, fundraising for scholarships, working with inner city grassroot organizations. It is ironic that as nursing shortages worsen, the pool of Baby Boom retired nurses may become the "safety net" for our overworked profession.

Innovative Opportunities: Entrepreneurship and Intrapreneurship

Scientific and technological advances occur by quantum leaps. They are creating a complex landscape that futurists caution will be vastly different from our present or past. In terms of the health-care system, how the care will be delivered and what will be required of its providers and consumers will differ (Kressley, 1998; Porter-O'Grady, 2000; Porter-O'Grady & Wilson, 1999). The work of providing care will also be altered, especially for nurses (Porter-O'Grady, 2000). Neuhauser, Bender, and Stromberg (2000) described today's world and its pace of the employment environment as "a jump to warp speed." Organizations are predicted to coalesce more on short-term teams of experts to accomplish specific goals and to deliver results. This new consultative way of working requires work to be channeled expediently through technological communications, which paradoxically will result in a greater demand for relationship building (Neuhauser, Bender, & Stromberg, 2000). Also in an era that points to the national and global nursing shortage, organizational leaders will need to seek nurses to fulfill organization capacity. They will need to attract nurses who can build top-notch teams and who are clinically advanced, technologically smart, and relationship advanced.

Supply and demand shortages lead to demand-based pricing. More now than ever, the nursing shortage brings the highest priority to nursing leaders and educators to retain those experts in the profession and to attract the brightest and best into the field. This calls for leaders with innovative product/service ideas and an eclectic repertoire of people skills who can make, have, and address more critical decision making and conceptualized ideas. Equally important will be to attract nurses who are politically astute, have negotiating skills, are well-versed in the art of compromise, and are tuned into the values of a growing culturally diverse nation. These qualities are present in the people with entrepreneurial and intrapreneurial spirit. Motivated by opportunities and driven by increasing consumer power, the promise of genetic research (Human Genome Program, 2005) and new drug and medical advancement, global trade and investment in system technology, today's RNs work in an

Practice to Strive For 24-1

Amongst nursing academics today, various top-ranked institutions with entrepreneurial programs (Entrepreneur.com, 2005) are identified, with curricula ranging from limited to comprehensive courses designed for nursing entrepreneurship. One of the comprehensively designed entrepreneur curricula is the first-of-its-kind New Center for Nursing Entrepreneurship (NCNE, 2005). The NCNE of the University of Rochester advertises that it "melds the essence of nursing with inventive business concepts, opening doors to career opportunities and responding to the evolution of health care." NCNE has also created a listserv and coined the word "nurspreneur" designed for "conversation and dissemination of information relevant to intrapreneurship and entrepreneurship in nursing." As an outgrowth of its recent symposium, Nursing Intrapreneurship and Entrepreneurship: Education, Practice, and Research, the nurspreneur listserv was established, sponsored in tandem with the Kaufmann Foundation Campus Initiative. Also, the Center for Nursing Entrepreneurs was established as an academic-business "think tank." It was developed for "people who have business ideas, designed to give nurses the resources and skills to get started, offering a way to stay in nursing and continue to provide health care to consumers" (NCNE, 2005).

incredible environment to enrich their professional development and carve out their **niches** in professional practice.

Career Planning and Development: Phases

Career planning follows a carefully designed, step-by-step method, whereas career development is a repetitive, continuous, and evolving nonlinear process. Both begin with an assessment of where the nurse has been experientially as well as a look at the current work environment. Donner and Wheeler (2001) described these bidirectional influences of self and environment as a "life skill, one that nurses can apply in their workplace, and in their personal life" (p. 8). Relating it to a series of phases of self-assessment, the career development process integrates the knowledge of self with the existing environmental opportunities. Donner and Wheeler broke these two basic interactive forces into five phases, "scanning your environment, completing your self-assessment and reality, creating your career vision, developing your strategic career plan, and marketing yourself"(p. 9). These discrete and yet fluid processes can be expanded relative to the process of becoming an entrepreneur or intrapreneur. For example, it is important to build personal characteristics that promote the entrepreneurial mindset, take control of self-knowledge gained, become aware of the dynamic forces that may ultimately shape your career, integrate the knowledge of self with the existing environmental opportunities, and then to take the risk and take action. Finally, the nurse is ready to use **critical thinking** and **decision making** to build a strategic plan that includes self-marketing.

CAREER ASSESSMENT

Career assessment as a part of career development is key to finding career satisfaction while maintaining ethical integrity. Nurses need to take a SWOT (Strengths, Weaknesses, Opportunities, Threats) analysis of their job situations and their individual characteristics and values to ascertain if they are congruent or divergent. Why do they like their chosen areas of work? What are the strengths and weaknesses of their professional areas? When and where are there opportunities? What are the threats to success? Assessing your current status is the first step of planning a career. Remember the adage, "If one fails to plan, one plans to fail." Perhaps there is still a chance to maintain ties within the organization yet meet career goals. McGillis-Hall, et al. (2004) noted, "Nurses who are committed to the organization in which they work and have the skills and flexibility to link personal effectiveness and satisfaction with achievement of the organization's strategic objectives" (p. 232) may continue to prosper. Currently, viewing supply and demand economics of nurses willing to work within an institution, nurses can see that this can work in their favor. Contino (2001) noted, "Accepting that hospital revenues are somewhat fixed, nurses need to find ways to help hospitals control costs, increase profitable service lines, and meet staff's scheduling and income needs." (p. 21). To assess the career development process, you need to ask the following questions:

- What are the basic values in nursing?
- How do nurses merge these core values to address the environmental needs?

- What forms of nursing bring greatest satisfaction in meeting the needs of their patients and society?

Answering such questions can help the nurse determine whether it is possible to continue to work within the status quo or go in the direction of change. Two areas that many nurses identify as basic career needs are the ability to feel in control of their practice and to have flexibility in their work. Autonomy in decision making, as long as it is within the scope of the organization's policies and procedures, allows nurses the flexibility to individualize care, think critically, and set patient priorities according to established standards of practice. Comparing one's own practice standards with those observed in the work environment will supply vital data that the nurse can use to decide whether to continue to practice in that setting.

PERSISTENCE: PUSHING THE ENVELOPE

Bellack and O'Neil (2000) described nursing as being at its "crossroads" with a chance to grow and develop its own vision of its professional practice. As entrepreneurial "free agents," notable nursing leaders such as Florence Nightingale, Lillian Wald, and Mary Breckinridge all carved out their own missions beyond their immediate **callings** to help patients or address community needs. They took

chapter star

Mary Seacole, referred to as the "Black Nightingale," was a daughter of a well-respected "doctress" who practiced Creole medicine in Jamaica. Guided by her mother, Mary was repeatedly rejected (due to the social constraints of the times and the color of her skin) in her quest to join Florence Nightingale in aiding the soldiers during the Crimean war. After many rejections, she funded her own trip and established an innovative entrepreneurial way of responding to battle-fatigued and injured soldiers by opening a comfort and recovering center In a British hotel. Returning to England destitute and ill, the press came to her aid by publishing her plight; this resulted in a grand military festival to raise money for her efforts and led to her being decorated with some of the highest medals of honor: the Crimean Medal, the Legion of Honour, and a Turkish medal (Florence Nightingale Museum, 1997).

action to reach beyond their usual practice, to create nontraditional nursing roles, to publish, to use epidemiological methods to address populations at risk, to lobby for health-care reform, to raise philanthropic funds, and to bring awareness of the plight of the poor and their lack of access to health care. These quests all stemmed from personal values about which they felt passionate, and they all channeled their voices through their professional practice (Carper, 1978). These entrepreneurial spirits pushed their goals and stirred up the social, political, and policy status quo to bring new standards to health care and nursing practice (Bellack & O'Neil, 2000).

Not unlike our predecessors, today's cyberworld requires nurses to challenge their old beliefs and assumptions of the way the nursing profession is envisioned. It will require nurses to break loose from worn-out thinking and to dream of new ways of practicing the profession. Porter-O'Grady (2000) noted the difficulties of change; however, humans naturally prefer the familiar and resist change. The greatest challenge for nurses will be to leave the familiar industrial era model of task-oriented nursing care, which served organizations well but left nurse/patient interactions to suffer.

Roy (2000) illustrated the power of entrenched minds and the strength of resistance: A major hospital chain in the 1980s hired a futurist firm to envision what changes the hospital should make by the 1990s, given the changing trends in society. The futurist predicted accurately, but with the hospital operating at its peak of financial growth the hospital administration failed to respond and so missed opportunities that would have benefited the organization. The lesson to be learned here is two-fold: what may be working today will not necessarily work in the future, and the time to change is when things are going well. Pushing the envelope necessitates getting out of your comfort zone and being proactive rather than reactive to change.

TAKING CONTROL: QUEST FOR A VISIONARY CHANGE

Donner and Wheeler (2001) urged "nurses to be proactive, to assert more control over their careers" (p. 80). Yet traditionally nurses have not articulated their expertise well, especially in health-care settings where high levels of accountability and evidenced-based practice were concerned (Hardy, et al., 2002). Whereas nurses are people-skilled and interface with a large network of disciplines, such as medicine, business, policy, and government, their core competencies in communication and group interactive skills have gone unrecognized. Furthermore, beyond their expert clinical skills in delivering patient care, their role in successes in patient outcomes has also not been acknowledged. As a result, nursing has allowed others to direct its own job redesign whenever hospital chief executive officers (CEOs) have sought operation efficiency or cost-cutting tactics; nurses have been treated as no more than dispensable production task-oriented workers. Such lack of recognition has suppressed nurses' ability to contribute actively to the goals of improving patient care. Short-term downsizing business tactics have phased out lifelong employment tenure and ignored the benefits of nurses' contributions and loyalty to institutions. These trends have damaged nurses' morale, led to shortages of nursing supply through professional attrition, and threatened patient safety.

In response to skyrocketing costs of health care in the United States over the last three decades, various forms of structural funding and payment mechanisms evolved, fundamentally changing treatment of patients. With decreasing length of costly hospital stays and a shift toward treating more acute care in the ambulatory and home settings, the need for experienced, highly skilled nurses dramatically increased outside hospital settings. Many nurses who remained committed to in-hospital settings found themselves unemployed and having to shift toward community-based care. Even for those who deemed themselves lucky to remain employed within their chosen setting, the heavy demands began to take a toll.

For nurses to take control of their careers, they will need to steer away from the old assembly-line shift-work mentality and to take active responsibility in managing their careers and actively marketing themselves. This will require nurses to identify their core competencies and to gain confidence in articulating to others (and to themselves) what they can market beyond their tenured process-oriented care. Regularly, nurses are faced with complex decision making, both in managing acutely ill patients and working collaboratively with multidisciplinary professionals and business organizations. Yet for nurses to take credit for their innovative care, they will need to show evidence that such interventions are proven to bring successes, especially when it comes to patient outcomes. This will be a challenge, as nursing care has traditionally been viewed as an extension of medicine, a tool in which medical care is provided, and not as a distinct profession in which the art of caring is founded on empirically based scientific principles.

Asoh, et al. (2005) noted, "Nursing presents an excellent opportunity for entrepreneurial activities since they (nurses) are trained in a holistic manner to care for patients rather than treat specific diseases" (p. 218). Beyond nurses' expertise in caring for patients, Roggenkamp and White (1995) found that nurses exhibited entrepreneurial characteristics of "commitment to service, desire to stay close to their customer, and had risk-taking, assertive and strong leadership skills" (p. 8). Above all other factors, the most dominant motivating factor was their "love for nursing" (p. 8). The biggest challenge in this visionary transformation may be the process of change in the image of self and instilling the image of nursing as innovative intrapreneurs. The first step toward gaining control of your career is becoming aware of one's valued contribution in bringing successful patient outcomes. Once the transformation has begun, nurses need to identify the value of their product (their expert ability), to take control of their careers, to shape them, and actively market so that other professionals and consumers will recognize nursing's unique knowledge base and innovative care. Only then can nurses expect to become valued players and be invited into the circle of caregiver experts.

Gaining control of your career entails defining the value of your product in the marketplace. To build a valued product line (or career specialty), nurses will need to recognize what knowledge and specialty skills they can offer to either fulfill or create a market demand so as to create career opportunities that will grow. Finally, for nurses to develop their careers and identify marketable expertise, they will need work environments and leaders who will be supportive of the nurse's intrapreneurial ventures. In selecting where the nurse will market her wares, it will be important to select organizations that promote a culture that rewards shared and creative ideas, translates creative ideas into action, acknowledges successes, and puts failures into perspective. Failures are lessons that improve ideas and help build an even better product. Therefore, gain-

ing control requires an environment that is supportive of your professional practice and career goals and personal goals.

Broscio, Paulick, and Scherer (2005) warn that careers will need to be more responsive to the free-market ideology; there will be a need to employ free agents with specialized skills. Paradoxically, working in a virtual world, what one presumes as a greater emphasis for autonomous and independent work will actually require greater emphasis on interconnected relationships and communication (Neuhauser, Bender, & Stromberg, 2000). Moreover, effective communication is strongly influenced by previous experiences, culture, and relationships. For example, as in a global interface, without face-to-face contact, without language fluency, more emphasis is placed on communication in both the transmission and feedback loop. There will need to be a check and balance between parties in communication and a greater reliance on the nonverbal communication that requires being sensitive to diverse human beliefs, values, and modes of communication. Nurses are people-skilled and interface with a variety of multidisciplinary teams, regularly implementing and utilizing collaboration, negotiating, and building partnerships in their collaborative interactions with a highly educated network of professionals.

Complex environments require complex decision making; therefore, a bureaucratic hierarchy model of top-down communication does not fit the needs of today's dynamic, unstable environment. Where environmental boundaries have become blurred, our response to such complex dynamic forces requires decentralized decision making that is flexible and rapid-response. Popularized by the profit center concept developed during World War II, decentralized decision making allows for those who are closest to the operations to exert greater freedom to take control. Decisions need to be made closer to the operational level or at the point of patient care. Whereas physicians and other health professionals have expertise in the disease management or various elements of the human body, it is the nurse who has the greatest patient contact in hospitals and in the home. Knowledgeable about human responses to illnesses during the most vulnerable times in people's lives, nurses have unique caring ways to bring patients back to health through their expert clinical skills and human interactions. Again, nurses' expertise in "knowing the patient" brings unique skills that help motivate clients with their self-care; thus, nurses have a unique ability to carve out patient education niches within the marketplace.

DYNAMIC FORCES: SHAPING NURSES' FUTURE CAREERS

Amidst the optimism of scientific and technological advances, health care is under the shadows of a growing socioeconomic crisis: issues of the growing uninsured and entitlement costs of the soon to retire **Baby Boomers** (Robert Wood Johnson Foundation, 1999). Such opposing forces create a complex landscape, vastly different from that of the past. In terms of the health-care system, how the care will be delivered, what will be required of its providers and consumers, and what provider roles will be expected to address in terms of institutional capacity needs will also differ (Kressley, 1998; Porter-O'Grady, 2000; Porter-O'Grady & Wilson, 1999). For nurses, the work of providing care will be greatly altered as well (Porter-O'Grady, 2000).

Clearly, nurses' skills and career paths will need to mirror the changing health-care environment (Porter-O'Grady, 2000). Taking stock of the world in which we live is the first step to shaping our careers. Porter-O'Grady (2000) outlined three major converging forces that are changing our health-care landscape, which directly and indirectly affect nursing: economic, sociopolitical, and technological forces.

National Forces: Economic and Sociopolitical

Today's U.S. health-care system is faced with some daunting challenges. Economic forces drive the health-care delivery system to monitor its service use and patient health outcomes. Closely related to economics are sociopolitical forces as the health-care industry shifted its focus of care from costly curative hospital-based care to a less costly preventive consumer-accountable community-based care. The change from cost-based to prospective pay has brought managed care to its third decade of maturity; yet the great hope of curbing escalating health-care costs has still not been fully realized. To improve U.S. health-care shortfalls, U.S. health-care leaders are now rethinking forms of funding and mechanisms for health-care alternatives, even learning from other countries.

Accompanying such sociopolitical forces is the change in America's demographic topography in terms of age and ethnicity: fewer young productive citizens to support aging Baby Boomers, increased ethnic diversity, with growing economic gaps leading to even greater disparities. The "wide-angle image" shows inadequate insurance coverage that is inching up toward middle class Americans, along with an insecure entitlement reimbursement for the retired. In the next decade, our nation is projected to have one of the highest dependency ratios of younger ethnically diverse underemployed to older retired citizens.

The close-up brings to view images of the plight of the nursing and labor shortages, which create a patient dependency ratio that exceeds that of hospital capacity. The current nursing shortage is said to be unlike that in the past; it is deemed more dire and enduring (Nevidjon & Erickson, 2001). Fueled by the aging demographics, its primary shortfall is the result of attrition, both in nurses and nursing educators. According to Nevidjon and Erickson, "from an economic perspective, this shortage is being driven more by the supply side of the supply/demand equation" (p. 1). Adding to the nursing shortfall are the shortages in allied health professionals and ancillary staff, such as secretaries and support staff. Thus, this is a more complex shortage, which promises to worsen during the next decade as more health-care professionals and educators retire. Such shortages all adversely affect the health-care delivery system. Early in the 1990s, for cost-cutting reasons, hospital executives increased the use of unlicensed assistive personnel; however, these models failed due to increasing patient acuities, higher patient nurse ratios, concerns over medical errors, and the declining numbers of ancillary personnel. The impact was felt by the patients as well, as nurses are deemed to have the most continuous contact and develop the closest relationships with the patients and their families.

Global Forces: Sociopolitical Economy, Nursing Shortage, Unintended Consequences

With globalization, today's world has become interdependent, yet highly competitive. International boundaries have become more fluid, especially in terms of U.S. interdependency in global trading. The blurring of domestic and international boundaries has shaped the environment in which we work and live. Its impact has filtered down to everyday American lives and work (Hall, 2002; Riverin-Simard, 2000). Our social sphere is growing smaller, with tightly interwoven diversity, both racially and ethnically. Partly the result of the American's insatiable consumerism, our link with foreign labor markets is much more visible. The 2000 U.S. Census indicated that, between 1990 and 2000, 33 million people were added to the total U.S. population, with the fastest and second fastest racial/ethnic groups being Hispanics and Asians, respectively. Such dramatic demographic change can be viewed positively as an enriched cultural mix for our society, or it can be viewed by others as a menacing mix of clashing values that threaten our society. In our country's efforts to assimilate our newcomers into society quickly, there is a demand not only for bilingual nurses but also a greater demand for employees who are sensitive to the nuances of working within a racially/ethnically mixed culture. Culture has a significant impact on how people interpret health and illness (Spector, 2000). This provides nurses greater career opportunities. Nurses are inherently people-sensitive, which fits the required portrait of the type of leader that is needed for tomorrow's culturally diverse employees (Vicere, 2004). Indeed, nurses are not only advocates and **care experts** to individuals, families, populations, and communities, but their leadership skills often include mentoring employees of diverse cultures. So in terms of expertise, nurses have a wealth of possible career development options that could be carved into a specialty niche to fit the needs of a growing international community.

With the increasing size and mobility of the human population, there are direct and unintended consequences of emerging diseases that pose a continuing threat to global health. Historically, the United States had come to see open trading as "a means not only of advancing its own economic interests but also as a key to building peaceful relations among nations" (Garrett, 1998, p. 787). Yet even with economic incentives and peaceful motivations, there are subtle political ideologies promoted. This can create ideological clashes between diverse nations, which can surface as trade disputes and power struggles. Ideological clashes have caused America (and other nations) to be targeted for terrorist attacks as protests against American policy.

Global unrest and international instability can have overreaching effects on countries and their people. The global outreach in nursing is extensive, and it encompasses a full spectrum of expertise and services, from policy-making, capacity-building efforts to point-of-service primary health-care delivery. International organizations, such as the World Health Organization (WHO) and the International Council of Nurses (ICN), provide opportunities for nurses to work abroad and to mix their expertise with their love of travel and learning about diverse populations. With growing global disputes, traveling outside the United States has become increasingly risky for Americans, especially to the most severely economically depressed, war-torn countries. Such global unrest has curbed the activities of many nurses and medical volunteers who otherwise would reach out with humanitarian efforts to serve where the nursing (and medical) shortages are the greatest.

International trade agreements have transformed the capacity of governments to monitor and to protect public health by regulating occupational and environmental health conditions, exporting and importing food products, and ensuring affordable access to medications (Shaffer, et al., 2005). Proposals are under way for the World Trade Organization's General Agreement on Trade in Services (GATS) and the regional Free Trade Area of the Americas (FTAA) agreement to seek coverage of a wide range of health services, health facilities, sanitation services, and clinician licensing. Linkages among global trade, international trade agreements, and public health will no doubt open new opportunities for global exchange, especially for nurses to participate overseas in a wide spectrum of entrepreneurial-type services.

Linkages among global trade, international trade agreements, and public health deserve greater attention. The effects of interdependency in trade of products can be seen in human resources as well. Shortages in the health workforce, especially nurses, present a major challenge for health-care policy makers nationally and internationally. The nursing shortage is worldwide, even in developed countries such as the United Kingdom, Canada, and Sweden. International exchanges, especially in nursing resources, could become an area of dispute. Working under North American Free Trade Agreement (NAFTA) status, current trade of foreign market is keenly felt in the area of nursing shortages;

recruitment continues from various foreign countries such as the Philippines, Canada, Mexico, and others. But while there has been an increasing trend to recruit foreign-born nurses to increase the U.S. labor market, the shift in supply to the United States does little for the global shortage of nurses and the demand it creates within the countries they left (Booth, 2002; Zurn, Dolea, & Stilwell, 2005). More recently, South Korean nurses have been proposed as an answer to the current shortage of nursing educators. Living in a highly competitive Korean job market, many Korean faculties are already doctorally prepared nurses and English-proficient and have taken the NCLEX International (2005) examination administered by the National Council of State Boards of Nursing (NCSBN). In the Western Pacific, Korea is among three nations that have reported a surplus of nurses at present (Socio-Economic News, 2003).

With the potential influx of nurses into the United States from diverse countries, the most poignant question that U.S. nursing professionals ask is, "Do foreign nurses hold similar professional nursing values and practice models as nurses in the United States?" Flynn and Aiken (2002), in their secondary analysis of nearly 800 nurses surveyed (with nearly a third from 34 other countries), challenged the prevailing sentiment that foreign nurses would have different nursing values and professional practice models compared with U.S. nurses. The findings also revealed that in the absence of a professional practice environment, foreign-born nurses would experience similar high levels of burnout as U.S. nurses. Although one answer to the nursing shortage might be to recruit from foreign countries, health-care administrators will still need to ensure that organizational and leadership attributes are congruent with a professional nursing practice environment.

With blurred boundaries, the world has become increasingly vulnerable to both (re)emerging infectious diseases, once thought controlled or never experienced before, and to natural disasters, such as earthquakes and hurricanes. Given the current size and mobility of the global community, the world is at risk for pandemic outbreaks and increasing climatic disasters. For example, increasing contact between humans and animal disease reservoirs contributed to the emergence of severe acute respiratory syndrome. Ecological changes, such as habitat fragmentation by deforestation, may increase the contact between people and reservoir species, all contributing to zoonoses (e.g., hemorrhagic fever virus). Early recognition of cases and application of appropriate infection control measures will be critical in controlling future outbreaks. Moreover, global warming has been identified as contributing to the spread of dengue beyond tropical regions and possibly contributing to the global climatic and typological turbulence.

Technological Forces and Unintended Consequences

Scientific and technological advances promise revolutionary changes in the health-care system. Yet such promises of technology and its ability to fix human ills may need to be balanced with cautious optimism. Beyond the impact on global communication capabilities, technology promises to offer resources to improve the quality and length of people's lives. It promises to transform the way diseases are diagnosed and treated. The technology presents new possibilities to design innovative methods for (1) preparing future generations of nurses, (2) addressing the issues of medical errors and the nursing shortage, and (3) satisfying and extending the requirements for entry-level RN practice in terms of knowledge, skills, and abilities.

One exciting example for nursing education and practice is the ability "to practice" low-frequency high-risk patient events through the use of simulation technology. Such technology has multiple applications in helping to reduce nursing and medical errors, advancing nursing skills, and improving teamwork without putting real patients in harm's way. Not unlike the military field training for combat, the simulation laboratories can be created as virtual hospital rooms and clinical settings with physiologically/verbally responsive mannequins for nurses, students, and other medical teams to act out realistic scenarios that simulate actual events. The impact of this technological training tool is enormous as it addresses multiple educational, nursing, and organizational issues. It provides a safe environment in which novice nurses and students can train; allows for errors to take place without putting an actual patient in harm's way; permits organizations to gather data and develop system changes to protect patients and adjust policies to improve patient safety; provides new possibilities for preparing novice nurses to expert level in a shorter time;

promotes teamwork by helping the health-care team to communicate with each other (where the majority of medical errors occur); and trains nurses and other medical members to improve their communication with patients/families (Institute of Medicine, 2000).

The flip side of technology is its unintended consequences. With any new technological advances, we need to scrutinize and critically think through what the unintended effects might be on the greater whole: the world. Without getting into the philosophical debate about the benefits/risks of reliance on technology, William Barrett (1979), in his classic *The Illusion of Technique,* warned about placing such high reliance on technology to solve human problems. Similarly, Ehrenfeld (1981) critiqued society's reliance on humanistic power to solve the world's problems. Some questions that need to be asked are:

- How is the technology to be applied?
- Who will be applying it?
- To whom is it being applied?
- What are alternate uses of such technology?
- How and whom might it harm?

The Human Genome Program (2005) is an example that illustrates the cost of technology. It affects myriad social and clinical applications, but there are a number of ethical dilemmas attending its use, ranging from ensuring privacy to informed consent.

CREATIVITY AND INNOVATION: THINKING AND PRODUCING

Rollo May (cited in Driver, 1971b) wrote, "out of the creative act is born symbols and myths. It brings to our awareness what was previously hidden and points to new life. The experience is one of heightened consciousness—ecstasy." Creative expression is vital to quality life, and everyone has the creative potential if they follow their interests. Although "creativity" continues to elude empirical measurement, we can see creativity in a person's affective "act of doing," seeing their spark through their being in the world/nature-at-large, and discovering their interactions with us and exploring their effect on us. Because creativity is an intrinsically motivating trait, its action may be associated with nonconformity, independence, persistent questioning, and persistent in-depth inquiry. This internal drive is what pushes entrepreneurs and intrapreneurs toward excellence. The adage, "time flies when you're having fun" can be applied to the process and outcomes of creativity. Csikszentmihalyi (1997) identified the spark as the heightened consciousness, or the creative *flow,* an energy that is not necessarily an isolated experience but can result as a synergy working with others. To learn how creativity worked, Csikszentmihalyi (1995) interviewed 90 leaders in various disciplines and discovered that they regularly experienced this state of *flow,* a heightened state of pleasure experienced when one is engaged in physical or mental challenges that absorb us and give us joy. Based on these interviews with some of the most creative people in the world, Csikszentmihalyi (1995) listed the steps that individuals could take to cultivate one's creativity. Furthermore, he recommended (1995) that one needs "to acquire many interests, abilities, and goals and to use them in such a way they harmonize with one another" (p. 30).

Creativity and innovation reflect "thinking and producing" respectively; both share in creating something new. Merriam-Webster (2005) describes creativity as a reflection of these two parts: creativity as "the ability or power to create something new" and innovation as "the power that puts the creative inspiration into action." The three key personality elements required to build a new vision of oneself as creative include having a high tolerance for ambiguity, being comfortable with the unknown, and having faith in yourself to handle any outcome.

CREATING VISIONARY CHANGE: SELF-REFLECTING AND REALITY CHECKS

Sister Callista Roy (2000), renowned theorist on adaptive nursing theory, wrote that nursing faces a great challenge: to create a visionary change within its own profession. However, Carper, Chinn, and Kramer (cited in Roy, 2000) revealed that nurses all too often struggle to find effective strategies for developing integrated knowledge, defined as a way of knowing that comes with synthesizing "the personal, ethical, aesthetic, and sociopolitical knowledge" (p. 118). Self-reflective thinking brings the "invisible" knowledge of self into clearer view. This process requires a nurse to assess what in his current position gives him joy and what he believes and values about life and the people around him (White, 1995).

Guided by the Professional Standards of Nursing Practice, nurses' core values and practice of nursing are centered on people and serving the good of society, which is unchanging and timeless (Strader & Decker, 1999; White, 1995). Conversely, nursing skills evolve to reflect the context of the time and environment (Williams-Evans & Carnegie, 2002). Specialized skills evolve over time, as one can see with many **nurse practitioner** skills. Their skills of assessment, diagnosing, and prescribing medications evolved from both the greater push for nursing practice and to fill the need of the primary care physician shortage. Yet the core of nursing values remains immutable, to advocate for the needy populace and to promote the good of society; thus, these values are embedded in each nurse's personal values and beliefs.

Creating the vision for career necessitates self-reflective thinking, a process that requires nurses to assess what in their position gives them joy and what they believe and value about life and the people around them. Nurses can then bring this self-reflection and compare it with how others perceive them (Donner & Wheeler, 2001). This process helps to identify the "invisible" personal and professional values (Roy, 2000). This vision of self is then linked to how you fit into the environment, how your values fit with the organization and whether the organization fits with your values, a reality check. This begins the "self-reflective" process of wondering and thinking:

- Where am I?
- Where do I want to be?
- Where have I been?
- How can I use my experience, and what else do I need to know?
- Who do I go to for more information and direction?
- How do I get there?
- How can I salvage what I already know?

INTEGRATING THE SELF WITH THE ENVIRONMENTAL OPPORTUNITIES

Nurses too often struggle to find strategies for integrating the self into the environmental opportunities (Carper, et al., 1978; cited in Roy, 2000). After completing a career self-assessment, you need to repeat the environmental assessment discussed earlier in the chapter. Through this repetitive process of self-assessing and seeking feedback from colleagues, the level of self-awareness deepens. With

an accurate picture of your values, strengths, and desires, you can immerse yourself in the offerings within and outside the health-care field.

It is vital to scope the environment and keep abreast of the surrounding marketplace, to view the trends in business and organizations, both related and unrelated to the health-care system. Scanning the environment means following the technological development and immersing yourself in the global news and local and national current events: identifying the sociopolitical and economic issues that directly or indirectly affect our nation and our profession. For example, topics of importance to hospital industry, business, and global news can easily be identified and collected by simply typing in the subject of interest through a search engine, such as Google. For example, a search of hospital CEOs concerning the financial outlook for health care resulted in a survey of hospital CEOs done by Deloitte and Touche, USA (2005). It reported that the industry was taking a more optimistic outlook of its financial future (Deloitte and Touche, USA, 2005). With a consumer-empowered market, it reported that the United States offers a more interconnected economy, which offers consumers greater advances in new drugs and medicine, promises of genetic research and its potential curative application to chronic diseases, greater investment in telemedicine, and new cyber- and biomedicine technology (Deloitte & Touche, USA, 2005).

Sources of information need to be widespread and diverse. Both online and library sources can bring a wealth of literature information. Also important is networking with a variety of people both inside and outside the field of nursing. Attending national conferences to learn about the national and global trends and ongoing issues and to meet others within and outside the field can be energizing and valuable. Information can be gathered easily online by signing up on a listserv, such as KaiserFoundation.org, which provides continuous legislative and policy information and updates relevant to one's interest area. Other access to information may be through a live or archival recorded Webcast of national and international conferences. Searching professional journals within and outside nursing, and even searching popular magazines, would give insight into current events and what the public is reading.

Once the environmental search is completed, sift through the materials identifying similar, related, and dissimilar issues within diverse disciplines. Analyzing the dissonance and the interconnectedness between various disciplines allows one to bring the pieces together, the parts brought together to bring a new whole, a synthesis of new ideas. Pulling this together, one can begin to identify the gaps, view the needs within the environment, and bring one's strength of expertise to develop a strategic plan, a blueprint of actions.

OPPORTUNITY SEEKING AND RISK TAKING: TAKING THE ENTREPRENEURIAL LEAP

Taking the "entrepreneurial leap" is the same for the intrapreneur as it is for the entrepreneur. Taking the leap requires the entrepreneur and intrapreneur to view themselves as opportunity seeking (Gordon, 1985; cited in Hisrich, 1990) and as having the ability to recognize opportunity (Paterson, 1985; cited in Hisrich, 1990). For the entrepreneur, that means seeking the opportunity outside the current employment; whereas, for the intrapreneur it means seeking an opportunity within the current workplace. In fact, many budding entrepreneurs arise from having evolved as intrapreneurs (Manion, 2001). Brugleman (cited in Hisrich, 1990) integrated these two traits of seeking opportunity and recognizing opportunity to describe entrepreneurship as "seeking to find and recognizing when opportunity knocks."

These traits give entrepreneurs and intrapreneurs the leading edge in developing and diversifying their businesses. For the nurse entrepreneur and intrapreneur, this can mean developing new skills to create a new role outside and inside of nursing. It is the discovery of something new, the creativity that ignites the entrepreneur's (and intrapreneur's) innovative ideas and propels her forward to the opportunity (Gordon, 1985; Paterson, 1985; cited in Hisrich, 1990).

Beyond the risk-bearing attributes, entrepreneurs and intrapreneurs themselves are known to have other unique personality attributes. They quest for quality, a willingness to move beyond the standard solution in preference for creating a new "original idea." McClelland (1965) noted that entrepreneurs had a need for high achievement, and Roscoe (cited in Bird, 1989) found they had a strong drive for independence and an exceptional belief in themselves. Smilor (cited in Baum & Locke, 2004)

suggested that passion is "perhaps the most observed phenomenon of the entrepreneurial process" (p. 342). Locke (cited in Baum & Locke, 2004) identified, in a qualitative analysis, core characteristics of famous wealth creators, such as Bill Gates and Michael Bloomberg: their zeal and their love for their work. Moreover, Lackman (cited in Bird, 1989) found that entrepreneurs held the personal values of honesty, integrity, duty, responsibility, and ethical behavior constant and applied them toward their life and work. Consistent with these values, Cunningham and Lischeron (cited in Bird, 1989) deemed high self-esteem as a notable characteristic of entrepreneurs. As leaders, they were found to be more flexible and adapted their leadership style to the needs of the people (Katz and Brockhaus, 1995).

BUILDING A STRATEGIC PLAN: CRITICAL THINKING AND DECISION MAKING

As discussed earlier, one of the first steps for a nurse considering the role of an entrepreneur or intrapreneur is to look within herself to see whether she has the ambition, fortitude, and inner strength needed to venture outside the role definitions that have been used in the past. As nurses begin to imagine what their professional lives could be, they need to do some critical thinking about their present environment. Can their goals and professional achievements be fostered from within their current organization, or must a break be made? A nursing process model, combined with critical thinking, is an excellent framework to use as a problem-solving method of career analysis. Nurses are expert at assessing, planning, synthesizing data to form diagnoses, setting goals, creating interventions, and evaluating. Nurses can immediately evaluate a plan of action according to its risk-benefit probability and can use critical thinking to develop a short-term evaluation of the consequences, both positive and negative.

The assessment includes looking at the organization in which nurses are employed; the organizational structure and leadership style should support decentralized decision making. As they survey their present organization, nurses should make judgments regarding its culture of human respect, its value of autonomy, and its ability to accept new ideas and discard old ones. Another important point to consider is whether the organization will thrive and grow or stagnate. The question that needs to be answered is whether to stay in the present organization, move to another one, or move outside of any organization. Or even whether to remain in the role of a nurse. McLees (1988) stated, "Former nurses developed careers in other professions that offered them greater outlets to express their individuality, creativity and freedom." The intrapreneur can work effectively within an enlightened organization, whereas an entrepreneur is destined to work from the outside, often with many different organizations. After the decision for a role change has been reached, the nurse needs to look at what needs to be done and what advantages can be gained from a strategic plan for marketing the idea or product. The environment needs to be assessed relative to the networking possibilities and the availability of potential mentors.

Marketing, Networking, and Mentoring

A nurse considering a move to intrapreneur or entrepreneur must become familiar with the concepts of marketing, networking, and mentoring; these are vital to a successful intraprise or enterprise.

MARKETING

Marketing lets potential users know about a product's existence and advantages. The dictionary defines marketing as "the process or technique of promoting, selling, and distributing a product or service" (Merriam-Webster, 2005). For nurses, marketing often becomes indistinguishable from self-marketing, which involves promoting who they are and what they do. Having a business plan will allow the nurse to answer objective questions about the product or service as to what it is, the advantages of it relative to its competitors, the innovation of it in relation to the status quo, the worth or value in monetary terms, the break-even point, the potential buyers, what might motivate them to purchase, and what the contractual obligations should entail. In order to sell the product or service, the nurse needs to become an expert on the needs of the organization. This involves research and tapping into people who may be able to help within the pertinent network as well as soliciting the advice of a mentor. Nurses are experts in picking up on behavioral cues and applying them to outcome criteria for their patients. Many of the same skills are useful in negotiating with potential clients. Reading books on selling and practicing with others who might agree to pose as "buyers" will help to bolster confidence and allow the nurse to anticipate questions and formulate confident answers beforehand.

Competition and the task of constantly proving one's worth to organizations can be emotionally draining. The independent contractor must be politically savvy within his current organization and able to apply these skills to new situations and people. Even though the **nurse entrepreneur** can, in theory, choose his own clients, when one is just beginning to get established this is usually not a reality. The nurse needs to please as many new clients as possible and follow up on other potential clients while they are still interested. The role of nurse entrepreneur brings the potential for increasing income, but at first there is often meager remuneration. Many unpaid work hours will be necessary to get the business started. Sometimes the fledgling entrepreneur must provide services and consultation almost for free just to get started Once the nurse has an established a reputation, fees can be increased and cancellation clauses introduced into written contracts. The business plan will include some of the start-up costs; typical needs are a computer with fax and color printer, file cabinets, and copier. Also important are business cards describing the nurse and the services available as well as a mailer or cover letter that can be given to prospective clients. Mailings and Web-site design may become eventual investments. Keeping the overhead down can do a lot to keep a fledgling business afloat. The nurse entrepreneur may need to borrow money to compensate for business setbacks or to fulfill orders that are not affordable within the current budget. Much depends on the type of service or product that the nurse entrepreneur intends to provide.

NETWORKING

Another important concept to consider in order to become a successful intrapreneur or entrepreneur is networking. The word "network" literally means a framework of nets. It has recently been used as a verb, referring to meeting people for the purpose of establishing links or contacts to further a goal. Hisrich (1990) found that "the density of the entrepreneur's business contacts or linkages" was important to start a new business and that "maintaining contacts were a significant predictor for early profit" (p. 6). For the nurse, it means becoming visible, getting to know people in other areas of the job site, finding out what they do and who they know. A more formal definition is offered by Benton (1997): "a way of establishing and using contacts for information, support and other assistance to further career goals, or as a way of building relationships" (p. 58). Most networks are made up of people who are receptive to communicating with one another. Benton sees the benefit of networks as a vehicle to gather "feedback" on a particular issue or on the nurse's performance. It may be a way for the nurse to "influence" or be influenced by a particular point of view. One of the more traditional reasons to network is to act on or procure a "referral" (p. 59). A network can also act as an excellent advertising vehicle (Hisrich, 1990): "satisfied customers help establish a winning business reputation and promote goodwill" (p. 6). Many individuals network to test the job market or to help secure a position outside of the organization. For the intrapreneur or entrepreneur, it may help to locate an area of need within the organization. This can serve as a springboard to fill the vacancy either permanently or temporarily as a consultant.

Some nurses are afraid to network because they think that it will involve small talk and taking advantage of a colleague or friend. Networking should be mutually advantageous for both parties involved. It is important that this give-and-take be implied at the outset. It may be difficult to see the immediate monetary or career rewards to networking because some contacts take more than one meeting in order to cultivate useful information. But at the very least a foundation has been formed. Beck and Utz (1996) sees the benefits as "increasing contacts, sharing resources, and gaining peer support to contribute to an ultimate goal" (p. 786). Networking is also "an effective means of fulfilling [the] responsibility of collegiality, while at the same time achieving personal and professional goals" (p. 786). Benton (1997) advises that successful networking is a "dynamic process," so it is important to strike a balance, keeping in touch with contacts but not becoming a nuisance. Follow up promptly on a promise of information or help, as reciprocity of a favor may be important in the future. It is important not to ask for favors or information that the person is unable to provide. Discretion is also extremely important as comments made to one person about another are bound to reach the ears of the one discussed, especially if the network is small (p. 52).

It is always advantageous to carry a good supply of business cards. Some nurses carry more than one type; one may describe the current job, and another highlights the nurse's intrapreneurial or entrepreneurial abilities. Obviously, this is also a good way of marketing one's skills or product. Within an organization, it is important to approach people who work in unfamiliar areas and get information on what their jobs entail and how their departments function. The nurse can approach a staff member whom she would like to know better and offer to treat the person to lunch in exchange for some information about how that person does an assigned job. The colleague will probably be flattered if the nurse is diplomatic. Benton (1997) recommends getting on mailing lists of professional organizations so that follow-up is possible with members related to newsletter submissions and advises the nurse to write or e-mail journal authors to establish contact and "open up a new network connection" (p. 53).

West (1997) offers many useful networking strategies, particularly if a new position is sought. When attending a large professional conference, circulate and meet as many new contacts as possible, disseminating business cards and collecting them from all. When a new contact asks, "What do you do?" it is best to describe it in behavioral terms to highlight particular skills. It is advisable to write notes on the back of the person's business card so that pertinent information is not forgotten. Even if a new permanent position is not being sought, finding out from contacts and nursing journals about vacant jobs will give useful information about where professional expertise may be needed and consultation opportunities exist. Whenever there is a chance to meet new people, it is also a good idea to have an updated résumé. Sometimes, a potential client is so enthusiastic that he will ask for one.

It is beneficial to join professional organizations and volunteer to serve on committees or task forces (Benton, 1997). West (1997) advises "diversification of the networking group by adding social acquaintances, college classmates, alumni, professors, church ministers, church members, and local business and social club officials. Even the family lawyer, doctor, dentist, insurance agent, and banker may be in a position to help" (p. 334). Web logs, known as blogs, are an emerging writing tool that is easy to use and that can enhance health professionals' communication, collaboration, and information-gathering skills and help to manage information, diminish medical error, and support decision making (Maag, 2005). Nurses can read and comment on others' blogs as well as starting blogs themselves. Maag noted that "Daily blogging will enhance positive writing skills, instill self-confidence in voicing personal opinions, and promote reflective thinking that, in turn, will allow the writer to appreciate his or her personal opinions or ideas" (p. 2). Bloggers must be careful about what they write online; a number of bloggers have been fired for criticizing their employers or presenting themselves in an unprofessional way online. Getting in touch with a wide range of global information and insight will facilitate knowing and becoming known. Having a perspective on worldwide nursing issues gives the professional an ability to interpret situations with greater accuracy.

MENTORS

The other concept that is vital to a successful career as an intrapreneur or entrepreneur is mentorship. The term "mentor" is originally from the Greek legends and "refers to Mentor, the loyal friend and wise advisor to Odysseus and the teacher and guardian of Odysseus' son Telemachus" (Merriam-Webster, 2005) (p. 920). The individual needs a personal moral support and a morale-building system and a professional network of contacts and advisors. A role model who will agree to give counsel and act as a sounding board for potential career plans and activities is an invaluable resource, particularly at the inception of a new business venture or even at the beginning of a nursing career. Byrne and Keefe (2002) describe a shift "in the nursing literature from an early emphasis on mentoring primarily for executive leadership roles to a current emphasis on special mentorships for clinician, researcher and other roles" (p. 391). Recommendations for mentoring of clinicians include support of new RN graduates (Andrews and Wallis, 1999; cited in Byrne and Keefe, 2002), novice nurse prac-

titioners (Hayes, 1998, and Hockenberry-Eaton & Kline, 1995; cited in Byrne and Keefe, 2002), and nurses making specialty transitions (Esper, 1999; cited in Byrne and Keefe, 2002). Byrne and Keefe noted, "Within nursing the experience of mentoring has sometimes been perceived as a learning continuum which extends from peer support and role modeling, through instructive preceptorship, self-initiated and guided networking, and finally the intense and personal occurrence of focused mentorship" (p. 396). Nursing is unique in that newly acquired knowledge, whether evidence-based or hypothesis-related, can almost immediately be put into practice. Nurses can immediately evaluate a plan of action according to its risk/benefit probability and, by using critical thinking, develop a short-term evaluation of the consequences, both positive and negative. If new nurses burn out because of the lack of available support and advice, they will not survive the rigors of the initial practice environment to become advanced practitioners, intrapreneurs, and entrepreneurs. Nurses are cognizant of the need to support, encourage, and teach new graduates and novice practitioners and are committed to helping them become competent, self-confident, and enthusiastic nurses.

Having a mentor within an organization can help a budding intrapreneur to gauge the advisability of assuming a new role. Finding someone who has worked in the same place for a number of years is a bonus; he knows the history of various programs and people. He can give a synopsis of what has been tried and why it was dropped or changed. This is vital information for the nurse who is planning to offer a "unique" and important service in order to occupy a niche within the hospital, healthcare center, or community facility. A mentor can give helpful feedback on ideas and proposals before they are presented. Temporary setbacks can be analyzed and a new plan theorized. For the nurse entrepreneur, it is advisable to seek a mentor with a business background as well as another within the health-care sector.

Nurse Intrapreneurs

A comprehensive perspective on the development of intrapreneurs and entrepreneurs in nursing involves looking at the qualities, roles, options, and successes of each designation.

QUALITIES

As described by Gifford Pinchot in 1986 relating to the corporate sector, "intrapreneur" refers to a person who wants to be entrepreneurial but does not want to change his/her workplace. "Behind most successful nurse leaders, executives, and entrepreneurs winds a long road of successful intrapreneurship, or innovation within an organization" (Manion, 2001, p. 5). The **nurse intrapreneur** develops skills that are needed by the organization, thus creating a visible, marketable, talent niche. "These professionals are continually seeking and recognizing opportunities for personal growth and development and are undeterred by typical organizational barriers to innovation" (Manion, 2001, p. 5). Because many of the intrapreneur's skills and internal innovations save the facility money, the organization directly benefits from the service. Intrapreneurs are loyal to the organization and want to be useful and feel appreciated. They are also confident, assertive, and willing to speak up when they see a situation that could be ameliorated or made more efficient. They are open to exploring new ideas, not mired in traditional mindsets or bound by convention. They can take two "old" environmental objects and synthesize a new one that becomes more than the sum of its parts. This nurse is also typically talented, innovative, and proactive; the facility wants to keep this valuable nurse on its payroll rather than lose the intrapreneur to a competitor.

ROLES

How can a nurse become an intrapreneur? Having a creative outlook is the first step. "The greatest obstacle to workplace creativity is the we-always-do-it-this-way mentality" (Cohen, 2002, p. 10). Intrapreneurs may recognize systems that need changing, skills that will become necessary to master new equipment, better ideas for organizing or sorting data or personnel—the possibilities are endless. By becoming a valued contributor to an organization, the nurse can build job security and increase professional and personal satisfaction with her career trajectory. One of the first steps is to get to know people in the organization and find out what they do. Having a network of individuals will help to identify problems and how they may have been solved in other departments. Finding multiple mentors is also important; they may all have expertise in different areas and may offer many possibilities for innovation. It is also important to look at the strategic plan and see where the organization will go in the future. An important tactic involves volunteering for task forces and committee assignments. It is both a good way to meet people and will acquaint the budding intrapreneur with the way the organization solves problems with its people and who has the power to make change. It is also important to adopt a philosophy of lifelong learning, to stay current in the newest innovations in nursing, and to be aware of what is happening in other fields. The intrapreneur needs to research what therapies are innovative and how they are being implemented at the facility; the next step would be to write an article for publication or make a presentation to other facilities. Entrepreneurs may be competitive with an established company, but the nurse intrapreneurs can maintain their security within the facility. Koch (1996) noted intrapreneurs "capitalize on the reputation of the organization and can readily access a diverse network of professionals who are crucial for answering questions, giving assistance and helping make ideas become realities" (Koch, 1996, p. 2). Nurse intrapreneurs can also utilize the facilities' meeting areas, copying, and Internet services, saving them the financial outlay that entrepreneurs must absorb as part of the cost of doing business on their own. Intrapreneurs have the relative safety to discuss new ideas as a means to a possible "intraprise" without worrying that someone from within the organization will steal their innovation.

What kind of culture would welcome the nurse intrapreneur? There must be a dynamic mindset with "networking, teamwork, sponsors, and mentors abounding; trust and close working relationships where tasks are viewed as fun activities (not chores) with participants gladly putting in the amount of hours necessary to get the job done. Instead of building barriers to protect turf, advice and cross-fertilization freely occur within and across functional areas and even divisions" (Hisrich, 1990, p. 7). The environment, including top **management**, needs to be open to new ideas and willing to experiment. Of course, some hypotheses do not work, and failure needs to be tolerated.

NURSE INTRAPRENEUR OPTIONS AND SUCCESSES

For the umbrella organization, the nurse intrapreneur is visible as a change agent and a role model for other staff members who may also have good ideas, inspiring and influencing others to become innovators "while advancing the science of nursing through clarifying, refining, and expanding the nursing knowledge base" (Koch, 2004, p. 9). One example is an operating room nurse who designed the "first hospital-based surgical recycling program in the country, a newly-created position of waste reduction specialist, and eventually into a national consulting business" (Manion, 2001). A nurse with demonstrated excellence in sterile technique and wound management might float from one hospital unit to another, helping nurses change complicated dressings or manage wound vacuum systems. Keeping before-and-after pictures and showing how patient days and money were saved may make the hospital realize that a wound care nurse is an asset. The hospital pays to send this nurse for an advanced certificate or to become a wound care specialist. Similarly, a nurse with experience with colostomies or ileostomies might become an enterostomal therapist. A nurse with a combination of computer and clinical expertise can become the in-house informatics consultant, responsible for orienting new staff, troubleshooting system glitches, and formulating new ways to use technology at the bedside. Some health-care facilities will have computers with Internet capabilities available at the bedside. It will be important for a nurse with computer expertise to help patients select and navigate the many health-care consumer Web sites for information, to be someone who can integrate the education according to the disease and wellness needs of the patient.

Nursing job niches are only limited to the imagination of the nurse intrapreneur. A nurse with children may create a job where there is the possibility of working at home or at an adjacent day-care site. Perhaps self-staffing began with nurses deciding that they could do it better. Traveling nurses, with experience in many cities and job sites, may bring new ideas about doing things to each site, making them very desirable as permanent hires should they decide to stay. A nurse who enjoys animals may volunteer while a pet visits its owners who are hospitalized or living in a rehabilitation center and may eventually convince her supervisor that a resident dog or cat needs her constant services as a pet-patient liaison. Facilities are always looking for an idea that they can promote to capture a particular market and become more competitive. It may just take a nurse intrapreneur to point them in a promising direction.

Nurse Entrepreneurs

It is important to compare the previously discussed qualities, roles, and options of the nurse intrapreneur with those of the nurse entrepreneur. There are many similarities but also some marked differences.

QUALITIES

It is important to look at the component parts of the nurse entrepreneur definition and assess whether the individual has what it takes to become self-made and successful. The definition speaks to a talented, independent, and experienced nurse who sees an available health-care business niche and decides to fill it. Consider what the individual does well professionally as well as what she likes and wants to do. Many entrepreneurs were once intrapreneurs with a particular talent that was recognized within an organization; subsequently, they embellished and magnified this talent so that other organizations would find it valuable also. Sullivan and Christopher (1999) describe many of the characteristics that are desirable in order to become a successful nurse entrepreneur. It is important to be a creative thinker and be willing to assume the leadership role to get an idea from concept to reality. Being a decision maker who is action-oriented rather than deliberative is essential to make change happen quickly. Having a high tolerance for ambiguity and knowing that there is always a transition period from the inception of an innovation until it finally takes a cohesive shape are integral to the role of entrepreneur. It is important to include nurse entrepreneurial activities as a part of the educational curriculum for management courses (really, at any level) to foster innovative ways to approach traditional patient care activities (Sullivan & Christopher, 1999). Sullivan noted, "Thus, it is possible to learn the basics of entrepreneurship while studying management, including strategic planning, continuous quality improvement, business plan development, marketing, management information systems, leadership, and financial management" (p. 329). Although it is vital to practice nursing according to principles and care standards, it is also important to forgo rigidity and a procedural mindset.

ROLES

Merriam-Webster defines entrepreneur as a "person who organizes and manages a business undertaking, assuming the risk for the sake of profit" (Merriam-Webster, 2005). The term commonly refers to a self-made individual with a good idea who, despite many setbacks, perseveres and becomes successful and wealthy. The term has been used often in the business community. The number of successful entrepreneurs and new companies has steadily increased, despite the high rate of failure for a fledgling business. The American culture is particularly supportive of the process. Hisrich (1990) noted, "Although dissatisfaction with various aspects of one's job—challenge, promotional opportunities, frustration, and boredom—often motivates the launching of a new venture, previous technical and industry experience is important once the decision to launch has been made" (p. 210). Whether a person possesses the qualities necessary for success in this venture may be determined by family support, education, personal motivation and, to some extent, age. Hisrich (1990) noted, "Generally, male entrepreneurs tend to start their first significant venture in their early 30s whereas female entrepreneurs tend to do this in their middle 30s." Although independence is usually the primary motivating factor, "money is the second reason for starting a new venture for men, whereas job satisfaction, achievement, opportunity, and money are the reasons in rank order for women" (p. 212).

If the job that an entrepreneur desires is not attainable with current skills, then it is necessary to find out what is needed and acquire it. Sometimes education will open the door to a new market. Education does not have to occur in a traditional manner, but having a baccalaureate, master's degree, or doctorate will open doors to previously unattainable positions or establish the credibility necessary for consulting. This will obviously be a longer-term goal, but with careful planning, the present company or hospital may actually pay for that credential as part of its employee benefits. One or more certifications and practice in another area may pave the way for a different career path. Accomplishing these things while still employed is time-consuming but may allow the nurse time to save money; extra start-up money may be necessary later when beginning to work as an entrepreneur. Perhaps a degree or certificate in law, hospital management, marketing, or business would complement the assets of a health-care background. The nurse must consider what will make her unique and sought as an entrepreneur. Sometimes working in the desired area part-time or in an entry-level position will help identify what is needed and how it can be supplied. Working with or observing a person who already has the desired type of job will supply invaluable experience, especially if it can be used as an apprenticeship. Often a lack of experience is a stumbling block to moving into a new job. Orientation and training are expensive for any organization, and if nurse entrepreneurs can "hit the ground running" they will have an advantage over the competition.

OPTIONS AND SUCCESSES

There are many ways in which a nurse can make the leap to an entrepreneurial role. For instance, a nurse who demonstrated excellence as a patient educator could become a corporate wellness coordinator. The nurse who had a position as an educator could subcontract to other health-care agencies without educators. Some hospitals and geriatric facilities have eliminated their educator positions as cost-cutting measures and now find that an educational consultant is cheaper than paying one full-time. A nurse manager who has coordinated care for multiple units has proven leadership ability; would-be coordinators might prove a marketable commodity. "Current research on complementary therapies, such as music therapy, guided imagery, and relaxation, can provide a springboard for the nurse entrepreneur who wants to apply research to practice and/or education" (Sullivan & Christopher, 1999, p. 332). A **care manager** or **case manager** may deliver registry or agency services to insurance companies or health-care management agencies. "With the aid of videoconferencing, fax, and e-mail transmission, practitioners can participate in operations, review laboratory data, and even perform a virtual physical exam. Telehealth is a major factor [that is] forcing state and federal regulatory bodies to reexamine their antiquated regulatory systems" (Shaffer & Sheets, 2001, p. 40). The nurse considering multistate consulting or giving advice via health-care information hotlines that cross state lines or country borders must consider the necessity and impact of multistate licensure.

Nurses have succeeded in their own businesses as business and health-care writers; educational consultants to hospitals, universities, and corporations; legal nurse consultants; health care and nursing Web design; state board examination tutoring; and home care nursing. Bensing (2005) illustrated a story about Richard C. Thompson in "How I Became a Nurse Entrepreneur" (pp. 36–37). Thompson started an agency that supplied nurses to hospitals and extended care facilities and guaranteed that shifts would be covered; if necessary, he replaced the ill nurse scheduled at the facility himself. This made his agency very attractive to hospitals. He also paid more money to his nurses than his competitors did, which made his agency very popular with his employees. There are many other opportunities for nurse entrepreneurs. Many nurses have begun agency staffing services for hospitals and home health. Other nurses have acted as their own brokers of services to hospitals and traveling nurse agencies. A nurse who found publishers unwilling to print submissions from nurses started her own publishing company (Lowder, 1997; cited in Bensing, 2005). Another nurse organized educational cruises. Still another became a financial consultant specializing in the nursing market. Some became cost-containment experts, able to market their services to facilities and families. Many nurse practitioners have set up independent practices in rehabilitation services and in as many areas as there are specialties.

In the last 10 years, as the "sandwich generation" has had to deal simultaneously with raising children and arranging for services for aging parents, nurse-run businesses have sprung up in the popular retirement states. These businesses arrange for extended care or nursing home placement of aging parents of children living at opposite ends of the country. They also make sure to provide follow-up care and regular updates if the adult children are unable to visit frequently. Nurses have also invented and patented useful products. Downey and Freidin (1997) invented communication vehicles for ventilator patients. Dr. Laura Gasparis Vonfrolio is a well-known nurse entrepreneur who began her first business with corporate cardiopulmonary resuscitation and professional education and eventually owned many businesses. Dr. Leslie Nicoll is an RN who has written "The Nurses' Guide to the Internet" and is editor-in-chief of *CIN: Computers, Informatics, Nursing* and the *Journal of Hospice and Palliative Nursing.* She is also "the principal and owner of Maine Desk, an entrepreneurial venture that helps nurses become published" (Bensing, 2005, p. 12).

All Good Things...

The future of nursing is largely unexplored; the required expertise and what the new roles will be are vastly different from how we envision nursing and its practice today. It will be increasingly important for nurses to develop and articulate their expertise in a growing global health-care environment. To develop this expertise, nurses will first need to be firmly grounded with their core values; second, they will need to be vigilant in scouting the dynamic environment; and third, they will need to merge their core values with environmental needs to bring together an expertise, a marketing niche. Developing new models of care will require nurses to craft themselves creatively and then take action to sell their product. Taking it to action will require nurses to articulate their nursing expertise in terms of unique care models and as "value of their product" and to speak a common language to market, to partner with other sellers, and to trade with buyers. In an ever-expanding trading market, nurses will interface with a variety of people, locally, nationally, and internationally. Thus, one no longer can view nursing in isolation or within one setting; the impact of one's action is now felt worldwide. Therefore, any action taken must be within nursing's social consciousness, considering the unintended consequences.

The focus on the process of nursing care rather than the outcome of nursing care has buried nurses' contribution in bringing successful patient outcomes. The current importance we place on evidence-based practice promises to link the nursing delivery process to its successful client outcomes. In turn this "product-line designing" advances nurses toward developing standards of practice and moves nursing toward greater competency.

Nurses will need to learn a new way to measure their successes; no longer will professional satisfaction be gained through traditional hierarchical advancement. The vertical structure that supports promotion of one administrative step at a time no longer fits the expert nursing model of care. Such a bureaucratic decision-making structure does not allow for that quick decision making required in the fast-paced, dynamic environment in which we live. Decision making will need to be streamlined to bring authority to those care experts who are at the point of care. Recently, nurses have begun to advance laterally within organizations as care experts and care managers and even through advanced practice into expanded roles as **nurse practitioners** and **clinical nurse specialists**.

The future of nursing and the work of providing care will be greatly altered and open doors to many new opportunities. Matched to keep pace with tomorrow's environment, the opportunities for practice will open from local to global. Organizations will coalesce to gather teams of experts, to accomplish specific goals and deliver results quickly. If nursing is to gain membership within this team of experts, it will need to articulate clearly its expertise to others on the health-care team. In addition to clinical knowledge, nurses offer expertise in top-notch team building, technological savvy, and the ability to foster many different types of relationships. This new consultative way of working offers nurses great entrepreneurial and intrapreneurial opportunities within an unstable environment. The phases in career development offer nurses ways to develop a clearer vision of their expertise as they develop expert practice models that fit a unique marketing niche. Expert models of care will provide nurses greater autonomy, respect, and career satisfaction.

Let's Talk

1. What is unique about the mentor role?

2. How is the mentor role different from the teaching role?

3. Define entrepreneur and intrapreneur. What are the key differences between the two professionals?

4. List four personal qualities that help the nurse entrepreneur to succeed.

5. Discuss the process of networking. Who might be important people or organizations that might be included in a nurse's network?

6. Compare and contrast the various advanced practice roles and discuss how they could become intrapreneurs and entrepreneurs.

7. Relate critical thinking, decision making, and creativity to the process of career management. The nurse intrapreneur or entrepreneur needs to look at situations objectively and insightfully to come to one or more conclusions. This information needs to be infused with creativity and incorporate the potential for innovation into the eventual decision. Several scenarios need to be hypothesized, and the selection process should include a risk/benefit analysis.

8. Describe the process of completing a SWOT analysis.

9. List the phases of career development.

10. Name five economic, sociopolitical, and technological forces that face the health career industry and will influence nursing career choices.

11. What are the global forces that influence health care and nursing practice choices?

NCLEX Questions

1. A nurse entrepreneur attends a national nursing convention and hears from a colleague that her hospital is in need of educational consulting

services that the entrepreneur can provide. This information was obtained by utilizing the process of:

A. Mentoring
B. Assimilation
C. Marketing
D. Networking

2. The term "marketing" is best defined as:
A. The process or technique of promoting, selling, and distributing a product or service
B. Counseling related to products and services
C. Using advanced practice knowledge to determine patient care needs
D. Health-care budgeting

3. A beginning nurse entrepreneur lists the phases of career development. One phase that is not in accord with most theories is:
A. Integrating the self with the environment
B. Opportunity-seeking and risk-taking
C. Leaving nursing to pursue the dry-cleaning business
D. Building a strategic plan

4. A quality that may only pertain to the role of nurse entrepreneur is:
A. Working within an established organization
B. Establishing an organizational niche
C. Being financially responsible for supporting a business
D. Utilizing the employer's equipment and expertise

5. A new nurse intrapreneur consults with a nurse from another facility who occupies a role to which the intrapreneur aspires. The second nurse agrees to coach and evaluate her progress in moving into the new role. The second nurse is acting as a (an):
A. Mentor
B. Marketer
C. Teacher
D. Orientee

6. The term "niche" is often associated with the position of a nurse intrapreneur. The best description of this word is:
A. A place, employment status, or activity for which a person or thing is best fitted
B. A mentoring role
C. A way to market a product

D. A calling, vocation, or employment requiring specialized knowledge and often long and intensive academic preparation

7. "Innovator" is a word that:
A. Applies only to a nurse intrapreneur
B. Applies only to a nurse entrepreneur
C. Could apply to both a nurse intrapreneur and entrepreneur
D. Is not a requirement for either the intrapreneur or entrepreneur role

8. The best definition of "networking" as it is used by a nurse entrepreneur is:
A. A group of networks
B. Using people for fiscal gain
C. Meeting people for the purpose of establishing links or contacts
D. A group that functions as a unit

9. The term "mentor" is best defined as:
A. Role model or counselor
B. A mental process of analyzing or evaluating
C. Selecting a course of action
D. Promoting or selling

10. A nurse entrepreneur sends pamphlets outlining products and services to the managers of cost centers at all of the area hospitals. This is an example of:
A. Networking
B. Mentoring
C. Educating
D. Marketing

REFERENCES

American Nurses Association. (1999). ANA to focus on core issues. *American Nurse,* Nov/Dec, 17–19.

American Nurses Association (2005). *Code of Ethics.* Retrieved March 12, 2005, http://www.nursingworld.org/ancc/magnet.html

American Nurses Association. (1975). *Standards for nursing education.* Kansas City, MO: Author.

American Nurses Association. (1991). *Standards of clinical nursing practice.* Kansas City, MO: Author.

American Nurses Credentialing Center. (2005). *NCC magnet recognition program recognizing excellence in nursing services;* retrieved March 13, 2005, http://www.nursingworld.org/ancc/magnet.html

Asoh, D.A., et al. (2005). Entrepreneurial propensity in health care: Models and propositions for empirical research. *Health Care Management Review, 30*(8), 212–230.

Barrett, W. (1979). *The illusion of technique.* New York: Anchor Press/Doubleday.

Baum, J.R., & Locke, E.A. (2004). The relationship of entrepreneurial traits, skill, and motivation, to subsequent venture growth. *Journal of Applied Psychology, 89*(4), 587–598.

Beck, S.M., & Utz, P.K. (1996). Perioperative educators network promotes collegiality. *AORN Online, 64*(5), 786–791.

Bellack, J.P., & O'Neil, E.H. (2000). Recreating nursing practice for a new century: Recommendations and implications of the Pew Health Professions Commission's final report. *Nursing Health Care Perspective, 21,* 14–21.

Bensing, K. (2005). Five star nurse. *Advance for Nurses: Greater Chicago/Wisconsin/Indiana, 3,* 12.

Benton, D.C. (1997). Networking. *Nursing Standard, 11*(35), 47–56.

Berg, J. (2004). Active reserves: Retired RNs prove a valuable resource in time of nursing shortage. *Nurse Week News.* Retrieved March 13, 2005, from http://www.nurseweek.com/edNote/04/0920004

Bird, B. (1989). *Entrepreneurial behavior.* Glenview, IL: Scott Foresman & Co.

Booth, R.Z. (2002). El déficit de la enfermería: Un problema mundial. *Revista Latino-Americana Enfermagem;* retrieved December 13, 2005, from http://www.scielo.br/pdf/rlae/v10n3/13348.pdf

Broscio, M., Paulick, S.S., & Scherer, J. (2005). New ways of thinking about career success. *Careers,* 6–11.

Byrne, M.W., & Keefe, M.R. (2002). Building research competence in nursing through mentoring. *Journal of Nursing Scholarship, Sigma Theta Tau International, 34*(4), 391–396.

Carper, B.A. (1978). Fundamental patterns of knowing in nursing. *Advances in Nursing Science, 1*(1), 13–23.

Center for Nursing Entrepreneurship. (2005). Great career and care delivery ideas have a place to grow. Retrieved December 31, 2005, from http://www.urmc.rochester.edu/son/CNC/pdf/New_center_Entre.pdf

Chinn, P.L., & Kramer, M.K. (1999). *Theory and nursing: Integrated knowledge development* (5th ed.). St. Louis: Mosby.

Cohen, S. (2002). Manager's fast track: Don't overlook creative thinking. *Nursing Management, 33*(8), 9–10.

Contino, D.S. (2001). Supply and demand: It's your business. *Nursing Management, 32*(12), 20–21.

Coombs, M.W. (1987). Measuring career concepts: An examination of the concepts, constructs, and validity of the career concept questionnaire. Unpublished doctoral dissertation. University of Southern California.

Csikszentmihalyi, M. (1995). *Creativity.* New York: HarperCollins.

Csikszentmihalyi, M. (1997). *Finding flow.* New York: Basic Books.

Deloitte & Touche USA (2005). Hospital CEOs more optimistic in financial outlook but face daunting decisions for the future: Deloitte survey finds U.S. hospital CEOs cite uninsured and government's involvement as upcoming challenges. Retrieved December 9, 2005, from http://www.deloitte.com/dtt/cda/doc/content/US_LSHC_Study_Highlights.pdf

Donner, G., & Wheeler, M. (2001). Career planning and development for nurses: The time has come. *International Nursing Review, 48*(4), 279–285.

Downey, J., and Freidin, M. (1997). *How I became a nurse entrepreneur: Tales from 50 nurses in business.* Staten Island, NY: Power Publications.

Driver, M.J. (1979). Career concepts and career management in organizations. In Cooper, C.L. (ed.). *Behavioral problems in organizations.* Englewood Cliffs, NJ: Prentice-Hall.

Driver, M.J. (1971). Individual decision making and creativity. In Kerr, S. (ed.). *Organizational behavior.* Columbus, OH: Grid Publishing.

Ehrenfeld, D. (1981). *The arrogance of humanism.* Oxford: Oxford University Press.

Ellis, J.R., & Hartley, C.L. (2005). Advancing your career. In *Managing and coordinating nursing care* (4th ed.). Philadelphia: Lippincott, Williams & Wilkins.

Entrepreneur.com: Solutions for growing business (2005). Ranking of 100 university and colleges in the nation with the best entrepreneurial programs. Retrieved December 31, 2005, from http://www.entrepreneur.com/topcolleges/0,6441,,00.html

Erikson, E., & Erikson, J.M. (1997). *The life cycle completed.* New York: W.W. Norton.

Florence Nightingale Museum Trust (1997). *The Florence Nightingale museum's school visit pack.* London: Author.

Flynn, L., & Aiken, L.H. (2002). Does international nurse recruitment influence practice values in U.S. hospitals? *Journal of Nursing Scholarship, 34*(1), 67–72.

Gardner, D.L. (1992). Career commitment in nursing. *Journal of Professional Nursing, 8*(3), 155–160.

Garrett, G. (1998). Global markets and national politics: Collision course or virtuous circle? *International Organization, 52*(4), 787–824.

Hall, D.T. (1986). *Career development in organizations.* San Francisco: Jossey-Bass.

Hall, D.T. (2002). *Careers in and out of organizations.* Thousand Oaks, CA: Sage, 2002.

Hardy, S., et al. (2002). Exploring nursing expertise: Nurses talk nursing. *Nursing Inquiry, 9*(3), 196–202.

Hisrich, R.D. (1990). Entrepreneurship/intrapreneurship. *American Psychologist, 45*(2), 209–222.

Holland, J. (1985) Making vocational choices: A theory of vocational personalities and work environments. (2nd ed.). Englewood Cliffs, NJ: Prentice-Hall.

Human Genome Program of the U.S. Department of Energy Office of Science. (2005). Ethical, legal, and social issues. Retrieved December 10, 2005, from http://www.ornl.gov/sci/techresources/Human_Genome/elsi/elsi.shtml

Institute of Medicine. (2000). *To err is human: Building a safer health system.* Washington, D.C.: National Academy Press.

Ireland, R.D., Hitt, M.A., & Sirmon, D.G. (2003). A model of strategic entrepreneurship: The construct and its dimension. *Journal of Management, 29*(6), 963–989.

Katz, J.A. (2003). Core publications in entrepreneurship and related fields: A guide to getting published. Retrieved December 31, 2005, from http://eweb.slu.edu/booklist.htm

Katz, J.A. (1991). The institution and infrastructure of entrepreneurship. *Entrepreneurship: Theory & practice, 15*(3), 85–102.

Katz, J.A., & Brockhaus, Sr. (1995). *Advances in entrepreneurship, firm emergence, and growth.* Greenwich, CT: JAI Press.

Koch, R. (1996). Intrapreneurship: Bloom where you're planted. *Tennessee Nurse, 59*(2), 1–2.

Kressley, K. (1998). *Living the third millennium.* New York: Factor Press.

Lancaster, L., & Stillman, D. (2003). *When generations collide.* New York: First HarperBusiness.

Maag, M. (2005). The potential use of blogs in nursing education. *Computer Information Nursing, 23*(1), 16–24.

MacArthur, D. Quotes.com. Retrieved March 8, 2005, from http://www.military-quotes.com/Macarthur.htm

Manion, J. (2001). Enhancing career marketability through intrapreneurship. *Nursing Administration Quarterly, 25*(2), 5–10.

May, R. (1975). *The courage to create.* New York: W.W. Norton.

McClelland, D.C. (1965). Achievement and entrepreneurship: A longitudinal study. *Journal of Personality and Social Psychology, 1,* 389–392.

McGillis-Hall, L. et al. (2004). Outcomes of a career planning and development program for registered nurses. *Nursing Economics, 22*(5), 231–238.

McLees, M.A. (1988). *The career patterns and orientation of nurses.* Doctoral dissertation, University of Alberta, Canada, 1988.

McMaster, G.E., Voorhis, D., & Anderson, C.W. (1997). The formation and management of teams: A proposed quantitative approach. *Proceedings of the Western Decision Sciences Conference, Seattle, Washington.*

Merriam-Webster Dictionary on-line (2005) http://www.m-w.com/cgi-bin/dictionary. Retrieved March 11, 2005.

Moen, P. (1998). Recasting careers: Changing reference groups, risks, and realities. *Generations, 22*(1), 40–45.

Moore, K., & Coddington, D. (1999). The next wave of innovation. *Health Forum Journal, 42*(6), 45–51.

NCLEX-RN, International. (2005). *Testing services.* National Council of State Board of Nursing. Retrieved March 8, 2005, from http://www.ncsbn.org/testing/index.asp

Neuhauser, P., Bender, R., & Stromberg, K. (2000). *Culture.com: Building corporate culture in the connected workplace.* Toronto: John Wiley & Sons Canada.

Nevidjon, B., et al. The nursing shortage: Solutions for the short and long term *Online Journal of Issues in Nursing.* Retrieved March 14, 2005, from http://www.nursingworld.org/ojin/topic14/tpc14_4.htm

New Center for Nurse Entrepreneurship. Retrieved December 31, 2005, from http://www.urmc.rochester.edu/son/CNC/index.cfm

Nicholson, P. (1996). *Gender, power, and organization: A psychological perspective.* New York: Routledge.

Orr, E.L. (1991). Career orientations, career patterns, and career satisfaction of nurses. Doctoral dissertation, Boston University, 1991.

Pinchot, G. (1986). *Intrapreneuring: Why you don't have to leave the corporation to become an entrepreneur.* New York: Harper-Collins.

Porter-O'Grady, T. (2000). Visions for the 21st century: New horizons, new health care. *Nursing Administration Quarterly, 25*(10), 30–38.

Porter-O'Grady, T., & Wilson, C. (1999). *Leading the revolution in health care.* Gaithersburg, MD: Aspen Publishers.

Ray, M.A., Turkel, M.C., & Marino, F. (2002). The transformative process for nursing in workforce redevelopment. *Nursing Administration Quarterly, 26*(2), 1–14.

Riverin-Simard, D. (2000). Career development in a changing context of the second part of working life. In Collin, A., & Young, R.A. (eds.). *The future of career.* Cambridge, UK: Cambridge University Press.

Robert Wood Johnson Foundation. (1999). *The Robert Wood Johnson Annual Report, Americans without health insurance: Myths and realities.* Princeton, NJ: Author.

Roggenkamp, S.D., & White, K.R. (1998). Four nurse entrepreneurs: What motivated them to start their own business? *Health Care Management Review, 23*(3), 67–75.

Roper. (2002). *Staying ahead of the curve: The American association of retired people (AARP work and career study.* Washington, D.C.: Roper Starch Worldwide & AARP.

Roy, C., Sr. (2000). The visible and invisible fields that shape the future of the nursing care system. *Nursing Administration Quarterly, 25*(1), 119–131.

Shaffer, E.R., et al. (2005). Global trade and public health. *American Journal of Public Health, 95*(1), 23–34.

Shaffer, F.A., & Sheets, V.(2001) Multistate licensure: opportunities for nurses to practice in new ways. *Nursing Administration Quarterly, 25*(2), 38–42.

Socio-Economic News (2003, January-March). Global issues in the supply and demand of nurses. Retrieved December 27, 2005, from http://www.icn.ch/sewjan-march03.htm

Spector, R.E. (2000). *Cultural diversity in health and illness* (5th ed.). Stamford, CT: Appleton & Lange.

Strader, M.K., & Decker, P.J. (1999). *Role transition to patient care management.* Norwalk, CT: Appleton & Lange.

Sullivan E.J., & Christopher, M.J. (1999). Ethical issues. In Sullivan, E.J. (cd.). *Creating nursing's future: Issues, opportunities, and challenges.* St. Louis: Mosby.

Super, D.E. (1980). A life span, life space approach to career development. *Journal of Vocational Behavior, 13,* 282–298.

U.S. Census Bureau. (2005) *Foreign trade statistics.* Retrieved December 12, 2005, from http://www.census.gov/foreign-trade/www/

Vicere, A. (2004). Entrepreneurs on the inside. *Leader values.* Retrieved March 15, 2005 from http://www.leader-values.com/Content/detail.asp?ContentDetail ID=89

West, J. S. (1997) Networking can lead to new career opportunities in perioperative nursing. *AORN Online, 66*(2) 334–335

White, J. (1995). Patterns of knowing: Review, critique, and update. *Advances in Nursing Science, 17*(4), 73–86.

Williams-Evans, S.A.A. & Carnegie, M.E. (2002). The evolution of professional nursing. In *Contemporary nursing: Issues, trends, & management (Barbara Cherry and Susan R. Jacob, Eds.).* St. Louis, MO: Mosby, Inc.

Zurn, P., Dolea, C., & Stilwell, B. (2005). Nurse retention and recruitment: Developing a motivated workforce. *The Global Nursing Review Initiative.* Issue Paper 4. Geneva, Switzerland: International Council of Nurses.

BIBLIOGRAPHY

Aidemark, L., & Lindvist, L. (2004). The vision gives wings: A study of two hospitals run as limited companies. *Management Accounting Research, 15,* 305–318.

American Association of Colleges of Nursing (2005). *Commission on collegiate nursing education moves to consider for accreditation only practice doctorates with the DNP degree title.* Retrieved December 11, 2005 from http://www.aacn.nche.edu/Media/NewsReleases/2005/CCNEDNP.htm

American Association of Colleges of Nursing (2003). *Position statement: Nursing education's agenda for the 21st century,* Washington, D.C., ACCN, www.accne.nche.edu

American Association of Colleges of Nursing (2005). *The clinical nurse* leader. Retrieved December 15, 2005. from http://www.aacn.nche,edu/cnl

American Association of Occupational Health Nurses (2005). *A tool for business professionals to assess their company's bottom-line healthcare costs.* Retrieved December 6, 2005. http://www.bizhealthcheck.com/

American Nurses Association (2005b) *Nursing Facts: Today's Registered Nurse – Numbers and Demographics.* Retrieved March 12, 2005. http://www.ana.org/readroom/fsdemogrpt.htm#Gender

Benner, P. (2005). *Patricia Benner's nursing theories.* Retrieved February 20, 2005 from Rutgers University. Website: http://www.eden.rutgers.edu/ ~ kmckee/description.html

Buerhaus, D. (2004). *New signs of a strengthening U.S. nurse labor market?* Retrieved December 12, 2005. http://content.healthaffairs.org/cgi/content/full/hlthaff.w4.526/DC1

Bruner, J.S. (1966). *Toward a theory of instruction.* New York, NY: W.W. Norton & Company, Inc.

Bureau of Labor Statistics, U.S. Department of Labor, (2004) *Occupational Outlook Handbook, 2004–2005 Edition, Entrepreneurship.* Retrieved June 8, 2004 from http://www.bls.gov/oco/ocos083.htm

Griffith, J. (1998). *Designing 21st century heath care.* Gaithersburg, MD: Aspen Publishers

Harrison, J.P. and Sexton, C. (2004). The paradox of the not-for-profit hospital. *The Health Care Manager,* 23(3), 192–204.

Health Resources and Services Administration (2001). The registered nurse population: National sample survey of registered nurses – March 2000. HRSA Bureau of Health Professions Division of Nursing.

Hess, R. (1994). Shared governance: Innovation or imitation? *Nursing Economics, 12*(1), 28–34.

Institute of Medicine (2003). *Health professions education: A bridge to quality.* Washington D.C.: National Academy Press.

National League of Nurses (2005). *Transforming nursing education.* Retrieved December 14, 2005, from http://www.nln.org/aboutnln/PositionStatements/transforming052005.pdf

Nursing Facts. Retrieved March 12, 2005, from http://www.nursingworld.org/readroom/fsdemogrpt.htm

Phillips, Kelly (2005). Hospitals must make accommodations to retain, recruit older RNs *NurseZone.com* Retrieved March 13, 2005. http://www.nursezone.com/stories/SpotlightOnNurses.asp?articleID=12579

Shanteau, J. (1992). Competence in experts: The role of task characteristics. *Organizational Behavior and Human Decision Processes, 53,* 252–266. Retrieved December 27, 2005, from http://www.k-state.edu/psych/cws/pdf/obhdp_paper91.PDF

Simpson, R.L. (1998) Making the Move from Nurse to Nursing Informatics Consultant. *Nursing Management, 29*(5)22, 24–25

U.S.Info.state.gov (2005). *Foreign trade and global economic policies.* Retrieved December 12, 2005 from http://usinfo.state.gov/products/pubs/ooecn/chap10.htm

Valanis, B. (1999). *Epidemiology in health care.* Stamford, CT: Appleton & Lange.

Von Bertalenffy, L. (1972). *General systems theory: Foundations, development, and applications.* New York, NY: George Braziller, Inc.

Von Stamm, B. (2003). Managing Innovation, Design & Creativity. NY: John Wiley & Sons, 2003.

Williamson, M.H.R. (1990). *Factors affecting the nursing career choice.* (Doctoral dissertation, The University of Texas at Austin, 1990). *Dissertation Abstracts International,* 179.

Wolf, G.A. (2000). Vision 2000: The transformation of professional practice. *Nursing Administrative Quarterly 24*(2), 45–51.

chapter
25

Managing Your Professional and Financial Future

GEORGIANNA THOMAS, EDD, RN
MARY E. HORTON ELLIOTT, DNSC, RN

CHAPTER MOTIVATION

Professionalism is knowing how to do what you want to do, when to do it, and getting it done.

CHAPTER MOTIVES

- Relate the unique position that the nursing profession possesses in the diversity of its educational paths to licensure.
- Identify the importance of advanced education to a profession.
- Define the purpose and importance of licensure and certification to the profession and the public.
- Relate the importance of professional organizations to the profession.
- Recognize the importance of scholarship opportunities available in nursing.
- Recognize methods of planning for retirement.

Nursing is regarded as a profession, and its members are expected to demonstrate evidence of professional characteristics. These characteristics have developed from the study of professionalism by Greenwood in 1957, which proposed five characteristics or attributes of a profession. These attributes can be applied to any functioning profession to defend its status, including nursing. The attributes are:

1. Systematic knowledge base, including a theoretical foundation unique to the profession as well as those adapted from other disciplines
2. Authority, which occurs through education and experience and gives the nurse knowledge and skill to make professional judgments
3. Community sanction, which occurs through statutes, rules, and regulations defining practice and role expectations
4. Code of ethics applicable to the practice area
5. Culture, which consists of formal and informal groups representing the profession

Individuals in nursing must demonstrate a high level of personal, ethical, and skill-related characteristics and career orientation to be considered professional. Performing the responsibilities should not be considered "just a job." To become a professional, one has to be appropriately qualified, licensed, credentialed, committed to lifelong learning, and career-oriented. To achieve this goal requires financial means, time, commitment, and caring.

The challenge of making the right educational choice begins now. Once licensed, many avenues exist for professional advancement. Examples include formal coursework that would lead to another degree, certification following a specialized study in an area, and continuing education. Continuing education involves updating knowledge needed for an individual's work environment or certification maintenance.

Education is only one element of a nurse's career, however. Learning how to function as a professional is also critical. By being involved in professional and community organizations and sharing information through scholarly activity such as making presentations, writing for publications, and/or performing research to help build the evidence-based scientific foundation for nursing practice, a nurse comes to realize that nursing is more than just "a job."

This chapter is meant to help readers plan their careers. It includes levels of nursing education, certifications after graduation from a formal program, pursuit of scholarship in nursing, and financial planning to secure a comfortable retirement for the nurse professional.

Nursing Education

Nursing is unique in that it has multiple related educational paths that lead to licensure and professional status. These paths, however, have led to a great deal of public consternation and confusion about the profession.

"The origins of the present diversity in education stem from its historic roots" (Catalano, 1996, p. 68). Starting as an apprentice-like system in early society, nursing was further developed by religious orders during the Middle Ages in Europe. These programs were independent in nature and varied by culture. The student learned what was believed to be of importance for practice in the culture. No formal plans for content or study existed. It was under these religious influences that Florence Nightingale obtained her education. She was also influenced by the secular health-care practices of her native England. From her work in the Crimean War, the earliest "best practices" were set for a formal systematic education in both the theoretical and practice arenas.

From the beginning of nursing education (hospital-based diploma schools) to its current status (in college settings), the scope of knowledge required for practice has grown continuously. This growth includes the development of standardized nursing curricula with variations by individual colleges. In the educational community, there was a belief as early as the early 1900s that nursing education should be housed in an academic environment, such as a college. The earliest nurse training school in America was started in 1871 (Worcester, 1927).

In 1949, the National Nursing Accrediting Service, working with the National League for Nursing Education, became the licensing body for all nursing schools. The first formal accreditation of schools came about in 1952. The accreditation of a school of nursing required that specific criteria, standards, and curricula be adopted and followed.

From the 1950s through the 1970s, an increased awareness of nursing as a profession was evident. During that time, nursing strove to align public perception of nursing with its reality. The events of a growing society after World War II—the population explosion during and after the war; the need for more health-care workers (especially nurses); political, economic, and educational changes—contributed to the development of the multiple entry levels into the profession (Bullough & Bullough, 1984; Schorr & Kennedy, 1999). Table 25-1 shows the various levels of nursing education.

Diploma programs have been phased out in many parts of the country. Most nurses today initially become licensed attending associate degree or baccalaureate degree programs and work in a variety of clinical settings. Presently, advanced practice nurses acquire their license through graduate study and passing certification examinations. Many nurses with this degree work as nurse practitioners, teach, and serve as administrators in hospitals or as clinical nurse specialists at the bedside. The highest level of education available is the doctorate. Many nurses prepared at this level perform research, teach, or continue in clinical practice.

Choosing the path of nursing study requires examining many factors in planning for the long-term goal. These factors include length of program, cost of education, distance learning, travel and selection of clinical sites for use in the program, pass rate of the students of the program on the National State Board for Nursing examination, personal and work time commitments needed, and student financial needs.

Certification

Certification has been utilized in many professions and is the process to acquire formal recognition as having expertise in a given area. It signifies knowledge beyond the minimum required for licensure. The process is believed to determine and maintain specific standards, knowledge, and skills to ensure the safety of the clients in a specified area of practice. Becoming certified helps to build confidence professionally and serves as a testimonial to one's dedication and accountability to a profession. Health-care consumers are familiar with this process when they seek physicians; however, that is not necessarily the case when working with nurses. Educating the public on this issue is one mechanism to help the public understand that certified nurses are available for consultation and care management/teaching.

Organizations that provide certification status usually do so on a voluntary basis and are not controlled by the government. Therefore, the certification credential may have a more professional than legal value. Individuals acquiring a credential are believed to be good for consumers by protecting the public and enabling the public to identify competent practitioners more readily.

Registered nurses (RNs) seeking certification must present evidence of an RN license, appropriate education, and experience in the area of specialization for which certification is requested. Requirements vary with the level of certification requested. The roles and responsibilities for advanced practice nursing, for example, are determined through many sources, beginning with each state's nurse practice act. The RN must contact the American Nurses Credentialing Center (ANCC) and the specialty practice organization of interest to determine the requirements for certification for both the basic and advanced practice levels. On September 1, 2004, ANCC began providing certification candidates with a handbook: the *General Testing Information* booklet, which includes key information on planning for certification and scheduling the computer–based examination. The test is administered by authorized testing agencies. Manual paper-and-

TABLE 25-1	**Nursing Educational Programs**	
PROGRAM TYPE	**OUTCOME MEASURE**	**DURATION OF STUDY**
Registered nurse	Diploma	1–3 years
Associate degree nurse	Associate degree	2+ years
Baccalaureate nurse	Baccalaureate degree	4+ years
Master's-prepared nurse	Master's degree	1–2 years post-baccalaureate
Doctoral degree	Doctoral degree	Up to 8 years post-master's

pencil examinations can also be taken and are generally given twice a year. Examination dates are provided by the authorized testing agencies when an individual registers for the examination. A test content outline and sample examination questions may be obtained through the ANCC Web site. Making and following a plan of action for the examination process will assist the individual in assessing, implementing, and completing the certification process. Table 25-2 provides information regarding certification opportunities.

Professional Organizations

The existence of professional organizations is considered to be a defining characteristic of a profession, as noted earlier in the chapter. Professional organizations are developed to meet the needs of their members and their common interests. Whereas state governments have legal control over licensure issues, these organizations provide professional standards of practice and ethical conduct to ensure the public of the availability of high-quality services (Mancino, 2001). Governed by members through bylaws and protocol derived from a board of directors and approved by members, professional organizations work to fulfill varied missions for nursing service in society. It is through organizations that the power of the professional can be recognized and consolidated to perform a variety of services and to provide leadership development opportunities.

Nursing associations have three major constituents: the public, the nursing profession, and the individual members (Mancino, 2001, p. 102). The public is served by the development of standards for

TABLE 25-2	Examples of Certification Opportunities	
ORGANIZATION	**CERTIFICATION**	**CREDENTIAL**
American Nurses Credentialing Center (part of ANA) www.nursingworld.org	Advanced Practice Registered Nurse, Board Certified	APRN, BC
	Registered Nurse, Board Certified (For Baccalaureate Nurses)	RN, BC
	Registered Nurse, Certified (For Associate Degree Nurses)	RN,C
	Clinical Nurse Specialists	APRN, BC
	Informatics	RN, CAN, BC
	Administration	RN,
	See Web site for others	CNAA,BC
National League for Nursing www.nln.org/faculty	Academic Nurse Educator Certification Program: Certified Nurse Educator	CNE
American Association of Critical Care Nursing certcorp@aacn.org	Critical Care Nursing Certification	CCRN
National Certification Board for Diabetes Educators www.ncbde.org	Certified Diabetes Educator	CDE
Board of Certification for Emergency Nursing www.ena.org/bcen	Certified Emergency Nurse	CEN
Rehabilitation Nursing www.rehabnurse.org	Certified Rehabilitation Nurse	CRRN
For a comprehensive overview, see www.nursingcenter.com		

practice and education and by ethical codes to ensure protection of human rights in practice. Professional organizations serve their members collectively to help define the role of the nurse and politically by helping to define actions of the nurse. This can be accomplished through continuing education courses and certifications to keep the nurse up to date with theory and research in caring for clients. In addition, the organizations provide leadership opportunities, such as serving as an officer, performing as an accrediting surveyor, assuming the role of project director on a local or national issue, becoming a board member, working with or becoming a lobbyist, or serving as a volunteer. These opportunities are available at the national, state, and local level.

Nurses have a responsibility to join professional organizations, to serve in a professional capacity, and to help define and better the profession. In general, there are three types of associations available: broad-purpose, specialty practice, and special interest. Deciding on the association that will best serve you may be difficult. Review the purpose, opportunities for involvement, benefits of membership, cost-effectiveness of membership, success of the political arm and issues it covers, and your personal goals before making a choice.

THE AMERICAN NURSES ASSOCIATION

The American Nurses Association (ANA) was established in 1896 by a group of nurses. In its early years, it focused primarily on standardizing nursing education and licensure. Today, the welfare of nurses and the public they serve is a cornerstone of the organization. The Code of Ethics helps guide practice and research policy, and clinical standards guide care and practice measures. This is evidenced in all settings by professional nurses. Public policy plays an integral role in monitoring and lobbying for measures to be adopted for practice, leading to quality and safe care. Membership is open to all nurses in each state of the country and in U.S. territories. Membership dues are used to maintain the organization and its programs. Joining and participating are carried out through national, state, and local district avenues. The ANA offers its members major programs and services, including legislative involvement, standards setting, formal and continuing education, and maintenance of quality practice.

In 1992, an International Nursing Center was established to collaborate with nurses internationally and to work for the common good.

NATIONAL STUDENT NURSES' ASSOCIATION

Created in 1952 through the ANA, the National Student Nurses' Association provides a means for all students in RN programs to develop as responsible, accountable, and career-oriented members of the profession. This organization allows students to have a voice in nursing. This is accomplished by working with faculty and students who network with each other and the ANA. The main purpose is to "help maintain high standards of education in schools of nursing with the ultimate goals of educating high quality nurses who will provide excellent health care" (Catalano, p. 180).

NATIONAL LEAGUE FOR NURSING (NLN)

Established in 1952, this organization claims to be the oldest nursing organization in this country (Mancino, 2001). The NLN is concerned with the quality of all nursing education, from practical nursing through master's degree programs. In 1917, the precursor to this organization drafted and disseminated the first standard curriculum for nursing schools. In 1952, the National Organization for Public Health Nursing and the Association of Collegiate Schools of Nursing joined to establish the NLN. This organization is utilized by all levels of nurses in practice today Membership is open to all nurses interested in the purpose of the organization—professional and public—at the state and national levels.

SIGMA THETA TAU (STT)

Sigma Theta Tau (STT) was established in 1922 by six students from Indiana University Training School for Nurses. STT has become the national honor society of nursing and recognizes the value of scholarship and excellence in nursing practice, technology, and research, striving to improve nursing care and health worldwide. Programs involved in this organization include mentoring programs in leadership, encouraging members to become involved in chapter, regional, and international efforts of study, task forces, and work.

Membership in STT is acquired through organized chapters within accredited schools of nursing that grant baccalaureate and higher degrees. Students usually enter the organization through their college chapter. Community leaders are also eligible and can apply through these same chapters. They must also meet requirements of a baccalaureate degree in nursing, and they must demonstrate marked achievement in education, practice, research, administration, or publication for membership. Being a member of this organization is considered an honor and creates many new opportunities in professional development, scholarship, and leadership.

SPECIALTY ORGANIZATIONS

There are multiple specialty organizations available for nurses to join: the American Association for Critical Care Nursing, the American Heart Association, the Emergency Nursing Organization represent a few. The area of nursing in which the RN practices might be of assistance when determining the most appropriate specialty organization. Every possible specialty in the nursing profession is represented by an organization. The work setting, the Internet, or a library search will help you locate the most appropriate organization. Dues are expected in most.

Scholarship

Scholarship is the culmination of activities that advance teaching, research, and the practice of a profession through rigorous study (Boyer, 1990). Nursing scholarship, like scholarship in other disciplines, also includes presentations and service. Even though the practice of nursing has been in existence since before Florence Nightingale, it was not considered to be a profession until much later. Concept, theory, and knowledge development continue today, as they must if nursing is to maintain its relevance and achieve its purpose. For some, nursing is too practical, too pragmatic, and too ordinary to be paired with the ancient, lofty, traditional, and self-disciplined idea of scholarship (Kitson, 1999). According to a position statement by the American

Association of Colleges of Nursing: "Scholarship in nursing can be defined as those activities that systematically advance the teaching, research, and

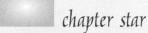 *chapter star*

Valerie J. Matthiesen, RN, DNSc, APRN, BC
Professor and Associate Dean
Graduate Nursing and Research
West Suburban College of Nursing
Oak Park, Illinois

Dr. Matthiesen began her journey as a nurse by attending a hospital school of nursing, receiving a diploma, and becoming a licensed RN. In addition to completing a bachelor's degree in sociology, she completed a baccalaureate in nursing degree. After working as a staff nurse in orthopedic nursing, she desired a specialty practice in geriatric nursing. She completed a master's degree with a clinical specialty in geriatric nursing (CNS). After practicing as a CNS in a geriatric hospital and teaching in a baccalaureate nursing program, she completed a doctorate in nursing science at Rush University Medical Center in Chicago. In addition, she completed postgraduate work, which allowed her to become certified as a nurse practitioner (NP) in both geriatric and adult health advanced practice nursing. After practicing in women's health as an NP for 2 years, she also became certified as a primary care NP in the subspecialty of Gynecology and Reproductive Health.

In addition, Dr. Matthiesen has more than 25 years of progressive teaching and educational administrative experience in nursing. She presently serves as the Associate Dean of Graduate Programs and Research in a specialty college of nursing. She as also served as a coordinator for NP educational programs.

Dr. Matthiesen has been active in a number of professional nursing organizations, including the ANA, STT, and the National Conference of Gerontological Nurse Practitioners, in which she served on the national executive board of directors. In regard to scholarship, her research, presentations, posters, and publications have focused on geriatric clinical problems of pressure sore prevention, physical restraint use by nurses, and Alzheimer's disease. In addition, she has been a regional speaker for caregivers of Alzheimer's patients. Presently, she is doing collaborative research on pain management in adults with sickle cell disease.

Dr. Matthiesn's journey as a professional nurse exemplifies a career pathway of lifelong learning in nursing. Her achievements require a continual commitment of time, energy, and responsibility to professional nursing.

practice of nursing through rigorous inquiry that 1) is significant to the profession, 2) is creative, 3) can be documented, 4) can be replicated or elaborated, and 5) can be peer-reviewed through various methods" (AACN, 1999, p. 373)

Nursing practice is rooted in the scientific principles of scholarly research. Nursing education, certification, and organizations, as described in the earlier sections of this chapter, rank nursing as a profession among its peers. It is important to understand that, until recently, scholarship was measured by the following:

- Significance of research questions asked
- How productively the results of the investigation are communicated
- Strictly followed research methods; how answers are found
- The soundness of the theoretical base
- How significant the answers are to the field and to humanity (Meleis, 2001).

The competition to obtain grant funding for research is stringent. Research is now being measured by the standards of grant funding, "indirect cost returns, evidenced-based practice, and outcome measures" (Meleis, 2001). Scholarship is a means by which the registered nurse's career can be advanced while advancing the profession of nursing. The nurse engaging in scholarship gains the opportunity to delve into areas of nursing science of interest to the nurse as well as share those areas of interest as they apply to others and the field of nursing. There is also motivation for the RN to engage in scholarship through the monetary and promotion incentives maintained by colleges and universities that employ nursing professionals.

WRITING AND PUBLISHING SCHOLARSHIP IN NURSING

Nursing, along with other disciplines, is in the process of redefining scholarship as it relates to itself as a discipline (Edwards, et al., 2000). Scholarship is pertinent to the individual members of the profession, whether faculty, administrator, or practitioner. Publishing, which includes writing articles, editorials, and books; integration and application of knowledge; curriculum development; and teaching methods and techniques, is another vital aspect of scholarship (Box 25-1).

Box 25-1

Writer Assistance From Experts

Writing is time-consuming, complex, and exacting; however, much has been written about the "how-to" of writing and publishing that will be of use to the interested nurse writer. Institutions have employed writing coaches to aid faculty through the writing process to publication (Baldwin & Chandler, 2002). The "mentor-guided analytical thinking method" is a method used to guide the novice writer in nursing to identify issues important to nursing, how to "make finer distinctions in a topic" that will aid the nurse writer to make writing and thinking changes (Lang, 2002). Whatever the method used to encourage and support nurses to write for publication, if the results increase scientific and professional publications, then that method is appropriate.

Good writing consists of at least four elements: readability, correctness, appropriateness, and thought. *Readability* refers to the process of stating complex ideas in an understandable way (Henry, 2002). It is important for the reader to be able to read the work with some ease. The second element is *correctness*, which is as much about coherency and logical thought as it is about correct punctuation and grammar. If sentences and paragraphs do not flow in an orderly fashion, manuscripts will be too difficult to follow. The third element is *appropriateness*. A tone that would insult or demean or preach must be avoided. The fourth element is *thought*. It is important to write from an outline and to think before, while, and after writing (Henry, 2002; Sullivan, 2002).

Plagiarism seems to be the most difficult concept to grasp. Plagiarism is the presentation of any substantial portion of the work of another without giving the other author credit by citing the work (APA, 2001). A publishing professional from any discipline respects other writers by giving them credit for their work by citing those writers in the body of the work (APA, 2001). Plagiarism causes harm to the one whose work is plagiarized, to the one committing plagiarism, to the institutions of both, and to the journal publishing the article (APA, 2001). If it is at all possible to find the original work, that work must be given credit. Prospective authors must research potential publishers or journals for particular requirements prior to submission of any work.

General Writing Guidelines

A shopping list of errors exists for which a work might be rejected. Many authors submit their work before they have closely scrutinized it for errors. Authors of any type of scholarly work—print, computer, or film—must make sure they have chosen the appropriate medium and ensure that the material will meet the needs of their audience. Some media will appeal to a limited clinical audience, whereas others will have a larger, more general audience. In some cases, the work may be well written, but the content may be too old, or the material does not supply new information, or the work does not make a specific point. Sloppy work does not represent scholarship.

SCHOLARSHIP IN PRESENTATIONS

Presentations may be made in on-unit in-services, hospital grand rounds, case studies, classroom lectures, professional meetings, and the community. There are several methods by which scholarship can be presented. Two methods discussed here will be speaking and poster presentations because they are the methods used most often at conferences and workshops. When the professional nurse has developed a specific idea or conducted research, it is the responsibility of the nurse to share that new knowledge with the discipline of nursing and/or other interested parties.

Speaking Presentations

Presenting papers and projects to large and small audiences, from national conferences to unit meetings, is a skill learned by doing and is perfected over time. After deciding the broad area of focus for the presentation (e.g., in-patient psychiatric care) and narrowing the focus to something manageable (comparing care for eating disorders—anorexia nervosa and bulimia), it always helpful to develop an outline (Strickland, 1999). The outline will serve two functions: it will guide the writer by delineating specific sections and details to be covered, and it will provide the conference attendees with a guide to follow at the actual presentation (Gregg & Pierce, 1994).

Walker prepared a "Survival Guide" to assist the professional with presentations. It includes the development of a title, an abstract, and audiovisual materials (Walker, 1997). The title of the presentation introduces the attendees to the session and tells them what it will be about. The title should be well considered. Clever titles are usually not informative and should be avoided in lieu of a clear and concise title that will invite people to attend the presentation.

An abstract is a concise statement that introduces and summarizes the work. The abstract should be accurate, comprehensive, and self-contained. It is used to present the pertinent information about the work to the reader. The conference committee will use the material to determine the suitability of the work for presentation at the conference. Unless otherwise specified, an abstract should be only up to 250 words; if it is more, it might be shortened by the service requiring the abstract (APA, 2001).

Much of what is read, seen, or heard is forgotten; however, when visual and audio media are combined, 70% is retained (Rawlins, 1993). Even in today's world of the computer and PowerPoint presentations, it continues to be important that all audiovisuals be prepared with care and thought to the material they will represent. Audiovisual materials include everything from PowerPoint slides, charts, posters, videotapes, and clips from movies to handouts. Overhead transparencies continue to be used as well. The type of media chosen is at the discretion of the presenter and should be determined by size of the room and audience, availability of equipment, availability of resources to develop the media, type of presentation, and time available for presentation (Gregg & Pierce, 1994).

Depending on resources and ability, the presenter may decide to personally develop the media or to have it professionally developed. No matter how the media are developed, they must represent and support the presentation. It is important to note here that slides/media should never be read to the audience. The speaker should highlight the presentation—points that can help the audience recall details long after the presentation has ended. The media can be considered an annotated outline, making points upon which the presenter will expound. When parts of videos or films are used, they must be chosen and prepared carefully. Only a specific portion of these media will be of importance to the presentation, and it must be absolutely pertinent (Gregg & Pierce, 1994). It is better to have too little than too much of a film because the presenter can always add what might have been omitted. See Table 25-3 for helpful hints when preparing and making presentations.

Presenting a Poster

Posters are the other main type of presentations used to disseminate information at conferences.

TABLE 25-3	Helpful Hints for Presentations

HELPFUL HINTS	RATIONALE
1. Be prepared. Come early, stay late. Know the room.	It will reduce your anxiety and allow for a more polished presentation. Your audience may want to know more about your research and presentation.
2. Know the equipment. Know how to use it. Know who will assist in setup.	Familiarity with equipment will help reduce anxiety. The technician will know how to assist where needed.
3. Ensure media can be seen and heard from every angle of the room.	Prevents audience from straining to see and hear and losing interest. Allows time for adjustments to be made.
4. Bring two sets of slides.	In case of loss or damage to a set.
5. Make sure slides are in proper sequence; number or tag slides.	Prevents uncomfortable pauses, makes smoother presentation, reduces anxiety.
6. Prepare PowerPoint carefully. Not too many slides, not too much material on one slide.	Crowded slides are difficult to read and points may get lost in the wordiness. Too many slides might prevent all materials from being presented. Presenter might use too much time. Slides must act to highlight the presentation.
7. Try out different colors for the background and font on the slides.	Some colors and combinations of colors make slides difficult to read or see.
8. Make PowerPoint printout with space available for note-taking.	Can use as outline for presenter, and handout for audience.
9. Insert blank slides for spaces when slides not being addressed.	Aids audience to focus on presenter's words versus words on slide
10. Choose topic carefully. It should be a topic you know and love.	Your knowledge and love will be demonstrated in your presentation.
11. Dress professionally for the occasion. Do not buy new shoes or clothes.	New clothes and shoes may prove uncomfortable before the presentation is over.
12. Bring many business cards.	Your audience may want to contact you.
13. Practice relaxation techniques—deep breathing, progressive relaxation.	These activities will enhance your presentation.
14. Make eye contact with each person in the audience; don't stare straight ahead or only in one place.	Prevents boredom and holds the interest of the audience.
15. Stand behind the podium.	If you feel anxious or feel your legs will shake, it will give you something on which to hold.
16. Do not try to memorize your presentation. Make note cards to which you can refer.	You might forget, lose your place, and cause a hitch in your otherwise smooth presentation. (Gregg & Pierce, 1994; Walker, 1997)

Poster presentations are less formal than oral presentations and usually require less discussion from the presenter. Posters are primarily visual and are expected to "stand alone" in their ability to depict the message of the researcher or presenter (Ryan, 1989). The poster might include photographs, bullet points, and tables and graphs because these methods allow much information to be communicated quickly.

Even though there is no formal verbal presentation, the researcher may be expected to remain in the vicinity of the poster during poster sessions. As attendees enjoy the posters, the researchers will be available to present specific information about the poster and research and to answer any questions the attendees might have. Poster sessions are also prime opportunities for professional networking with clinicians and researchers (Polit & Beck, 2006: Ryan, 1989).

Poster presentations generally follow the **IMRAD format—I**ntroduction, **M**ethods, **R**esults, **a**nd **D**iscussion (Polit & Beck, 2006, p. 68). The introduction presents the rationale for the study by describing the research problem, its significance, and the framework in which it was developed. The literature review is usually included in the introduction section. The method section gives a detailed description of how the researcher conducted the research, facilitating another researcher to be able to replicate the work. The method section will usually include a description of the research design, the setting and sample, how data were collected and instruments used, and how data were analyzed and/or processed. In a quantitative study, results of the study give a factual summary of the statistical analysis. Results in qualitative studies may include the emergence of themes and new theory; the report of data and the interpretation of the data may be intertwined. Actual edited quotes of the participants may also be included to tell the story of the research. The discussion section allows the presenter to include the main findings and what those findings mean, the validity of the results and the interpretations, comparison of results with prior knowledge, and implications of the finding to nursing and nursing research. The name and institution of the investigator and a brief abstract would also be included on the poster (Burns & Grove, 1993).

The appearance of the poster is very important because it must stand alone and draw spectators. The conference committee will determine the size of the poster and whether it will have one, two, three, or four panels. The title must be descriptive of the research as well as large enough to be seen easily from a distance. Keep in mind that some colors do not promote clarity and visibility of the poster. It is important to make a mock poster before completing the final copy; finances of the presenter determine whether the poster is produced by a professional artist. Some of the helpful hints in Table 25-3 may also be applicable with poster presentations.

In the process of making a name for yourself in the professional nursing community, you must consider financial planning for the future.

Practice to Strive For 25-1

1. Nurses must decide early to advance in the profession beyond the undergraduate degree.

2. Becoming an active member in a professional organization early in one's nursing career indicates a probable commitment to continued growth and involvement toward shaping the future of nursing.

3. It is the commitment to scholarship—through education, research, and service—that will maintain high standards of care to advance the profession and give evidence for the actions of the nurse.

4. Nursing is a very demanding profession, and the members must plan early for their financial future so their retirement years may afford them some stability in an ever-changing world.

Future Financial Planning

Nursing, a helping profession, is also a traditionally female profession. Helpers and women are not usually the groups that plan for their financial futures. In many instances, nurses tend to neglect their own future financial affairs (La Plante, 2003). According to Bartruff (2003), nurses tend to be too busy with their jobs for financial planning; or they change employment for greater financial benefits before they can build a substantial portfolio with any one employer. Nevertheless (and for these and perhaps other reasons), nurses should plan for their financial futures.

In people's early working years, ages 20–30, nurses, like many other professionals, are concerned with building a career, paying off college loans, and establishing an initial savings plan. The focus shifts toward preparing for retirement when the employee reaches the late 30s and 40s (Hawke, 2000). It has been found that increased salaries and career ladders greatly influence job satisfaction (Bruce, 1990); many health-care organizations are improving their benefits packages in other ways. According to a survey by the American Hospital Association, many health-care organizations are "reworking their retirement plans to recruit and retain healthcare workers," thus hoping to assist in slowing the trend of nurses changing jobs in search of better benefits, better pay, and better retirement before they can develop a substantial portfolio (*The American Nurse,* September/October, 2003; Runy, 2003).There is a need for nurses to recognize that retirement plans are necessary. Too large a percentage of nurses do not take advantage of employer-provided retirement plans. Nurses must require of their employers a retirement plan explanation and, with assistance, must develop goals for their financial retirement plans (Cook, 1997). Health-care organizations are increasing their spending on retirement plans and are offering ancillary services such as investment advice and flexible account spending services (Reilly, 2003).

Retirement planning includes planning for finances as well as health care. It also includes psychological adjustment to and acceptance of the aging process, the transition from an active working lifestyle to one which is, in many instances, far less active (Lee, 2003). According to MacEwen, et al. (1995), retirement preparation affects the individual's anxiety level. Financial savings must begin years before the psychological planning is needed if the individual is to accomplish the emotional state of one Canadian nurse who took an early retirement; she says she is not bored, but pleasantly busy and glad to be retired (Leeson, 2003).

EDUCATE YOURSELF

Nurses already multitask, but they must add another task to the list: gaining knowledge of retirement planning. It would simplify the process if all necessary information on retirement planning could be found in one place, but that is not the case. Therefore, nurses must actively search for the knowledge they require (Lewis & Hounsell, 2003). The nurse can also seek advice from the human resources department in the individual's place of employment.

PSYCHOLOGICAL KNOWLEDGE

According to La Plante (2003), each individual must determine what retirement means personally. At retirement, some may want to travel; others may plan to work longer and/or even part-time and do special interest activities. Others may want to pursue more education in areas in or outside of the nursing field. Whatever the retired nurse may do,

planning the finances for those activities is a vital part of retirement financial planning.

DOLLARS AND SENSE

There are many formulas for determining the finances required for retirement. Lewis and Hounsell (1999) have suggested a general rule of planning for the individual to maintain the same lifestyle in retirement as before retirement. These authors suggest that 65 % to 80 % of one's pre-retirement income is needed. Therefore, if the individual earned $50,000 annually, the retirement income would need to be $32,000 to $40,000 annually. It is possible that, given the present state of the economy and the current rate of inflation of about 4 %, the same amount of income may be required after retirement as before. They also suggest that nurses know their:

1. Savings on hand
2. Value of Social Security benefits
3. Current pension plan in detail
4. Rights to a spouse's pension
5. Values of other savings plans. Those plans may include: 401(k), 403(b), 503(c), 401(a), 457(b), and 457(f). See Box 25-2.

La Plante (2003) cautions the reader to maintain insurance, have emergency savings, and live a relatively debt-free lifestyle. Other advice includes changing from saving to investing because of more

---

Box 25-2

Various Retirement Plans

1. **401(k)**—Participants save for retirement by making pre-tax contributions to a profit-sharing, target benefit, or stock bonus plan. Sponsors can also make contributions into the fund for the contributor. Funds are not taxed until withdrawn.
2. **403(b)**—A tax-deferred plan for employees of educational institutions. Funds are not taxed until withdrawn.
3. **503(c)**—Employer-determined plan for amount contributed, benefits earned, requirements for receipt on contributions, and circumstances under which money can be made available.
4. **457**—Plan designed as a benefit for public employees to supplement other existing plans (Runy, 2003; Ward, 2005).

rapidly increased returns. When nurses control their future financial plans, they are participating in the control of their destinies.

401(k)

According to Cook (1997), the 401(k) [the 403(b) in non-profit organizations] plan quickly became the retirement vehicle of choice for financial planning in the 1990s and possibly into the 21st century as well. There are proposals, however, to replace public and private contribution plans with investment savings accounts that are sponsored by the employer (Ward, 2005).

Cook stated that hospital employees will have a greater advantage when choosing financial retirement plans if they understand **risk** and **diversification**. Diversification must not be confused with having a number of investment options (Cook, 1997). A clear understanding of risk and return is vital when making investment decisions.

Asset Allocation Strategies

Decisions regarding **risk tolerance** and the amount of **time** required to invest before the funds are acquired at retirement are at the discretion of the individual. There are at least four strategies for allocating assets for retirement funds. The conservative strategy is for individuals who have only a few years to invest (fewer than 4) and who cannot tolerate investment risk (experiencing their invested funds increase and decrease as the stock market loses and gains). The balanced strategy is for the individual who can tolerate only a moderate amount of investment risk and has at least 6 years to invest before retirement. The individual's funds will be distributed equally between rapidly growing investments and safer investments, which grow at a much slower rate. The growth strategy is for the individual who has at least 6 years to invest before retirement and who has a fairly high tolerance for investment risk. In this instance, the rapidly growing, more risky investments will consume more of the person's funds, and fewer funds will be attributed to the slower-growing safer investments. The last strategy, the aggressive growth strategy, is for the individual who has at least 7 to 10 years to invest, who wants a high rate of return, and who can tolerate greater investment risk. There are spe-

cific formulas that delineate this philosophy (Keefe, 2005).

Another concept to consider regarding investment plans is what to do with your funds when you leave one job for another. Nurses tend to change jobs frequently; thus, nurses may have investment funds in several different places. Four choices have been suggested for handling retirement assets in previous accounts. The individual can roll over the invested funds from the previous position into an individual retirement account (IRA), transfer previously invested funds to the new employer's 401(k) plan, allow the previously invested funds to remain in the former employer's plan, or take the previously invested funds in cash. One serious problem with "cashing out" investment funds is the considerable amount of taxes due for those funds because they are saved as pretax funds, and there are penalties for early withdrawal (Kohrmann, 2003). Another problem is the temptation to use the funds to pay for present financial responsibilities. This temptation should be resisted in lieu of a brighter financial future in retirement.

Changes in society, in nurses, and in the nursing profession are reflected in the way nurses are viewing and participating in financial planning for the future. Although acceptance of the aging process, transitioning from the working lifestyle to a much less active lifestyle, and planning for health care during retirement are extremely important, it is vital that the working nurse plan financially for retirement. The financial retirement once available for individuals through Social Security will no longer meet the needs of a population that is living longer and is more active. Time and risk tolerance might (in some cases) seem prohibitive in financial planning; however, the invested funds are the property of the individual, and the decision about how to manage them is for the individual to plan and make wisely.

All Good Things...

Professions demonstrate five attributes to defend their status. Nursing has declared itself to be a profession. To defend this status, nursing has met the attributes in the following manner: (1) it functions from a systematic knowledge base unique to the profession based on scholarship activities as well as knowledge from other disciplines; (2) it has authority, through education and experience, allowing the nurse to make professional judgments; (3) it demonstrates community sanction through licensing, certification, and defining practice through rules and regulations set at the state level; (4) it has a code of ethics for practice to protect both the nurse and the client; and (5) it has been identified as a culture through licensing, professional organizations, community organizations, and the educational programs in place for students and licensed nurses.

Scholarship is a key foundation to the basis for nursing practice. Commonly thought of as purely the research process, this is not scholarship's only component. Scholarship also includes dissemination of the information gained through study via writing (editorials, articles, books) and presenting (speaking, papers, or posters) related to the information. Guidelines for these activities include reviewing reading/writing level, using visuals (pictures, backgrounds, color schemes), using formats (PowerPoint IMRAD), and monitoring personal appearance (dress, eye contact, voice). Like the research process, time and planning are crucial for any of these activities to have a positive outcome.

Finally, it is never too late for planning one's financial future in retirement. Although this was not on the minds of many individuals in the past, now is believed to be a good time to start investing, even a small amount, toward this goal. Nurses must consider this fact and educate themselves through their employer's human resource department or select a financial advisor to assist them in this process, no matter where they are in their career presently.

There are many formulas for determining finances required for retirement. Factors to help determine a plan include one's savings, the value of Social Security benefits, detailed information on current pension plan, and rights related to a spouse's pension. Once known, it is important to review other savings plans, such as the 401(k), 403(b), 503(c), 401(a), 457(b), and 457(f), along with their risks and diversification. Based on the understanding of this information, a decision can be made.

Let's Talk

1. *Identify the barriers one should consider when deciding which paths to take in planning for a nursing career.*

2. *How does the level of nursing education relate to the standards of a profession, and does nursing meet the standard?*

3. *Although certification is considered of value to the consumer in selecting a physician, why is this not demanded from the public for nursing?*

4. *Professional organizations in nursing are not unlike those of other professions. Why are these organizations beneficial to their members, and why do the organizations in nursing have difficulty in attracting/maintaining members?*

5. *Scholarship opportunities take on a myriad of possibilities for one to practice. Why are these opportunities valuable to nursing, and how can we encourage nurses in practice to pursue these possibilities?*

6. *Retirement notes the end of the journey of a lifetime in professional practice. When is the best time to begin thinking about this aspect of life, and how do various opportunities for saving compare?*

NCLEX Questions

1. Functioning as a professional nurse involves which of the following EXCEPT:
   A. Being involved in community and nursing organizations
   B. Sharing information through scholarly activity such as research and publications
   C. Thinking of nursing as a job
   D. Obtaining specialty certification

2. Defining characteristics of a profession are exemplified through their organizations. These characteristics include:
   A. Attaining a common body of knowledge
   B. Practicing with agreed-upon performance standards

C. Providing a certification process

D. All of the above

3. The American Nurses Association describes some of the characteristics of the nursing profession as:
   A. Attaining a common body of knowledge
   B. Practicing with agreed-upon performance standards
   C. Having a representative professional organization
   D. Possessing a certification procedure
   E. All of the above

4. When assessing one's career, nurses need to take a SWOT test of their job situation. An identification and description of which letter is correct?
   A. S—Satisfaction with one's current situation
   B. W—Wellness assessment of patients in one's care
   C. O—Opportunities available for nurse to pursue
   D. T—Thinking as a part of decision making

5. Opportunities for nurse entrepreneurial activities continue to be necessary to advance nursing in today's world. Some activities engaged in by previous nurse entrepreneurs and appropriate for present-day nurses include all EXCEPT:
   A. Creating nontraditional nursing roles
   B. Use of epidemiological methods to address populations at risk
   C. Raising funds for the plight of the poor or underserved
   D. Working within known parameters

6. The profession of nursing has allowed others to usurp its recognition for many of the functions. This situation has caused many problems for the profession and has:
   A. Revealed nurses' contributions to patient care
   B. Improved nurses' morale
   C. Led to shortages in nursing supply
   D. Improved patient safety

7. Forces that determine the shaping of the nursing profession include:
   A. Technological forces such as simulation and computer technology
   B. Dynamic forces such as the aging of the "baby boomers"
   C. National forces such as the need for national health-care reform

D. Global forces that affect the cultural mix for our society

E. All of the above

8. Marketing is one of the concepts to be considered by nurses in the process of planning and developing a career in nursing. Marketing is:
   A. The meeting of people for the purpose of establishing links to meet specific goals
   B. The establishing of relationships for personal and professional support
   C. The promotion of self and of personal and professional abilities
   D. Making small talk and taking advantage of a colleague

9. The nurse intrapreneur is beneficial to the organization and possesses all of the following traits EXCEPT:
   A. Wants to change his/her workplace
   B. Develops skills needed by the organization
   C. Saves the institution money
   D. Is loyal to the institution

10. The value of an entrepreneur in nursing is:
    A. They are nursing's action-oriented decision makers
    B. They are able to make change in nursing happen quickly
    C. They are able to find innovative ways for resolution of traditional patient problems
    D. They promote formal education as the only way to attain their goals

REFERENCES

American Association of Colleges of Nursing. (1999). Position statement: Defining scholarship for the discipline of nursing. *Journal of Professional Nursing, 15*(6), 372–376.

American Nurse. (2003). September/October.

Baldwin, C., & Chandler, G.E. (2002). Improving faculty publication output: The role of a writing coach. *Journal of Professional Nursing, 18*(1), 8–15.

Bartruff, B. (2003). A financial wake-up call. *The Nursing Spectrum.*

Boyer, E.L. (1990). *Scholarship reconsidered: Priorities of the professorate.* Princeton, NJ: Carnegie Endowment for the Advancement of Teaching.

Brown, S., et al. (1995). Nursing perspective on Boyer's scholarship paradigm. *Nurse Educator, 20*(5), 26–30.

Bruce, J.A. (1990). *Reward strategies for the retention of professional nurses.* Doctoral dissertation, University of Massachusetts, 1990.

Bullough, V.L., & Bullough, B. (1984). *History, trends, and politics in nursing.* CT: Appleton-Century-Croft.

Burns, N., & Grove, S.K. (1993). *Understanding nursing research* (3rd ed.). Philadelphia: W.B. Saunders.

Catalano, J.T. (1996). *Contemporary nursing.* Philadelphia: F.A. Davis.

Cook, M.F. (1997). *The human resources yearbook: 1997/1998.* Prentice Hall.

Edwards, J., et al. (2000). Position statement on defining scholarship for the discipline of nursing. *Journal of Child and Family Nursing,* May/June, 244–248.

Fidelity Investments Tax-Exempt Services Company. (2003). Understanding the basics of investing. *Fidelity Investments,* 3–4.

Gregg, M.M., & Pierce, L.L. (1994). Developing a paper for conference presentations. *Gastroenterology Nursing, 17*(1), 6–10.

Greenwood, E. (1957). Attributes of a profession. *Social Work, 2*(3),45–55.

Hawke, M. (2000). Building a secure financial future: Part 2. *Nursing Spectrum.*

Henry, B. (2002). Writing for scientific publication. *Acta Paul Enf. Sao Paulo, 15*(1), 59–71.

In Brief. (2003). Reworking retirement plans. *The American Nurse,* 9.

Keefe, J. (2005). High time. *Plansponsor, 11*(5), 120–123.

Kitson, A. (1999). The relevance of scholarship for nursing research and practice. *Journal of Advanced Nursing, 29*(4), 773–775.

Kohrmann, J. (2003). Teach your old 401(k) assets new tricks. *Physical Therapy (PT) Magazine,* 35–36.

Lang, T.A. (2002). Mentor-guided analytical thinking (MAT): A method for training medical writers and editors. *American Medical Writers' Association Journal, 17*(1), 26–27.

La Plante, C. (2003). The basics of retirement planning. *Massage Therapy Journal,* 44–55.

Lee, W.K.M. (2003). Women and retirement planning: Towards the "feminization of poverty" in an aging Hong Kong. *Journal of Women & Aging, 15*(1), 31–53.

Leeson, E. (2003). Ode to retirement. *Hand in Hand,* 115–123.

Lewis, J.R., & Hounsell, C. (1999). Planning for retirement. *Physical Therapy Magazine,* 34–37.

MacEwen, K.E., et al. (1995). Predicting retirement anxiety: The role of parental socialization and personal planning. *Journal of Social Psychology, 135,* 203–213.

Mancino., D. (2001). Professional associations. In Chitty, K. *Professional nursing: Concepts and challenges* (3rd ed.). Philadelphia: W.B. Saunders.

Meleis, A.I. (2001). Scholarship and the RO1. *Journal of Nursing Scholarship,* 104–105.

National League of Nursing. 1992. Characteristics of associate degree education in Nursing. Council of Associate Degree Programs. National League of Nursing, New York.

Polit, D.F., & Beck, C.T. (2006). *Essentials of nursing research: Methods, appraisal, and utilization.* (6th ed.). Philadelphia: Lippincott, Williams & Wilkins.

Publication Manual of the American Psychological Association. (2001). (5th ed.). Washington, DC: American Psychological Association.

Rawlins, K. (1993). *Presentations communication skills: A handbook for practitioners.* Basingstoke: Macmillan Magazines.

Rawlins, K. (2004). Reap the benefits of joining NSNA. *American Nursing Student, 56*(2):19.

Reilly, P. (2003). Sweetening the offer: Organizations adding retirement, ancillary benefits to lure workers. *Modern healthcare,* 12.

Reworking retirement plans. (2003). *American Nurse. 35*(5), 9.

Riley, J.M., et al. (2002). Revisioning nursing scholarship. *Journal of Nursing Scholarship, 34*(4), 383–389.

Robinson, R. (2003). Don't send it yet! Getting your manuscript ready to submit. *Nurse Author and Editor* 1–7.

Runy, L.A. (2003). Retirement benefits as a recruitment and retention tool. *American Hospital Association Magazine,* www.ahamag.com.

Ryan, N.M. (1989). Developing and presenting a research poster. *Applied Nursing Research, 2*(1), 52–55.

Scherubel, J. 2005. Nursing licensure and certification. In Cherry, B., & Jacob S. *Contemporary Nursing: Issues, trends and management.* (3rd ed). St. Louis: Elsevier Mosby.

Schorr, T.M., & Kennedy, M.S. (1999). *100 years of American nursing: Celebrating a century of caring.* Philadelphia: Lippincott.

Strickland, T. (1999). Conference presentations with confidence. *The Case Manager,* 68–70.

Stromborg, M.F., et al. (2005). Specialty certification: More than a title. *Nursing Management,* 36–46.

Sullivan, E.J. (2002). Top 10 reasons a manuscript is rejected. *Journal of Professional Nursing, 18*(1), 1–2.

Walker, M. (1997). A survival guide to paper presentation. *British Journal of Occupational Therapy, 60*(1), 26–28.

Ward, J. (2005). Beside themselves. *Plansponsor,* 108–112.

Webster. (2004). *Miriam Webster Dictionary.* (11th ed.). Springfield, MA: Merriam-Webster.

Worcester, A. (1927). *Nurses and nursing.* Cambridge: Harvard University Press.

Page numbers followed by b indicate boxed material
Page numbers followed by f indicate figures
Page numbers followed by t indicate tables